T0248980

Encyclopedia of Hemodialysis: Complications

Volume I

Encyclopedia of Hemodialysis: Complications Volume I

Edited by **Frank Kesley**

FOSTER
ACADEMICS

New Jersey

Published by Foster Academics,
61 Van Reypen Street,
Jersey City, NJ 07306, USA
www.fosteracademics.com

Encyclopedia of Hemodialysis: Complications
Volume I
Edited by Frank Kesley

© 2015 Foster Academics

International Standard Book Number: 978-1-63242-153-1 (Hardback)

Printed in the United States of America.

Contents

Preface

This book presents reviews of several aspects of Hemodialysis therapy, especially focused on the complications in dialysis therapy. Earlier, many books on this discipline have been published but they were written by only a couple of authors. However, in this book several experts have discussed similar subjects, producing vital and fruitful suggestions. It will help readers to grasp and carry out HD practice. The information provided in this book will be of help for those who are interested in the field of HD therapy.

All of the data presented henceforth, was collaborated in the wake of recent advancements in the field. The aim of this book is to present the diversified developments from across the globe in a comprehensible manner. The opinions expressed in each chapter belong solely to the contributing authors. Their interpretations of the topics are the integral part of this book, which I have carefully compiled for a better understanding of the readers.

At the end, I would like to thank all those who dedicated their time and efforts for the successful completion of this book. I also wish to convey my gratitude towards my friends and family who supported me at every step.

Editor

Complications in Dialysis Therapy

Rare Inherited Diseases Among Hemodialysis Patients

Ane Cláudia Fernandes Nunes,
Fernanda de Souza Messias and
Elvino José Guardão Barros

Additional information is available at the end of the chapter

1. Introduction

Several diseases can be observed in patients submitted to hemodialysis treatment. Besides all variants of renal failure, hypertension and diabetes are the most common disorders that can be observed among these patients.

On the other hand, diagnosis of rare inherited diseases is more difficult and often done too late, because knowledge about them is limited, included among medical staff. It is estimated that 6-8% of the population in general will lead to some kind of rare disease and about 80% of that have a genetic background.

Although this is an extensive theme, the goal of this chapter is describe briefly two group of rare inherited conditions observed in patients submitted to hemodialysis: (1) tubular and (2) glomerular diseases. The major clinical features, genetic and molecular aspects and the management of the patient will be presented in the next pages.

2. Tubular diseases

2.1. Polycystic Kidney Diseases (PKD)

Up to 10-15% of the patients in hemodialysis can present cystic kidneys and different diseases with several phenotypes should be considerate in these situations. The autosomal dominant (ADPKD) and recessive (ARPKD) polycystic kidney diseases are the most important examples of these clinical conditions.

Approximately 50% of patients with ADPKD progress to End Stage Renal Disease (ESRD). In most cases, regular clinical monitoring is essential and the adoption of a method of renal replacement therapy (RRT - hemodialysis, peritoneal dialysis or transplantation) becomes indispensable in the treatment.

Reference	Year	Etnicity	% ADPKD
Iglesias *et al.*	1983	Euro-descendant	2.75
Gabow	1993	Euro-descendant	8-10
Sesso *et al.*	1994 ·	Euro-descendant	3
Higashira *et al.*	1998	Asian	2.5
Glassberg *et al.*	1998	Caucasian	10
Hwang *et al.*	2000	Asian	3.2
Nunes *et al.*	2008	Euro-descendant	7.5
Harris < Torres	2009	Euro-descendant	4.4

Table 1. Percentage of ADPKD among hemodialysis patients.

Although an apparent 100% penetrance, is considered to ADPKD heterogeneous genetic viewpoint, caused by mutations in one of two genes known to be associated with the disease: PKD1 (polycystic kidney disease 1), located in chromosome 16p13.3 and PKD2 (polycystic kidney disease 2), mapped on 4q21. Most cases (80-85%) results from mutations in PKD1, causing ADPKD type 1 ADPKD1. In the remaining patients (15-20%) mutations are identified in PKD2 and give rise to ADPKD type 2 ADPKD2.

The PKD1 gene encompasses 46 exons distributed over a genomic segment of about 52kb to produce a 14.2 kb mRNA and associated with an open reading frame of approximately 12.9 kb. The PKD1 gene encoding polycystin-1 (PC1), an integral membrane glycoprotein of 4303 amino acids. The PC1 has a large extracellular amino-terminal portion with approximately 3000 amino acids, 11 transmembrane domains and a short intracellular carboxy-terminal portion. The extracellular portion has a complex combination of fields, apparently involved in protein-protein and protein-carbohydrate bindings. This group comprises many domains types, like 16 copies of a repeat of 80 amino acids to similar regions of immunoglobulin domains PKD, a signal sequence segments of the leucine-rich repeats, a domain WSC, lectin-binding domains of type-C and LDL-A plus a field REJ (receptor for egg jelly) domain and a GPS domain.

PKD2 gene, in turn, expresses a 5.4 kb mRNA which encodes a polypeptide of 968 amino acids, polycustin-2 (PC2). The PC2 has six transmembrane domains and the two tails, amino and carboxy terminals, are intracytoplasmic.

Furthermore, PC2 shows homology with the last six transmembrane domains of PC1. Together, the polycystins form a subfamily to the part TRP channels (transient receptor potential). The PC2 works also as a channel of non-selective cation permeable to Ca^{++}, whose activity is regulated by PC1. Note also the presence of a field EF hand in the carboxy-terminus of PC2, involved in binding to Ca^{++}.

Of clinical point of view, although both forms are similar in their phenotypes, the greater severity ADPKD1 shows that ADPKD2, and the median age at diagnosis and progression to ESRD are lower. In addition, the patient is more likely to ADPKD1 hypertension, hematuria and urinary tract infections. The early development of a greater number of cysts in patients with ADPKD1 explain the fact seems to be virtually thus more serious than ADPKD2, since there seems no difference between these two forms on the rate of formation and/or cystic expansion. In terms of phenotype, ADPKD presents a great variability between different families and between members of one family. Cases of infants born to families living with ADPKD, with signs of established disease are good examples of this variability.

Several studies agree that this model of two events, also known as 'second hit', might explain the heterogeneous and focal mechanism of cyst formation of ADPKD kidney and liver. This process, which can be applied to both forms of genetic disease (ADPKD1 and ADPKD2) has the first blow the germline mutation inherited from one parent and all present in the patient's renal tubular cells, while the second event is represented by a somatic mutation in allele previously normal gene.

In addition to the genetic *locus* involved in the disease, the position of intragenic germline mutation and the nature of some mutations may account for the variation clinical interfamily, but cannot explain how a germline mutation subjects with common phenotype can significantly different. The specific type of this mutation does not appear to correlate with the phenotype of a decisive manner, but mutations located at the 5' portion of the PKD1 gene have been associated with progression to ESRD earlier than other positioned at the 3' portion of the same gene. Furthermore, the presence aneurysm also was more prevalent in patients with mutations in the 5' PKD1.

Recently, some studies in animal models are supporting the hypothesis that there is still a 'third hit' involved in the evolution of ADPKD. According to this hypothesis, the genetic basis associated events to accelerate cystogenesis in adult kidney may contribute to the clinical variability of ADPKD and its prognosis. Experiments carried out in animal models of ischemia/reperfusion demonstrated that the ischemic insult can be considered as additional blow to the formation of kidney cysts.

In fact, comparative observations between identical twins and siblings show that the regular course of renal disease is heterogeneous even among individuals with similar genetic heritage. Another important aspect is the fact that mechanisms of different nature, can influence the rate of somatic mutations on renal tubular epithelial cells, can potentially interfere with the severity of renal phenotype, also contributing to the observed variability in ADPKD.

Family history is essential for the diagnosis of ADPKD. For preparation of the interview should be alert to family history of cystic disease, with or without renal impairment. By presenting a pattern of dominant inheritance, are expected to be found members of ADPKD patients in all generations. However, the occurrence of new cases should be considered in those genealogies where prior registration is not found in polycystic kidney disease or kidney disease.

In the absence of a family history, which occur about 10% of all cases, the presumptive diagnosis may be done with evidence of bilateral renal cysts, according to criteria recently standardized by Pei *et al.* (2009). The adoption of more specific criteria relating to age of the patient increased the predictive value of diagnostic imaging. Furthermore, the inclusion of genetic tests, such as genetic linkage studies or direct DNA sequencing also allowed the identification of new cases with more accuracy and robustness. Besides that, the existence of one or more of the following criteria should also be considered: bilateral enlargement of the kidneys, hepatic, pancreatic or spleen cysts, brain aneurysm, cyst arachnoid alone in the pineal gland and diverticulitis.

The imaging examination is also essential for the diagnosis. In this sense, ultrasonography (US) is very useful in the diagnosis and can detect cysts from 1.0 to 1.5 cm. The presence of liver or pancreatic cysts helps confirm the diagnosis. The US diagnostic criteria include the number of cysts for each kidney and age of patients, as described in Table 2. In terms of sensitivity, computed tomography (CT) is the imaging test that can detect cysts from 0.5 cm. However, this test is not as the first choice is to use radiation or by having a higher cost. Finally, magnetic resonance imaging (MRI) is considered a more accurate tool than the US and must be requested in cases in which the distinction between carcinoma and renal cysts becomes necessary. The MRI examination allows detection of cysts from 0.3 cm in diameter and is able to assess more accurately the size of the kidneys.

Age	Diagnostic criteria for Inclusion
15-39 years	3 or more cysts unilaterally or bilaterally
40-59 years	2 or more cysts in each kidney
≥ 60 years	4 or more cysts in each kidney
	Diagnostic Criteria for Exclusion
≥ 40 years	Less than 2 cysts

Table 2. Diagnostic criteria for ADPKD.

The goal of treatment for patients with ADPKD is to preserve renal function and blood pressure control. In this context it is important to reduce progression to chronic kidney disease and monitor the risk of rupture of intracranial aneurysms and subarachnoid hemorrhage. Another important practice is to guide the patient to avoid sporting activities in which there is possibility of trauma in the lower back or abdominal in felt to minimize the risk of rupture of the cysts.

In normotensive patients with normal renal function annual US tests and renal function must be regular, keeping intervals not exceeding 12 months between assessments. For the control of blood pressure, angiotensin I to angiotensin converting (ACE), or receptor Antagonists of angiotensin II (ATII) are the drugs of choice, as the system renin-angiotensin system plays a central role in the pathophysiology of hypertension in this clinical situation.

Inhibition of vasopressin receptor also occupies a significant challenge as a therapeutic agent for ADPKD, since the increase of these receptors may directly contribute to increase the concentration of cAMP and interact with many other proteins associated with cyst formation. Studies with drugs specific to this scenario are underway and their results may help in clinical management soon.

Abdominal pain is managed with analgesics and rest. Avoid nonsteroidal anti-inflammatory effect due to the nephrotoxic potential of these drugs. When the cysts become infected patients should be hospitalized and monitored. It is recommended in this situation, administer antibiotics able to penetrate the cyst, such as ciprofloxacin, clindamycin, chloramphenicol and trimethoprim-sulfamethoxazole.

Surgical intervention may be needed in the following cases: *(1)* Pain: Acute pain can be caused by intracystic hemorrhage or renal obstruction, either by clot or lithiasis. Decompression of cyst is effective in relieving pain in approximately 60-80% of cases. One option is the percutaneous drainage followed by instillation of sclerosing substance. Another possibility is the decortication of cysts by laparotomy. *(2)* Cysts infected: non-responsive to conventional antibiotic therapy. *(3)* Nephrectomy: cysts suitable for high volume (> 35cm), recurrent infections, uncontrolled hypertension and possibility of malignancy. *(4)* Massive polycystic liver disease: when liver cysts, due to the large volume, preclude the patient adequate nutrition or cause severe abdominal discomfort.

2.2. Bartter's Syndrome (BS)

Bartter syndrome (BS) was so named after Dr. Frederic Bartter, in collaboration with Dr. Pacita Pronove, describes the first case in 1960. BS is a rare inherited defect in the thick ascending limb of the loop of Henle. Hypokalemia (low potassium levels), alkalosis (increased of blood pH) and normal to low blood pressure and elevated plasma renin and aldosterone are the major features of this disorder. There are two types of BS: neonatal (NBS) and classic (CBS). A closely associated disorder, Gitelman's syndrome (described below) is milder than both subtypes of Bartter's syndrome.

NBS are observed between 24 and 30 weeks of gestation with polyhydramnios (excess amniotic fluid) in 90% of cases. In first time after birth, the newborn presents polyuria (excess of urine production) and polydipsia (excessive thirst). Life-threatening dehydration may result if the infant does not receive adequate fluids. About 85% of infants dispose of hypercalciuria (excess of calcium in the urine) and nephrocalcinosis (excess of calcium in the kidneys), which may lead to kidney stones. In rare occasions, the infant may progress to renal failure.

Patients with CBS may have symptoms in the first two years of life, but they are usually diagnosed at school age or later. Like infants with the neonatal subtype, patients with CBS also have polyuria, polydipsia, and a tendency to dehydration, but normal or just slightly increased urinary calcium excretion without the tendency to develop kidney stones. These patients also have vomiting and growth retardation. Kidney function is also normal if the disease is treated, but occasionally patients proceed to ESRD.

Numerous causes of this syndrome probably exist. Diagnostic pointers include high urinary potassium and chloride despite low serum values, increased plasma renin, hyperplasia of the juxtaglomerular apparatus on renal biopsy, and careful exclusion of diuretic abuse. Excess production of renal prostaglandins is often found. Magnesium wasting may also occur.

The differential diagnosis should be made to avoid mistake with other identical symptoms like those observed in patients that use furosemide, for example. Although the major clinical findings characteristic of BS are hypokalemia, metabolic alkalosis, and normal to low blood pressure, these findings may also be caused by chronic vomiting, abuse of diuretic medications and magnesium and calcium deficiencies. These conditions should be available in all BS suspects.

Different mutations are associated to BS pathophysiology. These mutations are related to genes that encoding proteins with ions transporter role across renal cells in nephron, mainly in thick ascending limb.

BS type	Common name	Mutated gene	Deficiency
1	Neonatal Batter's Syndrome	SLC12A2 (NKCC2)	Na-K-2Cl symporter
2	Neonatal Batter's Syndrome	ROMK/KCNJ1	Thick ascending limb K^+ channel
3	Classic Batter's Syndrome	CLCNKB	Cl^- channel
4	BS with sensorineural deafness	BSND	Cl^- channel accessory subunit
5	BS associated with autosomal dominant hypocalcemia	CASR	Calcium-sensing receptor (activating mutation)

Table 3. Major characteristics of different types of BS.

In addition to hemodialysis the BS patient can received specific treatment to avoid the potassium loss. Spironolactone and potassium supplements can be required. Besides that, an increased sodium diet also can be associated. In specific cases, angiotensin-converting enzyme (ACE) inhibitors and nonsteroidal anti-inflammatory drugs can also be used, mainly in NBS patients.

In terms of prognostic, the limitation of knowledge about BS hampers any extrapolation on this field. In any case, early diagnosis remains the best predictor of successful treatment. For example, in CBS patients, the early treatment of electrolyte imbalances promotes good responses and patients tend to have few developmental failures.

2.3. Gitelman's Syndrome (GS)

Gitelman's syndrome (GS) was discovered in 1966 by Dr. Hillel Gitelman. It was discovered that some patients with BS showed a different myriad of symptoms. GS is also a renal salt wasting disorder but the defective tubule is in the thiazide-sensitive Na-Cl cotransporter in the distal convoluted tubule (DCT). Both disorders are associated with hypokalemia, renal potassium wasting, activation of the renin-angiotensin-aldosterone axis, and normal blood pressure. Unlike patients with Bartter's, patients with Gitelman's syndrome have hypomagnesemia, increased urinary magnesium and decreased calcium excretion.

GS is characterized by a milder and later clinical presentation. Often, this disorder is diagnosed in asymptomatic adults who present with unexplained hypokalemia. Pediatric cases typically present in the school age period with fatigue, muscle weakness, and symptoms of neuromuscular irritability. Growth retardation and polyuria-polydipsia are not prominent features of GS. Joint pain secondary to chondrocalcinosis has been described in this subset of patients and attributed to the hypomagnesemia.

Diagnosis of GS is distinguished by high plasma renin activity with normal aldosterone secretion rates, normal urinary prostaglandin excretion, hypocalciuria and usually marked hypomagnesemia.

Gitelman's is more common than Bartter's but is still a rare disorder. There is no racial predisposition for either BS or GS and both are inherited as autosomal recessive syndromes. Besides that, there is no gender preference and GS is often not easily diagnosed until adolescence or early adulthood.

The exact pathogenic mechanism of hypocalciuria and hypomagnesemia in GS is unclear. However, know that GS is an autosomal recessive kidney disorder caused by loss of function mutations of the thiazide sensitive sodium-chloride symporter (also known as NCC, NCCT or TSC) located in the distal convoluted tubule. This failure is associated to inactivating mutations in the *SLC12A3* gene. Until the distinct genetic and molecular bases of these disorders were identified Gitelman's syndrome was formerly considered a subset of Bartter's syndrome.

GS presents a great variability among patients. These phenotypic variations can be associated to genetic background and express specifics amino acid changes in the TSC mutated protein, which normally reabsorbs about 7% of the filtered NaCl load. This failure function cause defective Na and Cl reabsorption in the DCT.

Treatments to GS can be combine magnesium and potassium supplementation in association to spironolactone, amilioride and triamterene.

3. Glomerular diseases

3.1. Fabry Disease (FD)

Fabry disease (FD) is a lysosomal storage disorder caused by the deficient α-galactosidase A (α-gal A) activity. Fabry nephropathy typically progresses throughout the fifth decade to ESRD requiring hemodialysis and/or kidney transplantation. Except for ESRD development, a milder phenotype "renal variant" type is characterized with low plasma α-gal A activity.

FD low prevalence expresses the importance of this investigation among ESRD patients without known cause. Routine screening of male hemodialysis patients would enable earlier identification of other family members who might benefit from specific clinical treatment. The analysis of other epidemiological characteristics of regular FD could be used for the screening and detection of other kindred who might benefit from specific therapy as well as their offspring.

FD beginning in childhood, common symptoms include chronic or intermittent numbness; burning, tingling pain that can occur daily, usually in the fingers and feet; episodic pain that is incapacitating and may be brought on by stress, exercise, or temperature changes; recurring fever with elevated erythrocyte sedimentation rate; angiokeratomas that may appear in adolescence and increase as an adult; opacity of the corneal lens; inability to perspire; severe abdominal pain; and an intolerance to temperature (heat or cold) and exercise. The condition then progresses in adulthood to include renal, cardiovascular, cerebrovascular, and pulmonary complications that may lead to ESRD, stroke, myocardial infarction, breathing problems and obstructions, and more.

FD is a rare inborn error with a recessive X-linkage inherited pattern. The estimated FD incidence is between 1:40,000 and 1:117,000 in general population. The prevalence of end stage FD males on dialysis was estimated between 0.22% and 1.2% in several populations.

The enzymatic defect in FD results from the deficient activity of the α-galactosidase A (α-gal A), a lysosomal hydrolase encoded by a gene (*GLA*) localized to Xq22. The *GLA* gene is 12 kb long and consists of 7 exons encoding 429 amino acids including a 31-amino acid signal peptide. The mature form of α-gal A is a homodimeric glycoprotein with molecular weight of ~46kDa synthesized from that point on cleavage of the signal peptides with ~50kDa.

In FD this leads to progressive intracellular accumulation of glycosphingolipids, mainly in the form of globotriaosylceramide (Gb-3), in many cells, particularly in renal epithelial cells, endothelial cells, pericytes, vascular smooth muscle cells, cardiomyocytes, and neurons of the autonomic nervous system.

The genetic defect occurs in all cell types, but involvement differs greatly among different organs and cell types. This heterogeneity likely reflects different rates of sphingolipid metabolism. Thus the minimum threshold requirement for α-gal A activity to prevent Gb-3 accumulation varies across cell types due to the type and amount of substrates that are recycled by the different cells.

Clinical onset of the disease typically occurs during childhood or adolescence with recurrent episodes of severe pain in the extremities, characteristic cutaneous lesions know as angiokeratomas and a distinctive but asymptomatic corneal dystrophy. Proteinuria and chronic renal disease occur with increasing age. Severe renal impairment leads to hypertension and uremia. Without dialysis, transplantation or enzyme replacement therapy (ERT), progressive renal failure is the main cause of death in the 4th decade of life in most hemizygous males with FD. However, a number of variants with residual α-gal A activity with late-onset manifestations primarily limited to the heart or kidney have been described.

The 'classical phenotype' includes the pain and paresthesias in extremities, diffused angio-keratoma and hypohidrosis during childhood or adolescence, and also corneal opacities and renal failure. Fabry nephropathy typically progresses throughout the fifth decade of life to ESRD requiring hemodialysis and/or kidney transplantation. In view of this fact, hemodialysis patients represent an important target group for FD screening. Death usually occurs due to renal failure, cardiac or cerebrovascular disease. In addition, milder variants with residual α-gal A activity have been described. The cardiac and renal variants present with either late-onset manifestations primarily limited to the heart or kidney. The 'renal variant', a milder FD phenotype, can present late-onset manifestations primarily limited to the kidney.

While in an epidemiological point of view FD occurrence is low, on the other hand the FD diagnosis is very important for detection of family members. In view of this fact, dialysis patients represent an important target group for FD screening because they permit to identify FD patients and therefore others carriers among your family members. Each screened confirmed patient could allow early diagnosis of others related subjects, who can get treatment before or in the earlier symptoms manifestations. In these terms, FD screening among ESRD patients consists of an important tool for detection of FD patients and it could be followed by FD screening between family members of the index case. Both pedigree and population screening studies have been described and it can be carried out in subpopulations thought to be at higher risk of disease than the general population.

FD patients with proteinuria or CRI should have aggressive treatment of hypertension is present and should probably be treated preferentially with angiotensin antagonist therapy; the latter recommendation is based on theoretical considerations, as definitely proof of efficacy has not been obtained yet.

Two different recombination α-galactosidase-A preparations are in use for treating FD. One enzyme is produced by Chinese hamster ovary (CHO) cells with classic recombinant technology (agalsidase β, Fabrazyme – Genzyme Corporation), and the other enzyme is produced by cultured human skin fibroblast with an activated promoter of the α-gal A gene (Agalsidase α, Replagal – Shire Human Genetics Therapies). Both recombinant enzymes are quite comparable in properties and differ only alightly in glycan composition. The two enzyme preparations have independently been examined in clinical investigations. Although both enzyme therapies were found to result in the desired Gb-3 from endothelium, the clinical effects are not robust as anticipated. In some patients, stabilization of renal function and improvement in cardiac hypertrophy occurs upon therapy.

3.2. Alport's Syndrome (AS)

Alport syndrome (AS) or hereditary nephritis was first identified in a British family by Dr. Cecil Alport in 1927. It is a genetic disorder characterized by glomerulonephritis, ESRD and hearing loss. AS can also affect the eyes (lenticonus). Hematuria is almost always found in this condition.

This disorder is caused by mutations in COL4A3, COL4A4 and COL4A5 genes and/or in collagen biosynthesis genes. Mutations in any of these genes prevent the proper production or assembly of the type IV collagen network, which is an important structural component of basement membranes in the kidney, inner ear and eye. Basement membranes are thin, sheet-like structures that separate and support cells in many tissues. When mutations prevent the formation of type IV collagen fibers, the basement membranes of the kidneys are not able to filter waste products from the blood and create urine normally, allowing blood and protein into the urine.

The abnormalities of type IV collagen in kidney basement membranes cause gradual scarring of the kidneys, eventually leading to kidney failure in many people with the disease. Progression of the disease leads to basement membrane thickening and gives a "basket-weave" appearance from splitting of the *lamina densa*. Single molecule computational studies of type IV collagen molecules have shown changes in the structure and nanomechanical behavior of mutated molecules, notably leading to a bent molecular shape with kinks.

AS can have different inheritance patterns that are dependent on the genetic mutation. The pattern most common is X-linked, due to mutations in the COL4A5 gene. Mutations in both copies of the COL4A3 or COL4A4 genes, located on chromosome 2, confer an autosomal recessive pattern to mutation bearer. On the other hand, in rare situations (about 5%), some patients can have clinical features associated to AS autosomal dominant transmission. In these specific cases, renal failure tends to occur slowly.

The diagnosis of AS can be made according following observations:

1. family history of nephritis of unexplained hematuria in a first degree relative of the index case or in a male relative linked through any numbers of females;

2. persistent hematuria without evidence of another possibly inherited nephropathy such as thin Glomerular Basement Membrane (GBM) disease, polycystic kidney disease or IgA nephropathy;

3. bilateral sensorineural hearing loss in the 2000 to 8000Hz range. The hearing loss develops gradually, is not present in early infancy and commonly presents before the age of 30 years;

4. Mutation in one of the genes associated to disease (COL4A3, COL4A4 or COL4A5);

5. immunohistochemical evidence of complete or partial lack of the Alport epitope in glomerular, or epidermal basement membranes, or both;

6. widespread GBM ultrastructural abnormalities, in particular thickening, thinning and splitting;

7. ocular lesions including anterior lenticonus, posterior subcapsular cataract, posterior polymorphous dystrophy and retinal flecks;

8. gradual progression to ESRD in the index case of at least two family members;

9. macrothrombocytopenia or granulocytic inclusions, similar to the May-Hegglin anomaly and

10. diffuse leiomyomatosis of esophagus or female genitalia, or both.

Do not have a specific treatment to AS. In this case, treatments are symptomatic and patients are advised on how to manage the complications of kidney failure and the proteinuria that develops is often treated with ACE inhibitors, although they are not always used simply for the elevated blood pressure.

4. Conclusions

Many aspects can be considered in analysis of rare inherited diseases. In this chapter, we described only five different rare inherited disorders possible to observe among hemodialysis patients. However, is important to comment that other diseases with few population frequencies should be analyzed in patients with uncommon signals. Besides that, infection diseases and drugs dependent diseases also should be investigate in some cases. Genetic and molecular analysis also can be a relevant tool to use in situations of rare clinical presentations. A multidisciplinary approach, including the nephrologists and the geneticists besides others professionals, is the most important strategy to investigate any rare inherited disorder. For these specific uncommon conditions, the linkage between clinical and research staffs can be improve the diagnosis strategy.

Acknowledgments

This work was support by Genzyme Brazil, a Sanofi Company.

Author details

Ane Cláudia Fernandes Nunes[1,2]*, Fernanda de Souza Messias[1] and Elvino José Guardão Barros[3]

*Address all correspondence to: nunes.acf@gmail.com

1 Laboratory of Cellular, Genetic and Molecular Nephrology (LIM-29), Division of Nephrology, São Paulo University Medical School, University of São Paulo, São Paulo, Brazil

2 Developmental and Cell Biology Department, University of California, Irvine, CA, USA

3 Service of Nephrology, Clinical Hospital of Porto Alegre, Federal University of Rio Grande do Sul. Porto Alegre, RS, Brazil

References

[1]   Alroy J, Sabnis S, Kopp JB. (2002). Renal Pathology in Fabry disease. *J Am Soc Nephrol* 13: S134–138, 2002

[2]   Ares GR, Caceres PS, Ortiz PA. Molecular regulation of NKCC2 in the thick ascending limb. Am j Physiol Renal Physiol 2011; 301(6): F1143-59.

[3]   Bastos AP, Piontek K, Silva AM, Martino D, Menezes LF, Fonseca JM, Fonseca II, Germino GG, Onuchic LF. *Pkd1* Haploinsufficiency Increases Renal Damage and Induces Microcyst Formation following Ischemia/Reperfusion. *J Am Soc Nephrol* 20(11): 2389–2402, 2009.

[4]   Blom D, Speijer D, Linthorst GE, et al. (2003) Recombinant enzyme therapy for Fabry disease: absence of editing of human alpha-galactosidase A mRNA. Am J Hum Genet 72: 23-31.

[5]   Cosgrove D. Glomerular pathology in Alport syndrome: a molecular perspective. Pediatr Nephrol 2012; 27(6):885-90.

[6]   Fremont OT, Chan JC. Understanding Bartter syndrome and Gitelman syndrome. World J Pediatr 2012; 8:25-30.

[7]   Harris PC, Torres VE. Polycystic Kidney Disease: *Annu Rev Med* 60: 321-37, 2009.

[8]   Kashtan CE, Segal Y. Genetic disorders of glomerular basement membranes. Nephron Clin Pract 2011; 118(1):c9-c18.

[9]   Nakao S, Kodama C, Takenaka T, et al. (2003) Fabry disease: detection of undiagnosed hemodialysis patients and identification of a "renal variant" phenotype. *Kidney Int* 64(3):801-7.

[10] Nakhoul F, Nakhoul N, Doman E, Berger L, Skorecki K, Magen D. Gitelma's syndrome: a pathophysiological and clinical update. Endocrine 2012; 41: 53-7.

[11] Noone D, Licht C. An update on the pathomechanisms and futire therapies of Alport syndrome. *Pediatr Nephrol* 2012; Aug 18 [Epub ahead of print].

[12] Nunes AC, Milani V, Porsch DB, Rossato LB, Mattos CB, Roisenberg I, Barros EJ: Frequency and clinical profile of patients with polycystic kidney disease in southern Brazil. *Ren Fail* 30(2):169-73, 2008.

[13] Pei Y, Obaji J, Dupuis A, Paterson AD, Magistroni R, Dicks E, Parfrey P, Cramer B, Coto E, Torra R, San Millan JL, Gibson R, Breuning M, Peters D, Ravine D: Unified criteria for ultrasonographic diagnosis of ADPKD. *J Am Soc Nephrol* 2009 20(1): 205-12, 2009.

[14] Porsch DB, Nunes ACF, Milani V, et al. (2008) Fabry Disease in Hemodialysis Patients in Southern Brazil: Prevalence Study and Clinical Report. *Renal Failure* 30:825-30.

[15] Qian F, Watnick TJ, Onuchic LF, Germino GG: The molecular basis of focal cyst formation in human autosomal dominant polycystic kidney disease type I. *Cell* 87(6): 979-87, 1996.

[16] Takakura A, Contrino L, Beck AW, Zhou J: Pkd1 inactivation induced in adulthood produces focal cystic disease. *J Am Soc Nephrol* 19(12):2351-63, 2008.

[17] Thofhern S, Netto C, Cecchin C, et al. (2009) Kidney Function and 24-Hour Proteinuria in Patients with Fabry Disease during 36 Months of Agalsidase Alfa Enzyme Replacement Therapy: A Brazilian Experience. *Renal Failure* 31: 773-778.

[18] Torres V. Vasopressin antagonist in polycystic kidney disease. *Seminars in Nephrology* 28(3):306-17, 2008.

[19] Torres VE, Harris PC, Pirson Y. Autossomal, dominant polycystic kidney disease. *Lancet* 2007; 369:1287-301.

[20] Warnock, D. (2005) Fabry disease: diagnosis and management, with emphasis on the renal manifestations. *Cur Opinion in Nephrol and Hypert* 14: p. 87-95.

[21] Iglesias CG, Torres VE, Offord KP, Holley KE, Beard CM, Kurland LT. Epidemiology of adult polycystic kidney disease, Olmsted County, Minnesota: 1935-1980. *American Journal of Kidney Diseases* 2(6):630-9, 1983.

[22] Gabow PA. Autosomal dominant polycystic kidney disease. *The New England Journal of Medicine* 329:332-42, 1993.

[23] Sesso R, Anção MS, Madeira AS. Aspectos Epidemiológico do Tratamento Dialítico na Grande São Paulo. *Revista da Associação Médica do Brasil* 40(1):10-14, 1994.

[24] Higashira E, Nutahara K, Kojima M, Tamakoshi A, Yoshiyuki O, Sakai H, Kurokawa K. Prevalence and Renal Prognosis of Diagnosed Autosomal Dominant Polycystic Kidney Disease in Japan. *Nephron* 80:421-7, 1998.

[25] Glassberg KI. Renal dysplasia and cystic disease of the kidney. In: Campbell's Urology, 7th edition, Vol, 2, *W,B Saunders Company*, Philadelphia, pp1757-1813, 1998.

[26] Hwang Y, Ahn C, Hwang D, et al. Clinical characteristics of end-stage renal disease in autosomal dominant polycystic kidney disease in Koreans. *J Am Soc Nephrol* 2000; 11 (suppl): 392A.

[27] Nunes AC, Milani V, Porsch DB, Rossato LB, Mattos CB, Roisenberg I, Barros EJ: Frequency and clinical profile of patients with polycystic kidney disease in southern Brazil. *Ren Fail* 30(2):169-73, 2008.

[28] Harris PC, Torres VE. Polycystic Kidney Disease: *Annu Rev Med* 60: 321-37, 2009.

Chapter 2

Cardiovascular Disease in Hemodialysis Patients

Han Li and Shixiang Wang

Additional information is available at the end of the chapter

1. Introduction

Cardiovascular disease (CVD) is a most common complication and a chief cause of death in patients with end stage renal disease (ESRD) accounting for 45% to 50% of causes of death in ESRD patients. In ESRD patients, mortality due to CVD is 10~30 times higher than in the general population. 80% patients on maintenance homodialysis (MHD) had cardiovascular complication. In Chinese patients, the prevalence of CVD in young MHD patients was as high as 63.8%, and its characteristics were similar to middle- and old-aged MHD patients. This is likely due to ventricular hypertrophy as well as nontraditional risk factors, such as chronic volume overload, anemia, inflammation, oxidant stress, homocysteine and other aspects of the uremic milieu. China collaborative study on dialysis: a multi-centers cohort study on cardiovascular diseases in patients on maintenance dialysis showed that cardiovascular morbidity during chronic dialysis was more prevalent in peritoneal dialysis (PD) than HD patients among those with old age and long-term dialysis. Metabolic disturbance-related risk factors were independently associated with CVD only in PD patients. Better understanding the impact of dialysis modality on CVD would be an important step for prevention and treatment [1]. In this chapter we focus on epidemiology and management of traditional and nontraditional CVD risk fators and on ischemic heart disease, heart failure and arrhythmia.

2. Traditional risk factors

2.1. Hypertension

2.1.1. Epidemiology and pathophysiology

Hypertension is a common complication in patients with chronic kidney disease. The incidence of hypertension grows along with the decrease in glomerular filtration rate (GFR). It was reported that the incidence of hypertension in patients with GFR less than 60 ml/min was 50%-75%. However, the incidence of hypertension was extraordinarily higher in MHD patients. In 69 dialysis units in the United States, almost 86% of MHD patients were suffering from hypertension, and the control rate for their BP was merely 30%[2]. Hypertension is a significant risk factor for cardiovascular disease in MHD patients. Foley et al [3] found that with each 10 mm Hg increase of BP in MHD patients, the risk of LVH increased by 48%, ischemic heart disease increased by 39% and congestive cardiac failure increased by 44%.

The causes of hypertension in MHD patients are miscellaneous, including volume overload [4], activation of the RAS [5], sympathetic hyperactivity [6] and increases in inhibitors of nitric oxide (NO) in the blood circulation, such as ADMA [7]- which result in a high incidence of hypertension and difficulties in BP control. MHD patients always need to be treated with combinations of 3 or more categories of antihypertensive drugs.

2.1.2. Definition and drug therapy

a. Definition: Predialysis systolic pressure >140mmHg and/or diastolic pressure >90mmHg when the patient is believed to be at so-called "dry weight".

b. Drug Therapy goal: Arterial pressure goals should be established individually, taking into account age, comorbid conditions, cardiac function, and neurologic status. In patients with raised systolic and diastolic pressure and few background cardiovascular complications, a reasonable predialysis BP goal is <130/80mmHg, that targeted by JNC7 for patients with chronic renal disease. In patients with isolated systolic hypertension and wide pulse pressure (usually elderly patients with atherosclerotic complications), excessive lowering of BP may be hazardous. For them a target predialysis systolic pressure of about 140-150mmHg is prudent.

2.1.3. Treatment

a. Sodium and fluid restricton. Most fluid ingestion is driven by salt ingeston. Sodium restriction of 2g per day(87mmol) should not be onerous, and of the patient is open to a more stringent sodium restriction and caloric and protein intake seem adequate, then this should be encouraged.

b. Longer and/or more frequent/longer dialysis sessions. In some ESRD patients, a regular dialysis schedule, three times per week using 4-hour session lengths will be insufficient to maintain euvolemia. In such patients, the choics are to increase the dialysis session length, or to switch to a four times per week, or even daily dialysis[8].

c. Antihypertensive drug use

The regular antihypertensive drugs in MHD patients include angiotensin-converting enzyme inhibitor (ACEI) or angiotensin receptor blocker (ARB), calcium channel blocker (CCB) and β-receptor blocker or α-receptor blocker. The Avoiding Cardiovascular Events through Combination Therapy in Patients Living with Systolic Hypertension (ACCOMPLISH) trial showed that initial antihypertensive therapy with benazepril plus amlodipine was superior to benazepril plus hydrochlorothiazide in reducing cardiovascular morbidity and mortality.

The ACCOMPLISH trial [9] was a 3-year multicenter, event-driven trial involving patients with high cardiovascular risk who were randomized in a double-blinded manner to benazepril plus either hydrochlorothiazide or amlodipine and titrated in parallel to reach recommended blood pressure goals. Of the 8125 participants in the United States, 1414 were of self-described Black ethnicity. The composite kidney disease end point, defined as a doubling in serum creatinine, end-stage renal disease, or death was not different between Black and non-Black patients, although the Blacks were significantly more likely to develop a greater than 50% increase in serum creatinine to a level above 2.6 mg/dl. They found important early differences in the estimated glomerular filtration rate (eGFR) due to acute hemodynamic effects, indicating that benazepril plus amlodipine was more effective in stabilizing eGFR compared to benazepril plus hydrochlorothiazide in non-Blacks. There was no difference in the mean eGFR loss in Blacks between therapies. Thus, benazepril coupled to amlodipine was a more effective antihypertensive treatment than when coupled to hydrochlorothiazide in non-Black patients to reduced kidney disease progression. Blacks have a modestly higher increased risk for more advanced increases in serum creatinine than non-Blacks.

A recent research in China showed that the nitrate can decrease BP, reduce the total categories and quantities of other antihypertensive drugs needed, reverse LVH modeling and reduce the rate of acute heart failure in MHD patients, with good tolerance and safety, by the release of NO which is probably antagonized by ADMA in ESRD subjects. It is, therefore, appropriate to consider sustained-release nitrates as the sixth category of antihypertensive drugs for MHD patients, in addition to ACEIs and ARBs, CCBs, β-receptor blockers and α-receptor blockers [10].

2.2. Smoking

Smoking is associated with progression early-stage CKD patients, and may well adversely impact residual renal function in dialysis patients [11]. Smoking strongly associates with incident heart failure, incident peripheral vascular disease, and all-cause mortality in the U.S. Renal Data System (USRDS). Post hoc analysis of the HEMO Study in patients with available comorbidity, clinical, and nutritional data. The results showed that 17% were current smokers and 32% were former smokers at baseline. After case-mix adjustment, compared with never smoking, current smoking was associated with greater infection-related mortality (hazard ratio [HR], 2.04; 95% confidence interval [CI], 1.32-3.10) and all-cause mortality (HR, 1.44; 95% CI, 1.16-1.79) and greater cardiovascular (incidence rate ratio [IRR], 1.49; 95% CI, 1.22-1.82) and all-cause (IRR, 1.43; 95% CI, 1.24-1.65) hospitalization rates. The population attributable fraction (i.e., fraction of observed deaths that may have been avoided) was 5.3% for current smokers versus never-smokers and 2.1% for current versus former smokers [12].

2.3. Diabetes

Diabetics are at higher risk for acute coronary syndromes. Additionally, there is increased prevalence of heart failure. Poor blood glucose control is associated with increased mortality in dialysis patients [13]. NKF-K/DOQI guidelines recommend a target HbA1c of <7% for patients with DM and CKD[14]. A prospective interventional study in patients with DM but without renal failure showed an increase in all-cause mortality in patients with HbA1c <6% attained by intensive therapy compared to the standard therapy group[15]. Nonetheless some small observational studies mostly performed in Asian populations indicate the importance of good glycemic control for survival in dialysis patients with DM [16·17·18]. One observational study from Germany found higher HbA1c values to be a risk factor for all-cause mortality and cardiovascular disease[19]. However, in several studies no association between HbA1c and neither patient survival[20·21·22] nor cardiovascular disease [23] could be shown in dialysis patients with DM. Most of these studies were based on a single measurement of HbA1c values. Only two studies considered time-dependent analyses using all available measurements of HbA1c during the whole observation period instead of using only a baseline measurement [24]. Insulin resistance (IR) is highly prevalent in MHD patients and is associated with poor cardiovascular outcomes. Hyperinsulinemic euglycemic glucose clamp (HEGC) is the gold standard for measuring IR. An observational study in USA found that eighty-three percent of the subjects displayed either glucose intolerance or overt insulin resistance by HEGC (GDR median, 5.71; interquartile range [IQR], 4.16, 6.81). LAR and HOMA-AD were the best correlates of IR measured by HEGC (r=-0.72, P<0.001, and -0.67, P<0.001), respectively. Fat percentage, interleukin-6, and adipokines (leptin, adiponectin, and resistin) were strongly associated with GDR. HEGC, LAR, and HOMA-AD had the best intraclass correlation coefficients [25].

2.4. Dyslipidemia.

Dyslipidemia is a well-established metabolic disorder in dialysis patients. A recent study [26] found that a significant increase of serum triglycerides (p= 0.002), lipoprotein (a) (p = 0.001) and C Reactive Protein (p = 0.008) was observed in patients when compared with healthy controls. A significant decrease of serum total cholesterol (p=0.01), HDLcholesterol (p<0.001), LDL-cholesterol (p=0.005) and apolipoprotein AI (p<0.001) was also observed in patients. A study of cholesterol metabolism in patients with hemodialysis in the presence or absence of coronary artery disease showed that HD patients showed lower cholesterol concentrations than non-HD patients, and, as compensation, their cholesterol absorption might be accelerated. However, higher cholesterol synthesis, which was correlated with higher BMI, might be an independent predictor for the presence of coronary artery disease in HD patients [27].

2.4.1. Cholesterol

In dialysis, the relationship of total or low-density lipoprotein (LDL) cholesterol to mootality is U-shaped; patients with LDL cholesterol levels above 100 mg/dL (2.6 mmol/L) are most likely at increased risk for adverse cardiovascular outcomes, but low levels, probably indicating malnutrition, also are associated with higher mortality rates. Despite frequently reduced levels total and LDL cholesterol, atherogenic lipoprotein remnants and lipoprotein (a) are generally increased and high-density lipoprotein (HDL) cholesterol levels are generally reduced, likely contributing to CVD risk. On the other hand, Dialysis per se have neutral effects on serum lipid profile, however, certain dialysis-related parameters may have significant affect on lipoprotein metabolism and modify the feature of dyslipidemia in hemodialysis (HD) patients. These parameters include; membrane used in dialyzer (high flux vs. low flux), type of dialyzate (bicarbonate vs. acetate), anticoagulant (heparin) and the phosphate-binder (sevelamer hydrochloride). The use of high-flux polysulfone or cellulose triacetate membranous instead of low-flux membrane is associated with a significant reduction in triglyceride levels and an increase in apolipoprotein Al and HDL-cholesterol levels[28].The use of bicarbonate dialyzate may result in higher HDL-cholesterol concentrations than the use of acetate dialysate[29]. Chronic use of heparin as an anticoagulant releases lipoprotein lipase from the endothelial surface which may result in lipoprotein lipase depletion and defective catabolism of triglyceride rich-lipoprotein. Finally sevelamer hydrochloride significantly reduces the concentration of total cholesterol and apolipoprotein-b in HD patients[30].

2.4.2. Hypertriglyceridemia

Nearly one third of dialysis patients have hypertriglyceridemia, defined by levels above 200 mg/dL (2.26 mmollL), with levels occasionally up to 600 mg/dL (6.8 mmol/L). The predominant underling cause is a deficiency of lipoprotein lipase, resulting in reduced lipolysis of triglyceride (TG)-rich very low-density lipoproteins (VLDLs) and yielding high quantities of atherogenic remnant lipoproteins. Enrichment of LDL particles with triglycerides also suggests partial deficiency of hepatic lipase.

2.4.3. Measurement

If possible, dialysis patients should be evaluated with a fasting (although perhaps recommended we know not practical) serum lipid panel that includes total and HDL cholesterol as well as triglycerides.

a. LDL cholesterol. LDL cholesterol is commonly computed by subtracting the serum triglyceride level divided either by 5 (when TGs are measured in mg/dL) or by 2.19 (when TGs are measured in mmol/L) as well as the HDL cholesterol level from the total cholesterol.

b. Atherogenic, remnant lipoproteins and non-HDL cholesterol. In persons without elevated triglyceride levels (TG<200 mg/dL or 2.26 mmol/L), levels of atherogenic remnant lipoproteins correlate well with the calculated LDL cholesterol. When 200 <TG <500 mg/dL (2.26 <TG <5.64 mmol/L), levels of atherogenic remnant lipoproteins correlate well with VLDL levels.

2.4.4. Treatment

a. Target lipid levels. Because dialysis patients the highest risk group for CVD events, current KDOQI guidelines recommend that dyslipidemia shouldbe more aggressively treated than in the general population, with an LDL cholesterol target level below 100 mg/dL (2.6 mmol/L). Even lower LDL targets (70 mg/dL or 1.8 mmol/L) have been advocated in diabetic patients during the earlier stages of CKD based on extrapolation from results in nonuremic individuals. However, there is no direct trial evidence to support these lower LDL targets in diabetic patients with any srage of CKD. Treatment of very high TG levels (>500 mg/dl or 5.7 mmol/L) is recommended to protect against TG pancreatitis.

b. Drug (statins) therapy. Statins (HMG-CoA Reductase inhibitor) are the most commonly prescribed agents for the treatment of hypercholesterolemia. Statins primarily inhibit hepatic cholesterol biosynthesis through inhibition of HMG-CoA reductase. The net effect of statins administrations are reduction in serum total cholesterol and LDL-cholesterol, modest reduction in serum TG and modest elevation in serum HDL. Statins have multiple pleiotropic effects beside their significant cholesterol lowering effect. They include; reduction of proteinuria in human[31], anti-inflammatory effect and reduction of fibrosis of tubular cells. Treatment with HMG-CoA reductase inhibitors is associated with the attenuation of progression of atherosclerosis and reduction in cardiovascular and cerebrovascular events. The beneficial effects of statins are observed at the endothelial level, displayed by atherosclerotic plaque stabilization and in some case plaque regression[32]. The potential adverse effects associated with statin therapy are important to consider in the management of dyslipidemia in patients with ESRD. An recent study of Heart and Renal Protection showed that reduction of LDL cholesterol with simvastatin 20 mg plus ezetimibe 10 mg daily safely reduced the incidence of major atherosclerotic events in a wide range of patients with advanced chronic kidney disease [33].

3. Nontraditional risk factors

3.1. Chronic volume overload

Volume overload is a common manifestation in MHD patients [34]. Volume overload can increase returned blood volume, cardiac afterload, LVDd/LVEDV, and left ventricle wall pressure [35.36]. In early stage, the cardiac changes of adaptive ventricular chamber enlargement and myocardial hypertrophy induced by volume overload maybe reversible. Removal and control of excess fluid with dialysis is considered critical for protection against cardiovascular sequelae. A recent Chinese study found that antihypertensive agents including beta-blockers may influence hemodynamics, which may limit fluid removal during hemodialysis [37].

3.2. Anemia

Anemia is predictive of morbidity and mortality from cardiovascular causes in patients with CKD or on dialysis [38]. It leads to reduced oxygen delivery to tissues, causing organ dysfunction. It also causes hemodynamic adaptations including a high cardiac output state to maintain adequate tissue oxygenation leading to left ventricular dilatation and hypertrophy [39]. However, at the present time, correction of anemia to hemoglobin levels above 13 g/dL (130 g/L) has not been associated with a cardiovascular or survival benefit. Maintenance of hemoglobin levels above 11 g/dL (110 g/L) is currently recommended and may prevent further progression of LVH. Guidelines for the management of anemia and iron deficiency in chronic hemodialysis (HD) patients have been developed to standardize therapy and improve clinical outcome. But a recent Dutch study found that compliance with anemia targets in stable HD patients was poor and showed a wide variation between treatment facilities [40].

3.3. Inflammation

The role of chronic inflammation as a putative cause of high mortality in ESRD has attracted considerable interest during the last decade. It has been hypothesized that in addition to its direct pro-atherogenic effects, chronic inflammation may serve as a catalyst and in the toxic uremic milieu may modulate the effects of concurrent vascular and nutritional risk factors [41]. ESRD has become a prototype for chronic inflammation. There is consistent evidence that CRP and pro-inflammatory cytokines such as IL-1, IL-6 and TNF-α are risk factors for atherosclerotic complications and predict death and adverse cardiovascular outcomes in these patients [42,43,44,45]. Schwarz et al. [46] have shown that coronary atherosclerotic plaques in ESRD patients are characterized by increased medial thickness, infiltration by and activation of macrophages and marked calcification. Available evidence suggests that heavily calcified and inflamed plaques contribute to excessive cardiovascular risk in ESRD patients [47]. Levels of CRP increase as the renal function deteriorates and are particularly high in patients with ESRD. As many as one third to one half of patients with ESRD have CRP levels in the very high-risk category, and CRP continues to be an excellent predictor of adverse outcome in this population [48]. Parekh et al. [49] prospectively studied a cohort of more than 1,000 ESRD patients followed for a median of 2.5 years and reported that the highest tertile of CRP was associated with a two-fold increased adjusted risk of sudden cardiac death compared to patients in the lowest tertile.

3.4. Oxidant stress

Numerous factors in the dialysis patient increase o xidative stress (OxStress). These include inflammation (as marked by elevated C-reactive protein), malnutrition (by reducing antioxidant defenses), uremic toxins, and, potentially, the dialysis procedure itself. Many protective mechanisms are impaired, including reduced plasma protein-associated free thiols such as glutathione. This may magnify the impact of OxStress in the dialysis population. OxStress is recognized as a critical factor in the development of atherosclerotic cardiovascular disease (ACVD) [50,51]. According to the oxidation hypothesis of atherosclerosis, low-density lipoprotein (LDL) in its native state is not atherogenic [52,53]. LDL must undergo oxidative modification before it can contribute to the initiation and progression of atherosclerosis. Data from animal models of atherosclerosis, both diet-induced and genetically altered models, have demonstrated the presence of oxidized LDL (oxLDL) in plasma as well as in atherosclerotic lesions. Presence of oxLDL, autoantibodies against malondialdehyde-modified LDL, and of LDL-IgG immune complexes has also been reported in human plasma and human atherosclerotic lesions [54,55]. The pathways involved in the formation of these oxidative markers and the relationship between these markers and disease progression remain to be elucidated. Advanced oxidation protein products (AOPP) accumulation is a marker of oxidative stress. A recent study in China [56] found that accumulation of AOPP was more significant in HD compared to CAPD patients. The level of AOPP was independently associated with ischaemic heart disease only in HD patients.

3.5. Hyperhomocysteinemia

3.5.1. Epidemiology

Hyperhomocysteinemia is much more common in dialysis patients than in the general population. Homocysteine is typically measured in the plasma and normal levels range between 5 and 12 mcmol/L. In the general population, hyperhomocysteinemia is an independent risk factor for adverse CVD outcomes and is commonly associated with deficiencies in folate and vitamins B_6 and B_{12}. B-vitamin and folate supplementation effectively reduce homocysteine levels in the general population and recent extensive folate supplementation in foods has lowered the overall prevalence of hyperhomocysteinemia in the nondialysis population. Homocysteine levels increase dramatically as kidney function declines, with as many as 80% of dialysis patients classified as having hyperhomocysteinemia. In dialysis patients, some but not all studies suggest that hyperhomocysteinemia is independently associated with CVD mortality. Nutritional status confounds these analyses, since better nourished patients tend to have higher homocysteine levels. The relationship between homocysteine levels and cardiovascular disease was described initially by observational studies, which may overestimate the effect of this relationship. Two meta-analyses of epidemiologic studies [57,58] suggested that reduced homocysteine levels could lower the risk of coronary heart disease, stroke, and cardiovascular disease. However, Bazzano et al [59] concluded that folic acid therapy did not significantly contribute to cardiovascular disease, stroke, or myocardial infarction.

3.5.2. Treatment

Folic acid supplementation may play an important role in carcinogenesis, because when it is administered to individuals with established cancers, it potentially promotes tumor growth [60·61]. It has also been reported that the introduction of folic acid may increase the risk of colorectal cancer [62]. According to our review, folic acid therapy resulted in an 8% increase in the risk of cancer, although this difference was not statistically significant. The reason for this increase in carcinogenesis can be explained by the fact that folic acid supplementation may affect endothelial function and support cell growth through mechanisms independent of homocysteine [63]. Importantly, folic acid and B vitamins are water-soluble and excreted by the kidney; therefore, therapy toxicity may be of great concern in patients with impaired renal function. In patients with end-stage renal failure who have hyperhomocysteinemia wherein homocysteine levels must be reduced, alternative, non-vitamin therapies are important. For example, enhancing urinary excretion can help to avoid a decrease in glomerular filtration rate and an increase in major cardiovascular events [64].

4. Ischemic heart disease

4.1. Epidemiology

Acute myocardial infarction(AMI) is common in the ESRD population. Outcomes for patients with AMI are poor, with 50% 1-year mortality. Both atherosclerosis and atheriosclerosis and arteriosclerosis contribute to pathogenesis; arteriosclerosis may cause LVH with increased myocardial oxygen demand and altered coronary perfusion with subsequent subendocardial ischemia.

4.2. Diagnosis

Routine screening is not currently recommended. There are no preoperative screening guidelines specific to dialysis patients, and it is reasonable to use general population guidelines, recognizing that the extent of comorbid conditions prevalent in the dialysis population is likely to place them into the highest cardiovascular risk group. Because many dialysis patients are unable to achieve adequate exercise levels for valid stress tests, pharmacologic stress test should be used in this population. Furthermore, because of the high incidence of baseline electrocardiogram abnormalities, either nuclear or echocardiographic imaging should be utilized in stress testing.

4.3. Prevention

Aspirin, beta-blockers, ACE inhibitors, and nitrate preparations are all appropriate for primary therapy of AMI and are likely appropriate for secondary prevention, although data on aspirin for secondary prevention of coronary artery disease remain inadequate to date. Observational studies suggest that medical therapies including aspirin, beta- blockers, and ACE inhibitors may be underutilized in dialysis patients. Using the ESRD database and the Cooperative Cardiovascular Project (CCP) database, Berger AK, et al [65]found that ESRD patients are far less likely than non-ESRD patients to be treated with aspirin, beta-blockers, and ACE inhibitors during an admission for AMI. The lower rates of usage for these medications, particularly aspirin, may contribute to the increased 30-day mortality.

4.4. Treatment

4.4.1. Management of angina pectoris

The pharmacologic approach to angina in dialysis patients is similar to that in the general population. The progressive introduction of sublingual nitrates, oral long-acting nitrates, beta-blockers, and calcium channel blockers is appropriate. The usual dosages of sublingual and oral nitrates can be given to dialysis patients.

4.4.2. Angina during the hemodialysis session

For patients whose angina manifests primarily during hemodialysis session, a number of therapeutic options available. Nasal oxygen should be given routinely. If the anginal episode is associated with hypotension, then initial treatment should include raising the blood pressure by elevating the feet and by cautiously administering saline. Sublingual nitroglycerin can be given as soon as the pressure has increased to a clinically acceptable value. Consideration should be given to reducing the blood flow rate and stopping ultrafiltration until the anginal episode subsides. Predialysis administration of 2% nitroglycerin ointment may be of benefit when applied 1 hour prior to a hemodialysis session, assuming that the blood pressure will tolerate this intervention.

5. Heart failure

Heart failure is the commonest manifestation of cardiac dysfunction in patients on maintenance dialysis. According to the cross-sectional survey by Harnett and coworkers, which included both hemodialysis and peritoneal dialysis patients, nearly one-third of the patients developed heart failure on initiation of dialysis, of which 56% had further recurrences [66]. Even among patients with no heart failure at baseline, around 25% of patients developed heart failure at a rate of 7% per year. In addition, the presence of heart failure was associated with a worse prognosis in that median survival was 36 months for patients with heart failure at baseline compared to 62 months for patients without heart failure. They also found that increasing age, diabetes mellitus and ischemic heart disease were associated with heart failure at initiation of dialysis, while ischemic heart disease, anemia, hypoalbuminemia and systolic dysfunction were important predictors of heart failure recurrence [67]. The presence of ischemic heart disease is associated with greater left atrial diameter, greater left ventricular end-systolic diameter, lower fractional shortening and, thus, more systolic dysfunction [68].In the Canadian Prospective Cohort Study, which included 433 incident dialysis patients, 74% had left ventricular hypertrophy at baseline, 30% had left ventricular hypertrophy with dilatation, and 15% had systolic dysfunction [69], indicating that much of the cardiac hypertrophy and dysfunction was already established by the time patients started their dialysis therapy. This may also explain why dialysis patients are prone to develop heart failure.

6. Arrhythmia

Paroxysmal atrial fibrillation attack is one of most common tachyarrhythmia in MHD patients. Paroxysmal atrial fibrillation attack not only can affect the dialysis to proceed smoothly, but also it can increase the death risk in MHD patients. In the Dialysis Outcomes and Practice Patterns Study [70], which analyzed 37,765 participants in 12 countries in the Dialysis Outcomes and Practice Patterns Study to explore the association of the following practices with sudden death (due to cardiac arrhythmia, cardiac arrest, and/or hyperkalemia): treatment time [TT] <210 minutes, Kt/V <1.2, ultrafiltration volume >5.7% of postdialysis weight, low dialysate potassium [K(D) <3 mEq/L]), and prescription of Q wave/T wave interval-prolonging drugs,indicating that identified modifiable dialysis practices associated with higher risk of sudden death, including short TT, large ultrafiltration volume, and low K(D). Because K(D) <3 mEq/L is common and easy to change, K(D) tailoring may prevent some sudden deaths. Individualized interventions may effectively reduce paroxysmal atrial fibrillation attack during dialysis in MHD patients. The general individualized intervention in MHD patients are, (1) individualized dialysis programmes, such as increasing the dialysis or hemodialysisfiltrition frequency or be changed to daily dialysis for atrial fibrillation with frequent seizure. Regular monitoring of serum potassium levels before and post dialysis, adjusting dialysate concentration of potassium ions in a timely manner, using different prescription of individualized dialysate for hemodialysis treatment. (2)Behavioral interventions, such as improving their way of life to develop good habits and patterns of dialysis. (3) Closely monitoring the patients' vital signs during hemodialysis, such as heart rate, blood pressure and pulse rate. (4) Controlling interdialytic weight gain (IDWG), strict volume policy including salt restriction and adequate ultrafiltration is fundamental to reach normovolemia/normotension together with regression of left atrial hypertrophy in patients on hemodialysis. In HD patients, IDWG is significantly associated with left atrial volume/diameter. Together with better volume control, left atrium volume must be decreased. Most importantly, they should focus on salt restriction not water restriction. (5) Psychological intervention to reduce sympathetic excitement to induce atrial fibrillation.

7. Conclusion

A high prevalence of cardiovascular disease is observed in ESRD patients receiving dialysis therapy. This usually constitutes a combination of vascular and myocardial disease related to both traditional and nontraditional risk factors. Most of these cardiovascular complications are already established and advanced by the time patients are started on dialysis treatment, thus indicating the need for earlier and more active screening for cardiovascular disease even before patients progress to end-stage kidney disease. More attention should be focused on improving cardiovascular outcomes in ESRD patients receiving maintenance dialysis therapy.

Author details

Han Li and Shixiang Wang*

*Address all correspondence to: wxy1988@263.net

Blood Purification Center, Beijing Chaoyang Hospital, Capital Medical University, Beijing, China

References

[1] Hou FF, Jiang JP. China collaborative study on dialysis: a multi-centers cohort study on cardiovascular diseases in patients on maintenance dialysis. BMC Nephrol. 2012;13(1):94.

[2] Agarwal R, Nissenson AR, Batlle D, et al. Prevalence, treatment, and control of hypertension in chronic hemodialysis patients in the United States. Am J Med. 2003;115:291-297.

[3] Foley RN, Parfrey PS, Harnett JD, et al. Impact of hypertension on cardiomyopathy, morbidity and mortality in end-stage renal disease. Kidney Int. 1996;49:1379-1385.

[4] Agarwal R. Volume-associated ambulatory blood pressure patterns in hemodialysis patients. Hypertension. 2009;54:241-247.

[5] Neutel JM. Choosing among renin-angiotensin system blockers for the management of hypertension: from pharmacology to clinical efficacy. Curr Med Res Opin. 2010;26:213-222.

[6] Zilch O, Vos PF, Oey PL, et al. Sympathetic hyperactivity in haemodialysis patients is reduced by short daily haemodialysis. J Hypertens. 2007; 25: 1285-1289.

[7] Mallamaci F, Tripepi G, Maas R, et al. Analysis of the relationship between norepinephrine and asymmetric dimethylarginine levels among patients with end-stage renal disease. J Am Soc Nephrol. 2004;15:435-441.

[8] Lorenzen JM, Thum T, Eisenbach GM, Haller H, Kielstein JT. Conversion from conventional in-centre thrice-weekly haemodialysis to short daily home haemodialysis ameliorates uremia-associated clinical parameters. Int Urol Nephrol. 2012;44:883-890.

[9] Weir MR, Bakris GL, Weber MA, Dahlof B, Devereux RB, Kjeldsen SE, Pitt B, Wright JT, Kelly RY, Hua TA, Hester RA, Velazquez E, Jamerson KA. Kidney Int. 2012;81:568-576.

[10] Li H, Wang SX. Improvement of hypertension and LVH in maintenance hemodialysis patients treated with sustained-release isosorbide mononitrate. J Nephrol. 2011;24:236-245.

[11] Nagasawa Y, Yamamoto R, Rakugi H, Isaka Y. Cigarette smoking and chronic kidney diseases. Hypertens Res. 2012;35:261-265.

[12] Mc Causland FR, Brunelli SM, Waikar SS. Association of Smoking with Cardiovascular and Infection-Related Morbidity and Mortality in Chronic Hemodialysis.Clin J Am Soc Nephrol. 2012 Aug 23. [Epub ahead of print]

[13] Dyck RF, Naqshbandi Hayward M, Harris SB. Prevalence, determinants and co-morbidities of chronic kidney disease among First Nations adults with diabetes: results from the Circle study. BMC Nephrol. 2012;13:57.

[14] KDOQI Clinical Practice Guidelines and Clinical Practice Recommendations for Diabetes and Chronic Kidney Disease. Am J Kidney Dis. 2007;49: S12–154.

[15] Gerstein HC, Miller ME, Byington RP, Goff DC, Jr., Bigger JT, et al. Effects of intensive glucose lowering in type 2 diabetes. N Engl J Med. 2008;358: 2545–2559.

[16] Ishimura E, Okuno S, Kono K, Fujino-Kato Y, Maeno Y, et al. Glycemic control and survival of diabetic hemodialysis patients–importance of lower hemoglobin A_{1C} levels. Diabetes Res Clin Pract. 2009; 83: 320–326.

[17] Oomichi T, Emoto M, Tabata T, Morioka T, Tsujimoto Y, et al. Impact of glycemic control on survival of diabetic patients on chronic regular hemodialysis: a 7-year observational study. Diabetes Care. 2006; 29: 1496–1500.

[18] Tsujimoto Y, Ishimura E, Tahara H, Kakiya R, Koyama H, et al. Poor glycemic control is a significant predictor of cardiovascular events in chronic hemodialysis patients with diabetes. Ther Apher Dial. 2009; 13: 358–365.

[19] Drechsler C, Krane V, Ritz E, Marz W, Wanner C. Glycemic control and cardiovascular events in diabetic hemodialysis patients. Circulation. 2009; 120: 2421-2428.

[20] Fukuoka K, Nakao K, Morimoto H, Nakao A, Takatori Y, et al. Glycated albumin levels predict long-term survival in diabetic patients undergoing haemodialysis. Nephrology (Carlton). 2008; 13: 278-283.

[21] Shurraw S, Majumdar SR, Thadhani R, Wiebe N, Tonelli M .Glycemic control and the risk of death in 1,484 patients receiving maintenance hemodialysis. Am J Kidney Dis. 2010; 55: 875-884.

[22] Shima K, Komatsu M, Kawahara K, Minaguchi J, Kawashima S. Stringent glycaemic control prolongs survival in diabetic patients with end-stage renal disease on haemodialysis. Nephrology (Carlton). 2010; 15: 632-638.

[23] Okada T, Nakao T, Matsumoto H, Shino T, Nagaoka Y, et al. Association between markers of glycemic control, cardiovascular complications and survival in type 2 diabetic patients with end-stage renal disease. Intern Med. 2007; 46: 807-814.

[24] Kalantar-Zadeh K, Kopple JD, Regidor DL, Jing J, Shinaberger CS, et al. A1C and survival in maintenance hemodialysis patients. Diabetes Care. 2007; 30: 1049-1055.

[25] Hung AM, Sundell MB, Egbert P, Siew ED, Shintani A, Ellis CD, Bian A, Ikizler TA. A comparison of novel and commonly-used indices of insulin sensitivity in African American chronic hemodialysis patients.Clin J Am Soc Nephrol. 2011;6:767-774.

[26] Kharrat I, Jmal A, Jmal L, Amira Z, Ben Cheikh W, Ben Bourouba F, Sahnoun L, Abdennebi M. Alterations in lipidic metabolism in hemodialysis patients. Tunis Med. 2012 ;90:537-41.

[27] Fukushima M, Miura S, Mitsutake R, Fukushima T, Fukushima K, Saku K. Cholesterol metabolism in patients with hemodialysis in the presence or absence of coronary artery disease. Circ J. 2012;76:1980-1986.

[28] Blankestijn PJ, Vos PF, Rabelink TJ, et al. High-flux dialysis membranes improve lipid profile in chronic hemodialysis patients. J Am Soc Nephrol. 1995;5:1703-1708.

[29] Jung K, Scheifler A, Schulze BD, Scholz M. Lower serum highdensity lipoprotein-cholesterol concentration in patients undergoing maintenance hemodialysis with acetate than with bicarbonate. Am J Kidney Dis. 1995;25:584-588.

[30] Chertow GM, Burke SK, Raggi P. Sevelamer attenuates the progression of coronary and aortic calcification in hemodialysis patients. Kidney Int. 2002;62:245-252.

[31] Fellstrom B, Holdaas H, Jardine AG, et al. Cardiovascular disease in patients with renal disease: the role of statins. Curr Med Res Opin. 2009;25:271-285.

[32] Bianchi S, Bigazzi R, Caiazza A, Campese VM. A controlled, prospective study of the effects of atorvastatin on proteinuria and progression of kidney disease. Am J Kidney Dis. 2003;41:565-570.

[33] Baigent C, Landray MJ, Reith C, Emberson J, Wheeler DC, Tomson C, Wanner C, Krane V, Cass A, Craig J, Neal B, Jiang L, Hooi LS, Levin A, Agodoa L, Gaziano M, Kasiske B, Walker R, Massy ZA, Feldt-Rasmussen B, Krairittichai U, Ophascharoensuk V, Fellström B, Holdaas H, Tesar V, Wiecek A, Grobbee D, de Zeeuw D, Grönhagen-Riska C, Dasgupta T, Lewis D, Herrington W, Mafham M, Majoni W, Wallendszus K, Grimm R, Pedersen T, Tobert J, Armitage J, Baxter A, Bray C, Chen Y, Chen Z, Hill M, Knott C, Parish S, Simpson D, Sleight P, Young A, Collins R; SHARP Investigators. The effects of lowering LDL cholesterol with simvastatin plus ezetimibe in patients with chronic kidney disease (Study of Heart and Renal Protection): a randomised placebo-controlled trial. Lancet. 2011;377(9784):2181-2192.

[34] Nerbass FB, Morais JG, Santos RG, Kruger TS, Koene TT, Filho HA. Factors related to interdialytic weight gain in hemodialysis patients. J Bras Nefrol. 2011;33(3): 300-305.

[35] Munoz Mendoza J, Bayes LY, Sun S, Doss S, Schiller B. Effect of lowering dialysate sodium concentration on interdialytic weight gain and blood pressure in patients undergoing thrice-weekly in-center nocturnal hemodialysis: a quality improvement study. Am J Kidney Dis. 2011;58(6): 956-963.

[36] Afsar B, Elsurer R, Huddam B, Erden C. Helicobacter pylori infection: protective against increased interdialytic weight gain in asymptomatic hemodialysis patients? J Ren Nutr. 2011;21(4): 322-328.

[37] Bi SH, Linke L, Wu J, Cheng LT, Wang T, Ahmad S. Effects of Beta-blocker use on volume status in hemodialysis patients. Blood Purif. 2012;33(4):311-316.

[38] Weiner DE, Tighiouart H, Vlagopoulos PT, Griffith JL, Salem DN, Levey AS, et al. Effects of anemia and left ventricular hypertrophy on cardiovascular disease in patients with chronic kidney disease. J Am Soc Nephrol. 2005;16:1803-1810.

[39] Weiner DE, Tighiouart H, Vlagopoulos PT, Griffith JL, Salem DN, Levey AS, et al. Effects of anemia and left ventricular hypertrophy on cardiovascular disease in patients with chronic kidney disease. J Am Soc Nephrol. 2005;16:1803-1810.

[40] van der Weerd NC, Grooteman MP, Blankestijn PJ, Mazairac AH, van den Dorpel
      MA, den Hoedt CH, Nubé MJ, Penne EL, van der Tweel I, Ter Wee PM, Bots ML
      Poor Compliance with Guidelines on Anemia Treatment in a Cohort of Chronic He-
      modialysis Patients. Blood Purif. 2012;34(1):19-27.

[41] Carrero JJ, Stenvinkel P. Persistent inflammation as a catalyst for other risk factors in
      chronic kidney disease: a hypothesis proposal. Clin J Am Soc Nephrol. 2009;4:S49-
      S55.

[42] Stenvinkel P, Barany P, Heimburger O, Pecoits-Filho R, Lindholm B. Mortality, mal-
      nutrition, and atherosclerosis in ESRD: what is the role of interleukin-6? Kidney Int
      Suppl. 2002;103:108.

[43] Zoccali C, Benedetto FA, Mallamaci F, Tripepi G, Fermo I, Foca A, Paroni R, Malatino
      LS. Inflammation is associated with carotid atherosclerosis in dialysis patients. Creed
      Investigators. Cardiovascular Risk Extended Evaluation in Dialysis Patients. J Hyper-
      tens. 2000;18:1207-1213.

[44] Stenvinkel P, Heimburger O, Jogestrand T. Elevated interleukin-6 predicts progres-
      sive carotid artery atherosclerosis in dialysis patients: association with Chlamydia
      pneumoniae seropositivity. Am J Kidney Dis. 2002;39:274-282.

[45] Yeun JY, Levine RA, Mantadilok V, Kaysen GA. C-Reactive protein predicts all-cause
      and cardiovascular mortality in hemodialysis patients. Am J Kidney Dis.
      2000;35:469-476.

[46] Schwarz U, Buzello M, Ritz E, Stein G, Raabe G, Wiest G, Mall G, Amann K. Mor-
      phology of coronary atherosclerotic lesions in patients with end-stage renal failure.
      Nephrol Dial Transplant. 2000;15:218-223.

[47] Stenvinkel P, Pecoits-Filho R, Lindholm B. Coronary artery disease in end-stage renal
      disease: no longer a simple plumbing problem. J Am Soc Nephrol. 2003;14:1927-1939.

[48] Stenvinkel P, Alvestrand A. Inflammation in end-stage renal disease: sources, conse-
      quences, and therapy. Semin Dial. 2002;15:329-337.

[49] Parekh RS, Plantinga LC, Kao WH, Meoni LA, Jaar BG, Fink NE, Powe NR, Coresh J,
      Klag MJ. The association of sudden cardiac death with inflammation and other tradi-
      tional risk factors. Kidney Int. 2008;74:1335-1342.

[50] Singh U, Jialal I. Oxidative stress and atherosclerosis. Pathophysiology. 2006;13(3):
      129-142.

[51] Madamanchi NR, Vendrov A, Runge MS. Oxidative stress and vascular disease. Ar-
      teriosclerosis, Thrombosis, and Vascular Biology. 2005; 25(1): 29-38.

[52] Witztum JL. The oxidation hypothesis of atherosclerosis. Lancet. 1994; 344(8925):
      793-795.

[53] Torzewski M, Lackner KJ. Initiation and progression of atherosclerosis—enzymatic or oxidative modification of low-density lipoprotein? Clinical Chemistry and Laboratory Medicine. 2006;44(12):1389-1394.

[54] Le N-A. Reducing oxidized lipids to prevent cardiovascular disease. Current Treatment Options in Cardiovascular Medicine. 2008;10(4):263-272.

[55] Le NA. Oxidized lipids and lipoproteins: indices of risk or targets for management. Future Lipidology. 2009;4(1):41- 45.

[56] Zhou Q, Wu S, Jiang J, Tian J, Chen J, Yu X, Chen P, Mei C, Xiong F, Shi W, Zhou W, Liu X, Sun S, Xie D, Liu J, Xu X, Liang M, Hou F. Accumulation of circulating advanced oxidation protein products is an independent risk factor for ischaemic heart disease in maintenance haemodialysis patients.Nephrology (Carlton). 2012;17(7): 642-649.

[57] Boushey CJ, Beresford SA, Omenn GS, Motulsky AG. A quantitative assessment of plasma homocysteine as a risk factor for vascular disease. JAMA. 1995;274:1049-1057.

[58] Homocysteine Studies Collaboration. Homocysteine and risk of ischemic heart disease and stroke: a meta-analysis. JAMA. 2002;288:2015-2022.

[59] Bazzano LA, Reynolds K, Holder KN, He J. Effect of folic acid supplementation on risk of cardiovascular diseases: a meta-analysis of randomised controlled trials. JAMA. 2006;296:2720-2726.

[60] Smith AD, Kim YI, Refsum H. Is folic acid good for everyone? Am J Clin Nutr. 2008;87:517-533.

[61] Ebbing M, Bønaa KH, Nygard O, Arnesen E, Ueland PM, et al. Cancer incidence and mortality after treatment with folic acid and vitamin B12. JAMA. 2009;302:2119-2126.

[62] Mason JB, Dickstein A, Jacques PF, Haggarty P, Selhub J, et al. A temporal association between folic acid fortification and an increase in colorectal cancer rates may be illuminating important biological principles: a hypothesis. Cancer Epidemiol Biomarkers Prev. 2007;16:1325-1329.

[63] Zhang SM, Cook NR, Christine MA, Gaziano JM, Buring JE, et al. Effect of combined folic acid, vitamin B6, and vitamin B12 on cancer risk in women: a randomized trial. JAMA. 2008;300:2012-2021.

[64] Potter K, Hankey GJ, Green DJ, Eikelboom JW, Arnolda LF. Homocysteine or Renal Impairment: Which Is the Real Cardiovascular Risk factors? Arterioscler Thromb Vasc Biol. 2008;28:1158-1164.

[65] Berger AK, Duval S, Krumholz HM. Aspirin, beta-blocker, and angiotensin-converting enzyme inhibitor therapy in patients with end-stage renal disease and an acute myocardial infarction.J Am Coll Cardiol. 2003;42(2):201-208.

[66] Harnett JD, Foley RN, Kent GM, Barre PE, Murray D, Parfrey PS. Congestive heart
      failure in dialysis patients-prevalence, incidence, prognosis and risk factors. Kidney
      Int. 1995;47:884-890.

[67] Harnett JD, Foley RN, Kent GM, Barre PE, Murray D, Parfrey PS. Congestive heart
      failure in dialysis patients — prevalence, incidence, prognosis and risk factors. Kid-
      ney Int. 1995;47:884-890.

[68] Parfrey PS, Foley RN, Harnett JD, Kent GM, Murray D, Barre PE. Outcome and risk
      factors of ischemic heart disease in chronic uremia. Kidney Int. 1996;49:1428-1434.

[69] Foley RN, Parfrey PS, Harnett JD, Kent GM, Martin CJ, Murray DC, Barre PE. Clini-
      cal and echocardiographic disease in patients starting end-stage renal disease thera-
      py. Kidney Int. 1995; 47:186-192.

[70] Jadoul M, Thumma J, Fuller DS, Tentori F, Li Y, Morgenstern H, Mendelssohn D, To-
      mo T, Ethier J, Port F, Robinson BM. Modifiable practices associated with sudden
      death among hemodialysis patients in the Dialysis Outcomes and Practice Patterns
      Study. Clin J Am Soc Nephrol. 2012;7(5):765-774.

Chapter 3

Medical Nutrition Therapy for Hemodialysis Patients

F. Esra Güneş

Additional information is available at the end of the chapter

1. Introduction

Nutrition in hemodialysis is very important in decreasing complications and improving quality life of patients. Nutrition program on patients with chronic renal failure on dialysis plays an important role in the process of treatment.

The purposes of medical nutrition therapy in dialysis patients are to promote the nutrition to correct patients' appetite, to correct systemic complications composed by the loss of nephrons in progress, to reduce of protein catabolism to the lowest level, to relieve or prevent the cardio-vascular, cerebrovascular, peripheral vascular diseases formation, to prevent increasing fluid and electrolyte disorders, to reduce uremic symptoms such as itching, nausea, vomiting, loss of appetite and to ensure optimum nutrition. In addition, medical nutrition helps to avoid high-potassium and sodium from the diet, to prevent pulmonary edema, hypertension and heart failure, to prevent renal osteodystrophy keeping the consumption of calcium and phosphorus under control, to prevent protein energy malnutrition with saving patients' food consumption and detecting nutritional status with methods such anthropometric measurements, laboratory findings, subjective global assessment (SGA) (Cianciaruso 1995, Kopple 2004, Mahan 2012). Negative changes (hyperkalemia, hiperfosfotemi, peripheral and pulmonary edema) in fluid-electrolyte balance occur in patients who do not comply to the diet.

In this chapter, assessment of nutritional status in hemodialysis patients and preparation of individual dietary training programs for patients will be discussed.

2. Assesment of the nutritional status

Regular assessment of nutritional status in hemodialysis patients is important and early de-tection of malnutrition can be helpful in improving this condition (Fouque 2003).

The results of studies indicate that hemodialysis patients are at risk of malnutrition. The evaluation methods used in the nutritional status showed that 18-75% prevalence of malnutrition in hemodialysis patients, malnutrition could cause a worse outcome and subsequent mortality(Dwyer 2005). Chazot's study was assessed the nutritional status of twenty hemodialysis patients receiving hemodialysis treatment more than 20 years and was showed that hemodialysis treatment caused to malnutrition the long period of time(Chazot 2001).

Malnutrition occurs depending on several factors in hemodialysis patients. Especially, there is reduction of protein-energy intake because of inappropriate dietary restrictions, anorexia, and taste alterations, promoting malnutrition in most patients entering dialysis (Lavılle 2000). Studies illustrate that there are two types of malnutrition in dialysis patients: The first type is specified by uraemic syndrome and reduction in serum albumin levels due to decreasing energy and protein intake. It should be provided improvement with adequate energy and protein intake. The second type is associated with inflammation and atherosclerosis, high cardiovascular mortalite(MIA Syndrome). Prominent features of this type, proinflammatory cytokines, increased oxidative stress, increased protein catabolism, increased resting energy expenditure, hypoalbuminemia (Stenvınkel 2000, Baltzan 1998). İn addition, malnutrition due to poor nutrition, chronic volume overload congestive heart failure and systemic hypertension, uraemic bone disease and extraskeletal metastatic calcification due to hyperphosfotemia development are other adverse conditions encountered as a result of the diet incompatibility.

In general, there are catabolic and inflammatory situation in patients with end-stage. Patients receiving dialysis treatment are seen in tissue loss in the course of time. At the start of dialysis treatment, having a high level adipocyte tissue can be advantageous for individuals. Dialysis patients who have excess body fat mass are being protected against this situation because of more energy storage. Recent data shows that patients who are overweight or obese had higher rates of survival than normal or in hemodialysis patients. Low serum albumin level (hypoalbuminemia) revealed that the obese are less in HD patients. Reduction in mortality in overweight patients was reported as well as indicators of nutritional status of overweight HD patients was significantly higher than underweight HD patients and to be shorter than the duration of hospital stay. (Glanton 2003, Guida 2004, Kalantar-Zadeh 2005)

Different methods are used in the evaluation of nutritional status in hemodialysis patients. Biochemical, anthropometric measurements, nitrogen and energy balance techniques, record of food intake, subjective global assessment, bioimpedance analysis (BIA), Dual-Energy X-ray Absorptiometry (DEXA), creatinine kinetics, neutron activation analysis and nuclear magnetic resonance spectrometry and serum markers: albumin, pre-albumin, insulin-like growth factor-1 (IGF-1) and transferrin; main proteins of the acute phase (C-reactive protein (CRP), serum amyloid A), secondary proteins of the acute phase (fibrinogen, ferritin, complement), cytokines (interleukin-6 (IL-6), tumour necrosis factor) are used to assess the nutritional status of patients with chronic renal failure (Basile 2003).

Some studies (Beddhu 2002, Panichi 2006) describe hypoalbuminemia in HD patients as a strong indicator for mortality and morbidity. As a result of malnutrition, albumin synthesis decreases and develops hypoalbuminemia. In fact, the serum albumin level is a powerful way directly correlated with dietary protein, but recent literature emphasizes that the effect of serum albumin concentration on the inflammatory response. Albumin is a negative acute phase protein, except nutritional status, and its synthesis is supressed during inflammation. For this reason, there are limitations in the use of serum albumin level in order to assess the nutritional status of patients due to be affected by malnutrition and inflammatory reactions (Santos 2003). Indeed, because of longer half life, it cannot be a sensitive indicator for nutritional therapy. In studies, significant negative correlation was found between prealbumin and CRP (Kaysen 1995, Owen 1998, Sathishbabu 2012). Prealbumin is a negative marker of inflammation level that correlates positively and significantly with other nutritional markers in ESRD patients on hemodialysis (Sathishbabu 2012). Because of the shorter half life of prealbumin, many authors consider prealbumin to be a better marker of nutrition than serum albumin (Mittman 2001, Kalantar-Zadeh 2003). That is considered one of the indicators of uremic malnutrition less than 29mg/dl of serum prealbumin levels in patients on dialysis, serial measurements are recommended in the evaluation of nutritional status (Pupim 2004). Serum creatinine concentration (less than 10 mg/dl) should be evaluated for PEM and skeletal muscle wasting, because it indicates reduced dietary protein intake and skeletal muscle mass(Janardhan 2011).

Subjective Global Assessment (SGA) is often preferred by experts to assess the nutritional status in chronic dialysis patients as relatively quick, easy, and cheaper than other methods (Mutsert 2009). İt is important that SGA was proposed by the National Kidney Foundation (NKF) Kidney Disease/Dialysis Outcomes and Quality Initiative (K/DOQI) for nutritional assessment in the adult dialysis patients(K/DOQI 2000).

Subjective Global Assessment (SGA) reveals that there are seven components to assess nutritional status; two components related to physical examination (indicator of fat and muscle loss and nutritional status-associated with changes in fluid balance) and five components of medical history (weight change, diet, gastrointestinal symptoms, functional capacity, disease and nutrition relationship needs) (Steiber 2004). While SGA scoring points are given in each section of 1-7 and are categorized as 1-2 points (bad), 3-5 points (moderate), 6-7 points (normal). If it is received from this SGA most 6 or 7 points refers mild malnutrition. Most of 3, 4 or 5 points show moderate malnutrition. Most of the findings of sections 1 or 2 points received are recognized as marked malnutrition and severe malnutrition (Janardhan 2011). European Best Practice Guidelines (EBPG) on diagnosis and monitoring of malnutrition proposed that the SGA can be used to determine malnutrition in hemodialysis patients (Fouque 2007).

Nutritional history and dietary record provide information about nutrition of patients and determine for malnutrition development at risk whether or not. Because of record of food intake is taken long-term, bored patients may cause to give false information. Therefore, record of food intake 3-day to get more accurate for patients (Kalantar-Zadeh 2003).

3. Energy

Enough energy should be taken for the effective use of dietary protein and the protection of the nutrients stores of body. Energy metabolism is impaired and is composed of negative energy balance because of disrupted cellular energy metabolism in hemodialysis patients (Mak 2011). Therefore, to consume enough energy identified by the daily energy requirements of ESRD patients provides a positive nitrogen balance and preventing tissue destruction and protein catabolism.

The anorexia nervosa was often encountered in patients in the next few months from the start of dialysis therapy. This is because, even though dramatic changes in their lives, psychological conditions, can not be adapted to a new and restricted diet. It has been reported if protein and energy intake are not increased in these patients, lost energy is stored with muscle mass of patients, and the amount of body fat is decreased (Fouque 2003). The studies have suggested that the dietary energy failure is more on dialysis treatment days than non dialysis treatment days (Burrowes 2003, Rao 2000). In a prospective multicenter clinical trial that included 1901 participants of the Hemodialysis Study, dietary energy intake was 1.02 kcal/kg/day less on dialysis treatment days than on nondialysis treatment days. (Burrowes 2003, Stark 2011).

Some studies indicated that energy intake was low in hemodialysis patients. Poor appetite and hypermetabolism fairly reduce food intake in hemodialysis patients (O'Keefe 2002, Nakao 2003, Morais 2005, İkizler 2002, Pumpkin 2002). When the recommended energy requirements compared with consumed amounts, it is concluded that energy intake is inadequate in 90% of patients (Rocco 2002)

When energy intake of hemodialysis patients was 32-38 kcal/kg/day, have not been reported any increasing or decreasing in nitrogen balance and anthropometric parameters, and developing a negative or a positive energy balance. (Kopple 2004).

Studies demonstrated that low-energy and with low protein diet cause weight loss and malnutrition in patients. For these reasons, sedentary, non-obese dialysis patients's requirements of energy coming from all sources should be determined, according to NKF-DOQI, ESPEN and EDTNA-ERCA 2002; respectively, 35 cal/kg/day (under the age of 60), 30-35 cal/kg/day(over the age of 60); 35 cal/kg/day and 30-35 cal/kg (ideal body weight)/day. (Kopple 2001, Kopple 2004, Cano 2006, Fouque 2003). In some studies, it was shown that hemodialysis patients should receive daily energy as 30-40 kcal/kg (Kalantar-Zadeh 2003, Stenvinkel 2000).

4. Protein

Protein requirement increases due to the dialysate losses and catabolism in hemodialysis patients. In research, it is emphasized that the inadequate protein intake increases mortality (Ohkawa 2004).

Raj et al's study showed that hemodialysis increases both protein synthesis and degradation. The net effect of hemodialysis is loss of nitrogen in skeletal muscle. Protein synthesis and degradation increases by 50-100% of normal values. Hemodialysis causes to increase in catabolic indicators such as interleukin-1 (IL-1), interleukin-6 (IL-6) and tumor necrosis factor alpha (TNF-α). This increasing in the production of cytokines causes in protein degradation. Reasons for increased protein requirement; amino acid losses into the dialysate, increased protein catabolism, metabolic and hormonal changes(Raj 2007).

There are 0.2-0.3 g/kg or 6-8 g/day of protein, amino acids (aa) and peptide losses with the dialysis fluid during hemodialysis. Protein catabolism increases with these losses due to metabolic disorders. The lost in amino acids needs to be replaced to avoid negative nitrogen balance. According to "National Kidney Foundation Dialysis Outcome Quality Initative (NKF-DOQI)" and studies by other investigators to compensate for residual renal losses, dietary protein should be adjusted at least 1.2 g/kg/day in hemodialysis patients as indicated (Kopple 2001, Mahan 2012, Kalantar-Zadeh 2003, Locatelli 2005).

According to ESPEN, adjusted diet protein should be consumed as 1.1-1.2 g / kg / day and should be high in the biological value (of animal origin) of 50 % protein in hemodialysis patients (Mehrotra 2001, Karalis 2002, Cano 2006). Furthermore, the amount of protein of the patient's diet is determined by considering the state of hydration adjusted body weight, glomerular filtration rate and with the course of illness (Nissenson 2008). To determine the adequacy of protein intake in dialysis patients, a good evaluation parameter is BUN value under 120 mg. When 1.2 g / kg / day protein intake, it was indicated protein catabolic rate is associated with low morbidity, provided adequate control of blood urea concentration, improved the nutritional parameters (anthropometric measurements) and biochemical findings (blood albumin, total protein, blood, blood cholesterol, etc.), provided a positive nitrogen balance in dialysis patients (Bergstrom 1993, Amanda 2010).

However, it is required that adequate caloric intake prevent the use of protein as an energy source with gluconeogenessis. Otherwise, a positive nitrogen balance can not be provided in spite of high protein intake. When patients were given a low protein diet, should be followed adequate energy intakes and adequate phosphorus intakes of patients to ensure optimal nutrition, and to prevent malnutrition (Locatelli 2005, Gribotto 2012).

Metabolic acidosis in hemodialysis patients increases protein catabolism, the branched-chain amino acid degradation and muscle glutamine release. Amino acids and glutamine metabolism allow the formation of ammonium and bicarbonate excretion. Changes at branched-chain amino acids levels of muscle and plasma occur in hemodialysis patients. As a result of hemodialysis treatment, plasma valine, muscle valine, plasma leucine are low, muscle leucine, plasma isoleucine, muscle isoleucine are normally observed (Cano, Fouque 2006). Branched-chain amino acids play a regulatory role against chronic acidosis. After acidosis subside is given a support and enriched with branched-chain amino acids and valine during hemodialysis, branched-chain amino acids level of plasma and intracellular are enhanced. (Raj 2000).

Branched-chain amino acids improve appetite in hemodialysis patients. 6.6-15.7 g daily intake of essential amino acids in hemodialysis patients corrected the their nutritional parameters. In patients who underwent 12 g oral branched-chain amino acid a day showed improvement in protein and energy purchases in one month, in the anthropometric measurements six months later. Consantrations of albumin increased 3:31 g / dL to 3.93 g / dL. (Cano, Fouque 2006) According to Raj, although amino acid repletion increased in muscle protein synthesis, no decrease in muscle protein breakdown during HD treatment was observed (Raj 2007)

There is a dynamic effect of animal protein (such as egg, dairy etc.) on renal function in short-term clinical trials. But long-term effects on the normal kidney functions are still unknown. There are mechanisms shown to reveal the different effects of animal and vegetable proteins on renal function including differences in hormones, protein metabolism and interaction with micronutrients. Healthy individuals with normal renal function, long-term consumed high-protein diet (whether of animal protein or vegetable protein) may cause kidney damage and accelerate chronic renal failure. However, long term studies are necessary to determine the different effect of the consumption of animal or vegetable protein diet on renal functions (Bernstein 2007).

5. Carbohydrate

Carbohydrate intake requires enough energy and to maintain reserve protein that can be used for the synthesis protein of tissue.

When dialysis fluid not containing glucose is used for 4 hours, 28 g glucose is lost in hemodialysis. However, when 11 mmol / L glucose was added to the dialysis fluid, the patient gained approximately 23 g of glucose. When glucose is removed by dialysis in the extracellular fluid, loss of the glucose is completed with absorbed carbohydrates, destruction of liver glycogen, and glyconeogenesis in order to avoid symptomatic hypoglycemia. Then, increased protein breakdown and urea synthesis begin. Glucose-free dialysis is reduced pyruvate. Pyruvate does not change with glucose dialysis. Glyconeogenesis may be stimulated with glucose-free dialysis. However, there are negative effects of glucose intake such as hyperglycemia, hyperinsulinemia, hyperlipidemia, obesity etc(Lindholm 1998).

Deterioration of glucose metabolism and insulin resistance develops in chronic renal failure. This situation results in rising levels of glucose and urea when coupled with increased hepatic gluconeogenesis. Insulin metabolism in uremia shows severe abnormalities. Basal insulin secretion is reduced and receives limited response to glucose infusion (Kopple 2004).

In one study, it was observed occurrence of the insulin resistance impaired, muscle glucose uptake and nonoxidative glucose metabolism, in the presence of chronic uremia, but recovered after dialysis (Foss 1996).

Uric acid is generated during fructose metabolism. Serum uric acid levels have been found to correlate with fructose intake. High serum uric acid was associated with hypertension, inflammation, chronic kidney disease and the intake of fructose and added sugars (Feig 2008, Brymora 2012). But fruits containing fructose have some beneficial substances such as anti-oxidants. Therefore, it is possible that fructose intake from natural fruits with regular diet. (Jalal 2010, Brymora 2012).

Carbohydrate from the diet should be higher to provide enough energy, to protect the back-up protein to be used for tissue protein synthesis, to cover the energy deficit. It should pro-vided 60-65% of daily energy from carbohydrates (Kopple 2004). Most patients have difficulty in meeting energy needs with low protein diets. For this reason, the energy gap can be covered by glucose polymers (starch), sugar, simple sugars, pure carbohydrate sour-ces. Patients with diabetes should avoid concentrated sweets (Mahan 2012).

6. Lipids

Recent evidence suggests that protein calorie malnutrition often begins incipiently when the glomerular filtration rate (GFR) is about 28 to 35 mL/min/1.73 m2 or even higher (Kopple 1994) and continues to fall gradually as the GFR decreases below these values (Laville 2000). Reduced quantity of GFH causes a significant increase in plasma lipid levels(Liu 2004). Es-pecially, hyperlipidemia consists when creatinine clearance is below 50 ml/min in patients. In Rutkowski's study, accumulation of triglycerides-rich lipoproteins was associated with increased lipogenetik gene expression of enzymes and the high quantity triglycerides pro-duction by renal deficiency (Rutkowski 2003, Liu 2004).

Usually, there are hypertriglyceridemia and hyperlipidemia in hemodialysis patients. Low-density lipoprotein (LDL) and very low density lipoprotein (VLDL) are high concentration, high density lipoprotein (HDL) cholesterol concentration is low. The main reason of hyper-triglyceridemia is the lack of removal of triglycerides from the circulation (Kwan 2007, Lac-quaniti 2010). In these patients, it has been reported decreased lipoprotein lipase, hepatic lipase enzyme activity.

Generally it is known to decrease in carnitine storages in hemodialysis patients with malnu-trition. In addition, carnitine leaves from the extracellular fluid during dialysis therapy and this situation causes a sudden drop in serum level of carnitine. Carnitine deficiency is caused by deterioration of long-chain fatty acid oxidation and thus deficiency of energy(Ma-tera 2003, Flanagan 2010). İt was determined to put on 750 mg/day carnitine supplementa-tion in diet of hemodialysis patients, reduced the level of plasma TG and LDL cholesterol and increased HDL cholesterol levels(Naini 2012).

Hyperlipidemia develops in a large part of dialysis patients, the amount of fat in the diet should not be higher. Saturated fat content of the diet should be reduced and unsaturated fat content should be increased (Vaziri 2006).

Hyperlipidemia progresses in the majority of patients with CKD; therefore, content of fat in the diet should not be high. Total energy from fat should not exceed 25% to 30. İt should be reduced saturated fat content of the diet and increased unsaturated fat content.

It is recommended reducing saturated fat intake (total energy <7%) and cholesterol intake (<200 mg / day). Total fat content of the diet should be between 25-35% of energy and monounsaturated fatty acids 15-20% of total energy, polyunsaturated fatty acids 10% of total energy of the diet (Nissesson 2008). Recommended foods for patients with a high biological value such as meat, eggs contain high cholesterol. Therefore assessment of serum cholesterol levels should be specific for each patient. If patients have hypertriglyceridemia and high cholesterol, regulation dietary fat content, weight control, increased physical activity, reducing the use of hypertonic solution, restriction of simple sugars of dietary intake are recommended.

Signs and symptoms of deficiency of essential fatty acids such as dry and itchy skin, hair loss, abnormal prostaglandin synthesis are observed in dialysis patients. EPA and DHA which replace arachidonic acid in cell membrane and prevents the formation of pro-inflammatory compounds are part of linolenic acid in fish oil (n-3 fatty acids). According to FDA, intake of n-3 fatty acid with food supplements should not exceed 3 g / day (Vergili-Nelsen JM 2003).

The studies were reported that omega-3 food supplementation reduced levels of triglyceride (Bouzidi 2010, Skulas-Ray 2008), LDL cholesterol and CRP (Saifullah 2007), as well as Omega-6 / omega-3 polyunsaturated fatty acids ratio was important for inflammation and mortality rate in hemodialysis patients(Noori 2011, Daud 2012).

7. Water and electrolytes

The fluid adjustment should be made according to edema and dehydration in the patient. In hemodialysis patients, if conditions such as swelling of the eyes, hands or feet, fluid weight gain, shortness of breath, increased blood pressure or tachycardia are observed, fluid consumption should be restricted (Hegel 1992, Saran 2003). Hemodialysis patients should reduce fluid intake and should limit food consumption such as tea, coffee, soda, water, fruit juices, ice cream, sherbet, gelatin, soups and heavy sauces.

Dietitians, especially renal dietitians, are most often cited as the trusted source on providing information on fluid management and delivering dietary advice (Smith 2010).Research about fluid balance dietician indicates that it is important to teach patients how to deal with thirst without drinking liquids. Proposals such as sucking on ice chips, cold sliced fruit, or sour candies and using artificial saliva are recommended (Mahan 2012).

Controlling sodium and fluid intake are important components of the HD diet. Extracellular volume expansion is the main pathophysiologic determinant of hypertension in HD patients. Water and sodium intake in hemodialysis patients are adjusted according to the amount of urine, fluid balance and blood pressure. With hemodialysis, potassium restriction is often necessary, but the measure of restriction depends on residual renal function (Stark 2011).

Body weight gain during hemodialysis is recommended and should not exceed 1.5-2 kg. A recommended daily amount of fluid of hemodialysis patients should be 500ml + the urinary output in a day or around 1000-1500 ml. Sodium restriction should be based on the amount of urine. A mild salt restriction as 3-4 g / day is sufficient in oliguric patients that have an amount of urine totaling more than 1 liter per day. Anuric hemodialysis patients may consume up to 1 liter of liquid 1-1.5-2 g / daily of salt. If hypertension or heart failure is present, salt and water restriction should be more monitored more delicately. Excess salt intake causes an increase for the feeling of thirst and liquid intake (Fouque 2003, Lindley 2009).

To reduce sodium intake in hemodialysis patients, olives, pickles, cured meats, garlic sauce, soy sauce, canned foods, sausages, processed meats, ham, chips, pretzels and instant soups should be removed from the diet. Different spices, such as vinegar and lemon, can be used for consumption of unsalted foods or as a salt substitute.

Potassium levels are affected by hemodialysis therapy with the degree of residual renal function and net tissue breakdown (e.g. due to infections) and acid-base status. In HD patients, serum potassium concentrations may change to net intestinal potassium absorption or excretion. An example of this change or excretion is diarrhea. Serum potassium is impressed by dietary potassium intake. It is thought this relationship is stronger when the potassium intake is very low or very high in diets of HD patients (Kaveh 2001, Noori 2010).

Potassium restriction is often required because hemodialysis patients are usually anuric. Anuric HD patients are recommended to restrict their potassium intake to 1600-2000mg daily. Hypokalemia may occur with symptoms such as severe vomiting, diarrhea, diuretic use, due to the reduction of potassium. In this case, the potassium content of the diet should be increased (Fouquo 2003).

When blood potassium levels in dialysis patients are high, treatment of the patient's diet should be reviewed as a priority. The food consumption should be limited to reduce the intake of potassium levels, such as milk, meat products, fruits, legumes, cereals, dried fruits and vegetables,etc.

8. Vitamin and minerals

Some studies demonstrate vitamin and mineral supplements for the long-term hemodialysis patients. Hemodialysis patients are potentially at risk of deficiency and excess of trace elements (Inamoto 2003). Given that essential trace elements play key roles in multiple biological systems, including immunological defense against oxidation and infection. It has been hypothesized that the increased morbidity and mortality seen in hemodialysis patients may in part be due to the imbalance of trace elements that has not yet been recognized (D'Haese 1996, Coombes 2012).

In HD patients, there are many problems associated with the lack of food intake. Poor nutrition, restriction of foods that are rich in water-soluble vitamins, foods that are rich in potassium, metabolic disorders caused by uremia, infection and diseases such as gastrointestinal diseases or complications associated with reduced intake of foods are some of the possible scenarios. The lack of foods containing vitamins leads to vitamin and deficiencies that could cause of further possible complications in dialysis patients. (Mahan 2012).

In dialysis patients, B6, folic acid and vitamin C deficiencies have been observed (Coveney 2011). Vitamin B6 deficiencies, especially as it plays in amino acid utilization and lipid metabolism and maintains a critical role as a coenzyme, are very important to monitor closely. Deficiencies in either folic acid, vitamin B6 or vitamin B12 can greatly affect to capacity of the others to function properly (Wierzbicki 2007). This bond requires all to work in synchrony for optimum performance of the metabolic pathway. İf Vitamin B6 and folic acid supplements are not used in dialysis treatment, pyridoxine and folic acid may often reduce red cells and plasma (Steiber 2011). In dialysis patients, an additional intake of vitamin B6 reduces plasma cholesterol and triglyceride levels and additional intake of folic acid can reduce the high levels of homocysteine, which has been determined to be a risk factor for cardiovascular disease (Dumm 2003). Vitamin B6 and folic acid intake in HD patients are higher than normal healthy subjects, and respectively, the recommended intake varied between 1 mg and 10mg per day in most studies (Steiber 2011).

In addition, the loss of vitamin C has been observed in HD patients. Increasing vitamin C in the diet to a recommended amount of 100-200 mg/daily was at once the standard suggestion of mending this problem. However, the intake of higher doses of ascorbic acid was found to possibly lead to the accumulation of oxalate, which is the metabolite of vitamin C. With oxalate accumulation, formation of calcium oxalate stones in the kidneys, the accumulation of calcium oxalate in internal organs and blood vessels, hypercalcemia and hiperoxalemia are all symptoms (Moyad 2009). Recently, the daily requirement of vitamin C in patients undergoing hemodialysis is suggested at 60-90 mg/daily (Kopple 2004). In addition, ascorbic acid supplementations, are composed of iron overload. In uremic patients, it is recommended to prevent resistance to erythropoietin. Vitamin C supplementation increased intestinal iron absorption in these patients, which may reduce the incidences of iron deficiency anemia (Handelman 2011).

Thiamine sources are whole grain and enriched bread and cereals, peas, beans, nuts, brown rice, and meats. It is absent in rice and some cereal products. Thiamine nutritional value is lost with cooking, polishing and purifying. Thiamine is not stored in the body and is excreted in the urine, because of a water-soluble vitamins (Steiber 2011). The addition of thiamin is controversial among some experts. However, 30 mg thiamine has been shown to support the improving of the activity of translocases red blood cells. Thiamine requirements should be 1.5 mg / daily, when dialysis patients have operations, infections have a high risk of developing, convulsions of the neurological symptoms can occur and large quantities of glucose adds to the diet(Fattal-Valevski 2011, Fouque 2003).

25 (OH) D3 levels of dialysis patients are known to be lower than the normal population. Treating vitamin D deficiencies shows the important contributions and progressions towards enhancing the quality of life with dialysis patients (Cheng 2007). The studies showed 25(OH)D3 levels significantly lower than 15 ng / mL (37 nmol / L) in patients. The lowest value of vitamin D is accompanied by high levels of secondary hyperparathyroidism (Gha-

zali 1999). There are several reasons for this a) The patient should have a specific catered diet, but this diet may incude the reduction of the intake of vitamin D foods (milk, fish, cream, butter, etc.). b) The endogenous synthesis of vitamin D3 decreases in individuals over 60 years, due to increased melanin and reduced contact with sunlight in the skin (Godar 2012, Holick 1987). c) Urinary path 25 (OH) D3 and vitamin D binding protein loss is high (Saha 1994). d) The decrease of glomerular filtration rate (GFR)(Kawashima 1995, Thadhani 2012).

Hemodialysis treatment does not provide a change for vitamin A levels. B-carotene, ubiquinol, and laykopen levels were lower in patients that didn't have renal failure. The intake of dietary vitamin A should not exceed the RDA in HD patients of 800-1000 mg/day(Koople 2004).

İncreased oxidative stress and cardiovascular risks are associated with hemodialysis patients. The antioxidant properties of vitamin E may be useful in preventing or reducing these risks. HD patients are recommended 400 IU/Daily intake of vitamin E (Galli 2004, Mann 2004, Kopple 2004).

Protein and phosphorus restriction, loss of appetite, and vitamin D deficiencies increase the need of calcium in HD patients. Support of calcium and control of serum phosphorus levels, by using calcium-containing phosphate-binding agents, are balanced simultaneously (Miller 2010). Calcium acetate or calcium carbonate are effective with reducing concentration of serum phosphorus, simultaneously, correcting hypocalcemia and negative calcium balance (Isakova 2009, Miller 2010). However, the use of vitamin D and calcium in hemodialysis patients concluded the risk for severe hypercalcemia and renal osteodystrophy (Tilman 2009). Increasing calcium during treatment should be done carefully. As a result, to ensure the positive balance of calcium levels in dialysis patients, 1000-1500 mg of calcium should be taken daily.

Lack of phosphorus excretion in the human body can be closely related to the glomerular filtration rate. Even if a single nephron loses its function, it may result in the accumulation of phosphorus in the plasma while showing an inability to the discharging of phosphorus (Kopple 2004). When GFR decreased 120 mL / min to 25 mL / min, the accumulation of phosphorus was observed very clearly in the plasma. In hemodialysis patients, the level of serum phosphorus 2.5-4.5 mg / dL, and patients who have a glomerular filtration rate (GFR) between 25 mL/min/1.73 m2 and 70 mL/min/1.73 m2, 8 mg/kg/d to 10 mg/kg/d of phosphorus may be given with the 0.55 g/kg/d to 0.60 g/kg/d of protein. High biological value protein sources including essential amino acids are rich foods from phosphorus, therefore there are difficulties on the limitation of phosphorus. For this reason, the absorption of phosphorus is prevented with the phosphorus binding agents from the outside. Egg white is a rich source of high biological value protein have one of the lowest phosphorus-protein ratios and is also deprived from cholesterol; therefore, it is a particularly healthy food source of protein for patients on dialysis (Noori 2010). Whole eggs instead of egg whites, whole bread instead of white bread, dried beans instead of peas and preferably fish (cod, tuna) that have a low phosphorus / protein ratio, should be consumed to reduce dietary phosphorus intakes in dialysis patients (Cupisti 2003). The active form of vitamin D is added in the treatment, this is an important step in the control of serum parathyroid hormone activity (Steiber 20109).

About 80% absorption of dietary phosphorus from the gastrointestinal tract requires the use of phosphorus-binding agents (Locatelli 2002, Guarneri 2003, Noori 2010, Noori 2010). Niacin working with a different mechanism than phosphate binders, is helpful to lower phosphate levels while causing a decrease transport of phosphate without interfering with the sodium-phosphate pump in the GI lumen (Mahan 2012, Cheng 2006).

Patients with kidney disease are more difficult to assess whether there is sufficient amount of trace elements in the body. Iron (Fe), calcium and zinc deficiencies are demonstrated in dialysis patients. Frequently anemia is shown in dialysis patients due to an iron deficiency (Tarng 1999, Vinay 2009). Because the amount of iron absorbed in the intestine is decreased, severe blood loss can be a symptom. In addition, the formation of erythropoietin decreases due to bone marrow suppression by urea (Mahan 2012). Adding iron is recommended after assessing the patient's serum ferritin and iron levels (Rambod 2008). Intravenous iron therapy can be applied to patients for the treatment of anemia. With this treatment, hemoglobin was shown to be removable at 5-7 g / dL to 10 g / dL. Due to the fact that erythropoietin therapy increases usage of iron, it is recommended for patients to take iron supplementation.

Uremic symptoms, such as anorexia, impaired taste sensation, reduced oxidative stress improved immune function and sexual dysfunction are associated with Zn deficiency in HD patients. CRP is a sensitive marker of inflammatory activity; an association between decreased plasma Zn concentrations with higher CRP levels in hemodialysis patients has been noted (Guo 2010). Concentrations of serum Zn may affected from medications used by hemodialysis patients such as calcium carbonate, calcitriol (Dashti-Khavidaki 2010), aluminum phosphate-binders. For these reasons, Zn, Fe, magnesium (Mg) are needed, respectively, 15 mg / day, 10-18 mg / day, 200-300 mg / daily in dialysis patients (Fouque 2003). In addition, good sources of zinc are meat, poultry, nuts, and lentils and fortified breakfast cereals (Rucker 2010).

Mild selenium deficiency also appears to increase susceptibility to oxidant stress (Klotz 2003, Rayman 2002), which may be especially relevant to HD patients in whom oxidative stress is markedly increased (Stenvinkel 2003) and may contribute to accelerated atherosclerosis. Selenium deficiency may contribute to the risk of infection (Field 2002) and perhaps to uremic cardiomyopathy, thus contributing to the increased risk of CVD in the HD population. The selenium content of grains and seeds is variable, and depends on the selenium content of the soil and the form in which selenium is present (Rucker 2010). Selenium is also present in some meats, seafood, and nuts (particularly brazil nuts); levels in these foods may again be influenced by ambient soil levels (Rayman 2000). Some studies demonstrated oxidative stress and atherosclerosis is associated with selenium deficiency, because of its link to infection and uremic cardiomyopathy. Selenium deficiency increases risk of cardiovascular disease in HD patients(Fujishima 2011).

Recommended dietary nutrient intake for hemodialysis patients are shown below in Table 1 (Nissesson 2008, Rucker 2010, Fouque 2007).

Macronutrients and Fiber	
Dietary protein intake (DPI)	• 1.2 g/kg/d for clinically stable patients (at least 50% should be of high biological value)
Daily energy intake (DEI)	• 35 kcal/kg/d if <60 years • 30–35 kcal/kg/d if 60 years or older
Total fat	25–35% of total energy intake
Saturated fat	<7% of total energy intake
Polyunsaturated fatty acids	Up to 10% of total calories
Monounsaturated fatty acids	Up to 20% of total calories
Carbohydrate	Rest of calories (complex carbohydrates preferred)
Total fiber	"/>20–25 g/d
Minerals and Water (Range of Intake)	
Sodium	750–2000 mg/d
Potassium	2000-2750 mg/d
Phosphorus	800-1000 mg/d
Calcium	<1000 mg/d
Magnesium	200–300 mg/d
Iron	10-18 mg/d
Zinc	15 mg/d
Selenyum	55 µq/d
Water	Usually 750–1500 mL/d
Vitamins (Including Dietary Supplements)	
Vitamin B1 (thiamin)	1.1–1.2 mg/d
Vitamin B2 (riboflavin)	1.1–1.3 mg/d
Pantothenic acid	5 mg/d
Biotin	30 µg/d
Niacin	14–16 mg/d
Vitamin B6 (pyridoxine)	10 mg/d
Vitamin B12	2.4 µg/d
Vitamin C	75–90 mg/d
Folic Acid	1–5 mg/d
Vitamin A	800-1000 µg/d
Vitamin D	1000-1500 IU
Vitamin E	400–800 IU

Table 1. Recommended Dietary Nutrient Intake for Hemodialysis Patients

9. Conclusion

To evaluate the amount of food intake and food preference, the patient's diet history should be taken. The patient's age, gender, social environment, economic, psychological, and educational status and history of the disease should be considered due to nutrition effect. Also, including weekends, during the 3-7 days whole foods is recorded by the patient along with the amount. Daily intake of calories and nutrients of the patients are calculated with information from those records. In addition, laboratory values and SGA as a scoring tool are very important for preparing a appropriate diet for HD patients.

The hemodialysis therapy should be dealt with by a multidisciplinary team, as recommended for other high risk populations (Morais 2005). A part of medical nutrition therapy is to provide nutrition education and periodic counseling by dietitians. For effective intervention, dietitians should present a guide for educating HD patients about individual nutritional needs. This guide should provide information about food sources, nutrients and usage exchange food lists. Adapting to patients requirements of intakes should be based on their laboratory values. Patients may be predisposed to receiving lower than recommended amounts of energy and macro-nutrients to the diet and patients who received information or counseling about their diet must be followed up closely by renal dietitians (Mahan 2012).

If a patient has diabetes, the control of blood sugar is required with a specialized diet therapy. Due to high serum glucose levels, osmolality increases, water and potassium are pulled out of cells. There are the relationship between glycemic control and survival of hemodialysis patients (Mahan 2012). Poor glycemic control causes to macrovascular complications and generation of advanced glycation end products (AGEs)(Ricks 2012). The diet for diabetes management can be modified for a patient on dialysis.

Recently, dialysis treatment is increasing in elderly patients with end-stage renal disease (ESRD) (Tamura 2009). Elderly hemodialysis patients have some diseases such as ischemic heart disease, diabetes mellitus, infectious diseases, bone fracture, cerebrovascular disease in common with ESRD. Specific prescriptions should prepare for elderly dialysis patients such as longer treatment time, nutritional support, and a personalized treatment schedule(Burns 2003). In addition, tube feeding and parenteral interventions may reinforce protein and energy intake among patients with malnutrition and anorexia.

Author details

F. Esra Güneş

Marmara University, Health Science Faculty, Department of Nutrition and Dietetic, Turkey

References

[1] Mahan K, Escott-Stump S, Raymond JL (2012) Krause's Food and the Nutrition Care Process, 13. Edition, Elsevier.

[2] Stark S, Snetselaar L, Hall B, Stone RA, Kim S, Piraino B, Sevick M A (2011) Nutritional Intake in Adult Hemodialysis Patients, Top Clin Nutr, Vol. 26, No. 1, 45–56.

[3] D'Haese PC, De Broe ME (1996) Adequacy of dialysis: trace elements in dialysis fluids. Nephrol Dial Transplant 11(Suppl. 2):92–97.

[4] Fouque D, Guebre-Egziabher F (2007) An update on nutrition in chronic kidney disease, Int Urol Nephrol, 39:239–246.

[5] Fouque D, Guebre-Egziabher F, Laville M (2003) Advances in anabolic interventions for malnourished dialysis patients. J Renal Nutr 13:161–165.

[6] Ohkawa S, Kaizu Y, Odamaki M, Ikegaya N, Hibi I, Miyaji K, Kumagai H: (2004) Optimum dietary protein requirement in nondiabetic maintenance hemodialysis patients. Am J Kidney Dis, 43:454–463.

[7] Coombes JS, Fasset RG (2012) Antioxidant therapy in hemodialysis patients: a systematic review, Kidney International (2012) 81, 233–246.

[8] Vaziri ND, Moradi H (2006) Mechanisms of dyslipidemia of chronic renal failure. Hemodial Int,; 10: 1–7.

[9] Inamoto H, Kata M, Suzuki K (2003) Deficiency of Vitamins and Minerals in the Dialysis Diet: The State of 33 Essential Nutrients. Nephrology Dialysis Transplantation. 18:448.

[10] Mutsert R, Grootendorst DC, Boeschoten EW, Brandts H, Manen JG, Krediet RT, Dekker FW (2009) Subjective global assessment of nutritional status is strongly associated with mortality in chronic dialysis patients, Am J Clin Nutr 2009;89:787–93.

[11] Laville M, FouqueD (2000) Nutritional aspects in hemodialysis, Kidney International, Vol. 58, Suppl. 76, pp. S-133–S-139.

[12] Steiber A, Kalantar-Zadeh K, Secker D, McCarthy M, Sehgal A (2004) Subjective Global Assessment in Chronic Kidney Disease: A Review, Journal of Renal Nutrition, Vol 14, No 4 (October): pp 191-200.

[13] K/DOQI (2000) National Kidney Foundation: Clinical practice guidelines for nutrition in chronic renal failure. Am J Kidney Dis(suppl 2)35:S1-140,

[14] Dwyer JT, Larive B, Leung J, Rocco MV, TOM Greene T, Burrowes J, Chertow GM, Cockram DB, Chumlea WC, Daugirdas J, Frydrych A, Kusek JW forthe hemo study group (2005) Are nutritional status indicators associated with mortality in the hemodialysis (HEMO) study?. Kidney nt Vol68: 1766-1776.

[15] Stenvınkel P, Heımbürger O, Lındholm B, Kaysen, GA, Bergström J (2000) Are There Two Types of Malnutrition in Chronic Renal Failure Evidence for Relationships Between Malnutrition, Inflammation and Atherosclerosis (MIA Syndrome). Nephrol Dial Transplant. 15:953-960.

[16] Baltzan MA, Shoker AS (1998) Malnutrition and Dialysis, Kidney Int.:53:999.

[17] Chazot C, Laurent G, Charra B, Blanc C, Vovan C, Jean G, Vanel T, Terrat J C, Ruffet M (2001) Malnutrition in Long Term Hemodialysis Survivors. Nephrol Dial Transplant. 16:61-69.

[18] Basile C (2003) The effect of convection on the nutritional status of haemodialysis patients, Nephrol Dial Transplant,18 [Suppl 7]: vii46–vii49.

[19] Burrowes JD, Larive B, Cockram DB, Dwyer J, Kusek JW, McLeroy S, Poole D, Rocco MV, (2003) For the HEMO Study Group. Effects of dietary intake, appetite, and eating habits on dialysis and nondialysis treatment days in hemodialysis patients: cross-sectional results from the HEMO Study. J Ren Nutr.;13(3):191-198.

[20] Rao M, Sharma M, Juneja R, Jacob S, Jacob CK (2000)Calculated nitrogen balance in hemodialysis patients: Influence of protein intake, Kidney International, Vol. 58, pp. 336–345.

[21] O'Keefe A, Daigle NW(2002) A new approach to classifying malnutrition in the hemodialysis patient, J Ren Nutr.;12:248-55.

[22] Morais AC, Silva MA, Faintuch J, Vidigal E J, Costa RA, Lyrio DC, Trindade CR, Pitanga KK (2005) Correlatıon of nutrıtıonal status and food ıntake ın hemodıalysıs patıents, Clınıcs, 60(3):185-92

[23] Nakao T, Matsumoto H, Okada T, Kanazawa Y, Yoshino M, Nagaoka Y, Takeguchi F (2003) Nutritional management of dialysis patients: balancing among nutrient intake, dialysis dose, and nutritional status. Am JKidney Dis.: 41(3 Suppl 1):S133-6.

[24] Beddhu S, Kaysen GA, Yan G, Sarnak M, Agodoa L, Ornt D, Cheung AK (2002) Association of serum albümin and atherosclerosis in chronic hemodialysis patients. Am J Kidney Dis: 40(4):721-7.

[25] Panichi V., Rizza, M.G., Taccola, D., Paoletti, S., Mantuano, E., Migliori, M., Frangioni, S., Filippi, C., Carpi, A. (2006) C reactive protein in patients on chronic hemodialysis with different techniques and different membranes. Biomed Pharmacother; 60(1):14-7.

[26] Santos NCJ, Draibe SA, Kaimmura MA, Canziani MEF, Cendoroglo M, Júnior AG, Cuppari L (2003)Is serum albumin a marker of nutritional status in hemodialysis patients without evidence of inflammation. Artificial Organs 27(8):681-686.

[27] Mittman N, Morell MA, Kyin KO, ChattapadhyayJ (2001) Serum prealbumin predicts survival in hemodialysis and peritoneal dialysis: 10 years of prospective observation. Am J Kidney Dis;38(6): 1358-64.

[28] Sathishbabu M , Suresh S (2012) A study on correlation of serum prealbumin with other biochemical parameters of malnutrition in hemodialysis patient, Int J Biol Med Res; 3(1): 1410-1412.

[29] Kaysen GA, Rathore V, Shearer GC, Depner TA (1995) Mechanisms of hypoalbuminemia in hemodialysis patients. Kidney Int 1995; 48: 510-16.

[30] Owen WF, Lowrie EG(1998)C-reactive protein as an outcome predictor for maintanence hemodialysis patients. Kidney Int; 54:627-636.

[31] Pupim LB, İkizler A.(2004) Assessment and monitoring of uremic malnutrition. Journal Of Renal Nutrition ,14,6-19.

[32] Janardhan V, Soundararajan P, Vanitha Rani N, Kannan G, Thennarasu P, Ann Chacko R, Maheswara Reddy CU (2011) Prediction of Malnutrition Using Modified Subjective Global Assessment-dialysis Malnutrition Score in Patients on Hemodialysis, Indian J Pharm Sci., Jan-Feb; 73(1): 38–45.

[33] Kalantar-Zadeh K,İkizler TA, Block G, Morrel M,Kopple JD (2003) Malnutrition-inflammation complex syndrome in dialysis patients:causes and consequences. American Journal Of Kidney Disease,42(5),864-881.

[34] Fouque D, Vennegoor M, Wee PT, Wanner C, Basci A, Canaud B, Haage P, Konner K, Kooman J, Martin-Malo A, Pedrini L, Pizzarelli F, Tattersall J, Tordoir J, Raymond Vanholder R (2007) EBPG guideline on nutrition. Nephrol Dial Transplant;22(2):ii45–87.

[35] Kalantar-Zadeh K, Abbott KC, Salahudeen AK, Kilpatrick RD, Harwich TB (2005)Survival advantages of obesity in dialysis patients. Am J Clin Nutr:81:543-54.

[36] Glanton CW, Hypolite O, Hshien PB, Agodoa LY, Yuan CM, Abott K(2003) Factors associated with improved short term survival in obeses end stage renal disease patients. Ann Epidemiol. 2003; 13: 136-143.

[37] Guida B, Trio R, Nastasi A, Lacetti R, Pesola D, Torneca S, Memoli B, Cianciaruso B (2004) Body composition and cardiovascular risk factors in pretransplant hemodialysis patients. Clin Nutr 23:363-72.

[38] Rocco MV, Paranandı L, Burrowes JD (2002) Nutritional Status in the HEMO Study Cohort at Baseline Hemodialysis. Am JKidney Dis. 39:245-256.

[39] Ikizler TA, Pupim LB, John R. Brouillette JR, Levenhagen DK, Farmer K, Hakim RM, Flakoll PJ (2002) Hemodialysis stimulates muscle and whole body protein loss and alters substrate oxidation. AmJ Physiol Endocrinol Metab; 282: E107-116.

[40] Pupim LB, Flakoll PJ, Brouillette JR, Levenhagen DK, Hakim RM, Ikizler TA(2002) İntradialytic parenteral nutrition improves protein and energy homeostasis in chronic hemodialysis patients. J Clin Invest;110: 483-492.

[41] Kopple JD, Massery CG(2004) Nutritional management of renal disease. Second edition, wiliams&wilkins, Lippincott.

[42] Raj DS, Adeniyi O, Dominic EA, Boivin MA, McClelland S, Tzamaloukas AH, Morgan N, Gonzales L, Wolfe R, Ferrando A (2007) Amino acid repletion does not decrease muscle protein catabolism during hemodialysis, Am J Physiol Endocrinol Metab 292: E1534–1542.

[43] Kopple JD(2001) The national kidney foundation k/doqı clinical practice guidelines for dietary protein ıntake for chronic dialysis pateints. Am. J. of Kidney Disease ,38 (4) Supplement 1, S68-S73.

[44] Canoa N, Fiaccadorib E, Tesinskyc P, Toigod G, Drumle W, DGEM: Kuhlmann M, Mann H, Horl WH(2006). ESPEN guidelines on enteral nutrition: adult renal failure. Clinical Nutrition,25,295-310.

[45] Fouque D (2003) Nutritional requirements in maintenance hemodialysis. Advances İn Renal Replacement Therapy, 10(3),183-193.

[46] Stenvinkel P, Lindholm B, Heimbürger M (2000) Elevated serum levels of soluble adhesion molecules predict death in predialysis patients:association with malnutrition, inflamation and cardiovascular disease, Nephr. Dialysis Transpl.,15,1624-1630.

[47] Mehrotra R, Kopple JD (2001) Nutritional management of maintance dialysis patients. why aren't we going better?, Annual Review of Nutrition,21, 343-379.

[48] Karalis M (2002) Ways to increase protein intake, J.Renal Nutrition, 13(3), 199-204.

[49] Cano N, Fouque D, Leverve X (2006) Application of Branched- Chain Amino Acids in Human Patological States: Renal Failure. J. Nutr, 136, 299- 307.

[50] Raj D, Ouwendyk M, Francoeur R and Pierratos A. (2000) Plasma amino acid profile on nocturnal hemodialysis. Blood Purif, 18, 97–102.

[51] Bernstein A,Treyzon L, Li Z (2007) Are high protein,vegetable-based diets safe for kid ney function? A review of the literature. Journal American Dietetic Association, 107,644-650.

[52] Locatellı F, Vecchıo LD, Pozzonı P (2005) Clinical benefits of slowing the progression of renal failure, Kıdney International , 68(99), S152- S156.

[53] Lim VS, Kopple JD(2000) Protein metabolism in patients with chronic renal failure.role of uremia and dialysis. Kıdney International, 58, 1-10.

[54] Gribotto G, Bonanni A, Verzola D (2012) Effect of kidney failure and hemodialysis on protein and amino acid metabolism, Curr Opin Clin Nutr Metab Car, 15:78–84.

[55] Foss MC, Gouveıa LM, Neto MM, Paccola GM, Pıccınato CE (1996) Effect of Hemodialysis on Peripheral Glucose Metabolism of Patients with Chronic Renal Failure. Nephron. 73:48-53.

[56] Rigalleau V, Combe C, Blanchetier V, Aubertin J, Aparicio M, Gin H (1997) Low protein diet in uremia: Effects on glucose metabolism and energy production rate, Kidney Int., 51:1222-27.

[57] Feig DI, Kang DH, Johnson RJ (2008) Uric acid and cardiovascular risk, N Engl J Med; 359: 1811–1821.

[58] Brymora A, Flisiniski M, Johnson RJ, Goszka G, Stefaniska A, Manitius J (2012) Low-fructose diet lowers blood pressure and inflammation in patients with chronic kidney disease, Nephrol Dial Transplant, 27: 608–612.

[59] Jalal DI, Smits G, Johnson RJ, Chonchol M (2010) Increased fructose associates with elevated blood pressure. J Am Soc Nephrol; 21: 1543–1549.

[60] Liu Y, Coresh J, Eustace JA, Longenecker J, Jaar B, Fink N, Tracy R, Powe NR, Klag MJ (2004) Association Between Cholesterol Level and Mortality in Dialysis Patients. JAMA. 291:451-459.

[61] Rutkowski B, Szolkiewicz M, Korczynska J, Sucajtys E, Stelmanska E, Niewoglowski T, Swierczynski J (2003) The Role of Lipogenesis in the Development of Uremic Hyperlipidemia. Am J Kidney Dis. 41:84-88.

[62] Lindley EJ (2009) Reducing sodium intake in hemodialysis patients.Semin Dialysis, May-Jun;22(3):260-3.

[63] Cianciaruso B, Brunori G, Kopple JD, Traverso G, Panarello G, Enia G, Strippoli P, Vecchi A, Querques M, Viglino G, Vonesh E, Maiorca R (1995) Crosssectional comparisons of malnutrition in continuous ambulatory peritoneal dialysis and hemodialysis patients. Am Journal of Kidney Disease, 26, 475-86.

[64] Lindholm B, Wang T, Heimburger O and Bergstrom J (1998) Influence of different treatments and schedules on the factors conditioning the nutritional status in dialysis patients. Nephrol Dial Transplant, 13 [Suppl 6], 66–73.

[65] Vergili-Nelsen JM (2003) Benefits of fish oil supplementation for hemodialysis patients. J Am Diet Assoc;103: 1174-1177.

[66] Noori N, Dukkipati R, Kovesdy CP, Sim JJ, Feroze U, Murali SB, Bross R, Benner D, Kopple JD, Kalantar-Zadeh K (2011)Dietary omega-3 fatty acid, ratio of omega-6 to omega-3 Intake, inflammation, and survival in longterm hemodialysis patients. Am J Kidney Dis.;58(2):248–256.

[67] Bouzidi N, Mekki K, Boukaddoum A, Dida N, Kaddous A, Bouchenak M(2010) Effects of omega-3 polyunsaturated fatty-acid supplementation on redox status in chronic renal failure patients with dyslipidemia. J Ren Nutr.;20(5):321–328.

[68] Skulas-Ray AC, West SG, Davidson MH, Kris-Etherton PM (2008)Omega-3 fatty acid concentrates in the treatment of moderate hypertriglyceridemia. Expert Opin Pharmacother.;9(7):1237–1248.

[69] Saifullah A, Watkins BA, Saha C, Li Y, Moe SM, Friedman AN(2007)Oral fish oil supplementation raises blood omega-3 levels and lowers C-reactive protein in haemodialysis patients – a pilot study. Nephrol Dial Transplant.;22(12):3561–3567.

[70] Daud ZA, Tubie B, Adams J, Quainton T, Osia R, Tubie S, Kaur D, Khosla P, Shey-man M(2012) Effects of protein and omega-3 supplementation, provided during reg-ular dialysis sessions, on nutritional and inflammatory indices in hemodialysis patients, Vascular Health and Risk Management,8: 187–195.

[71] Kaveh K, Kimmel PL(2001)Compliance in hemodialysis patients: multidimensional measures in search of a gold standard. Am J Kidney Dis;37:244–66.

[72] Noori N, Kalantar-Zadeh K, Kovesdy CP, Murali SB, Bross R, Nissenson AR, Kopple JD, (2010) Dietary Potassium Intake and Mortality in Long-Term Hemodialysis Pa-tients, Am J Kidney Dis., 56(2): 338–347.

[73] Aviva Fattal-Valevski (2011)Thiamine (Vitamin B1), Journal of Evidence-Based Com-plementary & Alternative Medicine, 16: 12.

[74] Ghazali A,Fardellone P, Pruna A, Atık A, Achard JM, Oprisiu R, Brazier M, Remond A, Moriniere P, Garabedian M, Eastwood J, Fournier A (1999) Is low plasma 25-(OH) vitamin D a major risk factor for hyperparathyroidism and Looser's zones independ-ent of calsitirol? Kidney Int, 55:2169-2177.

[75] Cheng S, Coyne D(2007)Vitamin D and outcomes in chronic kidney disease. Curr Opin Nephrol Hypertens;16:77–82.

[76] Holick MF(1987)Photosynthesis of vitamin D in the skin: effect of environmental and life-style variables. Fed Proc., 46(5):1876–1882.

[77] Godar DE, Pope SJ, Grant WB, Holick MF (2012) Solar UV doses of young americans and vitamin D₃ production, Environ Health Perspect 120:139–143.

[78] Saha H(1994)Calcium and vitamin D homeostasis in patients with heavy proteinuria, Clin Nephrol, 41:290–96

[79] Kawashima H, Kraut JA, Kurokawa K(1995) Metabolic acidosis suppresses 25-hy-droxyvitamin D3-1a-hydroxylase in the rat kidney. J Clin Invest, 70:135–140.

[80] Thadhani R, Appelbaum E, Pritchett Y, Chang Y, Wenger J, Tamez H, Bhan I, Agar-wal R, Zoccali C, Wanner C, Lloyd-Jones D, Cannata J,Thompson T, Andress D, Zhang W, Packham D, Singh B, Zehnder D, Shah A, Pachika A, Manning WJ, Solo-mon SD (2012) Vitamin D therapy and cardiac structure and function in patients with chronic kidney disease, JAMA, February 15,Vol 307, No.7.

[81] Rucker D, Thadhani R, Tonelli M (2010)Trace element status in hemodialysis pa-tients, Seminars in Dialysis, 23,4:389–395,

[82] Cheng S, Coyne DW(2006) Niacin and niacinamide for hyperphosphatemia in pa-tients undergoing dialysis, Int.Urol.Nephrol.,38,171.

[83] Mak RH, Ikizler AT, Kovesdy CP, Raj DS, Stenvinkel P, Kalantar-Zadeh K (2011)Wasting in chronic kidney disease, J Cachexia Sarcopenia Muscle, 2:9–25.

[84] Bergstrom J(1993). Nutritional requirements of hemodialysis patients. Mitch W,Klahr S (Ed.).Nutrition and Kidney, U.S.A:Little,Brown and Company, 2nd ed.:263-293.

[85] Kwan BC, Kronenberg F, Beddhu S, Cheung AK(2007) Lipoprotein metabolism and lipid management in chronic kidney disease. J Am Soc Nephrol; 18: 1246–1261.

[86] Lacquaniti A, Bolignano D, Donato V, Bono C, Fazio RM, Buemi M(2010) Alterations of Lipid Metabolism in Chronic Nephropathies: Mechanisms, Diagnosis and Treatment, Kidney Blood Press Res., 33:100–110.

[87] Matera M, Bellinghieri G, Costantino G, Santoro D, Calvani M, Savica V(2003)History of L-carnitine: implications for renal disease. J Ren Nutr, 13:2-14.

[88] Flanagan JL, Simmons PA, Vehige J, Willco MDP, Garrett Q (2010) Rol of carnitine in disease, Nutrition & Metabolism, 7:30.

[89] Naini AE, Sadeghi M, Mortazavi M, Moghadasi M,Harandi AA (2012) Oral Carnitine supplementation for Dyslipidemia in Chronic Hemodialysis Patients, Saudi J Kidney Transp., 23(3):484-498.

[90] Smith K, Coston M, Glock K, BS1, Elasy TA, Wallston KA, PhD4, Ikizler TA, Cavanaugh KL, (2010) Patient Perspectives on Fluid Management in Chronic Hemodialysis, Ren Nutr.; 20(5): 334–341.

[91] Dumm GN, Giammona A (2003) Variations in the lipid profile of patients with chronic renal failure treated with pyridoxine. Lipids in Health andDisease,2,1-7.

[92] Coveney N, Polkinghorne KR, Linehan L, Corradini A, Kerr PG (2011)Water-soluble vitamin levels in extended hours hemodialysis, Hemodialysis International, 15(1): 30-38.

[93] Wierzbicki AS(2007)Homocysteine and cardiovascular disease: a review of the evidence. Diab Vasc Dis Res.;4:143-50.

[94] Steiber AL, Kopple J(2011) Vitamin Status and Needs for People with Stages 3-5 Chronic Kidney Disease,J Renal Nutr,21(5):355-368.

[95] Galli F, Buoncristiani U, Conte C, et al: (2004)Vitamin E in uremia and dialysis patients. Ann N YAcad Sci 1031:348-351,

[96] Mann JFE, Lonn EM, Yı Q, Gerstein HC, Hoogwerf B J, Pogue J, Bosch J, Dagenais GR, Yusuf S (2004)Effects of vitamin E on cardiovascular outcomes in people with mild-to-moderate renal insufficiency: results of the HOPE study. Kidney Int 65: 1375-1380.

[97] Miller JE, Kovesdy CP, Norris KC, Mehrotra R, Nissenson AR, Kopple JD, Kalantar-Zadeh K (2010) Association of Cumulatively Low or High Serum Calcium Levels with Mortality in Long-Term Hemodialysis Patients, Am J Nephrol; 32:403–413.

[98] Isakova T, Gutie' rrez OM Chang Y, Shah A, Tamez H, Smith K, Thadhani R, Wolf M (2009) Phosphorus Binders and Survival on Hemodialysis, J Am Soc Nephrol 20: 388–396.

[99] Drueke TB, Touam M (2009) Calcium balance in haemodialysis—do not lower the dialysate calcium concentration too much(con part),Nephrol Dial Transplant,24:2990–93

[100] Locatelli F, Fouque D, Heimburger O, Drüeke TB, Canata- Andia JB, Hörl W, Ritz W (2002) Nutritional status in dialysis patients: a european concensus. Nephrology Dialysis Trasplantation, 17, 563-572.

[101] Guarneri R, Antonione G (2003) Mechanisms of malnutrition in uremia.Journal of Renal Nutrition,13(2),153-157.

[102] Noori N, Kalantar-Zadeh K, Kovesdy CP, Bross R, Benner D, Kopple JD (2010) Association of Dietary Phosphorus Intake and Phosphorus to Protein Ratio with Mortality in Hemodialysis Patients, Clin J Am Soc Nephrol 5: 683–692.

[103] Noori N, Sims JJ, Kopple JD, Shah A, Colman S, Shinaberger CS, Bross R, Mehrotra R, Kovesdy CP, Kalantar-Zadeh K (2010) Organic and inorganic dietary phosphorus and its management in chronic kidney disease, Iranian Journal of Kidney Diseases, 4:2

[104] Cupisti A, Morelli E, Alessandro C, Lupetti S and Barsotti G. (2003) Phosphate control in chronic üremia: Don't forget diet. J Nephrol, 16, 29-33.

[105] Moyad MA, Combs MA, Crowley DC, Baisley JE, Sharma P, Vrablic AS, Evans M(2009) Vitamin C with metabolites reduce oxalate levels compared to ascorbic acid: a preliminary and novel clinical urologic finding. Urol Nurs 29:95-102,

[106] Handelman GJ (2011) New insight on vitaminc in patients with chronic kidney disease, JRenal Nutr,21(1):110-112.

[107] Locatelli F, Andrulli S, Memoli B, Maffei C, Vecchio CD, Aterini S, Simone WD, Mandalari A, Brunori G, Amato M, Cianciaruso B, Zoccali C (2006) Nutritional-inflammation status and resistance to erythropotein therapy in haemodialysis patients, Nephrol Dial Transplant, 21:991.

[108] Tarng DC, Huang TP, ChenTW, Yang WC (1999)Erythropoietin hyporesponsiveness: from iron deficiency to iron overload. Kidney Int.; 55(suppl 69):S107-118.

[109] Deved V, Poyah P, James MT, Tonelli M, Mann BJ, Walsh M, Hemmelgarn BR (2009) Ascorbic acid for anemia management in hemodialysis patients: a systematic review and meta-analysis, Am J Kidney Dis 54:1089-1097.

[110] Rambod M, Kovesdy CP, Kamyar Kalantar-Zadeh K (2008) Combined high serum ferritin and low iron saturation in hemodialysis patients: the role of inflammation, Clin J Am Soc Nephrol 3: 1691–1701.

[111] Fujishima Y, Ohsawa M, Itai K, Kato K, Tanno K, Turin TC, Onoda T, Endo S, Okayama A, Fujioka T (2011) Serum selenium levels are inversely associated with death risk among hemodialysis patients, Nephrol Dial.Transp.,26:10,3331-38.

[112] Stennett AK, Ofsthun NJ, Kotanko P, Gotch FA (2010) Kinetic modeling as a route to rational dialysis prescriptions—urea, phosphorus, calcium, and more, US Nephrology, 5(2):18–20.

[113] Klotz LO, Kroncke KD, Buchczyk DP, Sies H(2003)Role of copper, zinc, selenium and tellurium in the cellular defense against oxidative and nitrosative stress. J Nutr 133:1448S–1451S.

[114] Rayman MP(2002)The argument for increasing selenium intake,Proc Nutr.Soc, 61:203–215.

[115] Stenvinkel P(2003) Interactions between inflammation, oxidative stress, and endothelial dysfunction in end-stage renal disease. J Ren Nutr, 13:144–148.

[116] Field CJ, Johnson IR, Schley PD(2002) Nutrients and their role in host resistance to infection. J Leukoc Biol 71:16–32.

[117] Saran R, Bragg-Gresham JL, Rayner HC, Goodkın DA, Keen M, Van Dıjk PC, Kurokawa K, Pıera L, Saıto A, Fukuhara S, Young EW, Held PJ, Port FK (2003) Nonadherence in hemodialysis: associations with mortality, hospitalization, and practice patterns in the DOPPS, KidneyInternational, vol. 64, no. 1, pp. 254–262,.

[118] Hegel MT, Ayllon T, Thiel G, Oulton B (1992) Improving adherence to fluid restrictions in male hemodialysis patients: a comparison of cognitive and behavioral approaches, Health Psychology, vol. 11, no. 5, pp. 324–330.

[119] Joni Ricks, Miklos Z. Molnar, Csaba P. Kovesdy, Anuja Shah, Allen R. Nissenson, Mark Williams, Kamyar Kalantar-Zadeh (2012) Glycemic Control and Cardiovascular Mortality in Hemodialysis Patients With Diabetes, A 6-Year Cohort Study, Diabetes March, 61:3, 708-715.

[120] Burns A(2003) Conservative management of end-stage renal failure: Masterly inactivity or benign neglect? Nephron Clin Pract 95: c37–c39.

[121] Tamura MK, Covinsky KE, Chertow GM, Yaffe K, Landefeld CS, McCulloch CE (2009) Functional status of elderly adults before and after ınitiation of dialysis, N Eng J Med, 361;16.

Chapter 4

Bleeding Diathesis in Hemodialysis Patients

Gülsüm Özkan and Şükrü Ulusoy

Additional information is available at the end of the chapter

1. Introduction

End-stage renal disease patients, particularly those treated with hemodialysis (HD), suffer from complex hemostatic disorders. Patients with uremia may experience two opposite hemostatic complications: bleeding diathesis and thrombotic tendencies. Bleeding diathesis in uremic patients is primarily seen due to abnormalities in primary hemostasis, particularly platelet function disorder and impairment of the platelet-wall interaction. Anemia, abnormal nitric oxide production and some drugs employed also contribute to bleeding diathesis.

In addition to bleeding diathesis, thrombotic complications are also frequently seen in uremic patients. Thrombotic complications play a significant role in cardiovascular events, the main cause of mortality in this patient group. Thrombotic hemostatic changes include increased platelet aggregability, increased plasma fibrinogen, factor VIII:C and vWF levels, a decrease in protein C and protein S anticoagulant activity, changes in fibrinolytic system activity and a rise in plasma lipoprotein and homocysteine levels.

In addition to hemostatic changes caused by uremia in the HD patient group, HD therapy itself leads to various hemostatic changes. These include coagulation cascade activation as a result of contact between the dialysis membrane and blood elements, the effect of anticoagulants used to prevent coagulation developing due to this cascade activation and a decrease in the negative effects on platelet functions of middle molecule uremic toxins, thought to be eliminated during HD.

Both hemorrhagic and thrombotic changes in this patient group can give rise to life-threatening consequences. For that reason, research is still continuing into identification and treatment of hemostatic abnormalities in this patient group. Here, we shall be discussing the pathogenesis and treatment of hemorrhagic and thrombotic complications in the light of new research.

2. Normal hemostasis

A knowledge of normal hemostasis is needed in order to understand hemostatic disorders in uremic patients. The normal hemostatic process establishes blood viscosity inside the vessel and rapid plaque formation as a result of vascular injury. Hemostasis consists of three phases; primary hemostasis, coagulation and fibrinolysis (Galbusera et al., 2009). Platelets assume the main role in primary hemostasis. Under normal conditions, it prevents vascular endothelium platelet aggregation and adhesion. In the event of vascular injury, platelet-mediated hemostatic plaque formation begins (Stassen et al., 2004). Two main platelet receptors, glycoprotein Ib (GPIb) and activation-dependent glycoprotein IIb–IIIa (GPIIb–IIIa) complex, and the adhesion molecule von Willebrand factor (VWF) and fibrinogen are involved in the adhesion process in hemostatic plaque formation. Various modifications take place in the platelets after the adhesion phase, and molecules assisting platelet activation and adhesion, such as ADP, serotonin, epinephrine, fibrinogen, thromboxane and VWF, are released from the platelet granules (Ruggeri et al., 2003). The coagulation phase consists of intrinsic and extrinsic coagulation pathways. A number of coagulation proteins are involved in these coagulation pathways, including Tissue Factor (TF), and factors VII, IX, X, V, VIII, XI and XIII. Natural inhibitors of the coagulation cascade are protein C, Tissue factor (TF) pathway inhibitor and antithrombin III (Stassen et al., 2004). The fibrinolytic system leads to plasmin-mediated dissolution of fibrin. Molecules serving in this system are the plasminogen activator inhibitors PAI-1 and PAI-2, the plasmin inhibitor alpha-1-antiplasmin, alpha-2-macroglobulin and thrombin activatable fibrinolysis inhibitor (TAFI) (Fay et al., 2007).

3. Bleeding diathesis in uremic patients

The relation between uremia and bleeding diathesis has been known for many years. Uremic patients used to be lost from bleeding from vital organs. Despite today's improvement in anemia with modern HD techniques and erythropoietin therapy, bleeding diathesis continues to represent a significant problem. There may be serious, life-threatening bleeding, and surgical procedures may be delayed or not performed at all out of concern over bleeding diathesis. This causes a rise in patient morbidity. The most common cause of uremic bleeding diathesis is impaired primary hemostasis. The most frequent complications seen as a reflection of primary hemostasis disorders are petechiae, purpura, and bleeding in the arteriovenous fistula puncture site and regions where the HD catheter is inserted (Galbusera et al., 2009; Remuzzi et al., 1989). In addition, bleeding in vital organs may also be seen in uremia, leading to less frequently observed but fatal complications. In HD patients in particular, various HD therapy-related factors mean that bleeding complications to be seen more frequently. Although various rates have been citied in HD patients in different publications, the bleeding diathesis rate is around 10%-15%, and bleeding-associated morbidity around 15% (Davenport et al., 1994, Martin et al., 1994; van de Wetering et al., 1996). Gastrointestinal (GIS) bleeding, particularly upper GIS bleeding, is seen in one third of uremic patients (Galbusera et al., 2009). Kutsumi et al. showed that 17% of patients presenting to the emergency department with GIS bleeding received HD therapy (Kutsumi et al., 1998). Other examples of vital organ bleeding include hemorrhagic stroke, subdural hematoma, spontaneous retroperitoneal hemorrhage, hepatic subcapsular hematoma intraocular hemorrhage and hemorrhagic pericarditis leading to cardiac tamponade (Galbusera et al., 2009; Remuzzi, 1989). Of these, hemorrhagic stroke and subdural hematoma are widely observed in HD patients. Incidence of hemorrhagic stroke is 5-10 times greater than in the normal population. (Seliger et al., 2003; Toyoda et al., 2005), while that of subdural hematoma has been put at 20 times greater. Mortality in this patient group has been determined at above 40% (Power et al., 2010). van de Wetering et al. observed 48 hemorrhagic complications in 78 HD patients. Forty of the patients with hemorrhagic complications had major bleeding and 8 minor bleeding. Six of the 40 major hemorrhages were intra-abdominal, 18 involved bleeding around the catheter, 3 were GIS bleeding, 12 were oronasopharyngeal and 1 intracerebral. One intracerebral case, 1 intra-abdominal case and 1 with gastrointestinal bleeding died (van de Wetering et al., 1996). As seen in all these studies, a not inconsiderable level of hemorrhagic complications with high mortality is seen in HD patients. It is therefore important to understand the pathogenesis of and treatment approaches toward bleeding diathesis in the HD patient group. While bleeding diathesis in HD patients is associated with uremia-related factors, HD therapy itself also creates a tendency to bleeding.

3.1. The pathogenesis of uremia-associated bleeding diathesis

Predisposition to bleeding in uremic patients has been known for years. While the pathogenesis of bleeding diathesis is not fully established, multifactorial causes are thought to be responsible. The most important of these factors are structural and functional defects in platelets. Other factors are abnormal platelet-vessel wall interaction, anemia, abnormal Nitric oxide (NO) production, drug use and HD therapy itself.

3.1.1. Platelet dysfunction

3.1.1.1. Thrombocytopenia

Moderate level platelet function disorder not sufficient to cause life-threatening bleeding is frequently seen in uremic patients (Galbusera et al., 2009). The cause of thrombocytopenia is generally decreased platelet production or an increase in consumption (Boccardo et al., 2004; Panicucci et al., 1983). Thrombocytopenia may be related to HD therapy itself or develop due to primary renal disease or various accompanying comorbid conditions. These conditions include systemic lupus erythematosus, thrombotic thrombocytopenic purpura, hemolytic uremic syndrome and disseminated intravascular coagulation (Barbour et al., 2012; Boccardo et al., 2004; Loirat et al., 2012). HD-related thrombocytopenia may be related to the membrane and anticoagulant used in dialysis therapy. Studies investigating the effect of HD on platelet numbers have generally looked at platelet numbers 15-30 min before HD and after HD (Daugirdas & Bernardo, 2012). Studies investigating the effect of type of HD membrane on platelet number have shown that greater thrombocytopenia develops in non-biocompatible cellulose membranes compared to biocompatible synthetic polymer membranes. Thrombocytopenia observed in non-biocompatible membranes has been associated with complement activation (Gutierrez et al., 1994; Hoenich et al., 1997; Verbeelen et al., 1991). Few studies have investigated the effect of membrane sterilization technique on platelet number. One such study, by Miller et al. analyzed the biocompatibility of the high-flux membrane steam sterilized F60S and ethylene oxide sterilized F60 and the low-flux membrane ethylene oxide sterilized F6, in other words, their effect on platelet and leukocyte numbers. The three different membranes had no different effects on platelet numbers, while the steam-sterilized membrane was shown to reduce leukocyte numbers less (Müller et al., 1998). Another effect of HD therapy on platelet number concerns the heparin used during therapy. Because of its low cost and short half-life, heparin is a frequently used anticoagulant in HD therapy. However, heparin-induced thrombocytopenia (HIT) is a complication that may limit its use and cause mortality. HIT is classified into types I and II. Type-I HIT is a widely seen form. It arises as the result of a direct reaction between heparin and thrombocytes. There is generally a slight fall in platelet numbers soon after heparin administration, and platelet numbers return to normal despite repeated administrations of heparin. Type-II HIT is less common, with an incidence of between 0.5% and 5% (Jang & Hursting, 2005). Etiology is attributed to platelet factor 4 and antibodies developing against heparin complex (Suranyi & Chow, 2010; Visentin et al., 1994). HIT generally appears with the development of thrombocytopenia, thrombosis, skin necrosis and gangrene accompanied by acute systemic reactions 5-30 min after administration of bolus unfractionated heparin (Syed & Reilly, 2009). HIT diagnosis is established by scoring the following criteria: thrombocytopenia appearing 5-10 days after commencement of heparin therapy, the presence of any thrombotic event, a normal platelet number before heparin, a 50% fall in platelet numbers compared to basal values in the absence of any other cause of platelet decrease and platelet numbers returning to normal when heparin therapy is stopped (Warkentin, 2004). The first procedure in treatment is cessation of heparin until HIT antibody results are obtained and the use of alternative anticoagulant methods to heparin. The use of warfarin as an alternative anticoagulant until platelet numbers return to normal is not recommended (Syed & Reilly, 2009). Saline flush, citrate anticoagulation, the direct antithrombin inhibitors lepirudin and argatroban or the Factor Xa inhibitor danaparoid can be used in heparin-free dialysis (Matsuo & Wanaka, 2008, Syed & Reilly, 2009). In conclusion, in the light of current knowledge, generally, although uremia and HD-associated thrombocyte numbers may decline slightly, no fall in platelet numbers that might cause fatal bleeding is observed in association with uremia itself or in association with HD therapy (excluding HIT2).

3.1.1.2. Platelet function disorder

3.1.1.2.1. Structural and functional platelet disorder

Structural and functional disorders have long been known in uremic patients. One structural impairment is a decrease in mean platelet volume, and this contributes to bleeding diathesis by leading to a decrease in platelet mass (Galbusera et al., 2009; Michalak et al., 1991). There are three main types or granule in platelets; dense granules, α granules and lysosomes (Kaplan & Owen., 1986). Various substances in these granules are involved in the hemostatic process by being released from platelets with activation. In uremic patients, both the content of these granules and defects in secretion during platelet activation contribute to bleeding diathesis. There are various studies of platelet granule content in uremic patients. Eknoyan et al. showed that a low level of adenosine diphosphate (ADP) and serotonin in chronic kidney disease patients parallels platelets' functional defects, and that these defects can be reversed with hemodialysis or transplantation (Eknoyan and Brown., 1981). Di Minno et al. determined a low platelet ADP level in uremic patients compared to normal individuals, and a decrease in thrombin-stimulated thromboxane B2 and adenosine triphosphate secretion (Di Minno et al., 1985). Vlachoyannis et al. determined a higher cyclic-AMP level in uremic patients compared to healthy individuals (Vlachoyannis & Schoeppe., 1982). There is a rise in cyclic-GMP (c-GMP) in uremic patients. The rise in c-GMP level is associated with increased production of NO, produced by platelets (Noris et al., 1993). A rise in platelet Ca content and abnormal Ca release as a response to stimuli is another structural defect (Gura et al., 1982; Ware et al., 1989). There are contradictory findings regarding defective arachidonic acid in uremic platelets (Boccardo et al., 2004). Remuzzi et al. reported defective arachidonic acid metabolism in uremic platelets and a decrease in thromboxane A2 production as a reflection of this (Remuzzi et al., 1983). Bloom et al. reported no cyclooxygenase defect in uremic patients, but determined a decrease in thrombin-stimulated thromboxane synthesis (Bloom et al., 1986). These structural and functional defects in uremic patients contribute to impairment in adhesion and aggregation and facilitate bleeding diathesis. In addition to these structural and functional defects, various uremic toxins are known to lead to platelet aggregation defect. The uremic toxins guanidosuccinic acid and phenolic acid lead to platelet aggregation defect by inhibiting ADP-induced platelet aggregation (Hedges et al., 2007).

3.1.1.2.2. Platelet-vessel wall interaction defect

Platelet-vessel wall interaction defect is one of the significant causes of bleeding diathesis, in addition to platelet morphology and function disorder. As discussed in the section on normal hemostasis, defective platelet adhesion to the vascular endothelium is mediated by two important proteins; fibrinogen and von Willebrand factor (vWF). Additionally, two important proteins on the platelet surface, GP Ib (vWF receptor) and activation-dependent GPIIb–IIIa complex (fibrinogen receptor), are also involved in adhesion. Platelet glycoprotein (GP) content is divided into the membrane and intracellular component. Studies of uremic patients have produced different results regarding GP content (Moal et al., 2003). Nomura et al. determined decreased GP Ib expression and normal GPIIb-IIIa expression in uremic patients (Nomura et al., 1994). In complete contrast, Sreedhara et al. determined normal GP Ib expression and a decrease in GPIIb–IIIa expression (Sreedhara et al., 1996). Salvati et al. determined low GP Ib expression and high GPIIb–IIIa expression (Salvati et al., 2001). Moal et al. determined low GP Ib expression in platelets at rest. They also reported higher GP Ib expression in stimulated platelets in the HD patient group compared to the control and CKD groups, while GPIIb–IIIa expression was lower in the CKD and HD patients compared to the controls (Moal et al., 2003). We think this may be attributed to the technique for measuring these differences in results, whether the patient group is pre-dialysis or dialysis, if dialysis, then whether it is HD or Peritoneal dialysis (PD) and when blood specimen is collected (before or after HD). However, the majority of studies suggest that these two platelet GPs decrease in uremic patients or that there is a decrease in response to stimulation. This leads to platelet-wall interaction defect and bleeding diathesis.

vWF is one of the main important proteins in platelet adhesion. For that reason, there have been many studies on both vWF level and function in uremic patients. However, these have produced controversial results in terms of both levels and functions. One such study was that by Zwaginga et al., which showed that platelet adhesion defect was not associated with abnormal vWF (Zwaginga et al., 1990). Escolar et al. reported platelet adhesion defect in uremic patients and that the defect may stem from defective interaction between vWF and the receptor (Escolar et al., 1990). Despite these conflicting results, the fact that no response is obtained to cryoprecipitate and desmessoprin in uremic bleeding diathesis suggests defective vWF involvement (Boccardo et al., 2004; Galbusera et al., 2009). vWF defect in uremia arises because of reduced interaction with GPIIb–IIIa receptor or reduced expression of this receptor (Mohri et al., 1988). Defective vWF GPIIb–IIIa receptor interaction reduces TXA2 and ADP production by leading to defects in phosphatidylinositol bisphosphate breakdown and cytosolic calcium concentration. As a result, it leads to impaired adhesion (Hedges, 2007).

3.1.2. Anemia

Anemia is known to be widely seen in chronic kidney failure patients and to lead to morbidity and mortality. The most important reason why it leads to morbidity and mortality stems from its negative effect on myocardial functions. Another negative effect of anemia is that it contributes to bleeding diathesis. It is thought to do this in two ways. The first is that under normal conditions in a non-anemic individual the flow of formed elements of blood inside the vessel is regular. Therefore, in the event of injury, in order for the platelets to be quickly able to form a clot, they act in the periphery near the vascular endothelium. In anemic individuals, however, this rheological order is defective. And this leads to bleeding diathesis (Hedges et al., 2007). Another reason is that erythrocytes release ADP and TxA2. But this secretion decreases in anemic individuals. Decreased levels of ADP and TxA2 lead to a reduction in platelet aggregation (Valles et al., 1991). Another mechanism concentrated on is the effect of anemia on NO. Erythrocytes are known to have a high affinity for NO. In anemia, however, the NO scavenger role declines because the erythrocyte mass decreases. An increase in NO level, on the other hand, leads to a rise in cGMP level and a decline in platelet aggregation (Martin et al., 1985, Galbusera et al., 2009). Improvement of anemia with both blood transfusion and erythropoietin therapy reduces bleeding time. And these are findings that support the hypothesis that anemia has an effect on bleeding diathesis (Livio et al., 1982; Moia et al., 1987, Viganò et al., 1991).

3.1.3. Abnormal NO production

There is an accumulation of uremic toxins as well as guanidosuccinic acid in uremic patients. Guanidosuccinic acid accumulation is associated with guanidine transfer from L-arginine to aspartic acid. L-arginine is the most important precursor of NO. NO has a modulator effect on vascular tonus. In addition, NO prevents platelet adhesion to the endothelium, lowers cAMP-mediated platelet aggregation and reduces platelet-platelet interaction by increasing cGMP levels. (Noris & Remuzzi, 1999). The administration of inhale has led to a prolongation of bleeding time in studies on healthy individuals (Högman et al., 1993). Abnormal NO production is therefore thought to contribute to bleeding diathesis in uremic patients.

3.2. Evaluation of bleeding diathesis

Evaluation of bleeding diathesis in uremia begins with the taking of a detailed history. The presence of other systemic disease, drugs used, if renal replacement therapy is administered whether this is HD or PD, and if HD what kind of membrane and which anticoagulant in what doses are used must all be established. At physical examination, petechiae, purpura, epistaxis and bleeding from the catheter or AVF puncture site, generally a reflection of platelet function effect, may all be seen. In addition, physical examination findings secondary to GIS bleeding or intracranial or subdural bleeding may also be encountered. Platelet numbers are generally normal or slightly low at laboratory analysis. The most frequently used clinical finding in evaluation of uremic bleeding diathesis is bleeding time (Steiner et al., 1979).

3.3. Treatment of bleeding diathesis

3.3.1. Hemodialysis

As previously discussed, while the HD process itself facilitates bleeding diathesis, in renal failure patients it is used as a therapeutic approach that reduces bleeding diathesis. HD's reductive effect on bleeding diathesis comes about through the removal of uremic toxins from the blood. More than 90 uremic toxins are known today. These are classified as small, middle or large molecular toxins based on their molecular weight. Large and/or protein-bound molecules in particular cannot be removed with HD techniques using classic low-flux membranes, but they can with high-flux membranes (Vanholder et al., 2005; Weissinger et al., 2004). Daily and long-term dialysis may be needed for the removal of uremic toxins and to reduce bleeding diathesis using traditional HD techniques (Hedges et al., 2007). Studies have shown that dialysis therapy produces an improvement in platelet functions by removing uremic toxins (Boccardo et al., 2004; Galbusera et al., 2009; Hedges et al., 2007). However, another point here that must not be forgotten is that HD therapy can lead to bleeding diathesis, due to both membrane interaction and to the anticoagulants used. Therefore, heparin-free dialysis must be performed, especially with patients with active bleeding or who have recently undergone major surgery. Various methods are currently applied for heparin-free HD. These include HD using low-dose heparin, regional heparinization with protamine, intermittent saline flush, regional citrate anticoagulation, prostacyclin infusion and other alternative techniques. Swartz et al. showed that regional heparinization had a lower bleeding reduction effect than low-dose heparinization (Swartz & Port, 1979). However, in another study by Swartz, a bleeding level as high as 26% was observed in patients with an active risk of bleeding using low-dose controlled heparinization (Swartz, 1981). In addition, there are studies showing that regional heparinization with protamine neutralization has an increasing effect on bleeding, probably associated with the delayed heparin effect (Hampers et al., 1966). Nagarik et al. investigated the effects on bleeding diathesis episode of dialysis performed with intermittent saline flush and anticoagulant dialysis in patients administered intermittent renal replacement therapy in intensive care. They observed fewer bleeding episodes in patients administered intermittent saline flush (Nagarik et al., 2010). Sagedal et al. showed that intermittent saline flush did not reduce clot formation in dialyzers and intravascular coagulation in stable HD patients (Sagedal et al., 2006). Citrate has been used as an anticoagulant for many years because of its Ca-binding effect. Several studies have shown that citrate anticoagulant can be used safely in uremic patients with bleeding (Davies et al., 2011; Jarraya et al., 2010 Kreuzer et al., 2010; Park et al., 2011). However, it must not be forgotten that severe metabolic alkalosis may develop in patients receiving citrate anticoagulation, especially continuous renal replacement therapy (Alsabbagh et al., 2012). Additionally, there are various difficulties and side-effects in citrate anticoagulation beyond continuous renal replacement. Two reliable pumps are needed for citrate and Ca infusion, and these difficulties and side-effects are that serious metabolic alkalosis and hypocalcemia may result. Prostacyclin administration is another heparin-free dialysis technique. However, this technique is not much used, because it leads to headache, flushing and hypotension (Sagedal et al., 2006). Because regional anticoagulation with heparin-protamine or citrate-calcium infusion or intermittent saline flush lead to a loss of personnel time and have a number of side-effects, new techniques are under development. One of these is the use of citrate-enriched dialysate. Cheng et al. showed that citrate-enriched dialysate is more effective than intermittent saline flush (Cheng et al., 2011). However, studies showing efficacy in patients with bleeding are needed. Yixiong et al. showed that effective and safe anticoagulation is provided in high-risk bleeding patients with low-dose argatroban (direct thrombin inhibitor) saline flush (Yixiong et al., 2010). Providing effective dialysis in HD patients with bleeding continues to be a major problem. Techniques permitting safe and effective HD need to be developed with technological advances.

3.3.2. Desmopressin

Desmopressin (1-deamino-8-d-arginine vasopressin [DDAVP]) is a drug frequently used in HD patients with bleeding diathesis. While its reductive effect on bleeding diathesis is not fully understood, it is thought to function by increasing Factor VIII levels through release from where it is stored and by reducing the effect of vWF on dysfunction (Prowse et al., 1979). DDAVP's reducing effect on bleeding time starts within 1 h and continues for 4-8 h. Bleeding time returns to normal in 24 h (Mannucci et al., 1983; Galbusera et al., 2009). DDAVP has been shown to effectively reduce bleeding time when administered intravenously (0.3 microg/kg) by the subcutaneous and intranasal routes (Mannucci et al., 1983; Shapiro & Kelleher, 1984; Ulusoy et al.,2004; Viganò et al., 1989). One of the things that must not be forgotten in desmopressin therapy is that efficacy may decline with increasing use, probably in association with a decline in endothelial vWF stores (Canavese et al., 1985). Flushing, headache and tachycardia may be observed during desmopressin use. But not at such a level as to prevent its use in uremic bleeding diathesis.

3.3.3. Cryoprecipitate

Cryoprecipitate is a blood product rich in factor VII, vWF and fibrinogen. Use takes the form of 10 bags of American-Red-Cross-prepared cryoprecipitate infusion in 30 min. Its effect begins in 4-12 h. The effect mechanism is not fully understood, though it is thought to be associated with its concentrated coagulation factor content (Janson et al., 1980; Triulzi et al., 1990). Its advantage is that its effect appears early, the disadvantage that it involves a risk of transferring transfusion-related diseases. Hypocalcemia may also develop during cryoprecipitate transfusion, as with the transfusion of other blood products. Additionally, it may rarely lead to pulmonary edema and anaphylactic reaction. Factors requiring attention during blood and blood product transfusion, must also therefore not be forgotten in cryoprecipitate transfusion (Galbusera et al., 2009; Hedges et al., 2007; Spinella & Holcomb, 2009). Although cryoprecipitate works very quickly, other approaches are preferred because of the risk of transference of transfusion-related diseases.

3.3.4. Conjugated estrogen

The bleeding diathesis-reducing effect of conjugated estrogen emerged on the basis of observational data (Liu et al., 1980). Following these observational data, the effect on uremic bleeding diathesis began being investigated. It has been shown that use of 0.6 mg/kg iv (4-5 days) in uremic patients lowers bleeding time (Viganò et al., 1988). Twenty-five milligrams of oral conjugated estrogen for 3-20 days has been shown to safely reduce bleeding time (Viganò et al., 1988). In addition, low-dose transdermal administrations two times a week (50–100 microg/24 h) have also been shown to effectively reduce bleeding (Sloand & Schiff., 1995). The bleeding diathesis-reductive effect is thought to come about by preventing NO synthesis (Zoja et al., 1991). In the light of these studies, since there is greater research into reducing uremic bleeding diathesis, iv administration of conjugated estrogen is recommended over the subcutaneous and transdermal routes (Hedges et al., 2006).

3.3.5. Erythropoietin

We have already discussed the effect of anemia on bleeding diathesis. Based on these data, researchers have investigated the effect on bleeding diathesis of erythropoietin (EPO), an indispensible element in anemia treatment in chronic kidney patients. Several studies have shown that correction of anemia with EPO therapy reduces uremic bleeding diathesis. EPO's bleeding diathesis-reductive effect may come about through several mechanisms. The first of these is that the erythrocyte mass that increases with EPO therapy serves as an NO scavenger and reduces NO's negative effect on platelet adhesion. Another is the disappearance of blood rheology impairment brought about by anemia (Martin et al., 1985; Viganò et al., 1991). EPO therapy is thought to reduce bleeding diathesis by increasing the number of reticulated platelets in bone marrow, with its greater metabolic efficacy, by increasing platelet aggregation and interaction with the vascular endothelium and, finally by increasing platelets' response to stimuli (Diaz-Ricart et al., 1999; Hedges et al., 2007; Tàssies et al., 1995; Zwaginga et al., 1991). In conclusion, anemia treatment brings about a significant improvement in bleeding diathesis, especially Htc, at a level of 27%-32% (Galbusera et al., 2009; Viganò et al., 1991)

In conclusion, despite advances in technology, bleeding diathesis continues to be a life threatening condition in HD patients. Although bleeding diathesis is not fully understood, it is thought to be associated with primary hemostasis, in other words, platelet structure and functions. Anemia should be corrected with EPO therapy and, most important of all, effective dialysis must be performed in order to prevent bleeding diathesis in these patients. Since its effect starts quickly, we think that the use of DDAVP will be appropriate in acute, life-threatening bleeding; and because its effect is long-lasting, conjugated estrogen may be used in patients without life-threatening bleeding but requiring long-term monitoring.

4. Hypercoagulability in uremia

Thrombotic complications are encountered as frequently as bleeding diathesis and are life-threatening in uremic patients. Thrombotic complications lead to mortality giving rise to cardiovascular events and can also cause morbidity by leading to AVF thrombosis. Understanding the pathogenesis of thrombotic events in uremic patients and the treatment is therefore of vital importance. A rise in platelet hyperactivity, adhesion and aggregation, coagulation cascade activation and a decrease in fibrinolysis are held responsible in the pathogenesis of the thrombotic process.

4.1. Increased platelet activation, aggregation and adhesion

The findings of studies analyzing platelet activation in HD patients are inconsistent. These inconsistent results may stem from differences in the patient population and sampling techniques or from differences in the platelet activation markers used. Various molecules expressed on the surface of activated platelets or various substances known to be released into plasma in the event of platelet activation are today used as platelet activation markers. Platelet surface markers are generally evaluated using flow cytometry and monoclonal antibody-based measurement. CD41 is a flow cytometric marker of activation-dependent GPIIb/IIIa receptor. PAC-1 is used to determine this receptor in its activated state. CD42b or GPIb are used in the determination of vWF receptor. CD62P is used in the determination of p selectin found in the membrane of platelet alpha granules and given off during platelet activation. CD63 is used similarly to CD62P in the determination of degranulation of platelet dense granules (Daugirdas & Bernardo., 2012; Michelson, 1996). Many studies to date have evaluated the effect of the HD procedure on platelet activation using one or more of these markers. These studies have also evaluated the effects on activation markers of the membrane used in the HD procedure, the site of blood collection (where blood enters or leaves the HD membrane) and time of collection. Studies showing differences depending on blood collection site and time and that activation markers are higher in blood samples collected at the HD membrane exit are in the majority (Aggarwal et al., 2002; Daugirdas & Bernardo., 2012; Reverter et al., 1994;). Additionally, these studies have also shown higher platelet activation markers in patients using cuprophan membrane (Cases et al., 1993; Daugirdas & Bernardo., 2012; Reverter et al., 1994). Today, in addition to the analysis of platelet activation using flow cytometry, various markers found in platelet alpha granules and released into plasma during platelet activation are determined using ELISA. One such marker is sCD40L. This is a transmembrane protein structurally related to the tumor necrosis factor-α (TNF α) family. sCD40L is a form of CD40L released into plasma from the active thrombocyte surface (Henn et al., 1998). There are studies showing that sCD40L is correlated with platelet activation in both the normal population and HD patients. In a study of 103 HD patients in our clinic we determined a significantly higher predialysis sCD40 L level compared to healthy individuals. There was a rise in sCD40 L level in blood specimen taken at the end of HD, though this was not statistically significant. Our study supported the presence of platelet activation independent of the HD procedure and that the procedure had an enhancing effect on that activation (Ulusoy et al., 2012). Signal peptide-CUB (signal peptide–CUB (complement C1r/C1s, Uegf, and Bmp1)-EGF(epidermal growth factor)- domain-containing protein 1 (SCUBE1) is a cell surface protein belonging to the SCUBE gene family. SCUBE1 has been shown to rise in parallel to platelet activation in acute ischemic events (Tu et al., 2006). However, the number of studies on this novel molecule is rather limited. The first of these limited studies in the HD patient group was performed in our clinic. We determined that a high SCUBE 1 level in HD patients, in a manner correlated with sCD40L, regarded as a platelet activation marker in HD patients. SCUBE 1 levels were significantly high in predialysis blood specimens and exhibited a significant rise in post-dialysis specimens. Gender, blood pressure, BUN, creatinine, hematocrit and high-sensitivity C-reactive protein (hsCRP) levels, hemodialysis membrane surface area, amount of ultrafiltration, blood flow rate, dialysis flow rate and carnitine use also significantly affected elevated SCUBE 1 in our study (Ulusoy et al., 2012). In conclusion, there are several studies showing platelet activation in HD patients, and it is a fact that the HD process affects this activation. Studies on the subject are continuing today. In addition to the effect of the HD procedure on platelet activation, there are also evaluating the effect on adhesion. Platelet adhesion during the HD procedure can be analyzed using the level of lactate dehydrogenase (LDH) released from the platelets (Daugirdas & Bernardo., 2012). Researchers have particularly evaluated membrane-specific platelet adhesion using this technique. One such study analyzed platelet adhesion in different membrane types by investigating LDH levels, and reported the lowest adhesion in a polysulfone membrane (Asai) (Hayama et al., 2004). In conclusion, HD therapy leads to an increase in platelet adhesion and degranulation. There is also an increase in platelet-platelet and platelet-leukocyte interaction during HD. For these reasons, as with uremic bleeding diathesis, platelets primarily involved in the hemostatic phase in the hypercoagulable process are held responsible for function defects.

4.2. Coagulation cascade activation and a decrease in fibrinolysis

A number of coagulation abnormalities associated with the HD procedure and uremia appear in HD patients. The effect of the HD procedure on coagulation cascade is by two routes. The first is blood passing through blood tubing sets and dialyzers coming into contact with the foreign surface during the procedure. The second is the anticoagulation used during the procedure. As already discussed, a rise in platelet activation and adhesion comes about during the passage of blood through blood tubing sets and contact with the dialyzer during the HD procedure (Sabovic et al., 2005). The HD procedure also leads to neutrophils adhering to the dialysis membrane and release of granular content. The most important molecule in granular content is TF, one of the natural initiators of the coagulation cascade (Fischer, 2007). Endothelial damage may occur in chronic kidney patients due to uremia, elevated homocysteine, oxidative stress, inflammation and a number of traditional risk factors (HT, DM, hyperlipidemia, cigarettes, etc.). Endothelial damage or dysfunction may cause coagulation activation by leading to a rise in TF in particular, vWF and thrombomodulin (Gris et al., 1994; Gordge & Neild, 1991; Hergesell et al., 1993; Ishii et al., 1991) There are also studies showing a rise in plasmin and thrombin formation in uremic patients (Mezzano et al., 1996; Mezzano et al., 2001). The presence of endothelial damage in uremic patients has been evaluated using various markers. These include intracellular adhesion molecule-1 (ICAM-1), thrombin–antithrombin complex (TAT), prothrombin fragment 1+2 (F1+2), plasmin–antiplasmin complex (PAP), fibrin degradation products (FDP), vWF and soluble thrombomodulin (Rios et al., 2010). A great many studies have shown a rise in these markers of endothelial dysfunction and coagulation cascade and alterations in the fibrinolytic system in uremic patients (Rabelink et al., 1994). One such study was performed by Kushiya et al., who demonstrated increased plasma levels of fibrinogen, plasmin-plasmin inhibitor complex (PIC), thrombomodulin (TM), and D-dimer pre-HD and decreased plasma levels of protein C (PC), antithrombin (AT), TAT and tissue plasminogen activator (tPA)-plasminogen activator inhibitor-I (PAI-I) complex (tPA-PAI-1 complex) (Kushiya et al., 2003). Vaziri et al. determined a decline in coagulation activities even though Factor XII, IX, X and II levels were normal or elevated. Additionally, they determined a significant increase in hyperfibrinogenemia and D-dimer, VWF, factor VII, and factor XIII antibody levels and a pronounced decrease in antithrombin III, free protein S, plasminogen and tissue-type plasminogen activator concentration in end-stage kidney failure patients (Vaziri et al., 1994). Sagripanti et al. determined TAT, fibrinopeptide A (FPA), D dimer, vWF, tumor necrosis factor alpha (TNF), beta-thromboglobulin (beta TG) and serotonin (5HT) levels in predialysis and HD patients compared to the controls. Erdem et al. determined high F1+2, TAT, t-PA, urokinase-plasminogen activator (u-PA), PAP, plasminogen and α2-antiplasmin and α2-macroglobulin levels in HD patients (Erdem et al., 1996). Studies have analyzed the clinical reflections of this coagulation cascade activation and decrease in fibrinolysis. One such determined high levels of fibrinogen, CRP, factor VIII, antiphospholipid antibody and anti-factor 4 platelet-heparin levels in patients with recurrent vascular access thrombosis (O'Shea et al., 2003). Knoll et al. showed that presence of FV Leiden and increased FVIII, Lp(a) and homocysteine levels were associated with vascular access thrombosis (Knoll et al., 2005). In conclusion, in addition to bleeding diathesis in HD patients, a decrease in fibrinolysis and Hypercoagulation, a diametrically opposed condition, is a fact that must not be ignored and continue to give rise to significant morbidity and mortality.

4.3. Treatment

As we have already discussed, in chronic kidney patients the HD procedure itself creates a tendency to thrombus formation due to formed elements in blood making contact with a foreign surface (blood tubing sets and dialyzers). Anticoagulant is used during HD in order to prevent clot formation and ensure the procedure can be completed. Anticoagulant has been used in HD for many years. Selection and dose adjustment of anticoagulant must be based on the patient's clinical condition. Classic unfractionated heparin (UFH) and low molecular weight heparin (LMWH) are the most commonly preferred anticoagulant techniques. Direct thrombin inhibitor (danaparoid) can be used in some selected cases, but the cost is very high (Fischer et al., 2007). UFH and LMWH provide effective anticoagulation in patients with no contraindication in the HD procedure.

Thrombotic complication of vascular access is a frequently encountered condition in the HD patient group. Thrombotic complication is more common in patients using graft as vascular access route in particular. Studies low dose aspirin, sulfinpyrazone and ticlopidine in the prevention of vascular access thrombosis have produced good results (Fiskerstrand et al., 1985; Harter et al., 1979; Kaegi et al., 1975) But these drugs are not frequently used, both because of a lack of sufficient studies and out of a concern they may increase bleeding diathesis in this patient group with a tendency to bleeding. Another important thrombotic complication and main cause of mortality is cardiovascular thrombotic complications (myocardial infarction, cerebrovascular event). Preventive measures against these possibly fatal thrombotic complications in the HD patient group resemble those in the normal population. However, we think that the most important means of preventing various risk factors that facilitate the development of cardiovascular events particular to the HD patient group (hyperhomocysteinemia, inflammation, uremic toxins, Ca-P metabolism disorder) is with adequate dialysis. The provision of effective HD and that this effectiveness is being maintained should be checked at regular intervals.

In addition, as well as the contribution of uremia in HD patients, bleeding diathesis and thrombotic complications are associated with the HD procedure itself. Reduction of these complications with advances in HD technology (biocompatible membranes, new anticoagulant methods, etc.) will contribute to a decrease in mortality and morbidity in HD patients. As with complications of all kinds in HD patients, adequate dialysis plays a key role in this area.

Author details

Gülsüm Özkan and Şükrü Ulusoy

Karadeniz Technical University, School of Medicine, Department of Nephrology, Turkey

References

[1] Aggarwal, A., Kabbani, S.S., Rimmer, J.M., Gennari, F.J., Taatjes, D.J., Sobel, B.E. & Schneider, D.J. (2002) Biphasic effects of hemodialysis on platelet reactivity in patients with end-stage renal disease: a potential contributor to cardiovascular risk. Am J Kidney Dis, 40, 2, 315-2

[2] Alsabbagh, M.M., Ejaz, A.A., Purich, D.L. & Ross, E.A. (2012) Regional citrate anticoagulation for slow continuous ultrafiltration: risk of severe metabolic alkalosis. Clinical Kidney Journal, 5, 3, 212

[3] Barbour, T., Johnson, S., Cohney, S. & Hughes, P. (2012) Thrombotic microangiopathy and associated renal disorders. Nephrol Dial Transplant, 27, 7, 2673-85

[4] Bloom, A., Greaves, M., Preston, F.E. & Brown, C.B. (1986) Evidence against a platelet cyclooxygenase defect in uraemic subjects on chronic haemodialysis. Br J Haematol, 62, 1, 143-9

[5] Boccardo, P., Remuzzi, G., Galbusera, M. (2004) Platelet dysfunction in renal failure. Semin Thromb Hemost, 30, 5, 579-89

[6] Canavese, C., Salomone, M., Pacitti, A., Mangiarotti, G. & Calitri, V. (1985) Reduced response of uraemic bleeding time to repeated doses of desmopressin. Lancet, 1, 8433, 867-8

[7] Cases, A., Reverter, J.C., Escolar, G., Sanz, C., Lopez-Pedret, J., Revert, L. & Ordinas, A. (1993) Platelet activation on hemodialysis: influence of dialysis membranes. Kidney Int Suppl, 41, 217-20

[8] Cheng, Y.L., Yu, A.W., Tsang, K.Y., Shah, D.H., Kjellstrand, C.M., Wong, S.M., Lau, W.Y., Hau, L.M. & Ing, T.S. (2011) Anticoagulation during haemodialysis using a citrate-enriched dialysate: a feasibility study. Nephrol Dial Transplant, 26, 2, 641-6

[9] Daugirdas, J.T. & Bernardo, A.A. (2012) Hemodialysis effect on platelet count and function and hemodialysis-associated thrombocytopenia. Kidney Int, 82, 2, 147-57

[10] Davenport, A., Will, E.J. & Davison, A.M. (1994). Comparison of the use of standard heparin and prostacyclin anticoagulation in spontaneous and pump-driven extracorporeal circuits in patients with combined acute renal and hepatic failure. Nephron, 66, 4, 431-7

[11] Davies, H., Leslie, G. & Morgan, D. (2011) Continuous renal replacement treatment and the 'bleeding patient'. BMJ Case Rep, doi: 10.1136/bcr.01.2009.1523.

[12] Diaz-Ricart, M., Etebanell, E., Cases, A., López-Pedret, J., Castillo, R., Ordinas, A. & Escolar, G. (1999) Erythropoietin improves signaling through tyrosine phosphorylation in platelets from uremic patients. Thromb Haemost, 82, 4, 1312-7

[13] Di Minno, G., Martinez, J., McKean, M.L., De La Rosa, J., Burke, J.F. & Murphy, S. (1985) Platelet dysfunction in uremia. Multifaceted defect partially corrected by dialysis. Am J Med, 79, 5,552-9

[14] Eknoyan, G. & Brown, C.H. 3rd. (1981) Biochemical abnormalities of platelets in renal failure. Evidence for decreased platelet serotonin, adenosine diphosphate and Mg-dependent adenosine triphosphatase. Am J Nephrol, 1, 1, 17-23

[15] Erdem, Y., Haznedaroglu, I.C., Celik, I., Yalcin, A.U., Yasavul, U., Turgan, C. & Caglar, S. (1996) Coagulation, fibrinolysis and fibrinolysis inhibitors in haemodialysis patients: contribution of arteriovenous fistula. Nephrol Dial Transplant, 11, 7, 1299-305

[16] Escolar, G., Cases, A., Bastida, E., Garrido, M., López, J., Revert, L., Castillo, R. & Ordinas A. (1990) Uremic platelets have a functional defect affecting the interaction of von Willebrand factor with glycoprotein IIb-IIIa. Blood, 76, 7, 1336-40

[17] Fay, W.P., Garg, N. & Sunkar, M. (2007) Vascular functions of the plasminogen activation system. Arterioscler Thromb Vasc Biol, 27, 6, 1231-7

[18] Fischer, K.G. Essentials of anticoagulation in hemodialysis. (2007) Hemodial Int, 11, 2, 178-89

[19] Fiskerstrand, C.E., Thompson, I.W., Burnet, M.E., Williams, P. & Anderton, J.L. (1985) Double-blind randomized trial of the effect of ticlopidine in arteriovenous fistulas for hemodialysis. Artif Organs, 9, 1, 61-3

[20] Galbusera, M., Remuzzi, G. &Boccardo, P. (2009). Treatment of bleeding in dialysis patients. Semin Dial, 22,3,279-86

[21] Gordge, M.P. & Neild, G.H. (1991) Platelet function in uraemia. Platelets, 2, 3, 115-23

[22] Gris, J.C., Branger, B., Vécina, F., al Sabadani, B., Fourcade, J. & Schved, J.F. (1994) Increased cardiovascular risk factors and features of endothelial activation and dysfunction in dialyzed uremic patients. Kidney Int, 46, 3, 807-13

[23] Gura, V., Creter, D. & Levi, J. (1982) Elevated thrombocyte calcium content in uremia and its correction by 1 alpha(OH) vitamin D treatment. Nephron, 30, 3, 237-9

[24] Gutierrez, A., Alvestrand, A., Bergström, J., Beving, H., Lantz, B. & Henderson, L.W. (1994) Biocompatibility of hemodialysis membranes: a study in healthy subjects. Blood Purif, 12, 2, 95-105

[25] Hampers, C.L., Balufox, M.D. & Merrill, J.P. (1966) Anticoagulation rebound after hemodialysis. N Engl J Med, 275, 14, 776-8

[26] Harter, H.R., Burch, J.W., Majerus, P.W., Stanford, N., Delmez, J.A., Anderson, C.B. & Weerts, C.A. (1979) Prevention of thrombosis in patients on hemodialysis by low-dose aspirin. N Engl J Med, 301, 11, 577-9

[27] Hayama, M., Yamamoto, K., Kohori, F. & Sakai, K. (2004) How polysulfone dialysis membranes containing polyvinylpyrrolidone achieve excellent biocompatibility? Journal of Membrane Science, 234, 1-2, 41-49

[28] Hedges, S.J., Dehoney, S.B., Hooper, J.S., Amanzadeh, J. & Busti, A.J. (2007) Evidence-based treatment recommendations for uremic bleeding. Nat Clin Pract Nephrol, 3, 3, 138-53

[29] Henn, V., Slupsky, J.R., Gräfe, M., Anagnostopoulos, I., Förster, R., Müller-Berghaus, G & Kroczek, R.A. (1998) CD40 ligand on activated platelets triggers an inflammatory reaction of endothelial cells. Nature, 391, 591-594

[30] Hergesell, O., Andrassy, K., Geberth, S., Nawroth, P. & Gabath, S. (1993) Plasma thrombomodulin levels are dependent on renal function. Thromb Res,72, 5, 455-8

[31] Hoenich, N.A., Woffindin, C., Stamp, S., Roberts, S.J. & Turnbull, J. (1997) Synthetically modified cellulose: an alternative to synthetic membranes for use in haemodialysis? Biomaterials, 18, 19, 1299-303

[32] Högman, M., Frostell, C., Arnberg, H. & Hedenstierna, G. (1993) Bleeding time prolongation and NO inhalation. Lancet, 341, 8861, 1664-5

[33] Ishii, H., Uchiyama, H. & Kazama, M. (1991) Soluble thrombomodulin antigen in conditioned medium is increased by damage of endothelial cells. Thromb Haemost, 65, 5, 618-23

[34] Jang, I.K. & Hursting, M.J. (2005). When heparins promote thrombosis: review of heparin-induced thrombocytopenia. Circulation, 111, 20, 2671-83

[35] Janson, P.A., Jubelirer, S.J., Weinstein, M.J. & Deykin, D. (1980)Treatment of the bleeding tendency in uremia with cryoprecipitate. N Engl J Med, 303, 23, 1318-22

[36] Jarraya, F., Mkawar, K., Kammoun, K., Hdiji, A., Yaich, S., Kharrat, M., Charfeddine, K., Ben Hmida, M., Mahfoudh, H., Ayedi, F. & Hachicha, J. (2010) Regional citrate anticoagulation for hemodialysis: a safe and efficient method. Saudi J Kidney Dis Transpl, 21, 3, 533-4

[37] Kaegi, A., Pineo, G.F., Shimizu, A., Trivedi, H., Hirsh, J. & Gent, M. (1975) The role of sulfinpyrazone in the prevention of arterio-venous shunt thrombosis. Circulation, 52, 3, 497-9

[38] Kaplan, K.L. & Owen, J. Plasma levels of platelet secretory proteins. Crit Rev Oncol Hematol. 1986;5(3):235-55.

[39] Knoll, G.A., Wells, P.S., Young, D., Perkins, S.L., Pilkey, R.M., Clinch, J.J. & Rodger, M.A. (2005) Thrombophilia and the risk for hemodialysis vascular access thrombosis. J Am Soc Nephrol, 16, 4, 1108-14

[40] Kreuzer, M., Bonzel, K.E., Büscher, R., Offner, G., Ehrich, J.H. & Pape, L. (2010) Regional citrate anticoagulation is safe in intermittent high-flux haemodialysis treat-

ment of children and adolescents with an increased risk of bleeding. Nephrol Dial Transplant, 25, 10, 3337-42

[41] Kushiya, F., Wada, H., Sakakura, M., Mori, Y., Gabazza, E.C., Nishikawa, M., Nobori, T., Noguchi, M., Izumi, K. & Shiku, H. (2003) Atherosclerotic and hemostatic abnormalities in patients undergoing hemodialysis. Clin Appl Thromb Hemost, 9, 1, 53-60

[42] Kutsumi, H, Fujimoto, S & Rokutan, K. (1998). Risk factors for gastrointestinal bleeding]. Nippon Rinsho, 56 , 9, 2309-13

[43] Liu, Y.K., Kosfeld, R.E. & Marcum, S.G. (1984) Treatment of uraemic bleeding with conjugated oestrogen. Lancet, 2, 8408, 887-90

[44] Livio, M., Gotti, E., Marchesi, D., Mecca, G., Remuzzi, G. & de Gaetano, G. (1982) Uraemic bleeding: role of anaemia and beneficial effect of red cell transfusions. Lancet, 2, 8306, 1013-5.

[45] Loirat, C., Saland, J. & Bitzan, M. (2012) Management of hemolytic uremic syndrome. Presse Med. Mar, 41, 3, 115-35

[46] Mannucci, P.M., Remuzzi, G., Pusineri, F., Lombardi, R., Valsecchi, C., Mecca, G. & Zimmerman, T.S. (1983) Deamino-8-D-arginine vasopressin shortens the bleeding time in uremia. N Engl J Med, 308, 1, 8-12

[47] Martin, P.Y., Chevrolet, J.C., Suter, P. & Favre, H. (1994). Anticoagulation in patients treated by continuous venovenous hemofiltration: a retrospective study. Am J Kidney Dis, 24, 5, 806-12

[48] Martin, W., Villani, G.M., Jothianandan, D. & Furchgott, R.F. (1985) Blockade of endothelium-dependent and glyceryl trinitrate-induced relaxation of rabbit aorta by certain ferrous hemoproteins. J Pharmacol Exp Ther, 233, 3, 679-85

[49] Matsuo, T. & Wanaka, K. (2008). Management of uremic patients with heparin-induced thrombocytopenia requiring hemodialysis. Clin Appl Thromb Hemost, 14, 4, 459-64

[50] Mezzano, D., Tagle, R., Panes, O., Pérez, M., Downey, P., Muñoz, B., Aranda, E., Barja, P., Thambo, S., González, F., Mezzano, S. & Pereira, J. (1996) Hemostatic disorder of uremia: the platelet defect, main determinant of the prolonged bleeding time, is correlated with indices of activation of coagulation and fibrinolysis. Thromb Haemost, 76, 3, 312-21

[51] Mezzano, D., Pais, E.O., Aranda, E., Panes, O., Downey, P., Ortiz, M., Tagle, R., González, F., Quiroga, T., Caceres, M.S., Leighton, F. & Pereira, J. (2001) Inflammation, not hyperhomocysteinemia, is related to oxidative stress and hemostatic and endothelial dysfunction in uremia. Kidney Int, 60, 5, 1844-50

[52] Michalak, E., Walkowiak, B., Paradowski, M. & Cierniewski, C.S. (1991) The decreased circulating platelet mass and its relation to bleeding time in chronic renal failure. Thromb Haemost, 65, 1, 11-4

[53] Michelson, A.D. (1996) Flow cytometry: a clinical test of platelet function. Blood, 87, 12, 4925-36

[54] Moal, V., Brunet, P., Dou, L., Morange, S., Sampol, J. & Berland, Y. (2003) Impaired expression of glycoproteins on resting and stimulated platelets in uraemic patients. Nephrol Dial Transplant, 18, 9, 1834-41

[55] Mohri, H., Fujimura, Y., Shima, M., Yoshioka, A., Houghten, R.A., Ruggeri, Z.M. & Zimmerman, T.S. (1988) Structure of the von Willebrand factor domain interacting with glycoprotein Ib. J Biol Chem, 263, 34, 17901-4

[56] Moia, M., Mannucci, P.M., Vizzotto, L., Casati, S., Cattaneo, M. & Ponticelli, C. (1987) Improvement in the haemostatic defect of uraemia after treatment with recombinant human erythropoietin. Lancet, 2, 8570, 1227-9

[57] Müller, T.F., Seitz, M., Eckle, I., Lange, H. & Kolb, G. (1998) Biocompatibility differences with respect to the dialyzer sterilization method. Nephron, 78, 2, 139-42

[58] Nagarik, A.P., Soni, S.S., Adikey, G.K. & Raman, A. (2010) Comparative study of anticoagulation versus saline flushes in continuous renal replacement therapy. Saudi J Kidney Dis Transpl, 21, 3, 478-83

[59] Nomura, S., Hamamoto, K., Kawakatsu, T., Kido, H., Yamaguchi, K., Fukuroi, T., Suzuki, M., Yanabu, M., Shouzu, A. & Nishikawa, M. (1994) Analysis of platelet abnormalities in uremia with and without Glanzmann's thrombasthenia. Nephron, 68, 4, 442-8

[60] Noris, M., Benigni, A., Boccardo, P., Aiello, S., Gaspari, F., Todeschini, M., Figliuzzi, M. & Remuzzi, G. (1993) Enhanced nitric oxide synthesis in uremia: implications for platelet dysfunction and dialysis hypotension. Kidney Int, 44, 2, 445-50

[61] Noris, M. & Remuzzi, G. (1999) Uremic bleeding: closing the circle after 30 years of controversies? Blood, 94, 8, 2569-74

[62] O'shea, S.I., Lawson, J.H., Reddan, D., Murphy, M. & Ortel, T.L. (2003) Hypercoagulable states and antithrombotic strategies in recurrent vascular access site thrombosis. J Vasc Surg, 38, 3, 541-8

[63] Panicucci, F., Sagripanti, A., Pinori, E., Vispi, M., Lecchini, L., Barsotti, G. & Giovannetti, S. (1983) Comprehensive study of haemostasis in chronic uraemia. Nephron, 33, 1, 5-8

[64] Park, J.S., Kim, G.H., Kang, C.M. & Lee, C.H. (2011) Regional anticoagulation with citrate is superior to systemic anticoagulation with heparin in critically ill patients undergoing continuous venovenous hemodiafiltration. Korean J Intern Med, 26, 1, 68-75

[65] Power ,A., Hamady, M., Singh, S., Ashby, D., Taube, D. & Duncan, N.(2010) High but stable incidence of subdural haematoma in haemodialysis--a single-centre study. Nephrol Dial Transplant, 25,7, 2272-5

[66] Prowse, C.V., Sas, G., Gader, A.M., Cort, J.H. & Cash, J.D. (1979) Specificity in the factor VIII response to vasopressin infusion in man. Br J Haematol, 41, 3, 437-47

[67] Rabelink, T.J., Zwaginga, J.J., Koomans, H.A. & Sixma, J.J. (1994) Thrombosis and hemostasis in renal disease. Kidney Int, 46, 2, 287-96

[68] Remuzzi, G. (1989) Bleeding disorders in uremia: pathophysiology and treatment. Adv Nephrol Necker Hosp, 18,171-86

[69] Remuzzi, G., Benigni, A., Dodesini, P., Schieppati, A., Livio, M., De Gaetano, G., Day, S.S., Smith, W.L., Pinca, E., Patrignani, P. & Patrono, C. (1983) Reduced platelet thromboxane formation in uremia. Evidence for a functional cyclooxygenase defect. J Clin Invest, 71, 3, 762-8

[70] Reverter, J.C., Escolar, G., Sanz, C., Cases, A., Villamor, N., Nieuwenhuis, H.K., López, J. & Ordinas, A. (1994) Platelet activation during hemodialysis measured through exposure of p-selectin: analysis by flow cytometric and ultrastructural techniques. J Lab Clin Med, 124, 1,79-85

[71] Rios, D.R., Carvalho, M.G., Lwaleed, B.A., Simões e Silva, A.C., Borges, K.B. & Dusse, L.M. (2010) Hemostatic changes in patients with end stage renal disease undergoing hemodialysis. Clin Chim Acta, 411, 3-4, 135-9

[72] Ruggeri, Z.M. (2003) Von Willebrand factor, platelets and endothelial cell interactions. J Thromb Haemost, 1, 7, 1335-42

[73] Sabovic, M., Salobir, B., Preloznik Zupan, I., Bratina, P., Bojec, V. & Buturovic Ponikvar, J. (2005) The influence of the haemodialysis procedure on platelets, coagulation and fibrinolysis. Pathophysiol Haemost Thromb, 34, 6, 274-8

[74] Sagedal, S., Hartmann, A., Osnes, K., Bjørnsen, S., Torremocha, J., Fauchald, P., Kofstad, J. & Brosstad, F. (2006) Intermittent saline flushes during haemodialysis do not alleviate coagulation and clot formation in stable patients receiving reduced doses of dalteparin. Nephrol Dial Transplant, 21, 2, 444-9

[75] Sagripanti, A., Cupisti, A., Baicchi, U., Ferdeghini, M., Morelli, E. & Barsotti, G. (1993) Plasma parameters of the prothrombotic state in chronic uremia. Nephron, 63, 3, 273-8

[76] Shapiro, M.D. & Kelleher, S.P. (1984) Intranasal deamino-8-D-arginine vasopressin shortens the bleeding time in uremia. Am J Nephrol, 4, 4, 260-1

[77] Salvati, F. & Liani, M. (2001) Role of platelet surface receptor abnormalities in the bleeding and thrombotic diathesis of uremic patients on hemodialysis and peritoneal dialysis. Int J Artif Organs, 24, 3, 131-5

[78] Seliger, S.L., Gillen, D.L., Longstreth, W.T. Jr., Kestenbaum, B. & Stehman-Breen, C.O. (2003) Elevated risk of stroke among patients with end-stage renal disease. Kidney Int, 64,2,603-9

[79] Sloand, J.A. & Schiff, M.J. (1995) Beneficial effect of low-dose transdermal estrogen on bleeding time and clinical bleeding in uremia. Am J Kidney Dis, 26, 1, 22-6

[80] Spinella, P.C., & Holcomb, J.B. Resuscitation and transfusion principles for traumatic hemorrhagic shock. Blood Rev, 2009,23, 6, 231-40

[81] Stassen, J.M., Arnout, J. & Deckmyn, H. (2004) The hemostatic system. Curr Med Chem, 11, 17, 2245-60

[82] Sreedhara, R., Itagaki, I. & Hakim, R.M. (1996) Uremic patients have decreased shear-induced platelet aggregation mediated by decreased availability of glycoprotein IIb-IIIa receptors. Am J Kidney Dis, 27, 3, 355-64

[83] Steiner, R.W., Coggins, C. & Carvalho, A.C. (1979) Bleeding time in uremia: a useful test to assess clinical bleeding. Am J Hematol, 7, 2, 107-17

[84] Suranyi , M. & Chow, J.S.(2010) Review: anticoagulation for haemodialysis. Nephrology (Carlton), 15,4,386-92

[85] Swartz, R.D. & Port, F.K. (1979) Preventing hemorrhage in high-risk hemodialysis: regional versus low-dose heparin. Kidney Int, 16, 4, 513-8

[86] Swartz, R.D. (1981) Hemorrhage during high-risk hemodialysis using controlled heparinization. Nephron, 28, 2, 65-9

[87] Syed, S. & Reilly, R.F.(2009) Heparin-induced thrombocytopenia: a renal perspective. Nat Rev Nephrol, 5,9,501-11

[88] Tàssies, D., Reverter, J.C., Cases, A., Escolar, G., Villamor, N., López-Pedret, J., Castillo, R. & Ordinas, A. (1995) Reticulated platelets in uremic patients: effect of hemodialysis and continuous ambulatory peritoneal dialysis. Am J Hematol, 50, 3, 161-6

[89] Toyoda, K., Fujii, K., Fujimi, S., Kumai, Y., Tsuchimochi, H., Ibayashi, S. & Iida, M. (2005) Stroke in patients on maintenance hemodialysis: a 22-year single-center study. Am J Kidney Dis, 45,6,1058-66

[90] Triulzi, D.J. & Blumberg, N. (1990) Variability in response to cryoprecipitate treatment for hemostatic defects in uremia. Yale J Biol Med, 63, 1, 1-7

[91] Tu, C.F., Su, Y.H., Huang, Y.N., Tsai, M.H., Li, L.T., Chen, Y.L., Cheng, C.J., Dai, D.F., & Yang, R.B. (2006) Localization and characterization of a novel secreted protein SCUBE1 in human platelets. Cardiovasc Res, 71, 486–495

[92] Ulusoy, S., Ovali, E., Aydin, F., Erem, C., Ozdemir, F. & Kaynar, K. (2004) Hemostatic and fibrinolytic response to nasal desmopressin in hemodialysis patients. Med Princ Pract, 13, 6, 340-5

[93] Ulusoy, S., Ozkan, G., Menteşe, A., Yavuz, A., Karahan, S.C. & Sümer, A.U. (2012) Signal peptide-CUB-EGF domain-containing protein 1 (SCUBE1) level in hemodialysis patients and parameters affecting that level. Clin Biochem, http://dx.doi.org/10.1016/j.clinbiochem. 2012.07.103

[94] Valles, J., Santos, M.T., Aznar, J., Marcus, AJ., Martinez-Sales, V., Portoles, M., Broek-
      man, M.J. & Safier, L.B. (1991) Erythrocytes metabolically enhance collagen-induced
      platelet responsiveness via increased thromboxane production, adenosine diphos-
      phate release, and recruitment. Blood, 78, 1, 154-62

[95] van de Wetering, J., Westendorp, R.G., van der Hoeven, J.G., Stolk, B., Feuth, J.D. &
      Chang, P.C.(1996) Heparin use in continuous renal replacement procedures: the
      struggle between filter coagulation and patient hemorrhage. J Am Soc Nephrol,
      7,1,145-50

[96] Vanholder, R., Glorieux, G. & Lameire, N. (2005) New insights in uremic toxicity.
      Contrib Nephrol, 149:315-24

[97] Vaziri, N.D., Gonzales, E.C., Wang, J. & Said, S. (1994) Blood coagulation, fibrinolyt-
      ic, and inhibitory proteins in end-stage renal disease: effect of hemodialysis. Am J
      Kidney Dis, 23, 6, 828-35

[98] Viganò, G., Gaspari, F., Locatelli, M., Pusineri, F., Bonati, M. & Remuzzi, G. (1988)
      Dose-effect and pharmacokinetics of estrogens given to correct bleeding time in ure-
      mia. Kidney Int, 34, 6, 853-8

[99] Viganò, G.L., Mannucci, P.M., Lattuada, A., Harris, A. & Remuzzi, G. (1989) Subcuta-
      neous desmopressin (DDAVP) shortens the bleeding time in uremia. Am J Hematol,
      31, 1, 32-5

[100] Viganò, G., Benigni, A., Mendogni, D., Mingardi, G., Mecca, G. & Remuzzi, G. (1991)
      Recombinant human erythropoietin to correct uremic bleeding. Am J Kidney Dis, 18,
      1, 44-9

[101] Verbeelen, D., Jochmans, K., Herman, A.G., Van der Niepen, P., Sennesael, J. & De
      Waele, M. (1991) Evaluation of platelets and hemostasis during hemodialysis with
      six different membranes. Nephron, 59, 4, 567-72

[102] Viganò, G., Benigni, A., Mendogni, D., Mingardi, G., Mecca, G. & Remuzzi, G. (1991)
      Recombinant human erythropoietin to correct uremic bleeding. Am J Kidney Dis,
      18,1,44-9

[103] Visentin, G.P., Ford, S.E., Scott, J.P. & Aster, R.H.(1994) Antibodies from patients
      with heparin-induced thrombocytopenia/thrombosis are specific for platelet factor 4
      complexed with heparin or bound to endothelial cells. J Clin Invest, 93,1,81-8

[104] Vlachoyannis, J. & Schoeppe, W. (1982) Adenylate cyclase activity and cAMP content
      of human platelets in uraemia. Eur J Clin Invest, 12, 5, 379-81

[105] Ware, J.A., Clark, B.A., Smith, M. & Salzman, E.W. (1989) Abnormalities of cytoplas-
      mic Ca2+ in platelets from patients with uremia. Blood, 73, 1, 172-6

[106] Warkentin, T.E.(2004) Heparin-induced thrombocytopenia: diagnosis and manage-
      ment. Circulation, 2,110,18

[107] Warkentin, T.E., Aird, W.C. & Rand, J.H.(2003) Platelet-endothelial interactions: sepsis, HIT, and antiphospholipid syndrome. Hematology Am Soc Hematol Educ Program, 497-519

[108] Weissinger, E.M., Kaiser, T., Meert, N., De Smet, R., Walden, M., Mischak, H. & Vanholder, R.C. (2004) Proteomics: a novel tool to unravel the patho-physiology of uraemia. Nephrol Dial Transplant, 19, 12, 3068-77

[109] Yixiong, Z., Jianping, N., Yanchao, L. & Siyuan, D. (2010) Low dose of argatroban saline flushes anticoagulation in hemodialysis patients with high risk of bleeding. Clin Appl Thromb Hemost, 16, 4, 440-5

[110] Zoja, C., Noris, M., Corna, D., Viganò, G., Perico, N., de Gaetano, G. & Remuzzi, G. (1991) L-arginine, the precursor of nitric oxide, abolishes the effect of estrogens on bleeding time in experimental uremia. Lab Invest, 65, 4, 479-83

[111] Zwaginga, J.J., Ijsseldijk, M.J., Beeser-Visser, N., de Groot, P.G., Vos, J. & Sixma, J.J. (1990) High von Willebrand factor concentration compensates a relative adhesion defect in uremic blood. Blood, 75, 7, 1498-508

[112] Zwaginga, J.J., IJsseldijk, M.J., de Groot, P.G., Kooistra, M., Vos, J., van Es, A., Koomans, H.A., Struyvenberg, A. & Sixma, J.J. (1991) Treatment of uremic anemia with recombinant erythropoietin also reduces the defects in platelet adhesion and aggregation caused by uremic plasma. Thromb Haemost, 66, 6, 638-47

Chapter 5

Lipid Abnormalities in Hemodialysis Patients

Şükrü Ulusoy and Gülsüm Özkan

Additional information is available at the end of the chapter

1. Introduction

Approximately 50% of hemodialysis (HD) patients die from cardiovascular events. One of the main risk factors for cardiovascular events is hyperlipidemia. Progressive renal failure is associated with lipoprotein abnormalities and dyslipidemia. However, dyslipidemia may not appear as hyperlipidemia (a rise in plasma cholesterol and/or low-density lipoprotein (LDL)) in the majority of HD patients. Uremic dyslipidemia has an abnormal apolipoprotein profile and composition. It is characterized by reduced concentrations of apo A-containing lipoproteins in high-density lipoprotein (HDL) and increased concentrations of intact or partially metabolized triglyceride-rich apo B-containing lipoproteins in very-low-density lipoprotein (VLDL), intermediate-density lipoprotein (IDL) and LDL.

Common lipid abnormality in HD patients is hypertriglyceridemia. Other lipid abnormalities seen in HD patients are high serum lipoprotein levels and a decrease in HDL levels. Hypertriglyceridemia is caused by increased production of Apo B protein and a marked decrease in the metabolism of VLDL, primarily as a result of decreased endothelial cell debilitation of VLDL.

The lipoprotein abnormalities in HD patients are thought to be a significant factor in increased atherosclerosis. Serum total cholesterol, and particularly LDL-cholesterol, is known to be correlated with increased cardiovascular mortality in the general population. A similar correlation has also been reported in dialysis patients. However, it is today generally agreed that in the HD patient group, a low LDL cholesterol level is correlated with malnutrition and increased mortality.

Until recently, the treatment of hyperlipidemia in the HD patient group was based on adult hyperlipidemia guidelines, and it was generally thought that the approach to treatment and results in the general population would yield similar results in the HD patient group. However, in the same way that lipid abnormalities in the HD patient group differ from the general population, there are also various differences in terms of medical treatment. Treatment of hypertriglyceridemia, the most frequently observed lipid abnormality in this patient group, is advised since at above 500 mg/dl it can give rise to complications such as pancreatitis. Lifestyle changes plus fibrate or nicotinic acid are recommended for treatment of hypertriglyceridemia. However, medical treatment must be provided on the basis of a profit and loss calculation, bearing in mind the side-effects (myositis and rhabdomyolysis). The calculation of non-HDL cholesterol, used to measure the level of remnant lipoproteins, is useful in situations where LDL cholesterol is normal and triglyceride levels high. Studies have been published suggesting that this can initially reduce the frequency of cardiovascular events associated with the use of statin in the treatment of a high LDL cholesterol level. However, the AURORA study, a large prospective, randomized study published in 2009, showed that although rosuvastatin lowered LDL cholesterol in the HD patient group it did not lead to a decrease in cardiovascular mortality. From this important study and other similar research, different approaches may be expected in both the adult hyperlipidemia guideline and in guidelines regarding the HD patient group from those in the general population.

1.1. Vascular calcification

Cardiovascular diseases are the principal cause of death in HD patients. Widespread vascular calcification especially in the coronary arteries is one of the main causes of cardiovascular disease (Braun et al., 1996; London et al., 2003, Sigrist et al., 2007). Vascular calcification can be observed in two regions of the arterial structure, the intima and the media (Shanahan et al., 1999). Arterial intimal calcification (AIC) is generally associated with atherosclerotic lesions, and with plaque formation and the development of occlusive lesions (Shanahan et al., 1999). AIC may also be observed in patients with normal renal function, and calcification of the atherosclerotic plaque increases the frequency of MI and thrombotic complications. Arterial medial calcification (AMC) is seen in muscular arteries and leads to a reduction in vascular wall elasticity more than to occlusive lesions (London et al., 2003). AMC is more associated with uremia. Both AIC and AMC may be observed in HD patients.

Although vascular calcification was determined in uremic patients many years ago, research into its etiopathology is still on-going. Factors held responsible in the etiopathology today include a rise in osteogenic proteins such as osteocalcin, osteonectin, alkaline phosphatase and collagen-I, low levels of calcification inhibitors such as matrix Gla-protein, osteopontin, fetuin, pyrophosphate and osteoprotegerin, genetic factors, use of high-dose vitamin D, high Ca-P levels, hyperparathyroidism, inflammation and hyperlipidemia (Fukagawa & Kazama, 2007; Rutsch et al., 2011; Shantouf et al., 2009; Slatopolsky et al., 1980; Tamashiro et al., 2001; Tukaj et al., 2000).

As previously discussed, while classic cardiovascular risk factors are more associated with development of AIC, uremia and associated factors are more involved in the development of AMC. London et al.'s study on the subject determined that high phosphorus and low albunim levels and excessive Ca consumption represented risk factors for AIC, in addition to classic risk factors such as advanced age, a history of atherosclerotic disease, cigarette use and a history of DM and high LDL and CRP levels. They also showed that in addition to these classic risk factors, parameters more associated with HD and prolonged HD were influential in the development of AMC. In addition, in contrast to AIC, AMC may also be observed at early ages (London et al., 2003)

While definitive diagnosis of vascular calcification is made with histopathological examination, since this is not possible in clinical practice, the K-DIGO guideline recommends x-ray imaging and echocardiographic examination in the diagnosis of vascular and valvular calcification (Kidney Disease: Improving Global Outcomes (KDIGO) CKD-MBD Work Group. 2010). In conclusion, the term vascular calcification is used for two different entities in HD patients, AIC and AMC. The reason why the term vascular calcification is used to refer to both these clinical conditions is that both AIC and AMC can frequently be seen in the HD patient group and that differentiation cannot be performed with routine examinations. However, what must not be forgotten is that although they appear to be similar, there are various differences in the etiology, clinical reflections and approaches to treatment in these two clinical conditions. While improvement of atherosclerotic risk factors (hyperlipidemia, etc.) and sufficient dialysis may be beneficial in AIC, sufficient dialysis is of particular benefit in the treatment and prevention of AMC

2. The relation between dyslipidemia and cardiovascular events

Chronic kidney disease (CKD) is a significant health problem, the prevalence of which is increasing all over the world. The main cause of death in this patient population is cardiovascular disease (CVD)-related mortality (K/DOQI Workgroup. K/DOQI clinical practice guidelines for cardiovascular disease in dialysis patients, 2005; Silva et al., 2012). As with the normal population, CVD can also be treated in CKD patients, representing a potentially preventable disease group. In 1998, the National Kidney Foundation (NKF) reported that CKD patients are a high-risk group for CVD. That report stated that a high prevalence of CVD had been determined in CKD patients, leading to mortality 10-30 times greater in the dialysis patient group in particular compared to the normal population. (Levey et al., 1998; Sarnak et al., 2003). Kidney function disorder is therefore a traditional risk factor held responsible in the development of CVD.

CVD risk factors in chronic kidney patients are divided into traditional and non-traditional (Sarnak et al., 2003). Traditional and non-traditional risk factors are given in the table. The main traditional risk factors are advanced age, diabetes mellitus, kidney disease, hypertension, family history, cigarette use, male gender, obesity, left ventricular hypertrophy and a sedentary lifestyle (Anderson et al., 1991; Mallamaci et al., 2002). However, there are studies showing that of the traditional risk factors known to be correlated with mortality in the normal population, the relationship between the mortality and HT and Hyperlipidemia in HD patients do not linear (Sarnak &Levey, 2000). The correlation between mortality and HT and elevated total cholesterol in this patient group is U-shaped (Lowrie & Lew, 1990; Zager et al., 1998). For this and similar reasons, a large number of studies have shown that traditional risk factors are inadequate in determining CVD risk in CKD (Cheung et al., 2000; Longenecker et al., 2002; Sarnak et al., 2003). Other studies have therefore investigated whether other factors may influence the development of cardiovascular events in the CKD patient group, and non-traditional risk factors have been developed. Hyperhomocysteinemia is the main non-traditional risk factor thought to affect the development of CVD in CKD. Several clinical studies have shown elevated homocysteine levels in the HD patient group and that hyperhomocysteinemia increases cardiovascular mortality (Bostom et al., 1997; Mallamaci et al., 2002; Manns et al., 1999; Sirrs et al., 1999). It is generally accepted today that oxidative stress and a progressive atherosclerotic process are correlated with development of cardio-vascular events. Studies have also shown that this correlation also applies in the HD patient group. Oxidative stress may therefore be regarded as a non-traditional risk factor in the HD patient group (Boaz et al., 1999; Boaz et al., 1999). Inflammation (a rise in CRP) has been shown to be correlated with cardiovascular events in healthy individuals in prospective studies (Ridker et al., 1997). Studies also exist showing this relationship in the HD patient group (Zimmermann et al., 1999). As shown in the table 1, uremia-associated factors (anemia, impaired calcium-phosphorus metabolism, fluid electrolyte metabolism imbalance and dyslipidemia) may be added to the non-traditional risk factors in the HD patient group. As shown, dyslipidemia appears among both the traditional and non-traditional risk factors in the HD patient group. The reason is that, in contrast to the normal population, there are various lipid metabolism abnormalities in uremic patients and their being referred to as uremic dyslipidemia.

Traditional Risk Factors	Nontraditional Risk Factors
Advanced age	Hyperhomocysteinemia
Diabetes mellitus	Oxidative stress
Kidney disease	Inflammation
Hypertension	Anemia
Family history	Impaired calcium-phosphorus metabolism
Cigarette use	Fluid electrolyte metabolism imbalance
Male gender	Malnutrition
Obesity	Altered nitric oxide/endothelin balance
Left ventricular hypertrophy	Elevated fibrinogen level
Sedentary lifestyle	Other thrombogenic factors
Dyslipidemia (Higher LDL cholesterol, Lower HDL cholesterol)	Dyslipidemia
Family history of CVD	

Table 1. Traditional and Nontraditional Cardiovascular Risk Factors in Hemodialysis Patients

3. Uremic dyslipidemia

Severe lipid metabolism disorders arise in patients with kidney failure, and the lipid metabolism disorder peculiar to this patient group is known as uremic dyslipidemia (Tsimihodimos et al., 2011). However, both the pathogenesis of uremic dyslipidemia and its relationship with the atherosclerotic process that leads to the development of cardiovascular events are debatable. Studies have shown that there is abnormality in all lipoprotein fractions in uremic patients. Factors influencing these abnormalities include the degree of kidney function impairment, primary disease, presence of nephrotic syndrome, whether renal replacement therapy is administered, and if so whether HD or peritoneal dialysis (PD), drugs used (antihyperlipidemic drugs, sevelamer, calcineurin inhibitors, steroid, etc.), and the presence of malnutrition and inflammation (Attman et al., 2011; Kaysen 2009; Tsimihodimos et al., 2008; Tsimihodimos et al., 2011; Vaziri and Moradi., 2006). Abnormality in lipid metabolism commences in the early stages of CKD and contributes to the development of cardiovascular complications by initiating the atherosclerotic process. Factors contributing to lipid metabolism in stage 1-4 CKD are known to include type of primary kidney disease, degree of proteinuria and use of drugs affecting lipid metabolism. The main lipid metabolism abnormalities seen in renal patients in these stages are hypertriglyceridemia, a rise in triglyceride remnant-rich lipoproteins and lipoprotein a (Lp (a)) levels, and a decline in HDL-cholesterol levels. Moreover, with the exception of nephrotic syndrome, Total (T) cholesterol and LDL-cholesterol levels are generally at normal limits in stage 1-4 CKD patients (Tsimihodimos et al., 2008; Vaziri & Moradi., 2006; Vaziri, 2006) A rise in LDL-cholesterol levels has been determined in patients with nephrotic syndrome (Tsimihodimos et al., 2008; Vaziri, 2006).

4. Dyslipidemia in hemodialysis patients

Before discussing specific lipid metabolism disorders in HD patients, some general information about lipid metabolism will assist understanding of dyslipidemia in this patient group.

Lipids are transported in plasma by means of water-soluble molecules known as lipoproteins. In addition to their transport characteristics, various enzymes in the lipid metabolism also serve as chemical reaction platforms converting transported lipids into one another. Lipoproteins possess a core consisting of non-polar lipids such as triglyceride and cholesterol and a surrounding structure consisting of polar lipids such as apolipoprotein and phospholipid. Thanks to the structural and catalytic functions of apolipoproteins in the structure of lipoprotein, by interacting with one another or various receptors they permit specific lipid species to be added to or removed from this lipoprotein. The main plasma lipoproteins are known as HDL, LDL, IDL and VLDL, depending on their functions and molecular structures (Dominiczak&Caslake., 2011; Vaziri, 2006).

Various changes take place in uremic dyslipidemia with the start of HD therapy. However, the lipoprotein and apolipoprotein profile in HD patients resembles that in pre-dialysis patients (Attman et al., 1993). The main lipid abnormality in this patient group is a rise in triglyceride and triglyceride-rich remnant lipoprotein levels. Other lipid abnormalities are a rise in Lp (a) levels and a decrease in HDL. LDL levels are generally within normal limits. However, as with other lipoproteins, LDL is not homogeneous and there are variations in size, density and composition (Tsimihodimos et al., 2008; Wiemer et al., 2002).

Studies have shown that HD therapy has various effects on lipid profile. This gives rise to various differences, even though pathogenesis and lipid profile phenotype in HD patients are similar to the pre-dialysis period. One factor associated with HD therapy is membrane type. In one study, six weeks after transition from low flux membrane to high flux membrane, Blankestijn et al. observed a decrease in triglyceride and VLDL levels and an increase in HDL levels (Blankestijn et al., 1995). Docci et al. showed that polysulfone membranes have a more positive effect on lipid profile compared to cuprophan membranes (Docci et al., 1995). There are also studies showing that high flux polysulfone membranes reduce oxidized LDL (Wanner et al., 2004). Schiffl and Lang analyzed the effect of dialysate purity on dyslipidemia. They showed that ultrapure dialysis fluids brought about an improvement in dyslipidemia (Schiffl & Lang, 2010). Apart from dialysate purity, the effects of acetate or bicarbonate use on lipid profile have also been evaluated. It has been shown that use of bicarbonate dialysate can have positive effects on lipid profile (Jung et al., 1995). Another parameter thought to affect lipid profile during HD is heparin use. Heparin is known to cause lipoprotein lipase to be released from the endothelial surface. Chronic heparin use therefore leads to a decrease in lipoprotein lipase. Lipoprotein lipase is known to serve in the catabolism of triglyceride-rich lipoproteins such as chylomicrons and VLDL. The decrease in lipoprotein lipase in chronic heparin use gives rise to impairment in triglyceride-rich lipoprotein catabolism (Tsimihodimos et al., 2008). Studies analyzing the effect of unfractionated (UF) heparin on lipoprotein metabolism have produced controversial results. Mahmood et al. reported that heparin use during HD has no effect on lipoprotein lipase levels (Mahmood et al., 2010). However, there are also studies reporting that use of heparin has negative effects on both lipoprotein lipase and on lipid parameters (Daubresse et al., 1976; Schrader et al., 1990; Shoji et al., 1992). Another contentious issue is whether there is a difference in the use of unfractionated (UF) heparin and low molecular weight heparin (LMWH) in the effect on lipid parameters. Leu et al. determined a significant fall in T. cholesterol, LDL and Apo B levels after a transition from UF heparin to LMWH in hyperlipidemic HD patients (Leu et al., 1998). Yang et al., on the other hand, showed that the use of LMWH in diabetic hyperlipidemic HD patients caused a decrease in triglyceride and VLDL levels (Yang et al., 1998). Wiemer et al. showed that the use of LMWH brought about a decrease in oxidized LDL and triglyceride levels (Weimer et al., 2002). However, in an evaluation of the effects on lipid parameters of type of HD membrane and heparin type used, Katopodis et al. showed that both membrane and type of heparin have no effect on lipid parameters (Katopodis et al., 2004). Today, the effect of both heparin use and type of heparin on lipid parameters is debatable. We think that there is a need for studies analyzing the effect of HD therapy on lipoprotein metabolism in the HD patient group.

4.1. Triglyceride and triglyceride-rich lipoprotein metabolism disorders

As previously mentioned, hypertriglyceridemia is the most commonly seen lipid abnormality in both pre-dialysis and dialysis patients. Triglyceride-rich lipoprotein metabolism disorders give rise to an increase in triglyceride in CKD patients. The main triglyceride-rich lipoproteins are chylomicron and VLDL. Chylomicron and VLDL transport cholesterol from the intestine and liver to regions where it will be stored (adipose tissue) or used for energy (muscle cells). However, in order for chylomicron and VLDL to be able to do this they are exposed to various maturation processes. One of these is taking Apo E from HDL 2. Apo E enables binding to lipoprotein lipase and VLDL receptors. Another maturation process is taking Apo C-II from HDL 2. Apo C-II is a lipoprotein lipase activator. Apo C-III is a lipoprotein lipase inhibitor. Lipoprotein lipase enables the hydrolysis of chylomicron and VLDL and the fatty acids in them to be used by tissues (Tsimihodimos et al., 2011; Vaziri & Moradi., 2006; Vaziri, 2006). Through lipoprotein lipase, VLDL leads to a 70% decrease in hydrolyzed triglyceride content and the formation of remnant VLDL (IDL). IDL transfers Apo E and Apo C-II in plasma to HDL. After the transfer of the remaining triglycerides to HDL through the mediation of cholesteryl ester transfer protein (CETP), they are lipolyzed through mediation of hepatic triglyceride lipase.

Triglyceride metabolism defects emerge because of a rise in synthesis and/or a decrease in clearance. Lipoprotein lipase is very important in triglyceride and triglyceride-rich lipoprotein clearance. Vaziri et al. showed a decrease in lipoprotein lipase gene expression in several tissues in uremic patients (Vaziri & Moradi., 2006). There may be several causes of a decrease in lipoprotein lipase levels and efficacy in HD patients. One is the heparin use discussed in detail above (Daubresse et al., 1976; Schrader et al., 1990; Shoji et al., 1992). UF heparin use leads to a decline in lipoprotein lipase levels. Another cause is a reduced lipoprotein lipase activator (Apo C-II) and inhibitor (Apo C-III) ratio in HD patients (Chan et al., 2009; Moberly et al., 1999). Studies have shown that impaired Ca-P metabolism and secondary hyperparathyroid lead to a decrease in lipoprotein lipase activity (Akmal et al., 1990; Vaziri et al., 1997). In addition, physical inactivity, insulin resistance and an abnormal T4 (thyroxin) to-tri-iodothyromin (T3) conversion contribute to a decrease in lipoprotein lipase activity (Vaziri & Moradi., 2006). Another cause of reduced clearance is a decrease in hepatic lipase activity. Studies have shown a decrease in hepatic lipase activity in uremic patients. A decrease in hepatic lipase activity causes a decrease in the clearance of chylomicron remnants and IDL and a rise in plasma levels (Klin et al., 1996). Down regulation of VLDL receptor in various tissues is one cause of increased VLDL in plasma (Vaziri & Liang., 1997). Apart from decreased clearance, a rise in synthesis from the liver also contributes to hypertriglyceridemia. Insulin resistance is thought to be one of the factors leading to hypertriglyceridemia in HD patients by increasing hepatic VLDL production (Tsimihodimos et al., 2011). Another reason for increased triglyceride synthesis is the use of acetate dialysate, even though this is not used today. The acetate in the dialysate represents the source for fatty acid synthesis by passing into the blood (Vaziri, 2006). In addition to the use of heparin in HD therapy, various therapy-related factors are thought to cause modifications in triglyceride and triglyceride-rich lipoproteins. Use of a high flux membrane has been shown to reduce triglyceride levels in some studies, and to have no effect in others (Ottosson et al., 2001; Wanner et al., 2004).

4.2. High density lipoprotein metabolism impairment

Another frequently seen impairment of lipid metabolism in the CKD patient group, which includes HD patients, is a reduction in HDL cholesterol and impaired HDL metabolism. Impairments in HDL metabolism appear in the form of decreased Apo AI, impaired HDL maturation, increased HDL triglyceride and a rise in plasma pre β HDL (Pahl et al., 2009; Quaschning et al., 2001; Vaziri, 2006). The main function of HDL is to collect excess cholesterol from peripheral tissues and transport it to be metabolized in the liver (Genest et al., 1999). In addition, the fact that HDL levels decrease as a response to information suggests that it has an inhibitor effect on inflammation (Quaschning et al., 2001; Vaziri 2006). This inhibitor effect also occurs on platelet adhesion and LDL oxidation (Navab et al., 2001). As previously mentioned, another function of HDL is to represent a source for Apo CII and Apo E, which occupy an important place in the metabolism of triglyceride-rich lipoprotein. The most important proteins in the structure of HDL are Apo AI and Apo AII. Apo AI is an activator of lecithin cholesterol acyl transferase (LCAT), which occupies an important place in HDL metabolism. LCAT performs an important function in HDL maturation and in the mediated uptake of HDL from the peripheral tissue to be metabolized in the liver (Kaysen, 2009; Guarnieri et al., 1978; McLeod et al., 1984). Apo AII is a hepatic lipase activator permitting the metabolism of HDL-origin triglyceride (Vaziri, 2006). Okuboet al. showed that the level of Apo AI and Apo AII is low in uremic patients, and that the fall in Apo AI is related to a rise in catabolism and the fall in Apo AII to a decrease in production (Okubo et al., 2004). Low levels of Apo AI and Apo AII are one of the causes of low HDL in HD patients (Attman et al., 2011; Attman et al., 1993) Another reason for lowered HDL and impairment in its metabolism is LCAT deficiency (Guarnieri et al., 1978; Kaysen 2009; McLeod et al., 1984). A decrease in hepatic lipase activity in uremic patients has already been discussed. The role of hepatic lipase in the metabolism of HDL is to assist the hydrolysis and removal of HDL triglyceride content. When it is deficient, a rise in HDL triglyceride takes place (Klin et al., 1996). Cholesterol ester transfer protein (CETP) takes triglycerides by transferring cholesterol esters from HDL to LDL (Davidson and Toth, 2007; Madeleine et al., 2009; Vaziri, 2006). Kimura et al. showed a high CTEP level in HD patients (Kimura et al., 2003). Elevated CTEP may cause a rise in HDL triglyceride in this patient group (Vaziri, 2006). Studies have shown that the HD procedure itself has an effect on HDL-cholesterol levels in HD patients. One such study was performed by Jung et al. Those authors evaluated the effect of citrate and bicarbonate dialysate use on HDL-cholesterol levels and showed that bicarbonate dialysate use increased HDL-cholesterol levels (Jung et al., 1995). Another parameter affecting HDL-cholesterol level is the use of a low flux or high flux dialyzer. Studies have shown that use of a high flux membrane increased Apo AI and HDL-cholesterol levels (Blankestijn et al., 1995; Docci et al., 1995). In conclusion, with both its relation with CKD and the effect of HD therapy, the level of HDL-cholesterol, which has antiatherogenic, anti-inflammatory and antiplatelet functions, declines in the HD patient group, and various impairments arise in the metabolism.

4.3. Low density lipoprotein (LDL) and cholesterol metabolism impairment

LDL is the major source of extracellular cholesterol. In HD patients, as with CKD patients without pre-dialysis proteinuria, cholesterol and LDL levels are normal or low (Kharrat et al., 2012; Shoji et al., 1992; Vaziri, 2006). Although the LDL level is normal or low, the level of small dense LDL with its atherogenic potential is high (Alabakovska et al., 2002; Kaysen, 2009). Additionally, there is an increase in oxidized LDL, thought to be correlated with atherogenic and cardiovascular mortality. As shown in several previous studies, Mahrooz et al. demonstrated high oxidized LDL levels in HD patients (Mahrooz et al., 2012, Samouilidou et al., 2012). However, the findings from studies regarding the relation between oxidized LDL levels and mortality and morbidity are controversial. Asamiya et al. showed that the oxidized LDL/LDL-cholesterol ratio is higher in patients with coronary artery calcification (Asamiya et al., 2012). Sevinç ok et al. reported that neither oxidized LDL nor non-oxidized LDL values are correlated with mortality (Sevinc ok et al., 2012). Pawlak et al. reported low oxidized LDL in HD patients but high antibodies against oxidized LDL, and that the oxidized LDL/oxidized LDL antibody ratio might be a new marker for cardiovascular events (Pawlak et al., 2012). Mention has already been made of studies showing that LDL is small and dense in HD patients. Noori et al. determined no correlation between conventional lipid parameters and mortality, but showed that very small LDL particle concentration is correlated with mortality (Noori et al., 2011). Kimura et al. showed that small size LDL is correlated with coronary artery disease (Kimura et al., 2011). In conclusion, LDL levels are normal or low in the HD patient group while LDL fractions (oxidized LDL, small dense LDL) with their atherogenic potential are higher in this patient group.

4.4. Lipoprotein(a) metabolism impairment

Lipoprotein (a) (Lp (a)) is a LDL-like particle. It is distinguished from LDL by the presence of apolipoprotein (a) (Apo (a)). Apo a binds to Apo B-100 with disulfide bonds. Because of Apo (a)'s similarity to plasminogen it is thought to contribute to thrombogenesis by inhibiting fibrinolysis of Lp (a) (Milionis et al., 1999; Tsimihodimos et al., 2011). There have been many studies regarding the correlation between elevated Lp (a) and cardiovascular events in the normal population (Rader &Brewer., 1992; Schaefer et al., 1994). There have also been several studies on the subject in HD patients, with high levels being shown in these (Dieplinger et al., 1993; Hirata et al., 1993; Kronenberg et al., 1995). Several clinical studies have evaluated the relation between Apo (a) size and Lp (a) level. Correlations have been determined between Apo (a) low molecular-weight (LMW) isoforms and elevated Lp (a) levels, and also between high-molecular-weight (HMW) isoforms and low Lp (a) levels (Boerwinkle et al., 1992; Kraft et al., 1992). The relationship between Apo (a) phenotype and elevated Lp (a) in HD patients is questionable (Hirata et al., 1993; Kronenberg et al., 1995). One of these studies, by Milionis et al., determined elevated Lp (a) and Apo (a) levels in HD patients (Milionis et al., 1999). Kronenberg et al.'s study supported these findings (Kronenberg et al., 1995). However, Kronenberg et al.'s 1999 study showed that LMW Apo (a) phenotype is an independent predictor for CAD (Kronenberg et al., 1999). The Choices for Healthy Outcomes in Caring for ESRD (CHOICE) study showed that Lp (a) levels are high in young, white patients and correlated with cardiovascular events. However, that study also stated that Apo (a) size is not correlated with elevated Lp (a) and cardiovascular events (Longenecker et al., 2002). In conclusion, while the correlation between elevated Lp (a) and Apo (a) size in the HD patient group is still unclear, elevated Lp (a) in particular is thought to be a cardiovascular risk factor.

4.5. Reverse epidemiology in hemodialysis patients

Hyperlipidemia is known to be one of the most important cardiovascular risk factors in the normal population (Gordon et al., 1977). However, the relationship between dyslipidemia and mortality in HD patients is controversial. Cheung et al. determined that several traditional risk factors, including T. cholesterol, were not correlated with mortality in HD patients (Cheung et al., 2000). A cross-sectional study by Stack et al. produced similar results (Stack & Bloembergen). However, some studies have reported a correlation between dyslipidemia and mortality (Hahn et al., 1983; Nishizawa et al., 2003). As already discussed, whether renal replacement is performed with CRD patients, and whether that replacement is HD, modifies lipid metabolism disorders. No dyslipidemia-mortality correlation has been determined in certain patient populations (cancer patients, hospitalized patients, etc.) including the HD patient group (Shoji et al., 2011). This reverse relationship is therefore known as 'reverse epidemiology' (Kalantar-Zadeh et al., 2004). Hypercholesterolemia, high body mass index (BMI) and hyperhomocysteinemia lead to shortening in long-term survey in the normal population. But in the HD patient these factors lead to an increase in short-term survey. Researchers have described this to malnutrition inflammation (MIA) syndrome (Stenvinkel et al., 1999). MIA syndrome is known to be correlated with atherosclerosis and mortality in HD patients. Presence of hypercholesterolemia, high BMI and hyperhomocysteinemia in this patient group shows that nutrition status may be good. Improvement in MIA in these patients may cause a decrease in mortality (Nurmohamed &Nubé, 2005). In conclusion, these traditional risk factors for HD patients should be reviewed and new treatment objectives set out.

4.6. Treatment

It is today recognized that there is a correlation between hyperlipidemia and cardiovascular events in individuals with normal renal functions and that cardiovascular mortality can be reduced by treating hyperlipidemia. It has been shown in several randomized, controlled meta-analyses that reducing LDL cholesterol with statin therapy brings about a significant decrease in CAD and myocardial infarction (MI) in the normal population (Baigent et al., 2005). However, in the same way that impairments in lipid metabolism in HD patients differ from those in individuals with normal renal functions, so there are various differences in dyslipidemia treatment in these patients. This section discusses dyslipidemia treatment and its effect on mortality and morbidity in the light of major studies.

4.6.1. The use of statin in dyslipidemia treatment

The use of statin has been shown to have a lowering effect on mortality and morbidity in hyperlipidemic patients without renal function disorder. Statin use in pre-dialysis CKD patients is known, with its LDL-cholesterol reducing effect and an effect independent of the lipid lowering effect known as pleotropic effect, to reduce mortality and morbidity and to slow renal progression (Deshmukh & Mehta., 2011; Olyaei et al., 2011). Statins' pleotropic effects may be listed as a decrease in endothelial cells' permeability to LDL, an increase in vasodilator response, a decrease in endothelial adhesion molecules and an antioxidant effect (Vaughan et al., 2000). The use of statin in HD patients is controversial. One study on the subject by Saltissi et al. showed that simvastatin significantly reduces non-HDL cholesterol levels (Saltissi et al., 2002). Chang et al. determined that simvastatin has an anti-inflammatory effect as well as a lipid-reducing one in HD patients (Chang et al., 2002). These and similar studies have shown that statins have a lipid-reducing effect in HD patients, as well as the presence of pleotropic effects (Nishikawa et al., 1999; Soliemani et al., 2011; van den Akker et al., 2003). One piece of research to investigate the effect on mortality of statin therapy was the Deutsche Diabetes-Dialyse-Studie (4D) study. This was a prospective, randomized study involving 178 HD centers. It included more than 1000 diabetic HD patients and observed 21% MI -associated mortality in the group receiving atorvastatin and the control group. However, sudden cardiac death-related cardiac mortality levels approaching 50% developed in both groups. The researchers suggested that sudden cardiac deaths might be related to arrhythmia and were not reduced by the use of statin (Wanner et al., 2005). Another major piece of research, the AURORA study published in 2009, included 2776 HD patients. That study showed that despite a significant fall in LDL cholesterol with rosuvastatin, there was no significant decrease in cardiovascular mortality (Fellström et al., 2009). Finally, the SHARP study was conducted with 9270 patients with CKD (3023 dialysis patients). In that study, simvastatin + ezetimibe (4193 simvastatin plus ezetimibe from the start, 457 beginning with simvastatin alone and then plus ezetimibe after one year) was administered to one arm, and placebo (4191 plus at the beginning, 429 plus one year after) to the other. Average duration of monitoring was 4.9 years. Major cardiovascular events (non-fatal myocardial infarction or coronary death, non-hemorrhagic stroke, or arterial revascularization) were observed in 11.3% of the simvastatin plus ezetimibe group, and in 13.4% of the placebo group. A 17% fall in major atherosclerotic events was observed with a decrease of 0.85 mmol/L in LDL. In addition, this decrease in risk did not alter depending on whether the patients enrolled received dialysis therapy or not. In other words, in contrast to the 4D and AURORA studies, a decrease in major cardiovascular events was brought about with statin therapy in that study (Baigent et al., 2011).

4.6.2. The use of ezetimibe in the treatment of dyslipidemia

Ezetimibe is a selective intestinal cholesterol absorption inhibitor. Prevention of cholesterol absorption in addition to inhibition of cholesterol synthesis has been shown to reduce cardiovascular mortality in recent years. For that reason, studies have begun being performed regarding the use of ezetimibe alone in patients with a high risk of side-effects from ezetimibe plus low-dose statin combinations or statin for the purpose of reducing side-effects frequently observed with statins, particularly at increased doses (myopathy/myositis, hepatitis, etc.). In the HD patient group, in which the effect of statin on mortality and morbidity is controversial, studies with low patient numbers have shown that ezetimibe produces a reliable and effective fall in cholesterol (Hattori & Hattori., 2010; Ahmed & Khalil., 2010). Finally, the SHARP study showed that simvastatin plus ezetimibe produced a significant decrease in atherosclerotic cardiovascular events (Baigent et al., 2011).

4.6.3. The use of fibrate in the treatment of dyslipidemia

Fibrates have been used for many years, particularly in the treatment of hypertriglyceridemia. In the HD patient group, hypertriglyceridemia exhibits a pronounced impairment of lipid metabolism. HD would therefore seem to represent a potential patient group for fibrate use. However, since fibrate metabolites are eliminated by the kidney, and since these metabolites give rise to serious side-effects such as myopathy and rhabdomyolysis by accumulating with a decrease in glomerular filtration rate, use in this patient group is limited. However, one study including some 9000 patients published in 2012 showed that fibrate use is quite safe and effective in diabetic patients with moderate renal damage. Patients with a GFR above 30 were included in that study, however (Ting et al., 2012). There are not many studies concerning the use of fibrate in HD patients. One such study is that by Makówka et al. The study included 27 chronic HD patients and lasted for 63 days. It determined a significant fall in T cholesterol, LDL and triglyceride with fenofibrate therapy and a significant rise in HDL. AST and ALT levels remained normal in patients receiving fenofibrate, while CPK levels rose significantly compared to basal values but then remained stable (Makówka et al., 2012). Prospective randomized studies involving large patient numbers evaluating the reliability and efficacy of fibrate use in the HD patient group are now needed.

4.6.4. Use of nicotinic acid in the treatment of dyslipidemia

Nicotinic acid is a water-soluble vitamin B complex (vitamin B3) that has been used in the treatment of hypertriglyceridemia for many years. It produces a fall in triglyceride, LDL and VLDL levels and a rise in HDL. However, hepatoxicity and flushing are side-effects that limit its use. While there have been pharmacokinetic studies in HD patients, studies showing its effectiveness in the treatment of dyslipidemia are restricted to a very small number of cases (Reiche et al., 2011). There are no studies showing its effect on mortality and morbidity. Restrepo Valencia and Cruz reported a fall in T. cholesterol and triglyceride levels and a rise in HDL after nicotinic acid therapy in 3 HD and 6 PD patients (Restrepo Valencia &Cruz., 2008). Shahbazian et al. reported a rise in HDL cholesterol in 48 HD patients after 8-week nicotinamide therapy (Shahbazian et al., 2011).

4.6.5. The use of sevelamer in the treatment of dyslipidemia

Sevelamer hydrochloride is a non-calcium containing phosphorus-binding resin used in the treatment of hyperphosphatemia in HD patients. The Dialysis Clinical Outcomes Revisited (DCOR) and Renagel in New Dialysis (RIND) studies showed that it provides a better sur-

vey that calcium-containing phosphorus-binders (Block et al., 2007; Suki et al., 2007). Sevelamer prevents the absorption of intestinal cholesterol. Studies have shown it has positive
effects on lipid parameters in HD patients (Yamada et al., 2005; Qunibi, 2005). Iimori et al.
showed that dyslipidemia improved significantly with treatment with sevelamer and that
mortality declined (Iimori et al., 2012). However, the use of sevelamer in the treatment of
dyslipidemia in HD patients has not been accepted due to the lack of wide-ranging and
long-term studies.

4.6.6. The use of carnitine in the treatment of dyslipidemia

Also known as trimethyl-aminobutyric acid, carnitine is a naturally-occurring vitamin-like
substance. Carnitine serves in several important metabolic pathways. One of the most important of these is that it lowers the level of free fatty acid necessary for triglyceride synthesis and beta-oxidation of fatty acids (Guarnieri et al., 2001). Since the kidneys are an
important site of carnitine synthesis, that synthesis decreases in the event of kidney failure
(Bellinghieri et al., 2003). Studies exist showing that carnitine therapy has a positive effect on
lipid parameters in HD patients, while others report no positive effect (Emami Naini et al.,
2012; Naini et al., 2012; Hurot et al., 2002; Guarnieri et al., 2007). For that reason, carnitine is
not definitively accepted in the treatment of dyslipidemia in HD patients.

4.6.7. Heparin-induced extracorporeal LDL precipitation

Heparin-induced extracorporeal LDL precipitation (HELP) is a form of lipid apheresis particularly used in the treatment of familial hyperlipidemia. The number of case reports in the
literature is limited, although a significant lipid decrease has been observed with HELP. One
of this limited number of studies in the literature is that by Bosch et al. A pronounced fall in
LDL was observed with 29 sessions of HELP in 5 HD patients (Bosch et al., 1993). Another
study by Bosch et al. reported quite good results with HELP in 3 HD patients (Bosch et al.,
1993). Eisenhauer et al. achieved a significant fall in LDL cholesterol with HELP in 6 HD patients (Eisenhauer et al., 1991). In the light of these case reports, we think that HELP may be
a useful form of treatment, especially in HD patients with familial hyperlipidemia and with
no response to drug therapy.

4.6.8. Guideline

The K-DOQI treatment of hyperlipidemia guideline was published in 2003 because of the
variation in dyslipidemia in HD patients (Kidney Disease Outcomes Quality Initiative (K/
DOQI) Group, 2003) Until then, there had been recommendations resembling an adult hyperlipidemia guideline in the studies performed. In essence, the recommendations of that
guideline are as follows;

In order to prevent serious complications such as pancreatitis in patients with a triglyceride
level above 500 mg/dl, primary focus must be on triglyceride-lowering therapy. Diet, fibrate
and nicotinic acid can be used in treatment.

If the triglyceride level is below 500 mg, treatment should be adjusted according to LDL levels. If LDL is above 100 mg/dl, LDL-lowering therapy (diet and statin) is recommended.

If LDL is normal while triglyceride is elevated, there is generally a rise associated with lipid remnants. The amount of remnant lipoprotein can generally be estimated with a calculation of non-HDL cholesterol. Non- HDL cholesterol is calculated as the difference between T. cholesterol and HDL cholesterol. Treatment is recommended in patients with non-HDL cholesterol above 130 mg/dl.

As already stated, because of the insufficient number of studies, the dyslipidemia treatment guideline in chronic kidney patients was adapted to the adult hyperlipidemia treatment guideline. However, it is clear that treatment in HD patients requires a different approach. We therefore think that this guideline published in 2003 should be updated in the light of more recent studies.

5. Conclusion and recommendations

The pathogenesis of dyslipidemia in the HD patient group, which has various impairments in lipid metabolism, has not yet been fully clarified. New studies regarding that pathogenesis are therefore needed. In addition, new studies regarding what the aim of treatment in dyslipidemia and the parameter to be targeted should be (triglyceride, LDL, IDL, VLDL or non-HDL cholesterol?). Finally, treatment adapted to the adult hyperlipidemia treatment guideline because of a lack of sufficient studies must clearly be turned into a lipid guideline aimed at HD patients in the light of newly published studies.

Author details

Şükrü Ulusoy and Gülsüm Özkan

Karadeniz Technical University, School of Medicine, Department of Nephrology, Turkey

References

[1] Ahmed, M.H. & Khalil, A.A. (2010) Ezetimibe as a potential treatment for dyslipidemia associated with chronic renal failure and renal transplant. Saudi J Kidney Dis Transpl, 21, 1021-9

[2] Akmal, M., Kasim, S.E., Soliman, A.R. & Massry, S.G. (1990) Excess parathyroid hormone adversely affects lipid metabolism in chronic renal failure. Kidney Int, 37, 854-8

[3]   Alabakovska, S.B., Todorova, B.B., Labudovic, D.D. & Tosheska, K.N. (2002) LDL and HDL subclass distribution in patients with end-stage renal diseases. Clin Biochem, 35,211-6

[4]   Anderson, K.M., Wilson, P.W., Odell, P.M. & Kannel, W.B. (1991) An updated coronary risk profile. A statement for health professionals. Circulation, 83, 356-62

[5]   Asamiya, Y., Yajima. A., Tsuruta, Y., Otsubo, S., & Nitta, K. (2012) Oxidised LDL/ LDL-cholesterol ratio and coronary artery calcification in haemodialysis patients. Nutr Metab Cardiovasc Dis. May 16.

[6]   Attman, P.O., Samuelsson, O. & Alaupovic, P. (1993) Lipoprotein metabolism and renal failure. Am J Kidney Dis, 21,573-92

[7]   Attman, P.O., Samuelsson, O. & Alaupovic, P. (2011) The effect of decreasing renal function on lipoprotein profiles. Nephrol Dial Transplant, 26,2572-5

[8]   Baigent, C., Landray, M.J., Reith, C., Emberson, J., Wheeler, D.C., Tomson, C., Wanner, C., Krane, V., Cass, A., Craig, J., Neal, B., Jiang, L., Hooi, L.S., Levin, A., Agodoa, L., Gaziano, M., Kasiske, B., Walker, R., Massy, Z.A., Feldt-Rasmussen, B., Krairittichai, U., Ophascharoensuk, V., Fellström, B., Holdaas, H., Tesar, V., Wiecek, A., Grobbee, D., de Zeeuw, D., Grönhagen-Riska, C., Dasgupta, T., Lewis, D., Herrington, W., Mafham, M., Majoni, W., Wallendszus, K., Grimm, R., Pedersen, T., Tobert, J., Armitage, J., Baxter, A., Bray, C., Chen, Y., Chen, Z., Hill, M., Knott, C., Parish, S., Simpson, D., Sleight, P., Young, A. & Collins, R. ; SHARP Investigators. (2011) The effects of lowering LDL cholesterol with simvastatin plus ezetimibe in patients with chronic kidney disease (Study of Heart and Renal Protection): a randomised placebo-controlled trial. Lancet, 377,2181-92

[9]   Baigent, C., Keech, A., Kearney, P.M., Blackwell, L., Buck, G., Pollicino, C., Kirby, A., Sourjina, T., Peto, R., Collins, R. & Simes, R. ; (2005) Cholesterol Treatment Trialists' (CTT) Collaborators. Efficacy and safety of cholesterol-lowering treatment: prospective meta-analysis of data from 90,056 participants in 14 randomised trials of statins. Lancet, 366,1267-78

[10] Bellinghieri, G., Santoro, D., Calvani, M., Mallamace, A. & Savica, V. (2003) Carnitine and hemodialysis. Am J Kidney Dis, 41,116-22

[11] Blankestijn, P.J., Vos, P.F., Rabelink, T.J., van Rijn, H.J., Jansen, H. & Koomans, H.A. (1995) High-flux dialysis membranes improve lipid profile in chronic hemodialysis patients. J Am Soc Nephrol, 5,1703-8

[12] Block, G.A., Raggi, P., Bellasi, A., Kooienga, L. & Spiegel, D.M. (2007) Mortality effect of coronary calcification and phosphate binder choice in incident hemodialysis patients. Kidney Int, 71,438-41

[13] Bosch, T., Samtleben, W., Thiery, J., Gurland, H.J. & Seidel, D. (1993) Reverse flux filtration: a new mode of therapy improving the efficacy of heparin-induced extracor-

poreal LDL precipitation in hyperlipidemic hemodialysis patients. Int J Artif Organs, 16,75-85

[14] Bosch, T., Thiery, J., Gurland, H.J. & Seidel, D. (1993) Long-term efficiency, biocompatibility, and clinical safety of combined simultaneous LDL-apheresis and haemodialysis in patients with hypercholesterolaemia and end-stage renal failure. Nephrol Dial Transplant, 8,1350-8

[15] Bostom, A.G., Shemin, D., Verhoef, P., Nadeau, M.R., Jacques, P.F., Selhub, J., Dworkin, L. & Rosenberg, I.H. (1997) Elevated fasting total plasma homocysteine levels and cardiovascular disease outcomes in maintenance dialysis patients. A prospective study. Arterioscler Thromb Vasc Biol, 17,2554-8

[16] Boaz, M., Matas, Z., Biro, A., Katzir, Z., Green, M., Fainaru, M. & Smetana, S. (1999) Serum malondialdehyde and prevalent cardiovascular disease in hemodialysis. Kidney Int, 56,1078-83.

[17] Boaz, M., Matas, Z., Biro, A., Katzir, Z., Green, M., Fainaru, M. & Smetana, S. (1999) Comparison of hemostatic factors and serum malondialdehyde as predictive factors for cardiovascular disease in hemodialysis patients. Am J Kidney Dis, 34,438-44

[18] Boerwinkle, E., Leffert, C.C., Lin, J., Lackner, C., Chiesa, G. & Hobbs, H.H. (1992) Apolipoprotein(a) gene accounts for greater than 90% of the variation in plasma lipoprotein(a) concentrations. J Clin Invest, 90,52-60

[19] Braun, J., Oldendorf, M., Moshage, W., Heidler, R., Zeitler, E. & Luft, F.C. (1996) Electron beam computed tomography in the evaluation of cardiac calcification in chronic dialysis patients. Am J Kidney Dis, 27,3, 394-401

[20] Chan, D.T., Dogra, G.K., Irish, A.B., Ooi, E.M., Barrett, P.H., Chan, D.C. & Watts, G.F. (2009) Chronic kidney disease delays VLDL-apoB-100 particle catabolism: potential role of apolipoprotein C-III. J Lipid Res, 50,2524-31

[21] Chang, J.W., Yang, W.S., Min, W.K., Lee, S.K., Park, J.S. & Kim, S.B. (2002) Effects of simvastatin on high-sensitivity C-reactive protein and serum albumin in hemodialysis patients. Am J Kidney Dis, 39,1213-7

[22] Cheung, A.K., Sarnak, M.J., Yan, G., Dwyer, J.T., Heyka, R.J., Rocco, M.V., Teehan, B.P. & Levey, A.S. (2000) Atherosclerotic cardiovascular disease risks in chronic hemodialysis patients. Kidney Int, 58,353-62

[23] Daubresse, J.C., Lerson, G., Plamteux, G., Rorive, G., Luyckx, A.S. & Lefebvre, P.J. (1976) Lipids and lipoproteins in chronic uraemia. A study of the influence of regular haemodialysis. Eur J Clin Invest, 6,159-66

[24] Davidson, M.H.&Toth, P.P. (2007) High-density lipoprotein metabolism: potential therapeutic targets. Am J Cardiol, 100,32-40

[25] Deshmukh, A. & Mehta, J.L. (2011) Statins and renal disease: friend or foe? Curr Atheroscler Rep, 13,57-63

[26] Dieplinger, H., Lackner, C., Kronenberg, F., Sandholzer, C., Lhotta, K., Hoppichler, F., Graf, H. & König, P. (1993) Elevated plasma concentrations of lipoprotein(a) in patients with end-stage renal disease are not related to the size polymorphism of apolipoprotein(a). J Clin Invest, 91,397-401

[27] Docci, D., Capponcini, C., Mengozzi, S., Baldrati, L., Neri, L. & Feletti, C. (1995) Effects of different dialysis membranes on lipid and lipoprotein serum profiles in hemodialysis patients. Nephron, 69,323-6.

[28] Dominiczak, M.H. & Caslake, M.J. (2011) Apolipoproteins: metabolic role and clinical biochemistry applications. Ann Clin Biochem, 48,498-515

[29] Eisenhauer, T., Müller, U., Schuff-Werner, P., Armstrong, V.W., Bosch, T., Thiery, J., Gurland, H. & Seidel, D. (1991) Simultaneous heparin extracorporeal LDL precipitation and hemodialysis. First clinical experience. ASAIO Trans, 37,494-6

[30] Emami Naini, A., Moradi, M., Mortazavi, M., Amini Harandi, A., Hadizadeh, M., Shirani, F., Basir Ghafoori, H. & Emami Naini, P. (2012) Effects of Oral L-Carnitine Supplementation on Lipid Profile, Anemia, and Quality of Life in Chronic Renal Disease Patients under Hemodialysis: A Randomized, Double-Blinded, Placebo-Controlled Trial. J Nutr Metab, 510483

[31] Fellström, B.C., Jardine, A.G., Schmieder, R.E., Holdaas, H., Bannister, K., Beutler, J., Chae, D.W., Chevaile, A., Cobbe, S.M., Grönhagen-Riska, C., De Lima, J.J., Lins, R., Mayer, G., McMahon, A.W., Parving, H.H., Remuzzi, G., Samuelsson, O., Sonkodi, S., Sci, D., Süleymanlar, G., Tsakiris, D., Tesar, V., Todorov, V., Wiecek, A., Wüthrich, R.P., Gottlow, M., Johnsson, E. & Zannad, F.; AURORA Study Group. (2009) Rosuvastatin and cardiovascular events in patients undergoing hemodialysis. N Engl J Med, 360,1395-407

[32] Fukagawa, M, & Kazama JJ. The making of a bone in blood vessels: from the soft shell to the hard bone. (2007) Kidney Int, 72, 5, 533

[33] Genest, J. Jr., Marcil, M., Denis, M. & Yu, L. (1999) High density lipoproteins in health and in disease. J Investig Med, 47,31-42

[34] Gordon, T., Castelli, W.P., Hjortland, M.C., Kannel, W.B. & Dawber, T.R. (1977) High density lipoprotein as a protective factor against coronary heart disease. The Framingham Study. Am J Med, 62,707-14

[35] Guarnieri, G.F., Moracchiello, M., Campanacci, L., Ursini, F., Ferri, L., Valente, M. & Gregolin, C. (1978) Lecithin-cholesterol acyltransferase (LCAT) activity in chronic uremia. Kidney Int Suppl, 8,26-30

[36] Guarnieri, G., Situlin, R. & Biolo, G. (2001) Carnitine metabolism in uremia. Am J Kidney Dis, 38:63-7

[37] Guarnieri, G., Biolo, G., Vinci, P., Massolino, B. & Barazzoni, R. (2007) Advances in carnitine in chronic uremia. J Ren Nutr, 17,23-9

[38] Hahn, R., Oette, K., Mondorf, H., Finke, K. & Sieberth, H.G. (1983) Analysis of cardi-
      ovascular risk factors in chronic hemodialysis patients with special attention to the
      hyperlipoproteinemias. Atherosclerosis, 48,279-88

[39] Hattori, S. & Hattori, Y. (2010) Efficacy and safety of ezetimibe in patients undergo-
      ing hemodialysis. Endocr J, 57,1001-5

[40] Hirata, K., Kikuchi, S., Saku, K., Jimi, S., Zhang, B., Naito, S., Hamaguchi, H. & Ara-
      kawa, K. (1993) Apolipoprotein(a) phenotypes and serum lipoprotein(a) levels in
      maintenance hemodialysis patients with/without diabetes mellitus. Kidney Int,
      44,1062-70

[41] Hurot, J.M., Cucherat, M., Haugh, M. & Fouque, D. (2002) Effects of L-carnitine sup-
      plementation in maintenance hemodialysis patients: a systematic review. J Am Soc
      Nephrol, 13,708-14

[42] Iimori, S., Mori, Y., Akita, W., Takada, S., Kuyama, T., Ohnishi, T., Shikuma, S., Ishi-
      gami, J., Tajima, M., Asai, T., Okado, T., Kuwahara, M., Sasaki, S. & Tsukamoto, Y.
      (2012) Effects of sevelamer hydrochloride on mortality, lipid abnormality and arterial
      stiffness in hemodialyzed patients: a propensity-matched observational study. Clin
      Exp Nephrol, May 12

[43] Jung, K., Scheifler, A., Schulze, B.D. & Scholz, M. (1995) Lower serum high-density
      lipoprotein-cholesterol concentration in patients undergoing maintenance hemodial-
      ysis with acetate than with bicarbonate. Am J Kidney Dis, 25,584-8

[44] Kalantar-Zadeh, K., Block, G., Horwich, T. & Fonarow, G.C. (2004) Reverse epidemi-
      ology of conventional cardiovascular risk factors in patients with chronic heart fail-
      ure. J Am Coll Cardiol, 43,1439-44

[45] Katopodis, K.P., Elisaf, M., Balafa, O., Nikolopoulos, P., Bairaktari, E., Katsaraki, A. &
      Siamopoulos, K.C. (2004) Influence of the type of membrane and heparin on serum
      lipid parameters during a dialysis session: a pilot study. Am J Nephrol, 24,469-73

[46] Kaysen, G.A. (2009) Potential restoration of HDL function with apolipoprotein A-I
      mimetic peptide in end-stage renal disease. Kidney Int, 76,359-61

[47] Kaysen, G.A. (2009) Lipid and lipoprotein metabolism in chronic kidney disease. J
      Ren Nutr, 19,73-7

[48] Kaysen, G.A. (2009) New insights into lipid metabolism in chronic kidney disease:
      what are the practical implications? Blood Purif, 27,86-91

[49] K/DOQI Workgroup. (2005) K/DOQI clinical practice guidelines for cardiovascular
      disease in dialysis patients. Am J Kidney Dis, 45,1-153

[50] Kharrat, I., Jmal, A., Jmal, L., Amira, Z., Ben Cheikh, W., Ben Bourouba, F., Sahnoun,
      L. & Abdennebi, M. (2012) Alterations in lipidic metabolism in hemodialysis patients.
      Tunis Med, 90,537-41

[51] Kidney Disease Outcomes Quality Initiative (K/DOQI) Group. (2003) K/DOQI clinical practice guidelines for management of dyslipidemias in patients with kidney disease. Am J Kidney Dis, 41, 1-91

[52] Kidney Disease: Improving Global Outcomes (KDIGO) CKD-MBD Work Group. (2009) KDIGO clinical practice guideline for the diagnosis, evaluation, prevention, and treatment of Chronic Kidney Disease-Mineral and Bone Disorder (CKD-MBD). Kidney Int Suppl, 113, 1-130

[53] Kimura, H., Miyazaki, R., Imura, T., Masunaga, S., Suzuki, S., Gejyo, F. & Yoshida, H. (2003) Hepatic lipase mutation may reduce vascular disease prevalence in hemodialysis patients with high CETP levels. Kidney Int, 64,1829-37

[54] Kimura, H., Miyazaki, R., Imura, T., Masunaga, S., Shimada, A., Mikami, D., Kasuno, K., Takahashi, N., Hirano, T. & Yoshida, H. (2011) Smaller low-density lipoprotein size as a possible risk factor for the prevalence of coronary artery diseases in haemodialysis patients: associations of cholesteryl ester transfer protein and the hepatic lipase gene polymorphism with low-density lipoprotein size. Nephrology (Carlton), 16, 558-66

[55] Klin, M., Smogorzewski, M., Ni, Z., Zhang, G. & Massry, S.G. (1996) Abnormalities in hepatic lipase in chronic renal failure: role of excess parathyroid hormone. J Clin Invest, 97,2167-73

[56] Kraft, H.G., Köchl, S., Menzel, H.J., Sandholzer, C. & Utermann, G. (1992) The apolipoprotein (a) gene: a transcribed hypervariable locus controlling plasma lipoprotein (a) concentration. Hum Genet, 90,220-30

[57] Kronenberg, F., König, P., Neyer, U., Auinger, M., Pribasnig, A., Lang, U., Reitinger, J., Pinter, G., Utermann, G. & Dieplinger, H. (1995)Multicenter study of lipoprotein(a) and apolipoprotein(a) phenotypes in patients with end-stage renal disease treated by hemodialysis or continuous ambulatory peritoneal dialysis. J Am Soc Nephrol, 6,110-20

[58] Kronenberg, F., Neyer, U., Lhotta, K., Trenkwalder, E., Auinger, M., Pribasnig, A., Meisl, T., König, P. & Dieplinger, H. (1999) The low molecular weight apo(a) phenotype is an independent predictor for coronary artery disease in hemodialysis patients: a prospective follow-up. J Am Soc Nephrol, 10,1027-36

[59] Leu, J.G., Liou, H.H., Wu, S.C., Yang, W.C., Huang, T.P. & Wu, S.C. (1998) Low molecular weight heparin in diabetic and nondiabetic hypercholesterolemic patients receiving long-term hemodialysis. J Formos Med Assoc, 97,49-54

[60] Levey, A.S., Beto, J.A., Coronado, B.E., Eknoyan, G., Foley, R.N., Kasiske, B.L., Klag, M.J., Mailloux, L.U., Manske, C.L., Meyer, K.B., Parfrey, P.S., Pfeffer, M.A., Wenger, N.K., Wilson, P.W. & Wright, J.T. Jr. (1998) Controlling the epidemic of cardiovascular disease in chronic renal disease: what do we know? What do we need to learn? Where do we go from here? National Kidney Foundation Task Force on Cardiovascular Disease. Am J Kidney Dis, 32,853-906

[61] London, G.M., Guérin, A.P., Marchais, S.J., Métivier, F., Pannier, B. & Adda, H. (2003) Arterial media calcification in end-stage renal disease: impact on all-cause and cardiovascular mortality. Nephrol Dial Transplant, 18,9,1731-40

[62] Longenecker, J.C., Coresh, J., Powe, N.R., Levey, A.S., Fink, N.E., Martin, A. & Klag, M.J. (2002) Traditional cardiovascular disease risk factors in dialysis patients compared with the general population: the CHOICE Study. J Am Soc Nephrol, 13,1918-27

[63] Longenecker, J.C., Klag, M.J., Marcovina, S.M., Powe, N.R., Fink, N.E., Giaculli, F. & Coresh, J. ; Choices for Healthy Outcomes in Caring for ESRD. (2002) Small apolipoprotein(a) size predicts mortality in end-stage renal disease: The CHOICE study. Circulation, 106,2812-8

[64] Lowrie, E.G. & Lew, N.L. (1990) Death risk in hemodialysis patients: the predictive value of commonly measured variables and an evaluation of death rate differences between facilities. Am J Kidney Dis, 15,458-82

[65] Mahmood, D., Grubbström, M., Lundberg, L.D., Olivecrona, G., Olivecrona, T. & Stegmayr, B.G. (2010) Lipoprotein lipase responds similarly to tinzaparin as to conventional heparin during hemodialysis. BMC Nephrol, 11:33

[66] Mahrooz, A., Zargari, M., Sedighi, O., Shaygani, H. & Gohari, G. (2012) Increased oxidized-LDL levels and arylesterase activity/HDL ratio in ESRD patients treated with hemodialysis. Clin Invest Med, 35,144-51

[67] Makówka, A., Dryja, P., Chwatko, G., Bald, E. & Nowicki, M. (2012) Treatment of chronic hemodialysis patients with low-dose fenofibrate effectively reduces plasma lipids and affects plasma redox status. Lipids Health Dis, 11,47

[68] Mallamaci, F., Zoccali, C., Tripepi, G., Fermo, I., Benedetto, F.A., Cataliotti, A., Bellanuova, I., Malatino, L.S. & Soldarini, A.; CREED Investigators. (2002) Hyperhomocysteinemia predicts cardiovascular outcomes in hemodialysis patients. Kidney Int, 61,609-14

[69] Manns, B.J., Burgess, E.D., Hyndman, M.E., Parsons, H.G., Schaefer, J.P. & Scott-Douglas, N.W. (1999) Hyperhomocyst(e)inemia and the prevalence of atherosclerotic vascular disease in patients with end-stage renal disease. Am J Kidney Dis, 34,669-77

[70] McLeod, R., Reeve, C.E. & Frohlich, J. (1984) Plasma lipoproteins and lecithin:cholesterol acyltransferase distribution in patients on dialysis. Kidney Int, 25,683-8

[71] Milionis, H.J., Elisaf, M.S., Tselepis, A., Bairaktari, E., Karabina, S.A. & Siamopoulos, K.C. (1999) Apolipoprotein(a) phenotypes and lipoprotein(a) concentrations in patients with renal failure. Am J Kidney Dis, 33,1100-6

[72] Moberly, J.B., Attman, P.O., Samuelsson, O., Johansson, A.C., Knight-Gibson, C. & Alaupovic, P. (1999) Apolipoprotein C-III, hypertriglyceridemia and triglyceride-rich lipoproteins in uremia. Miner Electrolyte Metab, 25,258-62

[73] Naini, A.E., Sadeghi, M., Mortazavi, M., Moghadasi, M. & Harandi, A.A. (2012) Oral carnitine supplementation for dyslipidemia in chronic hemodialysis patients. Saudi J Kidney Dis Transpl, 23,484-8

[74] Navab, M., Berliner, J.A., Subbanagounder, G., Hama, S., Lusis, A.J., Castellani, L.W., Reddy, S., Shih, D., Shi, W., Watson, A.D., Van Lenten, B.J., Vora, D. & Fogelman, A.M. (2001) HDL and the inflammatory response induced by LDL-derived oxidized phospholipids. Arterioscler Thromb Vasc Biol, 21,481-8

[75] Nishikawa, O., Mune, M., Miyano, M., Nishide, T., Nishide, I., Maeda, A., Kimura, K., Takahashi, T., Kishino, M., Tone, Y., Otani, H., Ogawa, A., Maeda, T. & Yukawa, S. (1999) Effect of simvastatin on the lipid profile of hemodialysis patients. Kidney Int Suppl, 71,219-21.

[76] Nishizawa, Y., Shoji, T., Kakiya, R., Tsujimoto, Y., Tabata, T., Ishimura, E., Nakatani, T., Miki, T. & Inaba, M. (2003) Non-high-density lipoprotein cholesterol (non-HDL-C) as a predictor of cardiovascular mortality in patients with end-stage renal disease. Kidney Int, 84,117-20

[77] Noori, N., Caulfield, M.P., Salameh, W.A., Reitz, R.E., Nicholas, S.B., Molnar, M.Z., Nissenson, A.R., Kovesdy, C.P. & Kalantar-Zadeh, K. (2011) Novel lipoprotein sub-fraction and size measurements in prediction of mortality in maintenance hemodialysis patients. Clin J Am Soc Nephrol, 6,2861-70

[78] Nurmohamed, S.A. & Nubé, M.J. (2005) Reverse epidemiology: paradoxical observations in haemodialysis patients. Neth J Med, 63,376-81

[79] Okubo, K., Ikewaki, K., Sakai, S., Tada, N., Kawaguchi, Y. & Mochizuki, S. (2004) Abnormal HDL apolipoprotein A-I and A-II kinetics in hemodialysis patients: a stable isotope study. J Am Soc Nephrol, 15,1008-15

[80] Olyaei, A., Greer, E., Delos Santos, R. & Rueda, J. (2011) The efficacy and safety of the 3-hydroxy-3-methylglutaryl-CoA reductase inhibitors in chronic kidney disease, dialysis, and transplant patients. Clin J Am Soc Nephrol, 6,664-78

[81] Ottosson, P., Attman, P.O., Knight, C., Samuelsson, O., Weiss, L. & Alaupovic, P. (2001) Do high-flux dialysis membranes affect renal dyslipidemia? ASAIO J, 47,229-34

[82] Pahl, M.V., Ni, Z., Sepassi, L., Moradi, H. & Vaziri, N.D. (2009) Plasma phospholipid transfer protein, cholesteryl ester transfer protein and lecithin:cholesterol acyltransferase in end-stage renal disease (ESRD). Nephrol Dial Transplant, 24, 2541-6

[83] Pawlak, K., Mysliwiec, M. & Pawlak, D. (2012) Oxidized LDL to autoantibodies against oxLDL ratio - The new biomarker associated with carotid atherosclerosis and cardiovascular complications in dialyzed patients. Atherosclerosis, Jul 16

[84] Quaschning, T., Krane, V., Metzger, T. & Wanner, C. (2001) Abnormalities in uremic lipoprotein metabolism and its impact on cardiovascular disease. Am J Kidney Dis, 38, 14-9

[85] Qunibi, W.Y. (2005) Dyslipidemia and progression of cardiovascular calcification (CVC) in patients with end-stage renal disease (ESRD). Kidney Int Suppl, 95, 43-50

[86] Rader, D.J. & Brewer, H.B. Jr. (1992) Lipoprotein(a). Clinical approach to a unique atherogenic lipoprotein. JAMA, 267, 1109-12

[87] Reiche, I., Westphal, S., Martens-Lobenhoffer, J., Tröger, U., Luley, C. & Bode-Böger, S.M. (2011) Pharmacokinetics and dose recommendations of Niaspan® in chronic kidney disease and dialysis patients. Nephrol Dial Transplant, 26, 276-82

[88] Restrepo Valencia, C.A. & Cruz, J. (2008) [Safety and effectiveness of nicotinic acid in the management of patients with chronic renal disease and hyperlipidemia associated to hyperphosphatemia]. Nefrologia, 28, 61-6

[89] Ridker, P.M., Cushman, M., Stampfer, M.J., Tracy, R.P. & Hennekens, C.H. (1997) Inflammation, aspirin, and the risk of cardiovascular disease in apparently healthy men. N Engl J Med, 336, 973-9

[90] Rutsch, F., Nitschke, Y., Terkeltaub, R. (2011) Genetics in arterial calcification: pieces of a puzzle and cogs in a wheel. Circ Res, 109, 5, 578-92

[91] Shanahan, C.M., Cary, N.R., Salisbury, J.R., Proudfoot, D., Weissberg, P.L., Edmonds, M.E. (1999) Medial localization of mineralization-regulating proteins in association with Mönckeberg's sclerosis: evidence for smooth muscle cell-mediated vascular calcification. Circulation, 100, 21, 2168-76

[92] Saltissi, D., Morgan, C., Rigby, R.J. & Westhuyzen, J. (2002) Safety and efficacy of simvastatin in hypercholesterolemic patients undergoing chronic renal dialysis. Am J Kidney Dis, 39, 283-90

[93] Samouilidou, E.C., Karpouza, A.P., Kostopoulos, V., Bakirtzi, T., Pantelias, K., Petras, D., Tzanatou-Exarchou, H.J. & Grapsa, E. (2012) Lipid abnormalities and oxidized LDL in chronic kidney disease patients on hemodialysis and peritoneal dialysis. Ren Fail, 34, 160-4

[94] Sarnak, M.J. & Levey, A.S. (2000) Cardiovascular disease and chronic renal disease: a new paradigm. Am J Kidney Dis, 35, 117-31

[95] Sarnak, M.J., Levey, A.S., Schoolwerth, A.C., Coresh, J., Culleton, B., Hamm, L.L., McCullough, P.A., Kasiske, B.L., Kelepouris, E., Klag, M.J., Parfrey, P., Pfeffer, M., Raij, L., Spinosa, D.J. & Wilson, P.W.; American Heart Association Councils on Kidney in Cardiovascular Disease, High Blood Pressure Research, Clinical Cardiology, and Epidemiology and Prevention. (2003) Kidney disease as a risk factor for development of cardiovascular disease: a statement from the American Heart Association Councils on Kidney in Cardiovascular Disease, High Blood Pressure Research, Clinical Cardiology, and Epidemiology and Prevention. Hypertension, 42, 1050-65

[96] Schiffl, H. & Lang, S.M. (2010) Effects of dialysis purity on uremic dyslipidemia. Ther Apher Dial, 14, 5-11

[97]   Schaefer, E.J., Lamon-Fava, S., Jenner, J.L., McNamara, J.R., Ordovas, J.M., Davis, C.E., Abolafia, J.M., Lippel, K. & Levy, R.I. (1994) Lipoprotein(a) levels and risk of coronary heart disease in men. The lipid Research Clinics Coronary Primary Prevention Trial. JAMA, 271,999-1003

[98]   Schrader, J., Andersson, L.O., Armstrong, V.W., Kundt, M., Stibbe, W. & Scheler, F. (1990) Lipolytic effects of heparin and low molecular weight heparin and their importance in hemodialysis. Semin Thromb Hemost, 16 ,41-5

[99]   Sevinc Ok, E., Kircelli, F., Asci, G., Altunel, E., Ertilav, M., Sipahi, S., Bozkurt, D., Duman, S., Ozkahya, M., Toz, H. & Ok, E. (2012) Neither oxidized nor anti-oxidized low-density lipoprotein level is associated with atherosclerosis or mortality in hemodialysis patients. Hemodial Int, Apr 13. doi: 10.1111/j.1542-4758.2012.00683.x.

[100] Shoji, T., Nishizawa, Y., Nishitani, H., Yamakawa, M. & Morii, H. (1992) Impaired metabolism of high density lipoprotein in uremic patients. Kidney Int, 41, 1653-61

[101] Shoji, T., Masakane, I., Watanabe, Y., Iseki, K. & Tsubakihara, Y. ; Committee of Renal Data Registry, Japanese Society for Dialysis Therapy. (2011) Elevated non-high-density lipoprotein cholesterol (non-HDL-C) predicts atherosclerotic cardiovascular events in hemodialysis patients. Clin J Am Soc Nephrol, 6, 1112-20

[102] Shoji, T., Nishizawa, Y., Nishitani, H., Yamakawa, M. & Morii, H. (1992) Impaired metabolism of high density lipoprotein in uremic patients. Kidney Int, 41,1653-61

[103] Shahbazian, H., Zafar Mohtashami, A., Ghorbani, A., Abbaspour, M.R., Belladi Musavi, S.S., Hayati, F. & Lashkarara, G.R. (2011) Oral nicotinamide reduces serum phosphorus, increases HDL, and induces thrombocytopenia in hemodialysis patients: a double-blind randomized clinical trial. Nefrologia, 31, 58-65

[104] Shantouf, R., Kovesdy, C.P., Kim, Y., Ahmadi, N., Luna, A., Luna, C., Rambod, M., Nissenson, A.R., Budoff, M.J., Kalantar-Zadeh, K. (2009) Association of serum alkaline phosphatase with coronary artery calcification in maintenance hemodialysis patients. Clin J Am Soc Nephrol, 4,6,1106

[105] Sigrist, M.K., Taal, M.W., Bungay, P., McIntyre, C.W. (2007) Progressive vascular calcification over 2 years is associated with arterial stiffening and increased mortality in patients with stages 4 and 5 chronic kidney disease. Clin J Am Soc Nephrol, 2, 6, 1241-8

[106] Silva, L.S., Oliveira, R.A., Silva, G.B., Lima, J.W., Silva, R.P., Liborio, A.B., Daher, E.F. & Sobrinho, C.R. (2012) Cardiovascular disease in patients with end-stage renal disease on hemodialysis in a developing country. Saudi J Kidney Dis Transpl, 23, 262-6

[107] Sirrs, S., Duncan, L., Djurdjev, O., Nussbaumer, G., Ganz, G., Frohlich, J. & Levin, A. (1999) Homocyst(e)ine and vascular access complications in haemodialysis patients: insights into a complex metabolic relationship. Nephrol Dial Transplant, 14, 738-43

[108] Slatopolsky, E., Martin, K. & Hruska, K. (1980) Parathyroid hormone metabolism and its potential as a uremic toxin. Am J Physiol, 239, 1, 1

[109] Soliemani, A., Nikoueinejad, H., Tabatabaizade, M., Mianehsaz, E. & Tamadon, M. (2011) Effect of hydroxymethylglutaryl-CoA reductase inhibitors on low-density lipoprotein cholesterol, interleukin-6, and high-sensitivity C-reactive protein in end-stage renal disease. Iran J Kidney Dis, 5, 29-33

[110] Stenvinkel, P., Heimbürger, O., Paultre, F., Diczfalusy, U., Wang, T., Berglund, L. & Jogestrand, T. (1999) Strong association between malnutrition, inflammation, and atherosclerosis in chronic renal failure. Kidney Int, 55,1899-911

[111] Stack, A.G. & Bloembergen, W.E. (2001) Prevalence and clinical correlates of coronary artery disease among new dialysis patients in the United States: a cross-sectional study. J Am Soc Nephrol, 12, 1516-23

[112] Suki, W.N., Zabaneh, R., Cangiano, J.L., Reed, J., Fischer, D., Garrett, L., Ling, B.N., Chasan-Taber, S., Dillon, M.A., Blair, A.T. & Burke, S.K. (2007) Effects of sevelamer and calcium-based phosphate binders on mortality in hemodialysis patients. Kidney Int, 72,1130-7

[113] Tamashiro, M., Iseki, K., Sunagawa, O., Inoue, T., Higa, S., Afuso, H., Fukiyama, K. (2001) Significant association between the progression of coronary artery calcification and dyslipidemia in patients on chronic hemodialysis. Am J Kidney Dis, 38, 1, 64

[114] Ting, R.D., Keech, A.C., Drury, P.L., Donoghoe, M.W., Hedley, J., Jenkins, A.J., Davis, T.M., Lehto, S., Celermajer, D., Simes, R.J., Rajamani, K. & Stanton, K.; FIELD Study Investigators.(2012) Benefits and safety of long-term fenofibrate therapy in people with type 2 diabetes and renal impairment: the FIELD Study. Diabetes Care, 35, 218-25

[115] Tsimihodimos, V., Mitrogianni, Z. & Elisaf, M. (2011) Dyslipidemia associated with chronic kidney disease. Open Cardiovasc Med J, 5, 41-8

[116] Tsimihodimos, V., Dounousi, E. & Siamopoulos, K.C. (2008) Dyslipidemia in chronic kidney disease: an approach to pathogenesis and treatment. Am J Nephrol, 28,958-73

[117] Tukaj, C., Kubasik-Juraniec, J., & Kraszpulski, M. (2000) Morphological changes of aortal smooth muscle cells exposed to calcitriol in culture. Med Sci Monit, 6, 4, 668

[118] Wanner, C., Bahner, U., Mattern, R., Lang, D. & Passlick-Deetjen, J. (2004) Effect of dialysis flux and membrane material on dyslipidaemia and inflammation in haemodialysis patients. Nephrol Dial Transplant, 19, 2570-5

[119] Wanner, C., Krane, V., März, W., Olschewski, M., Mann, J.F., Ruf, G. & Ritz, E. ; German Diabetes and Dialysis Study Investigators. (2005) Atorvastatin in patients with type 2 diabetes mellitus undergoing hemodialysis. N Engl J Med, 353,238-48

[120] Wiemer, J., Winkler, K., Baumstark, M., März, W. & Scherberich, J.E. (2002) Influence of low molecular weight heparin compared to conventional heparin for anticoagulation during haemodialysis on low density lipoprotein subclasses. Nephrol Dial Transplant, 17, 2231-8

[121] van den Akker, J.M., Bredie, S.J., Diepenveen, S.H., van Tits, L.J., Stalenhoef, A.F. & van Leusen, R. (2003) Atorvastatin and simvastatin in patients on hemodialysis: effects on lipoproteins, C-reactive protein and in vivo oxidized LDL. J Nephrol,16, 238-44

[122] Vaughan, C.J., Gotto, A.M. Jr. & Basson, C.T. (2000) The evolving role of statins in the management of atherosclerosis. J Am Coll Cardiol, 35, 1-10

[123] Vaziri, N.D. & Moradi, H. (2006) Mechanisms of dyslipidemia of chronic renal failure. Hemodial Int, 10:1-7

[124] Vaziri, N.D. (2006) Dyslipidemia of chronic renal failure: the nature, mechanisms, and potential consequences. Am J Physiol Renal Physiol, 290, 262-72

[125] Vaziri, N.D., Wang, X.Q. & Liang, K. (1997) Secondary hyperparathyroidism down-regulates lipoprotein lipase expression in chronic renal failure. Am J Physiol, 273,925-30

[126] Vaziri, N.D. & Liang, K. (1997) Down-regulation of VLDL receptor expression in chronic experimental renal failure. Kidney Int, 51, 913-9

[127] Yamada, K., Fujimoto, S., Tokura, T., Fukudome, K., Ochiai, H., Komatsu, H., Sato, Y., Hara, S. & Eto, T. (2005) Effect of sevelamer on dyslipidemia and chronic inflammation in maintenance hemodialysis patients. Ren Fail, 27, 361-5

[128] Yang, C., Wu, T & Huang, C. (1998) Low molecular weight heparin reduces triglyceride, VLDL and cholesterol/HDL levels in hyperlipidemic diabetic patients on hemodialysis. Am J Nephrol, 18,384-90

[129] Zager, P.G., Nikolic, J., Brown, R.H., Campbell, M.A., Hunt, W.C., Peterson, D., Van Stone, J., Levey, A., Meyer, K.B., Klag, M.J., Johnson, H.K., Clark, E., Sadler, J.H. & Teredesai, P. (1998) "U" curve association of blood pressure and mortality in hemodialysis patients. Medical Directors of Dialysis Clinic, Inc. Kidney Int, 54, 561-9

[130] Zimmermann, J., Herrlinger, S., Pruy, A., Metzger, T. & Wanner, C. (1999) Inflammation enhances cardiovascular risk and mortality in hemodialysis patients. Kidney Int, 55, 648-58

Chapter 6

Pathogenesis and Treatment of Chronic Kidney Disease-Mineral and Bone Disorder

Yasuo Imanishi, Yoshiki Nishizawa and
Masaaki Inaba

Additional information is available at the end of the chapter

1. Introduction

The prevalence of chronic kidney disease (CKD) is increasing, and CKD patients are at risk for severe adverse outcomes such as progressive loss of kidney function, cardiovascular (CV) disease, and premature death [1]. CKD-Mineral and Bone Disorder (CKD-MBD) is the clinical syndrome that develops as a systemic disorder of bone and mineral metabolism due to CKD, which is manifested by abnormalities in bone and mineral metabolism [1]. Alterations in calcium and phosphate metabolism that are frequently observed in secondary hyperparathyroidism of uremia (SHPT), particularly in patients with maintenance hemodialysis, contribute to ectopic calcification, CV disease, and the risk of death [2].

SHPT is associated with various bone diseases including osteitis fibrosa caused by excessive secretion of parathyroid hormone (PTH), osteomalacia, adynamic bone disease, and combinations thereof; these diseases are collectively called renal osteodystrophy (ROD). In addition, ectopic calcifications such as soft-tissue and vascular calcifications are observed in patients with long-standing CKD. These patients are characterized by calcification of the vascular media, which is called Mönckeberg medial calcific sclerosis, and vascular intima, which is typically triggered by abnormal calcium and phosphorous metabolism due to SHPT [3]. Calcification of the vascular media is a particularly important factor for predicting CV mortality in dialysis patients. Elevation of the serum calcium × phosphate product also increases the relative mortality risk. The abovementioned facts suggest that the pathology of CKD-MBD should be fully elucidated to prepare an appropriate treatment plan.

2. Calcium and phosphate homeostasis

Small changes in extracellular fluid calcium concentration have major effects on muscle contraction and neuronal excitability, as well as numerous cellular functions such as cell division, cell adhesion, plasma membrane integrity, and coagulation. However, the changes in serum phosphate concentration are asymptomatic in normally functioning kidneys. Severe chronic depletion may cause anorexia, muscle weakness, and osteomalacia. Hyperphosphatemia is also asymptomatic, although symptoms of hypocalcemia, including tetany, can occur when concomitant hypocalcemia is present.

Parathyroid hormone (PTH), the active form of vitamin D (1,25-dihydroxyvitamin D; 1,25-$(OH)_2D$), and fibroblast growth factor (FGF)-23, are the principal physiologic regulators of calcium and phosphate homeostasis in humans [4,5] (Figure 1). Feedback loops exist between ionized calcium (Ca^{2+}), phosphate, 1,25-$(OH)_2D$, FGF-23, and PTH.

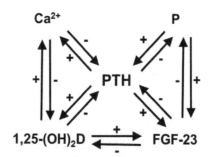

Figure 1. Feedback loops in calcium ion (Ca^{2+}) and phosphate (P) homeostasis [4,5], modified from a previous report [8]. Feedback loops exist between Ca^{2+}, P, 1,25-dihydroxyvitamin D (1,25-$(OH)_2D$), fibroblast growth factor 23 (FGF-23), and parathyroid hormone (PTH). Ca^{2+}, 1,25-$(OH)_2D$, and FGF-23 suppress PTH secretion, whereas P overload accelerates it. P overload does not always cause the elevation of serum phosphate, with the exception of some conditions such as chronic kidney disease.

2.1. Parathyroid Hormone (PTH)

The extracellular fluid Ca^{2+} concentration is the primary regulator of the rapid (in minutes) synthesis and secretion of PTH. An inverse relationship was observed between the extracellular fluid Ca^{2+} concentration and PTH secretion from parathyroid cells *in vitro* [6] (Figure 2). Hypersecretion of PTH causes hypophosphatemia due to hyperphosphaturia in normally functioning kidneys; however, it leads to hyperphosphatemia by mobilization of phosphate from skeletal tissues in CKD, particularly in hemodialysis patients.

2.2. 1,25-dihydroxyvitamin D (1,25-(OH)$_2$D)

In contrast to the rapid action of PTH, 1,25-(OH)$_2$D contributes to long-term calcium homeostasis. 1,25-(OH)$_2$D also elevates serum phosphate concentration by promoting incremental intestinal phosphate absorption.

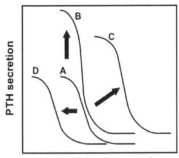

Serum calcium concentration

Figure 2. Pathogenesis of secondary hyperparathyroidism of uremia (SHPT) [56], modified from a previous report [26]. The analyses of PTH secretions inhibited by extracellular calcium in vitro revealed the sigmoidal relationship of the PTH–calcium relationship. Setpoint, the calcium concentration causing half-maximal inhibition of PTH secretion, is an indicator of sensitivity of parathyroid cells to extracellular calcium by CaR. (A) The relationship in healthy subjects was fitted to a symmetrical sigmoidal curve. (B) The normal sigmoidal curve will shift upward when the secretory cell number is increased, without changing its setpoint. (C) An altered sigmoidal curve is observed in human parathyroid adenomas, refractory SHPT, by changing the setpoint to the right. In the case of severe setpoint shift, PTH secretion is persistent even at high calcium concentration: so-called 'autonomous' PTH secretion. An altered PTH–calcium relationship was also observed in PTH-cyclin D1 transgenic mice [4, 52]. (D) Administration of cinacalcet or activating mutation of CaR observed in autosomal dominant hypocalcemia increases the CaR sensitivity to serum calcium. Activations of CaR result in the PTH–calcium relationship curve moving to the left.

2.3. Fibroblast Growth Factor 23 (FGF-23)

FGF-23, a member of the FGF family, is a major phosphaturic factor in the development of hypophosphatemic rickets/osteomalacia, including X-linked hypophosphatemic rickets (XLH) and oncogenic osteomalacia [7]. FGF-23 suppresses both PTH secretion and its expression in parathyroid cells [8]. PTH also stimulated FGF-23 expression and its secretion in bone [9], suggesting that a negative feedback loop exists between PTH and FGF-23 [4,5] (Figure 1).

3. Receptors in parathyroid cells

The 3 parathyroid cell receptors that are important in calcium and phosphate homeostasis include the calcium-sensing receptor (CaR) and the FGF receptor (FGFR)-Klotho complex located on the cell surface and nuclear vitamin D receptor (VDR) (Table 1). CaR and VDR are target molecules for the treatment of hyperfunctioning parathyroid diseases in CKD patients.

Receptor	Location
1. Vitamin D receptor; VDR	cell nucleus
2. Calcium-sensing receptor; CaR	cell membrane
3. FGFR-Klotho complex	cell membrane

Table 1. Receptors in parathyroid cells

3.1. Calcium-Sensing Receptor (CaR)

CaR contains a characteristic G protein-coupled receptor 7 membrane-spanning motif with an unusually large N-terminal extracellular domain, which was cloned in 1993 [10]. Positional cloning approaches have clarified that loss-of-function mutations in the *CaR* gene cause familial hypocalciuric hypercalcemia (heterozygous mutations) and neonatal severe hyperparathyroidism (homozygous mutations) [11].

Heterozygous *CaR* knockout mice exhibited a phenotype that was similar to that of familial hypocalciuric hypercalcemia [12]. Serum PTH levels were inappropriately elevated; however, the parathyroid glands were not enlarged in the heterozygous knockout mice. Homozygous knockout mice demonstrated markedly elevated serum calcium and PTH concentrations, retarded growth, and premature death [12]. These symptoms are similar to those of human neonatal severe hyperparathyroidism.

Synthetic allosteric modulators of CaR have been developed that act as either positive modulators (calcimimetics) or negative modulators (calcilytics). These ligands do not activate the wild-type receptor directly, but rather shift the PTH-calcium sigmoidal curves to the left or right, respectively (Figure 2).

3.2. Vitamin D Receptor (VDR)

$1,25-(OH)_2D$ is the major steroid hormone that plays a crucial role in calcium and phosphate homeostasis, and its actions are mediated by VDR. Hereditary hypocalcemic vitamin D-resistant rickets (HVDDR) is an autosomal recessive disorder that is caused by inactivating mutations in the *VDR* gene, resulting in target tissue insensitivity to $1,25-(OH)_2D$ [13].

VDR knockout mice exhibit hypocalcemia, hypophosphatemia, rickets, alopecia, and hyperparathyroidism with enlarged parathyroid glands, similar to HVDDR [14,15]. Tissue-specific ablation of *VDR* in parathyroid tissue results in decreased parathyroid CaR expression and moderately increased basal PTH levels; however, no significant abnormalities in PTH-calcium sigmoidal curves were observed [16], suggesting limited roles of *VDR* in parathyroid pathophysiology.

3.3. FGF Receptor (FGFR)-Klotho complex

Klotho, which is expressed in kidney and pituitary and parathyroid glands, converts FGFR1, a canonical receptor for various FGFs, into an FGF-23-specific receptor [17]. *FGF-23* null mice exhibit various senescence-like phenotypes such as a short lifespan, infertility, atrophy of the lymphopoietic and reproductive organs, decreased bone mineral density, and ectopic calcification. This phenotype is similar to that of Klotho-deficient mice [18], suggesting that FGF-23 signaling is Klotho dependent.

4. Chronic Kidney Disease – Mineral and Bone Disorder (CKD-MBD)

It is widely known that the progression of CKD increases mortality risk and the incidence of CV events [19]. Hyperphosphatemia is a critical electrolyte abnormality in patients with CKD-mineral and bone disorder (CKD-MBD) [20]. Even though hemodialysis or peritoneal dialysis is given to hyperphosphatemia patients with advanced CKD, these therapies are ineffective due to insufficient phosphorus-removal ability.

4.1. Calcium and phosphate metabolism in CKD-MBD

FGF-23 is involved in abnormal calcium and phosphate metabolism in CKD patients as the disease progresses. A cross-sectional study of 80 CKD patients revealed decreases in estimated GFR (eGFR), serum calcium, and $1,25\text{-}(OH)_2D$ levels as well as increases in serum P, fractional excretion of phosphate, PTH, and FGF-23 [21].

Further study of the abovementioned data revealed an increase in serum FGF-23 level (eGFR 45~60 mL/min), which is an independent predictor of the fractional excretion of phosphate, far earlier than the increase in serum phosphate levels (eGFR <30 mL/min). The increase in FGF-23 level is one of the greatest independent predictors of decreased $1,25\text{-}(OH)_2D$ level, independent of serum phosphate and eGFR. This suggests that the increase in FGF-23 level is the main reason for the decrease in $1,25\text{-}(OH)_2D$ level in CKD progression. Thus, the increase in FGF-23 level compensates for the increase in the serum phosphate levels caused by the decrease in nephrons associated with CKD progression by increasing the fractional excretion of phosphate. However, the increase in FGF-23 level also decreases the level of $1,25\text{-}(OH)_2D$, which promotes PTH secretion and accelerates the progression of SHPT.

4.2. Vascular calcification in CKD-MBD

In an experiment using human vascular smooth muscle cells, inorganic phosphate transport into the cells via type III Na-Pi co-transporter (Pit-1) increased as the extracellular phosphate concentration increased. The increase in the intracellular phosphate concentration induced the expression of marker genes of apoptosis and osteogenic/chondrogenic cells in the vascular wall cells, which resulted in calcification [22]. This finding also implies a relationship between blood vessel calcification and phosphate levels *in vitro*.

Maintenance hemodialysis patients often develop blood vessel calcification, which is directly proportional to the duration of dialysis, irrespective of their age; this condition is characterized by calcification of the vascular media called Mönckeberg sclerosis rather than calcification of the vascular intima. The onset of blood vessel calcification in dialysis patients is mainly caused by abnormal calcium and phosphate metabolism due to SHPT [3], which is one of the signs of CKD-MBD. Calcification of the iliac artery [23] and abdominal aorta [24] are critical predictors of CV mortality in dialysis patients.

4.3. Renal Osteodystrophy (ROD)

ROD is a mineral and bone disorder that occurs as a complication of CKD, which exacerbates bone fragility and fracture [1]. The serum phosphorus concentration was significantly related to hospitalization for fracture [2]. Old age, dialysis vintage, female gender, white race, and lower body weight were significantly associated with an increased risk of fracture-related hospitalization.

In CKD patients, ROD manifests as alterations in bone morphology, such as osteitis fibrosa cystica, mild hyperparathyroid-related bone disease, osteomalacia, adynamic bone disease, and mixed uremic osteodystrophy. ROD represents histopathologic changes observed in bone and is typically characterized by changes in bone turnover, volume, and mineralization (TMV) (Table 2). The TMV classification, assessed by histomorphometry, provides a clinically relevant description of the underlying bone pathology and helps define the pathophysiology of the disease.

Turnover	Mineralization	Volume
Low	Normal	Low
Normal	Abnormal	Normal
High		High

TMV: bone turnover, mineralization, and volume

Table 2. TMV classification for renal osteodystrophy (ROD) [1]

5. Pathogenesis of Secondary Hyperparathyroidism of uremia (SHPT)

PTH secretion increases when the glomerular filtration rate (GFR) of CKD patients decreases to 40–50 mL/min or less [25]. Renal impairment decreases urinary phosphate excretion, gradually leading to hyperphosphatemia. Phosphate accumulation in the body reduces 1α hydroxylase activity in the kidneys and suppresses vitamin D activation, which results in decreased serum active vitamin D ($1,25\text{-}(OH)_2D$) levels [26] (Figure 3). Hyperphosphatemia causes hypocalcemia by directly affecting the parathyroid glands; moreover, impaired vitamin D activation promotes PTH synthesis and secretion [27], which induces the proliferation of parathyroid cells and parathyroid hyperplasia. This change stimulates excessive PTH activity and allows phosphates of the bone to move into the blood, exacerbating the hyperphosphatemia. Even though hemodialysis or peritoneal dialysis is given to hyperphosphatemia patients with advanced CKD, these therapies are ineffective due to the patients' insufficient phosphate-removal ability.

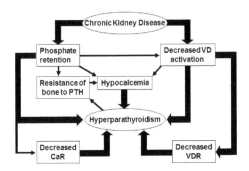

Figure 3. Pathogenesis of parathyroid tumorigenesis [4]. (A) A set of somatic mutations (hits) confers a growth advantage to an affected cell. Monoclonal growth renders the cells susceptible to more somatic mutations (hits), which leads to clonal evolution. (B) A uremic status such as chronic hypocalcemia, decreased levels of serum 1,25-(OH)₂D, and hyperphosphatemia stimulates parathyroid cell growth and leads to multi-glandular polyclonal hyperplasia. These hyperplastic parathyroid cells are susceptible to somatic mutations (hits), resulting in monoclonal growth.

In the earliest stages of CKD, the parathyroid glands undergo multi-glandular generalized hyperplasia, presumably a true polyclonal expansion, in response to stimuli that may include chronic hypocalcemia, decreased levels of serum 1,25-(OH)₂D, and hyperphosphatemia. However, in the late stage of this disease, usually after many years of dialysis treatment, a subset of patients develop refractory SHPT in which excessive PTH secretion no longer responds to physiological influences or standard medical therapy. Therefore, medically refractory SHPT is quite different from the readily managed SHPT, which is characterized by an abnormal PTH-calcium secretory relationship [28,29], is "autonomous," and is typically treated by surgical parathyroidectomy. VDR [30] and CaR [31] expression was reduced in the parathyroid tumors of these patients.

The majority of surgically removed uremic parathyroid glands were confirmed to be monoclonal neoplasms by X-chromosome inactivation analysis [32]. This monoclonality implies that somatic mutation of certain genes controlling cell proliferation occurred in a single parathyroid cell, conferring a selective growth advantage upon it and its progeny (Figure 4). Distinct chromosomal abnormalities in sporadic parathyroid adenomas [33] and uremia-associated parathyroid tumors [34] revealed that the molecular pathogenesis of tumorigenesis in these 2 categories of parathyroid tumors was different. However, the major genes involved in the pathogenesis of SHPT remain unknown.

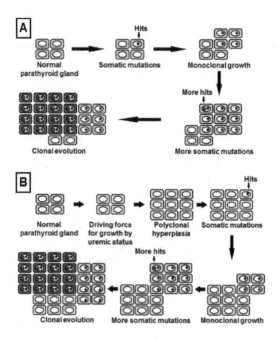

Figure 4. The sigmoidal curve of the PTH-calcium relationship [56]. The analyses of PTH secretions inhibited by extracellular calcium *in vitro* revealed a sigmoidal PTH-calcium relationship [6]. The setpoint, the calcium concentration causing half-maximal inhibition of PTH secretion, is an indicator of sensitivity of parathyroid cells to extracellular calcium by the calcium receptor (CaR). (A) This relationship in healthy subjects was fitted to a symmetrical sigmoidal curve. (B) The normal sigmoidal curve will shift upward when secretory cell number is increased without changing its setpoint. (C) An altered sigmoidal curve is observed in human parathyroid adenomas, refractory secondary hyperparathyroidism of uremia, with the setpoint shifting to the right. In the case of severe setpoint shift, PTH secretion is persistent even at high calcium concentrations, due to so-called "autonomous" PTH secretion. An altered PTH-calcium relationship was also observed in PHPT model mice [4,52]. (D) Administration of calcimimetics or the presence of an activating mutation of CaR in autosomal dominant hypocalcemia (ADH) patients [57] increased the sensitivity of CaR to serum calcium concentration in parathyroid cells. Activations of CaR result in a shift of the PTH-calcium relationship curve to the left.

Reduced expression of Klotho and FGFR1 was noted in the hyperplastic parathyroid glands of SHPT patients [35], suggesting that reduced FGF-23 signaling in parathyroid cells plays a role in the development of SHPT. However, some studies of Klotho expression in uremic animals reported conflicting results [36-38]. Further studies are necessary to clarify the role of FGFR-Klotho signaling in uremic parathyroid glands.

6. Guidelines for CKD-MBD

The National Kidney Foundation Kidney Disease Outcomes Quality Initiative (K/DOQI, USA) published the "K/DOQI clinical practice guidelines for bone metabolism and disease in chronic kidney disease" in 2003 as evidence-based clinical practice guidelines [39]. In

2005, according to "Definition and classification of chronic kidney disease: a position statement from Kidney Disease: Improving Global Outcomes (KDIGO)," the term CKD-MBD was proposed, stating that the importance of bone and mineral metabolism in CKD should be conceptualized in terms of prognosis [20]; this means that bone and mineral metabolism in CKD can be considered a systemic disease. In 2009, KDIGO proposed the current clinical practice guidelines [40], which have been adopted in clinical settings.

7. Treatment of CKD-MBD

The risk of all-cause mortality and CV events in patients with CKD-MBD on maintenance hemodialysis is well established. A greater mortality risk associated with phosphate, followed by calcium and PTH levels, was reported [41]. These 3 parameters are not only the best surrogate markers but also the best targets for CKD-MBD treatment.

7.1. Phosphate-binding agents

All-cause mortality increased regardless of whether serum phosphate levels were higher or lower than the reference value, exhibiting a U-shaped distribution [42]. However, maintenance dialysis patients in stable condition are likely to develop hyperphosphatemia, indicating that hyperphosphatemia treatment should be a primary target. Diet therapy is the first-line therapy that can sufficiently control serum phosphate levels. If it is insufficient, phosphate binders are administered orally. Calcium-containing phosphate binder (e.g., calcium carbonate) have been used for a long time. However, concomitant use of active vitamin D products can lead to the development of hypercalcemia and increase serum calcium × phosphate product levels. Therefore, non-calcium-containing phosphate binder such as sevelamer hydrochloride and lanthanum carbonate are widely used.

Although hyperphosphatemia is a risk factor for mortality in dialysis patients, the effects of restricting phosphorus intake in these patients are unclear. When oral phosphorus intake is controlled, serum phosphate levels decrease, but poor nutritional status occurs as well. Thus, it is difficult to judge the true effect of the restriction of phosphorus intake, although studies using phosphate binders have been performed.

The Accelerated Mortality on Renal Replacement (ArMORR) study is a 1-year observational cohort study of 10,044 hemodialysis patients in 1,056 medical institutions in the US. According to this study, the 1-year survival rate of 3,555 patients prescribed phosphate binders before or within 90 days of initiating dialysis was higher than that of 5,055 patients who were not treated with these agents during the same period [43]. That study also compared survival in a subcohort of patients treated and not treated with phosphate binders matched by their baseline serum phosphate levels (i.e., a propensity score matched cohort study) and concluded that the survival rate was greater in the treated group, demonstrating the positive effect of these agents on the survival rate (Figure 5).

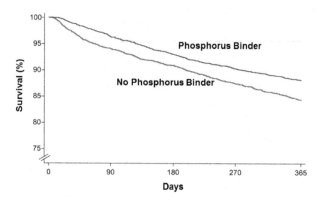

Figure 5. Survival of treated and untreated patients of the overall propensity score-matched cohort in the Accelerated Mortality on Renal Replacement (ArMORR) study [43]. A 1-year observational cohort study involving 10,044 dialysis patients in 1,056 medical institutions in the US studied the relationship between the effect of phosphate binders before and within 90 days of initiating dialysis and 1-year survival rate. The survival rate was greater in the group treated with phosphate binders. The subcohort study of patients treated and untreated with phosphate binders, matched by their baseline serum phosphate levels (i.e., the propensity score matched cohort), also demonstrated that the treated group had a better survival rate, demonstrating the positive effect of these agents on survival.

Many studies on maintenance dialysis patients have been performed. What about studies on patients who have just started dialysis? The Choices for Healthy Outcomes in Caring for End-Stage Renal Disease (CHOICE) study is a prospective cohort study of patients who just started hemodialysis or peritoneal dialysis [44]. That study included 1,007 subjects, 98% of whom were enrolled in the study within 4 months. The study was started at a median of 45 days after the patients started dialysis. The results obtained 2.5 years later indicated that higher serum phosphate levels were an independent predictor of all-cause mortality. In addition, the relative risk of all-cause mortality was also high in subjects whose serum phosphate levels were high at the start of dialysis but decreased 6 months later. The abovementioned results suggest that the serum phosphate level at the start of dialysis is an important prognostic factor.

7.2. Vitamin D Receptor Activators (VDRAs)

Active vitamin D products inhibit PTH gene transcription and secretion as well as parathyroid cell proliferation in the parathyroid glands. Daily oral administration of 1α-(OH)D_3 (alfacalcidol), $1,25$-(OH)$_2$D$_3$ (calcitriol), and/or $26,27$-hexafluoro-$1,25$-(OH)$_2$D$_3$ (falecalcitriol) is performed to prevent the progression of SHPT. However, the effect of this treatment is insufficient, because the expression of vitamin D receptor (VDR) decreases in uremia-associated parathyroid tumor.

A rapid increase in serum $1,25$-(OH)$_2$D levels due to intravenous administration of calcitriol can partly inhibit the synthesis and secretion of PTH in parathyroid cells, which express less VDR. Furthermore, $1,25$-dihydroxy-22-oxavitamin D$_3$ (maxacalcitol, OCT), an analog in which the carbon of calcitriol at position 22 is replaced with an oxygen atom, is character-ized by a weaker intestinal calcium absorption capacity than that with the inhibition of PTH secretion. Therefore, it is unlikely to cause hypercalcemia.

Among the subjects in the ArMORR study who were not treated with active vitamin D ana-logs, 25OHD level, which exhibits individual nutritional vitamin D status, was elevated, while both all-cause mortality and CV mortality decreased (Figure 6). Furthermore, all-cause mortality and CV mortality decreased significantly in the subjects administered VDRA, re-gardless of 25OHD level, indicating that the prognosis of VDRA improved in the mainte-nance dialysis patients [45].

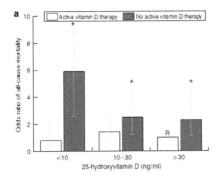 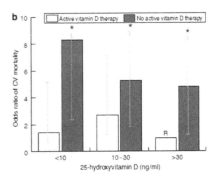

Figure 6. Multivariate-adjusted ORs of 90-day all-cause and cardiovascular (CV) mortality in the ArMORR study [45]. The ArMORR study involved 825 maintenance dialysis patients who were not treated with active vitamin D before or within 90 days of initiating dialysis to evaluate the effect of active vitamin D products on prognosis. 25OHD, which indicates the individual nutritional vitamin D status, was high in the subjects who were not treated with active vitamin D, while all-cause mortality and CV mortality decreased. Furthermore, all-cause mortality and CV mortality decreased significantly in the subjects administered with VDRA regardless of 25OHD levels.

7.3. Calcimimetics

Information on extracellular Ca^{2+} levels is transferred to parathyroid cells via CaR in the par-athyroid glands, which control PTH secretion. Multivalent cations including Ca^{2+}, Mg^{2+}, and Gd^{3+} act on CaR as agonists. However, calcimimetics do not act as agonists but allosterically increase the sensitivity of CaR to multivalent cations [46].

Calcimimetic cinacalcet suppressed PTH secretion in cultured human pathological parathy-roid cells obtained from primary hyperparathyroidism (PHPT) and SHPT patients, which exhibit reduced expression of CaR, the target molecule of cinacalcet [47]. These data support the clinical application of cinacalcet for PHPT and SHPT treatment.

Calcimimetic cinacalcet suppressed not only PTH secretion but also parathyroid cell prolif-eration, which prevented parathyroid hyperplasia *in vivo* in 5/6-nephrectomized rats, the an-imal model of SHPT [48]. Calcimimetic tecalcet also reversed the development of osteitis fibrosa in the SHPT rats [49]. In a relative hypocalcemic to normocalcemic environment, calcimimetics effectively suppress PTH secretion and parathyroid cell proliferation. Interestingly, cinacalcet suppressed aortic calcification in SHPT rats by decreasing serum PTH, calcium, and phosphate concentrations [50], suggesting that cinacalcet may be beneficial for the prevention of ectopic calcification as well as the improvement of morbidity and mortality in patients with CKD.

Cinacalcet also suppressed PTH secretion in *PTH-cyclin D1* transgenic mice [51]. *PTH-cyclin D1* transgenic mice are an animal model of PHPT that overexpress the *cyclin D1* oncogene in the parathyroid glands, which was accomplished by using a transgene that mimics the human *PTH-cyclin D1* gene rearrangement [52]. Tissue-specific overexpression of the *cyclin D1* oncogene not only resulted in abnormal parathyroid cell proliferation but, notably, also led to the development of biochemical hyperparathyroidism with characteristic bone abnormalities.

Hypercalcemia may stimulate considerable CaR activity, as the expression of CaR was suppressed in the parathyroid glands of these mice [52]. These conditions are compatible with the status observed in refractory SHPT patients undergoing maintenance hemodialysis. Although older transgenic mice exhibited advanced hyperparathyroidism caused by severely decreased CaR expression, cinacalcet suppressed both serum calcium and PTH concentrations [51] and parathyroid growth [53]. CaR is a potentially useful target for a therapeutic agent such as cinacalcet to suppress PTH secretion, despite the reduction in CaR expression observed in the parathyroid glands of patients with advanced PHPT and SHPT.

A meta-analysis of 8 randomized, double-blind, placebo-controlled trials (total number of subjects, 1,429) revealed that calcimimetics significantly decrease serum PTH, serum calcium, and serum phosphate levels, in turn significantly decreasing the serum calcium × phosphate product [54] (Figure 7). The improvements in the abovementioned serum parameters due to calcimimetics were clarified in the analysis. However, no improvement in all-cause mortality or decreased parathyroidectomy was observed, and the incidence of bone fracture was not studied.

An observational study was performed using the United States Renal Data System to determine all-cause and CV mortality. Time-dependent Cox proportional hazards modeling found that all-cause and CV mortality rates were significantly reduced in cinacalcet-treated patients relative to those that did not receive cinacalcet treatment. Although this study revealed a significant survival benefit associated with cinacalcet, randomized clinical trials are needed to confirm a survival advantage associated with calcimimetics [55].

7.4. Percutaneous Ethanol Injection Therapy (PEIT)

Percutaneous ethanol injection therapy (PEIT) is performed by directly injecting ethanol into a parathyroid tumor under ultrasound guidance to necrotize parathyroid tumor cells. Its merits include minimal invasiveness and multiple sessions. However, the technique sometimes induces recurrent laryngeal nerve paralysis, making it inapplicable in the presence of recurrent laryngeal nerve paralysis in the contralateral parathyroid gland.

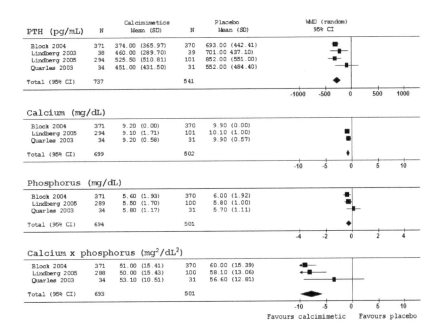

Figure 7. Positive effect of cinacalcet on serum parameters in the meta-analysis of 8 randomized, double-blind, placebo-controlled trials (total number of subjects, 1,429) [54] Cinacalcet significantly decreased serum PTH, calcium, and phosphate levels, thereby significantly decreasing the serum calcium × phosphate product; WMD: weighted mean difference, SD: standard deviation, CI: confidence interval

7.5. Parathyroidectomy (PTX)

PTX is recommended for the treatment of SHPT that is resistant to medical management. Isolation of the parathyroid glands always decreases serum PTH levels. However, there are often 5 or more parathyroid glands, and mediastinal or intrathyroid ectopic parathyroid tumors sometimes develop. Therefore, pre- and intraoperative detection of parathyroid glands is essential. The techniques for detecting them include subtotal extirpation, total extirpation, and total expiration followed by autotransplantation.

8. Conclusion

Clinical evidence regarding CKD-MBD is reported in the literature, and guidelines have been developed accordingly. Well-controlled serum phosphate, calcium and PTH levels improve the prognosis of dialysis patients. Many pharmaceuticals aiming to achieve this goal have been developed and launched. As the pathology of CKD-MBD is elucidated, the prognosis of dialysis patients and their quality of life will improve.

Author details

Yasuo Imanishi[1], Yoshiki Nishizawa[2] and Masaaki Inaba[1]

*Address all correspondence to: imanishi@med.osaka-cu.ac.jp

1 Department of Metabolism, Endocrinology and Molecular Medicine, Osaka City University Graduate School of Medicine, Osaka, Japan

2 Osaka City University, Osaka, Japan

References

[1] Moe S, Drueke T, Cunningham J, Goodman W, Martin K, Olgaard K, Ott S, Sprague S, Lameire N, Eknoyan G. Definition, evaluation, and classification of renal osteodystrophy: a position statement from Kidney Disease: Improving Global Outcomes (KDIGO). *Kidney Int* 2006;69: 1945-1953.

[2] Block GA, Klassen PS, Lazarus JM, Ofsthun N, Lowrie EG, Chertow GM. Mineral metabolism, mortality, and morbidity in maintenance hemodialysis. *J Am Soc Nephrol* 2004;15: 2208-2218.

[3] Goodman WG, Goldin J, Kuizon BD, Yoon C, Gales B, Sider D, Wang Y, Chung J, Emerick A, Greaser L, Elashoff R, Salusky IB. Coronary-artery calcification in young adults with end-stage renal disease who are undergoing dialysis. *N Engl J Med* 2000;342: 1478-1483.

[4] Imanishi Y, Inaba M, Kawata T, Nishizawa Y. Animal models of hyperfunctioning parathyroid diseases for drug development. *Expert Opin Drug Discov* 2009; 4: 727-740.

[5] Imanishi Y, Inaba M, Kawata T, Nishizawa Y. Cinacalcet in hyperfunctioning parathyroid diseases. *Ther Apher Dial* 2009;13 Suppl 1, S7-S11.

[6] Brown EM. Four-parameter model of the sigmoidal relationship between parathyroid hormone release and extracellular calcium concentration in normal and abnormal parathyroid tissue. *J Clin Endocrinol Metab* 1983;56: 572-581.

[7] Jonsson KB, Zahradnik R, Larsson T, White KE, Sugimoto T, Imanishi Y, Yamamoto T, Hampson G, Koshiyama H, Ljunggren O, Oba K, Yang IM, Miyauchi A, Econs MJ, Lavigne J, Juppner H. Fibroblast growth factor 23 in oncogenic osteomalacia and X-linked hypophosphatemia. *N Engl J Med* 2003; 348: 1656-1663.

[8] Ben-Dov IZ, Galitzer H, Lavi-Moshayoff V, Goetz R, Kuro-O M, Mohammadi M, Sirkis R, Naveh-Many T, Silver J. The parathyroid is a target organ for FGF23 in rats. *J Clin Invest* 1997;117: 4003-4008.

[9]   Kawata T, Imanishi Y, Kobayashi K, Miki T, Arnold A, Inaba M, Nishizawa, Parathyroid hormone regulates fibroblast growth factor-23 in a mouse model of primary hyperparathyroidism. *J Am Soc Nephrol* 2007;18: 2683-2688.

[10] Brown EM, Gamba G, Riccardi D, Lombardi M, Butters R, Kifor O, Sun A, Hediger MA, Lytton J, Hebert SC Cloning and characterization of an extracellular Ca^{2+}-sensing receptor from bovine parathyroid. *Nature* 1993;366: 575-580.

[11] Pollak MR, Brown EM, Chou YH, Hebert SC, Marx SJ, Steinmann B, Levi T, Seidman CE, Seidman JG. Mutations in the human Ca^{2+}-sensing receptor gene cause familial hypocalciuric hypercalcemia and neonatal severe hyperparathyroidism. *Cell* 1993;75: 1297-1303.

[12] Ho C, Conner DA, Pollak MR, Ladd DJ, Kifor O, Warren HB, Brown EM, Seidman JG, Seidman CE. A mouse model of human familial hypocalciuric hypercalcemia and neonatal severe hyperparathyroidism. *Nat Genet* 1995;11: 389-394.

[13] Haussler MR, Whitfield GK, Haussler CA, Hsieh JC, Thompson PD, Selznick SH, Dominguez CE, Jurutka PW. The nuclear vitamin D receptor: biological and molecular regulatory properties revealed. *J Bone Miner Res* 1998;13: 325-349.

[14] Li YC, Pirro AE, Amling M, Delling G, Baron R, Bronson R, Demay MB. Targeted ablation of the vitamin D receptor: an animal model of vitamin D-dependent rickets type II with alopecia. *Proc Natl Acad Sci USA* 1997;94: 9831-9835.

[15] Yoshizawa T, Handa Y, Uematsu Y, Takeda S, Sekine K, Yoshihara Y, Kawakami T, Arioka K, Sato H, Uchiyama Y, Masushige S, Fukamizu A, Matsumoto T, Kato S. Mice lacking the vitamin D receptor exhibit impaired bone formation, uterine hypoplasia and growth retardation after weaning. *Nat Genet* 1997;16: 391-396.

[16] Meir T, Levi R, Lieben L, Libutti S, Carmeliet G, Bouillon R, Silver J, Naveh-Many T. Deletion of the vitamin D receptor specifically in the parathyroid demonstrates a limited role for the receptor in parathyroid physiology. *Am J Physiol Renal Physiol* 2009;297: F1192-1198.

[17] Urakawa I, Yamazaki Y, Shimada T, Iijima K, Hasegawa H, Okawa K, Fujita T, Fukumoto S, Yamashita T. Klotho converts canonical FGF receptor into a specific receptor for FGF23. *Nature* 2006;444: 770-774.

[18] Shimada T, Kakitani M, Yamazaki Y, Hasegawa H, Takeuchi Y, Fujita T, Fukumoto S, Tomizuka K, Yamashita T. Targeted ablation of Fgf23 demonstrates an essential physiological role of FGF23 in phosphate and vitamin D metabolism. *J Clin Invest* 2004;113: 561-568.

[19] Go AS, Chertow GM, Fan D, Mcculloch CE, Hsu CY. Chronic kidney disease and the risks of death, cardiovascular events, and hospitalization. *N Engl J Med* 2004;351: 1296-1305.

[20] Levey AS, Eckardt KU, Tsukamoto Y, Levin A, Coresh J, Rossert J, De Zeeuw D, Hostetter TH, Lameire N, Eknoyan G. Definition and classification of chronic kidney dis-

ease: a position statement from Kidney Disease: Improving Global Outcomes (KDIGO). *Kidney Int* 2005;67: 2089-2100.

[21] Gutierrez O, Isakova T, Rhee E, Shah A, Holmes J, Collerone G, Juppner H, Wolf M. Fibroblast growth factor-23 mitigates hyperphosphatemia but accentuates calcitriol deficiency in chronic kidney disease. *J Am Soc Nephrol* 2005;16: 2205-2215.

[22] Jono S, Mckee MD, Murry CE, Shioi A, Nishizawa Y, Mori K, Morii H, Giachelli CM. Phosphate regulation of vascular smooth muscle cell calcification. *Circ Res* 2000;87: E10-17.

[23] London GM, Guerin AP, Marchais SJ, Metivier F, Pannier B, Adda H. Arterial media calcification in end-stage renal disease: impact on all-cause and cardiovascular mortality. *Nephrol Dial Transplant* 2003;18: 1731-1740.

[24] Okuno S, Ishimura E, Kitatani K, Fujino Y, Kohno K, Maeno Y, Maekawa K, Yamakawa T, Imanishi Y, Inaba M, Nishizawa Y. Presence of abdominal aortic calcification is significantly associated with all-cause and cardiovascular mortality in maintenance hemodialysis patients. *Am J Kidney Dis* 2007;49: 417-425.

[25] Bricker NS, Slatopolsky E, Reiss E, Avioli LV. Calcium, phosphorus, and bone in renal disease and transplantation. *Arch Intern Med* 1969;123: 543-553.

[26] Slatopolsky E, Brown A, Dusso A. Pathogenesis of secondary hyperparathyroidism. *Kidney Int* 1999; Suppl 73: S14-19.

[27] Russell J, Lettieri D, Sherwood LM. Direct regulation by calcium of cytoplasmic messenger ribonucleic acid coding for pre-proparathyroid hormone in isolated bovine parathyroid cells. *J Clin Invest* 1983;72: 1851-1855.

[28] Brown EM, Wilson RE, Eastman RC, Pallotta J, Marynick SP. Abnormal regulation of parathyroid hormone release by calcium in secondary hyperparathyroidism due to chronic renal failure. *J Clin Endocrinol Metab* 1982;54: 172-179.

[29] Goodman WG, Veldhuis JD, Belin TR, Van Herle AJ, Juppner H, Salusky IB. Calcium-sensing by parathyroid glands in secondary hyperparathyroidism. *J Clin Endocrinol Metab* 1998;83: 2765-2772.

[30] Carling T, Rastad J, Szabo E, Westin G, Akerstrom G. Reduced parathyroid vitamin D receptor messenger ribonucleic acid levels in primary and secondary hyperparathyroidism. *J Clin Endocrinol Metab* 2000;85: 2000-2003.

[31] Kifor O, Moore FD, Wang P, Goldstein M, Vassilev P, Kifor I, Hebert SC, Brown EM. Reduced immunostaining for the extracellular Ca^{2+}-sensing receptor in primary and uremic secondary hyperparathyroidism. *J Clin Endocrinol Metab* 1996;81: 1598-1606.

[32] Arnold A, Brown MF, Urena P, Gaz, RD, Sarfati E, Drueke TB. Monoclonality of parathyroid tumors in chronic renal failure and in primary parathyroid hyperplasia. *J Clin Invest* 1995;95: 2047-2053.

[33] Palanisamy N, Imanishi Y, Rao PH, Tahara H, Chaganti RS, Arnold A. Novel chro-
      mosomal abnormalities identified by comparative genomic hybridization in parathy-
      roid adenomas. *J Clin Endocrinol Metab* 1998;83: 1766-1770.

[34] Imanishi Y, Tahara H, Palanisamy N, Spitalny S, Salusky IB, Goodman W, Brandi
      ML, Drueke TB, Sarfati E, Urena P, Chaganti RS, Arnold A. Clonal chromosomal de-
      fects in the molecular pathogenesis of refractory hyperparathyroidism of uremia. *J
      Am Soc Nephrol* 2002;13: 1490-1498.

[35] Komaba H, Goto S, Fujii H, Hamada Y, Kobayashi A, Shibuya K, Tominaga Y, Otsuki
      N, Nibu K, Nakagawa K, Tsugawa N, Okano T, Kitazawa R, Fukagawa M, Kita T.
      Depressed expression of Klotho and FGF receptor 1 in hyperplastic parathyroid
      glands from uremic patients. *Kidney Int* 2010;77: 232-238.

[36] Canalejo R, Canalejo A, Martinez-Moreno JM, Rodriguez-Ortiz ME, Estepa JC, Men-
      doza FJ, Munoz-Castaneda JR, Shalhoub V, Almaden Y, Rodriguez M. FGF23 fails to
      inhibit uremic parathyroid glands. *J Am Soc Nephrol* 2010;21: 1125-1135.

[37] Galitzer H, Ben-Dov IZ, Silver J, Naveh-Many T. Parathyroid cell resistance to fibro-
      blast growth factor 23 in secondary hyperparathyroidism of chronic kidney disease.
      Kidney Int 2010;77: 211-218.

[38] Hofman-Bang J, Martuseviciene G, Santini MA, Olgaard K, Lewin E. Increased para-
      thyroid expression of klotho in uremic rats. *Kidney Int* 2010;78: 1119-1127.

[39] K/DOQI Work Group. K/DOQI clinical practice guidelines for bone metabolism and
      disease in chronic kidney disease. *Am J Kidney Dis* 2003;42: S1-201.

[40] Kidney Disease: Improving Global Outcomes (KDIGO) CKD-MBD Work Group.
      KDIGO clinical practice guideline for the diagnosis, evaluation, prevention, and
      treatment of Chronic Kidney Disease-Mineral and Bone Disorder (CKD-MBD). *Kid-
      ney Int* 2009; Suppl: S1-130.

[41] Covic A, Kothawala P, Bernal M, Robbins S, Chalian A, Goldsmith D. Systematic re-
      view of the evidence underlying the association between mineral metabolism distur-
      bances and risk of all-cause mortality, cardiovascular mortality and cardiovascular
      events in chronic kidney disease. *Nephrol Dial Transplant* 2009;24: 1506-1523.

[42] Young EW, Albert JM, Satayathum S, Goodkin DA, Pisoni RL, Akiba T, Akizawa T,
      Kurokawa K, Bommer J, Piera L, Port FK. Predictors and consequences of altered
      mineral metabolism: the Dialysis Outcomes and Practice Patterns Study. *Kidney Int*
      2005;67: 1179-1187.

[43] Isakova T, Gutierrez OM, Chang Y, Shah A, Tamez H, Smith K, Thadhani R, Wolf M.
      Phosphorus binders and survival on hemodialysis. *J Am Soc Nephrol* 2009;20: 388-396.

[44] Melamed ML, Eustace JA, Plantinga L, Jaar BG, Fink NE, Coresh J, Klag MJ, Powe
      NR. Changes in serum calcium, phosphate, and PTH and the risk of death in incident
      dialysis patients: a longitudinal study. *Kidney Int* 2006;70: 351-357.

[45] Wolf M, Shah A, Gutierrez O, Ankers E, Monroy M, Tamez H, Steele D, Chang Y, Camargo CA, Tonelli M, Thadhani R. Vitamin D levels and early mortality among incident hemodialysis patients. *Kidney Int* 2007;72: 1004-1013.

[46] Hammerland LG, Garrett JE, Hung BC, Levinthal C, Nemeth EF. Allosteric activation of the Ca^{2+} receptor expressed in Xenopus laevis oocytes by NPS 467 or NPS 568. *Mol Pharmacol* 1998;53: 1083-1088.

[47] Kawata T, Imanishi Y, Kobayashi K, Onoda N, Okuno S, Takemoto Y, Komo T, Tahara H, Wada M, Nagano N, Ishimura E, Miki T, Ishikawa T, Inaba M, Nishizawa Y. Direct in vitro evidence of the suppressive effect of cinacalcet HCl on parathyroid hormone secretion in human parathyroid cells with pathologically reduced calcium-sensing receptor levels. *J Bone Miner Metab* 2006;24: 300-306.

[48] Colloton M, Shatzen E, Miller G, Stehman-Breen C, Wada M, Lacey D, Martin D. Cinacalcet HCl attenuates parathyroid hyperplasia in a rat model of secondary hyperparathyroidism. *Kidney Int* 2005;67: 467-476.

[49] Wada M, Ishii H, Furuya Y, Fox J, Nemeth EF Nagano N. NPS R-568 halts or reverses osteitis fibrosa in uremic rats. *Kidney Int* 1998;53: 448-453.

[50] Kawata T, Nagano N, Obi M, Miyata S, Koyama C, Kobayashi N, Wakita S, Wada M. Cinacalcet suppresses calcification of the aorta and heart in uremic rats. *Kidney Int* 2008;74: 1270-1277.

[51] Kawata T, Imanishi Y, Kobayashi K, Kenko T, Wada M, Ishimura E, Miki T, Nagano N, Inaba M, Arnold A, Nishizawa Y. Relationship between parathyroid calcium-sensing receptor expression and potency of the calcimimetic, cinacalcet, in suppressing parathyroid hormone secretion in an in vivo murine model of primary hyperparathyroidism. *Eur J Endocrinol* 2005;153: 587-594.

[52] Imanishi Y, Hosokawa Y, Yoshimoto K, Schipani E, Mallya S, Papanikolaou A, Kifor O, Tokura T, Sablosky M, Ledgard F, Gronowicz G, Wang TC, Schmidt EV, Hall C, Brown EM, Bronson R, Arnold A. Primary hyperparathyroidism caused by parathyroid-targeted overexpression of cyclin D1 in transgenic mice. *J Clin Invest* 2001;107: 1093-1102.

[53] Imanishi Y, Kawata T, Kenko T, Wada M, Nagano N, Miki T, Arnold A, Inaba M. Cinacalcet HCl suppresses Cyclin D1 oncogene-derived parathyroid cell proliferation in a murine model for primary hyperparathyroidism. *Calcif Tissue Int* 2011;89: 29-35.

[54] Strippoli GF, Palmer S, Tong A, Elder G, Messa P, Craig JC. Meta-analysis of biochemical and patient-level effects of calcimimetic therapy. *Am J Kidney Dis* 2006;47: 715-726.

[55] Block GA, Zaun D, Smits G, Persky M, Brillhart S, Nieman K, Liu J, St Peter WL. Cinacalcet hydrochloride treatment significantly improves all-cause and cardiovascular survival in a large cohort of hemodialysis patients. *Kidney Int* 2010;78: 578-589.

[56] Imanishi Y. Molecular pathogenesis of tumorigenesis in sporadic parathyroid adeno-
      mas. *J Bone Miner Metab* 2002;20: 190-195.

[57] Pollak MR, Brown EM, Estep HL, Mclaine PN, Kifor O, Park J, Hebert SC, Seidman
      CE, Seidman JG. Autosomal dominant hypocalcaemia caused by a Ca^{2+}-sensing re-
      ceptor gene mutation. *Nat Genet* 1994;8: 303-307.

Chapter 7

Remnant Proteinuria in Chronic Hemodialysis

Hernán Trimarchi

Additional information is available at the end of the chapter

1. Introduction

Patients with end-stage renal disease are at high risk of developing cardiovascular events. In addition to the major traditional risk factors for cardiovascular disease (ie, advanced age, hypertension, diabetes mellitus, dyslipidemia, and smoking), recent studies suggest that chronic kidney disease is an independent risk factor [1]. Several groups have reported that coronary artery disease severity and lesion complexity are associated with a decrease in the estimated glomerular filtration rate [2,3]. Recent epidemiological studies and clinical trials have demonstrated that chronic kidney disease is associated with increased mortality rate in patients with cardiovascular disease [4,5]. Notwithstanding the deep deleterious effects chronic renal disease itself plays in endothelial and medial arterial wall, renal failure leads to both significant increases in morbidity and decreases in life survival, particularly in hemodialysis patients, who represent the most severe and advanced expression of renal disease.

The mechanisms that underlie the association between renal dysfunction and coronary artery disease have not been elucidated fully. Previous studies have shown that renal dysfunction is associated with low-grade inflammation and activation of the sympathetic nervous system and of the renin-angiotensin aldosterone system [6-8]. Other factors such as calcium-phosphate disbalance, oxidative stress, hyperglycemia, advanced glycosylated end-products, and abnormal apolipoprotein levels also were shown, among others, to promote renal dysfunction [9,10]. As such, these factors could also contribute to the pathogenesis of atherosclerosis.

As renal function deteriorates at early stages, the different organ systems start to experience subtle alterations. These initial disturbances that develop at the molecular level, encompass mainly chronic inflammatory pathways mediated by cytokines secreted by leukocytes and uremic retention toxins. In turn, and with different degrees of clinical and biochemical manifestations, the many culprits interact and cause systemic impacts. The most important, albeit not the one, harmful effect is evident at the cardiovascular level. This is due to the fact that the endothelium is a direct target of plasmatic toxins, free radicals and altered synthesized molecules, abnormal platelets, short-live erythrocytes and malfunctioning leukocytes, hyperglycemia, dyslipidemia and hypertension. The damaged endothelium interacts with both the plasmatic and cellular constituents of blood and the inner vessel wall cells, particularly smooth muscle cells, circulating monocytes and tissular macrophages and fibroblasts. The direct consequences are vascular thrombosis, calcification and lipid deposition, and tissue hypoxia. Although these mentioned vascular alterations exist in all organ systems, the central nervous system, the heart and the kidneys are the most important clinically involved organs. This situation finds its most critical exponent when kidney function reaches stage 5 and uremia is present [11]. At this stage, renal replacement therapy is mandatory. Among the therapeutic options, hemodialysis, peritoneal dialysis and kidney transplantation are available. These options are far from ideal, albeit transplantation offers the best results. With respect to the dialysis procedures, hemodialysis is the most frequent modality employed worldwide to treat end-stage renal disease. Among the factors that add morbidity and mortality to hemodialysis individuals are -as mentioned- comorbid conditions as diabetes mellitus, hypertension, aging, endocrine and electrolyte derangements, oxidative stress, volume overload, hyporexia and nutrient losses during the dialysis process, dialysis devices and vascular access-blood interactions, the predisposition to infections, and water quality. All these main factors will definitively result in a vicious cycle in which protein energy wasting, malnutrition, uremic toxins retention, inflammation, and a hypercatabolic state with grim and most frequently irreversible consequences harmfully interact. Cardiovascular disease, malnourishment and inflammation are the main roads that can merge or independently lead to premature death, the reality dialysis patients still face nowadays [11,12].

As mentioned before, many clinical, nutritional, and biochemical parameters may be indicating a chronic inflammatory state in these individuals. Conventional and non-traditional risk factors and metabolic alterations observed in the uremic milieu may contribute to the excessive risk of cardiovascular disease [12]. Both Framingham and the so called *non-traditional* risk factors as inflammation, endothelial dysfunction, sympathetic activation, protein-energy wasting, oxidative stress, vascular calcification, and volume overload may play relevant roles in the development of vascular disease in dialysis patients [13-15]. However, it has recently demonstrated that the addition of multimarker scores (including markers of inflammation and volume overload) to conventional risk factors resulted only in small increases in the ability to grade risk, at least in the general population [16,17].

An important factor in hemodialysis that is linked to survival is residual renal function, clinically assessed as the amount of daily urinary output. Many factors conspire against this important variable: Lifetime on dialysis, aging, the etiologies of end-stage renal disease and higher degrees of ultrafiltration. However, proteinuria, an important marker of progression of renal disease that is associated in time with decreased renal function and oliguria, is not assessed routinely in hemodialysis.

The aim of the present chapter is to consider remnant proteinuria as an active marker of inflammation and cardiovascular disease, and also as a cause of decrease of residual renal function and urinary output in hemodialysis. Although not yet assessed, it is reasonable to presume that also in hemodialysis patients, proteinuria should be associated with increased cardiovascular events, inflammatory processes and decreased life survival.

2. Residual renal function in dialysis

In recent years, there has been a greater focus on residual renal function of patients on chronic dialysis therapy. Although residual renal function is often used to indicate remaining glomerular filtration rate, it also reflects remaining endocrine functions such as erythropoietin production [18], calcium, phosphorus and vitamin D homeostasis [19,20], volume control, and removal of "middle molecules" or low molecular weight proteins [21,22]. It is assumed by some authors that an estimated urine volume < 200 ml/24 h should be considered as a cut-off to consider loss of residual renal function. However, several of the significant associations with residual renal function loss have generated testable hypotheses regarding potential therapies that may preserve renal function among dialysis patients that may be independent of the urinary volume, even at less than 200 ml daily. Renal replacement function is clinically important in that it can account for major differences in dialysis requirements, since it contributes to measures of adequacy, both Kt/V urea and creatinine clearance [23,24]. As mentioned before, residual renal function has also been shown to be associated with mortality. Analysis of the CANUSA study [25] has shown that every 0.5 ml/min higher glomerular filtration rate was associated with a 9% lower risk of death in subjects with renal disease but not still in dialysis [26]. It has been shown that clinically important and statistically significant decreases in nutritional parameters occur with residual renal function loss [25]. Furthermore, it has been demonstrated that small increments in it may account for major differences in quality of life [27,28]. It is therefore very important to determine and understand the predictors of loss of residual renal function in the dialysis patient. The importance of identifying factors that protect and preserve renal function has been recognized among patients with chronic renal failure and pre-end-stage renal disease (stages 3 and 4). Control of blood pressure, angiotensin-converting enzyme inhibition, decreasing proteinuria, dietary modification, avoidance of nephrotoxins, and glucose control have all been considered integral parts of the pre-stage 5 care [29]. However, few studies have comprehensively evaluated whether these or other factors are important in preserving residual renal function after initiation of dialysis. Also on a clinical level, evaluating and monitoring factors that preserve it in patients who have just started dialysis has not received the same level of care as among the chronic renal failure population. It is also probable that subjects with stage 5D (under dialysis) may be treated differently than stage 5 subjects not still in dialysis: In stage 5 not in dialysis, individuals may be under pharmacologic regimes to control proteinuria, that may be left aside when dialysis is started, or the beneficial effects of which are not carefully assessed or even considered.

Several authors have observed that preservation of residual renal function is prolonged with peritoneal dialysis compared to hemodialysis [30-32]. Others have noted a more rapid decline in renal function among patients on automated peritoneal dialysis versus continuous ambulatory peritoneal dialysis [33]. For hemodialysis patients, there has been debate in the literature about whether the type of dialyzer membrane has an effect on remnant renal function. Some have suggested that biocompatible membranes preserve renal function for a longer time period [34-36]. Cause of end-stage renal disease, level of blood pressure, rate and profile of fluid removal, contrast materials as iodide and gadolinium, and also various medications have all been implicated as having an effect on renal function [29,37,38]. However, the current knowledge about the factors that preserve renal function in end-stage renal disease is still very limited. Daily urinary volume recollection may be cumbersome and imprecise, but has proved to be a useful measure of residual renal function. It is interesting that patients are more likely to have the outcome variable, urine volume, reported if they are on peritoneal dialysis or if they are female. It has been recognized that residual renal function is important in continous ambulatory peritoneal dialysis due to its contribution to small solute clearance, and more attention may be paid to monitoring it in this population. The reason for the gender difference is not clear. Several studies about the progression of chronic renal disease have reported that the decline in renal function is either linear or exponential [29,39]. Thus, it is assumed that longer follow- up and lower levels of renal function at the start of dialysis would be associated with a greater likelihood of loss of residual renal function. It is therefore necessary to control for these factors when evaluating the effect of other potential predictors. Duration of time on dialysis is indeed a significant predictor of renal function loss in the overall population and among the peritoneal dialysis population, but, interestingly, not among the hemodialysis population. Among the peritoneal dialysis patients, there is an increasing risk of loss of residual renal function over time, suggesting that time on dialysis is an important variable. Likewise, higher estimated glomerular filtration rates at dialysis initiation is associated with lower risk of loss of residual renal function at follow-up among peritoneal dialysis-treated patients but not among hemodialysis-treated patients.

Increasing age may not be associated with residual renal function loss. This is consistent with data from the Modification of Diet in Renal Disease (MDRD) study [29], in which age was not an independent predictor of progression of renal disease among patients with chronic renal failure. Female gender independently predicted renal function loss loss in the overall analysis and in the analysis limited to peritoneal dialysis patients. This gender effect could not be explained by differences in body mass index, mean arterial pressure, albumin, estrogen use, or menopausal status because the effect remained despite controlling for these variables [40]. However, other studies have shown the opposite, in which a slower rate of progression of renal function decline was reported in females with chronic renal failure [41-44]. Data from the MDRD study indicated a slower mean glomerular filtration rate decline in women compared to men with chronic renal failure. However, gender differences were reduced and no longer significant after controlling for baseline proteinuria, mean arterial pressure, and HDL cholesterol [29]. Non-white race was associated with residual renal function loss in the overall analysis; however, this effect was found to be limited to peritoneal dialysis patients only. This was true of both blacks and the category "other non-white race." These relationships were independent of cause of renal disease and blood pressure at dialysis initiation, and also could not be explained by reported differences in pre-dialysis care. African-Americans are known to have a faster rate of progression of renal failure in the chronic renal failure population [29,45]. This analysis suggests that, at least among peritoneal dialysis-treated patients, this race effect may persist after dialysis initiation. The presence of diabetes predicts renal function loss particularly in both dialysis populations. Diabetic patients with hypertension and proteinuria have been shown to have an increased rate of loss of renal function in the chronic renal failure community. A history of congestive heart failure may also predict renal function loss, likely due to decreased blood flow to the compromised kidney. However, this statement has not been assessed properly in hemodialysis patients.

Several comparative studies of peritoneal dialysis and hemodialysis mortality have shown that the relative mortality risk favors peritoneal dialysis to the greatest degree early after end-stage renal disease start and the relative mortality risk increases for peritoneal dialysis with time on dialysis [46-49]. One reason that peritoneal dialysis may offer this early advantage may be the greater preservation of residual renal function. Higher postdialysis blood pressure at baseline appears to correlate with a lower risk of renal function loss loss in the hemodialysis-only population but may be an insignificant predictor in the peritoneal dialysis subjects. Several studies have observed a relationship of higher mortality associated with low predialysis blood pressure [50-52]. A similar phenomenon may exist for residual renal function. Previous studies have shown that use of cellulose dialyzer membranes among hemodialysis patients hastens residual renal function loss [34,36] due to blood and cellulose dialysis membrane interactions, which may induce potentially nephrotoxic inflammatory mediators [53].

Comparing peritoneal dialysis patients to hemodialysis patients using biocompatible membranes revealed that peritoneal dialysis patients are still significantly less likely to lose residual renal function than hemodialysis patients. Preservation of residual renal function is an important goal. In addition to identifying demographic groups at risk, it is also important to identify other potentially modifiable factors as calcium and phosphorus metabolism, blood pressure, hyperglycemia, PTH and vitamin D levels, dose of erythropoietin, use of iron, and therapies (dialysis modality, angiotensin converting enzyme inhibitors or angiotensin receptor blockers, calcium channel blockers, statins and aspirin) that are involved in residual renal function. There appear to be substantial differences in both the actual loss of residual renal function and the contributing risk factors among peritoneal dialysis compared to hemodialysis patients. Additional prospective studies, ideally clinical trials, are necessary to determine whether these possible interventions are efficacious. Proteinuria has not been assessed in any of both modalities as a marker of progression of residual renal function loss, and as a cause of cardiovascular disease and inflammation [40].

In peritoneal dialysis, the best means for assessing adequacy remain ill defined [54]. The concept of adequate dialysis should include some defined level of solute removal, adequate fluid removal to achieve normal volume homeostasis and blood pressure control, maintenance of adequate nutrition, normal acid–base balance, normal mineral metabolism, minimal anemia, normal lipid metabolism, and prevention of atherosclerosis. Small solute clearance has traditionally been an integral part of the overall definition of peritoneal dialysis adequacy; most other measures appear to parallel solute removal. The importance of small solute clearance in peritoneal dialysis has been confirmed by a variety of studies [55,56], most notably CANUSA, which showed that Kt/V and corrected creatinine clearance independently predict patient survival. All these studies have been confounded by residual renal function. Solute removal by peritoneal dialysis may not be clinically equivalent to an equal quantitated solute removal by residual renal function. For example, the increased fractional secretion of creatinine during declining glomerular filtration rate can be extremely misleading if other solutes do not show a fractional increase in excretion. Conversely, the increased secretion of organic solutes during chronic renal failure may far exceed the diffusive losses of the same solute during peritoneal dialysis. Hence, the relative effects of renal versus peritoneal clearance on survival remain to be elucidated. There is consensus that residual renal function has a major impact on the ability to achieve small solute clearance targets [57]. Residual renal function contributes to approximately 25% of total Kt/V and 40% of total weekly creatinine clearance. This numerical contribution is even greater for high and middle molecular weight solutes. As residual renal function deteriorates, failure to compensate for this loss will result in an increasing frequency of inadequate dialysis. Even with increasing dialysis prescription, as many as 40% of continuous ambulatory peritoneal dialysis patients fail to meet the target [58,59]. Small changes in residual renal function with time on peritoneal dialysis may account for major differences in quality of life and dialysis outcome. Data from the CANUSA study showed that the overall outcome was worse for patients who lost their residual renal function [60,61]. The adverse impact of loss of residual renal function on outcome in peritoneal dialysis patients could be due partly to loss of residual diuresis and difficulty in managing fluid status, hypertension, and left ventricular hypertrophy, all of which contribute to cardiovascular mortality [62].

Residual renal function has also been shown to have a greater influence on dietary protein intake and nutritional status than peritoneal clearance [63-65]. Following the initial observation of Rottembourg et al., a number of studies have shown that the decline in residual renal function is more protracted in patients on peritoneal dialysis than those on hemodialysis [31,66-69]. However, the changes in residual renal function with time are not uniform in all patients. The issue of which factors affect preservation of residual renal function in patients with chronic renal failure once dialysis is started has received very little attention [70-74]. There appears to be a gradual deterioration of residual glomerular filtration rate with time on peritoneal dilaysis, with 33% of patients developing anuria at a mean of 20 months after the start of dialysis, according to Singal et al data [75]. In that study, on comparison between patients in the highest and lowest quartiles of slope for residual glomerular filtration rate, male gender, presence of diabetes, higher grades of left ventricular dysfunction, and glomerular filtration rate higher 24-hour urine protein excretion corresponded with faster decline of residual renal function. Singal et al could not show a good correlation between the decline of urine volume and renal glomerular filtration rate. Urine volume was well maintained until 30 months after start of peritoneal dialysis. This was in contrast to previous studies, where the decline in creatinine clearance and urine volume in individual patients was significantly correlated [76]. A number of studies have shown that residual renal function is better preserved in peritoneal dialysis patients than in those on hemodialysis. However, all these comparisons were made between hemodialysis using conventional bioincompatible membranes and peritoneal dialysis. The advent of newer dialytic techniques such as automated peritoneal dialysis and biocompatible hemodialysis membranes may alter this relationship. It has also been suggested that peritoneal dialysis patients with rapidly falling residual renal function depart from therapy at a high rate, leaving those with better preservation of residual renal function on peritoneal dialysis after many months [77]. Previous studies have not clearly defined the factors that affect the rate of residual renal function loss in patients on dialysis. In hemodialysis patients, Iest et al. reported that the mean rate of decline of residual renal function was unaffected by weight, gender, age, hypertension status or medications, and by the original disease [78]. Lutes et al. also reported in 32 peritoneal dialysis patients no influence of age, diabetes, mean arterial pressure, peritonitis rate, and initial creatinine clearance at the start of peritoneal dialysis, on the rate of residual renal function loss [70]. Davies et al. looked at the half-life of loss of residual renal function in 303 patients started on peritoneal dialysis between 1990 and 1997 [32]. Patients with interstitial nephritis, renovascular disease and hypertensive nephrosclerosis had slower decline of residual renal function. Comorbid conditions did not influence rate of loss of residual renal function. Moist et al. studied predictors of loss of residual renal function in new dialysis patients [40]. As partially mentioned before, increasing age, female gender, and nonwhite race predicted faster loss, whereas peritoneal dialysis and use of angiotensin converting enzyme inhibitors and calcium channel blockers was associated with slower loss of residual renal function. However, the primary outcome variable was urine volume, not residual glomerular filtration rate, in that study. Singal et al evaluated the risk factors assumed to be associated with residual glomerular filtration rate [75]. There was no effect of age, race, or primary renal disease on the rate of decline of residual renal function. Presence of diabetes as a cause of renal disease or as a comorbidity was significantly associated with the rate of decline. Presence of peripheral vascular disease and higher degrees of left ventricular dysfunction on echocardiography may have a significant effect in patients in upper and lower quartiles of slope of residual glomerular filtration rate. Considering the 105 patients with diabetes, 38% had peripheral vascular disease and left ventricular dysfunction of grades I to IV in 60%, 13%, 15%, and 12% of patients respectively; compared to 137 patients with no diabetes where 12% had peripheral vascular disease and left ventricular dysfunction of grades I to IV in 77%, 13%, 7%, and 3% respectively. Similarly, 24-hour urinary protein excretion may also be associated with diabetic nephropathy as a cause of end-stage renal disease.

Therefore, residual renal function may contribute significantly to total solute clearance and fluid balance in patients on continuous peritoneal dialysis. Changes in residual renal function with time are not uniform in all patients. Faster decline of residual renal function corresponds with male gender, large body mass index, presence of diabetes mellitus, higher grades of congestive heart failure and higher 24-hour proteinuria. Higher rates of peritonitis and use of antibiotics for the treatment of peritonitis are also associated independently with faster decline of residual renal function. Whether the type of peritoneal dialysis and use of larger dialysate volume are associated with faster decline of residual renal function remains speculative [75]. In summary, loss of residual renal function and urinary output is an important risk factor of morbidity and mortality in dialysis patients. In predialysis patients, proteinuria is clearly associated with renal and cardiovascular disease progression. However, the link between proteinuria and residual renal function in dialysis is to be discussed next.

3. Proteinuria and chronic kidney disease

The incidence of end-stage renal disease is dramatically increasing worldwide [80]. Most patients with kidney problems visit their physicians in the late stages of the disease. Progression from mild to moderate kidney disease to end-stage renal disease may be halted or slowed when kidney damage is detected and appropriate treatment is started during the early stages. Kidney damage is frequently asymptomatic but can be suspected in the presence of proteinuria, hematuria, or a reduced glomerular filtration rate [81]. Due to increased awareness of people about chronic kidney disease and early detection and prevention programs implemented in developed countries, the incidence of end-stage renal disease has shown a small downward trend [82,83]. However the total number of individuals worldwide with chronic kidney disease is still high and estimated at 500,000,000 people [82-84].

Proteinuria is a major risk factor for renal disease progression [85-87]. Among the main causes that lead to dialysis, diabetes, hypertension and glomerular diseases account for more than 70% of the most frequent described etiologies in the adult population. All these entities display a marker of disease progression: Proteinuria. In this setting, proteinuria can be due to primary glomerulopathies, which is the third cause of end-stage renal disease in the adult population and an important cause of secondary hypertension, or could be the result of secondary glomerular damage due to primary hypertension, diabetes mellitus, hyperfiltration, metabolic syndrome, reduced renal mass, autoimmune or infectious diseases, vesicoureteral reflux, etc.

Proteinuria is another predictor of increased cardiovascular risk in the general population [88]. Numerous studies have shown that treating proteinuria in patients with diabetic or non-diabetic chronic kidney disease and proteinuria slows the progression of renal disease. It can also be stated that the greater the decrease in proteinuria, the greater the clinical benefit [89-91]. In addition to predicting kidney disease progression, proteinuria is a well-established risk marker for cardiovascular disease [86,92-94]. In chronic kidney disease individuals, reduction in proteinuria confers a significant decrease in cardiovascular events. For example, the RENAAL study showed that albuminuria is the most important factor in predicting the cardiovascular risk in patients with type 2 diabetic nephropathy, and at 6 months for every 50% reduction in albuminuria, a 18% reduction in cardiovascular risk and a 27% reduction in heart failure was reported[16]. It is evident that proteinuria presents an important predictive value in cardiac failure, both as a marker of future events and also as a therapeutic target. Patients with diabetic nephropathy and proteinuria greater than 3 g/g have a 2.7-fold higher risk for heart failure when compared with patients with low proteinuria (<1.5 g/g) [95]. A coexistent diagnosis of hypertension and diabetes increases the risk of adverse cardiovascular and renal outcomes. This increased risk extends to a diastolic blood pressure of 83 mmHg and a systolic of 127 mmHg [96,97]. Reduction of proteinuria by >30% within the first 6 to 12 months of treatment in patients with chronic kidney disease has also been shown to predict long-term renal and cardiovascular outcomes [86,88,98]. Moreover, the management of albuminuria in normotensive or hypertensive patients with diabetes may slow progression of diabetic nephropathy [99], and microalbuminuria itself, an early marker of kidney vascular dysfunction, is a strong prognostic indicator of mortality and cardiovascular disease in hypertension and diabetes mellitus [100,101]. Therefore, one of the main goals to slow the progression of renal disease is an adequate and not unusually aggressive control of blood pressure and the reduction of proteinuria to its lowest possible level [102]. Moreover, proteinuria has been shown to be the strongest predictor of cardiovascular outcomes, including hospitalization for heart failure. Extinguishing proteinuria by decreasing blood pressure, hyperfiltration states, sodium intake, and tight glycemia control are generally accepted potential strategies to reduce cardiovascular risk events [89]. Although the nature of the links between proteinuria and vascular disease may partly be due to endothelial dysfunction, persistent low-grade inflammation also plays a role. Indeed, inflammation is associated with both endothelial dysfunction and albuminuria [11,102-104].

4. Residual renal function and proteinuria

The past 20 years of research in nephrology have yielded substantial information on the mechanisms by which persisting dysfunction of an individual component cell in the glomerulus is generated and signaled to other glomerular cells and to the tubule. Spreading of disease is central to processes by which nephropathies of different types progress to end stage renal disease. Independent of the underlying causes, chronic proteinuric glomerulopathies have in common a sustained or permanent loss of selectivity of the glomerular barrier to protein filtration. Glomerular sclerosis is the progressive lesion beginning at the glomerular capillary wall, the site of abnormal filtration of plasma proteins. Injury is transmitted to the interstitium favoring the self-destruction of nephrons and eventually of the kidney. The underlying mechanisms of tubulointerstitial injury that are activated by ultrafiltered protein load of tubular epithelial cells continue during the entire process of the disease, which is accompanied by several clinical markers, as fluid and toxins retention, edema, hypertension, proteinuria, creeping creatinine and a continuous decrease in urinary output. It needs to be emphasized that this field is relevant to interpret clinical findings and to improve treatment of patients with non-diabetic or diabetic nephropathies.

The opinion among nephrologists that proteinuria could be a marker only of injury largely has been challenged. The strong predictive value of proteinuria in chronic nephropathies now is firmly established. Baseline proteinuria was an independent predictor of renal outcome in patients with type 1 diabetes and nephropathy [105]. and in patients who did not have diabetes and entered the MDRD study [86]. In the Ramipril Efficacy In Nephropathy (REIN) trial [92], urinary protein excretion was the only baseline variable that correlated significantly with glomerular filtration rate decline and progression of non-diabetic chronic proteinuric nephropathies to end-stage renal disease. Similar evidence was provided recently in patients with type 2 diabetes and overt nephropathy [87]. Other studies corroborated these data and extended the predictive value of proteinuria to risks for overall or cardiovascular mortality [106,107]. Clinical trials consistently showed renoprotective effects of proteinuria reduction and led to the recognition that the antiproteinuric treatment is instrumental to maximize renoprotection [86,92,94,108]. The MDRD study revealed tight association between reduction of proteinuria and decrease in rate of glomerular filtration rate decline [86]. Protection that was achieved by lowering blood pressure depended on the extent of initial proteinuria. The renoprotection that was conferred by angiotensin-converting enzyme inhibition in the REIN study was mediated by the drug's action of reducing urinary protein levels, to the extent that patients who were on ramipril had a better outcome paralleled by more reduction in proteinuria, whereas blood pressure was comparable to that of control subjects [92]. Angiotensin converting enzyme inhibitor–induced reduction in proteinuria was the strongest time-dependent covariate predicting slower progression to uremia. Finding that the rate of glomerular filtration rate decline correlated negatively with proteinuria reduction and positively with residual proteinuria provided further evidence for a pathogenetic role of proteinuria [109]. Likewise, trials in type 1 [94,110] and type 2 diabetes [111,112] documented that whenever proteinuria is decreased by treatments, progression to end-stage renal disease is reduced. As already mentioned, the Reduction of Endpoints in type 2 diabetes with the Angiotensin II Antagonist Losartan (RENAAL) study [111] in 1513 patients with type 2 diabetic nephropathy confirmed that more reduction in proteinuria by losartan invariably was associated with more renoprotection at comparable levels of blood pressure control. Beneficial cardiovascular effects of losartan also were driven by effects on urinary protein and largely depended on the amount of residual proteinuria. Similar results were found in the Irbesartan Diabetic Nephropathy Trial [112]. Finally, the Angiotensin-Converting-Enzyme Inhibition and Progression of Renal Disease study [113,114] confirmed that proteinuria is a strong risk factor for progression of chronic renal disease and that patients with more severe renal disease benefit most from angiotensin converting enzyme inhibitor therapy. Importantly, in no case from a was there a worsening in proteinuria that subsequently was associated with an improved outcome [115].

In progressive nephropathies, severe dysfunction of the glomerular capillary barrier to circulating proteins causes protein overload of tubular epithelial cells and intrarenal activation of complement that is responsible for spreading of injury to the tubulointerstitium. Drugs that block angiotensin II limit the abnormal passage of plasma proteins and are renoprotective. The podocyte is the primary site of antiproteinuric action through stabilization of podocyte–podocyte contacts and prevention of permselective dysfunction at the slit diaphragm. Although the abnormal passage of plasma proteins across the glomerular capillary wall is likely to be a factor that is responsible for further podocyte injury and progression to glomerulosclerosis [116], most of the available data highlight the mechanisms underlying proximal tubular cell activation and interstitial inflammation and fibrosis. The toxicity of albumin seems to be mediated by its initial endocytic uptake, although the importance of albumin itself *versus* protein-bound molecules in the induction of irreversible tubular damage is not clear. Other molecules, including ultrafiltered transferrin and immunoglobulins, and the intrarenal complement and ammonium interactions could play relevant roles. Developments in these areas yield further support to design protocols in which drugs against secondary pathways of injury should be tested in association with drugs that limit the abnormal passage of proteins across the glomerular capillary barrier [117]. This statement must be borne in mind when considering treatment of proteinuria as the patient enters dialysis, as the already triggered pathologic pathways are perpetuated.

In this regard, the pathophysiological process that leads to end-stage renal disease where proteinuria is a hallmark is crucial to be followed and treated. As long as urinary output is present, all the severely damaged nephron structures may be still abnormally working, as hypertension and proteinuria are two clinical evident markers of renal disease virtually present in the vast majority of dialysis individuals.

5. Hemodialysis: Is there a role of proteinuria as a marker of disease?

Noteworthy, despite this active attempt to reduce proteinuria in pre-dialysis patients to delay disease progression, proteinuria appears to be forgotten or even ignored by nephrologists once a patient enters dialysis. However, its existence may certainly continue conferring the well-known inflammatory, catabolic, fibrinolytic and toxic effects on the endothelium that has been exerting in the pre-dialysis period [104,118,119]. Our group determined that the higher degrees of proteinuria in chronic hemodialysis patients are associated with inflammatory and cardiovascular markers of disease [120]. These results may also be related to the nutritional status and mortality rates.

In chronic kidney disease patients, proteinuria is a common event, irrespective of cause, and virtually all patients with chronic kidney disease present variable degrees of proteinuria [121]. However, in dialysis patients, the prevalence of proteinuria is unknown. In the present study, proteinuria was present in 87% of the hemodialyzed population. Noteworthy, despite significantly differences in proteinuria among the three groups, these changes were not accompanied by significant alterations in albuminemia or in cholesterolemia. This phenomenon could be attributed to the similar nutritional status the three groups displayed and to the use of statins in virtually all patients. In patients with proteinuria > 3/day, the two main causes of end-stage renal disease were diabetes nephropathy and primary glomerulonephritis, although no significant differences in the amount the proteinuria could be observed between both subpopulations. However, there was a significant increase in diabetic patients with heavy proteinuria in comparison to the other two groups, and a relative increase in the diabetic population was observed as proteinuria augmented. Proteinuric levels did not correlate with body mass index, the type of vascular acceses, and could not be attributed to hypertension or to hemodynamic fluctuations, as Pro-Brain natriuretic peptide (Pro-BNP) measurements were not different among the groups. There was a significant difference in the ultrafiltration rates, but we could not associate it to any of the variables under consideration, particularly with Pro-BNP or adiponectin, between which important feedback regulations exist. Interestingly, as proteinuria worsened, a significant correlation developed between Troponin T, a cardiovascular biomarker, and C-Reactive Protein (CRP), an inflammatory marker. This interrelationship may suggest that proteinuria could interact as a covert and ignored culprit in the complex and chronic protein energy wasting syndrome dialysis patients live in, contributing to a higher risk of cardiovascular disease and inflammation as proteinuria rises.

In our own experience, in a one-year recruitment cross-sectional study where 265 chronic kidney disease patients were classified into the 5 stages according to K/DOQI guidelines, proteinuria was present in 204 subjects (76.98%) [122]. Interestingly, proteinuria significantly worsened as kidney function declined, and the highest rates of proteinuria were encountered in the most advanced stages of the cohort: Stage 3, 1.39±3.2 g/day (range: 0-21.6) in 80% of the 90 cases included vs stage 4, 1.87±0.99 g/day (range 0-5.1), which represented the 95% of the 37 individuals included in this group. In Stage 5D, proteinuria was present in 85% of the 60 patients included, and the mean level of proteinuria was 2.48±3.72 g/day (range 0-21.5). This level of proteinuria was significantly higher and different from stages 3 (p=0.001) and 4 (p=0.013). These findings underscore previous findings that demonstrated that proteinuria is associated with chronic kidney disease, that worsens renal function, and that it is highly prevalent in end-stage renal disease [89-91,121].

Cardiovascular disease in the main cause of death in the chronic population. However, cardiovascular disease can be the final pathophysiological pathway where many different entities may converge: Framingham factors, malnutrition, oxidative stress, calcium-phosphate metabolism, anemia, infections, inflammation. Although we have included many of the traditional Framingham risk factors in our study, only diabetes mellitus was significantly more frequent in patients with proteinuria > 3 g/day compared to the other groups. In chronic kidney disease, the main causes that lead to renal replacement therapies are diabetic nephropathy, hypertension and glomerulonephritis. In all these entities, cardiovascular disease is a major cause of morbidity and mortality, and proteinuria again plays a key role in these pathophysiological processes. In our study, higher degrees of proteinuria (> 3 g/day) significantly correlated with Troponin T and CRP, markers of cardiovascular stress and systemic inflammation. Which is the relationship among CRP, Troponin T and proteinuria in hemodialysis, if any?. Both CRP and Troponin T have been employed as markers of highly prevalent complications as inflammation and cardiovascular disease in dialysis subjects. CRP has been reported to be elevated in 30 to 60% of dialysis patients, and can be employed as a predictor of cardiovascular mortality in hemodialysis [123]. In addition, it has been established that troponin T levels are increased in subjects with renal failure, even in the absence of myocardial ischemia [124-125]. In fact, approximately 53% of patients with chronic kidney disease present with elevated troponin T without acute myocardial necrosis [126] As troponin T is normally cleared by the kidneys, it could be elevated in chronic kidney disease owing to delayed clearance [127]. However, other reasons could also explain the high troponin T levels, as left ventricular hypertrophy, congestive heart failure, and sepsis [125,126,128]. The combination of increased levels of CRP and troponin T levels are associated with an increased risk of death in chronic kidney disease [129]. Finally, Wong et al state that the positive correlation between Troponin T and CRP could be due to an inflammatory process that could induce a sub-clinical myocardial damage resulting from endothelial injury and athero-sclerosis [130]. How does proteinuria fit into this process?: In dialysis, proteinuria could be an important cause of inflammation and of endothelial dysfunction and atherosclerosis and peripheral vascular disease as in previous stages of chronic kidney disease [91, 117, 131], triggering CRP and troponin T elevations. This situation could justify that as proteinuria worsens, the correlation we found between troponin T and CRP rises significantly. It has re-cently been published that in a murine model of spontaneous albuminuric chronic kidney disease, the systemic endothelial glycocalyx is altered in its glycosylated components due to proteinuria itself. Therefore, it becomes reasonable to speculate that as this meshwork of surface-bound and loosely adherent glycosaminoglycans and proteoglycans modulates vas-cular function, its loss could contribute to both renal and systemic vascular dysfunction in proteinuric chronic kidney disease, including dialysis patients [132].

Therefore, it ought to be reasonable to focus on proteinuria as a target to treat, as its de-crease may portend a better care of residual kidney function and cardiovascular status in stage 5D subjects. However, once patients are started on dialysis, proteinuria generally ap-pears to be ignored and forgotten as a potential factor of morbidity and mortality, as it oc-curs in predialysis subjects. Proteinuria may contribute to the burden of cardiovascular disease and should be a parameter to pay attention to in dialysis individuals. Finally, de-spite being on dialysis, proteinuria should be controlled as its persistence may hasten the loss of residual renal function, a relevant item to preserve at any price in this population.

Moreover, proteinuria is not only important as a marker of progression of renal disease, but it is also associated with catabolic processes, protein-energy wasting, hypoalbumine-mia, and inflammation. All these processes are prevalent in the dialysis community [11,12,17]. However, the data relating proteinuria and hemodialysis is more than scant. In a work published by Goldwasser et al in 1999, in which they observed a rise in albumin and creatinine in those patients who entered dialysis after six months of treatment, they hypothesized that this phenomenon could be attributed, in part, to a better nutritional sta-tus, a gain in muscle mass, and to a decline in residual renal function [121]. This decrease in urinary output could consequently result in lower losses of protein in the urine. Final-ly, it is well known that as proteinuria progresses, and more importantly without any medical intervention focused specifically on it, parenchymal fibrosis ensues and residual renal function rapidly deteriorates.

One question that needs to be addressed for dialysis patients is the threshold above which proteinuria would be implicated in inflammatory processes and could have any implica-tion or contribution in the development of cardiovascular disease. Should the levels of proteinuria be interpreted in the same way as in pre-dialysis subjects?. Our study sug-gests that as proteinuria increases, cardiovascular stress and inflammatory processes are more prone to be encountered. No data exists whether proteinuria should be treated in di-alysis and, if that were the case, the level to pursue. Our data suggest that proteinuria should be treated, considering its association with inflammation and cardiovascular stress. Although, as mentioned above, angiotensin converting enzyme inhibitors or angiotensin II receptor blockers could have modified the results, these drugs were employed homogeneously in the three groups.

Finally, we have observed (data not published) that at higher degrees of proteinuria, urinary output deteriorates faster. At similar initial urinary output rates, patients with proteinria > 3 g/day performed differently from those < 3 g/day: After three years of follow-up, patients with proteinuria > 3 g/day when entering hemodialysis were anuric and therefore had no residual renal function. Patients with proteinuria < 3 g/day still had residual renal function, and proteinuria did not worsen significantly during the time of follow-up. Whether this was be due to a higher proportion of diabetic patients, to higher degrees of proteinuria, or to other cofactors as previous administration of contrast agents or exposure to nephrotoxic drugs cannot be concluded from our data. Besides, in patients with heavy proteinuria a shorter time on hemodialysis trend was observed. Again, whether this phenomenon should be ascribed to diabetes mellitus itself, or to proteinuria could not be concluded. Interestingly, as mentioned before, in non-dialysis patients proteinuria in diabetics is associated with an increased risk of cardiovascular events and mortality [85-87,95-97]. However, we underscore the critical importance proteinuria may play on hemodialysis as a forgotten, overlooked marker of cardiovascular and inflammation.

Our experience, albeit limited, calls the attention of nephrologists to take proteinuria into account when a hemodialysis patient is assessed. Due to the small number of cases included in our recently published study, conclusions must be drawn cautiously. In this respect, the significant correlation found between CRP and Troponin T may be associated with heavy proteinuria, but other factors not assessed in this study may also be involved. We were unable to measure other inflammatory molecules as interleukin-6 and Tumor Necrosis Factor, or endothelial and procoagulant molecules as Plasminogen Activator Inhibitor-1, which are more sensitive than CRP and would have certainly added more information to the data presented in this study. Finally, no vascular arteriosclerotic parameters as pulse wave velocity were evaluated in our patients, which would have certainly enriched our primary findings. Moreover, as an observational study in a cross-sectional cohort, no follow-up with regard to patient prognosis, to the evolution of proteinuria and its correlation with other biomarkers, and to mortality rates could not be obtained. All these results require validation [120]. However, we believe this work is a call of attention to nephrologists regarding another important aspect of the characteristics of urinary output and residual renal function in dialysis patients.

6. Conclusions

Proteinuria is a strong predictor of chronic kidney disease progression. It is also an important marker of cardiovascular disease, both in patients with or without kidney disease. In hemodialysis individuals, urinary output is associated with morbidity and mortality. At higher levels of diuresis, there is a trend to lesser rates of hospitalization and a higher mortality. Most of renal functions are better preserved if associated with higher volumes of urine. In this regard, proteinuria plays a critical role in renal fibrosis, stimulating sclerosis in the glomerular and in the interstitial compartments. This sclerosis causes in turn local is-chaemia and further deterioration of kidney function, which can be clinically assessed with creeping of serum creatinine and a final decline in urinary output. This phenomenon is ob-served throughout the chronic kidney disease process, even at the dialysis setting. We have found that in chronic hemodialysis patients, at higher degrees of proteinuria, systemic markers of cardiovascular disease and inflammation are elevated. Albeit not proven yet, as proteinuria causes an eventual decline in renal function, and preservation of residual renal function is associated with higher survival rates in dialysis patients, proteinuria may be also associated with a decrease in urinary output and an increase in morbidity events and mor-tality in chronic hemodialysis.

Author details

Hernán Trimarchi

Chief Nephrology Service, Hospital Británico de Buenos Aires, Buenos Aires, Argentina

References

[1] Culleton BF, Larson MG, Wilson PW, Evans JC, Parfrey PS, Levy D. Cardiovascular disease and mortality in a community-based cohort with mild renal insufficiency. Kidney Int 1999; 56: 2214 – 2219.

[2] Kilickesmez KO, Abaci O, Okcun B, Kocas C, Baskurt M, Arat A, et al. Chronic kid-ney disease as a predictor of coronary lesion morphology. Angiology 2010; 61: 344 – 349.

[3] Yagi H, Kawai M, Komukai K, Ogawa T, Minai K, Nagoshi T, et al. Impact of chronic kidney disease on the severity of initially diagnosed coronary artery disease and the patient prognosis in the Japanese population. Heart Vessels 2011; 26: 370 – 378.

[4] Go AS, Chertow GM, Fan D, McCulloch CE, Hsu CY. Chronic kidney disease and the risks of death, cardiovascular events, and hospitalization. N Engl J Med 2004; 351: 1296 – 1305.

[5] Kinoshita T, Asai T, Murakami Y, Suzuki T, Kambara A, Matsubayashi K. Preopera-tive renal dysfunction and mortality after off-pump coronary artery bypass grafting in Japanese. Circ J 2010; 74: 1866 – 1872.

[6] Schiffrin EL, Lipman ML, Mann JF. Chronic kidney disease: Effects on the cardiovas-cular system. Circulation 2007; 116: 85 – 97.

[7] Manabe I. Chronic inflammation links cardiovascular, metabolic and renal diseases. Circ J 2011; 75: 2739 – 2748.

[8] Iwanaga Y, Miyazaki S. Heart failure, chronic kidney disease, and biomarkers: An integrated viewpoint. Circ J 2010; 74: 1274 – 1282.

[9] Foley RN, Collins AJ, Ishani A, Kalra PA. Calcium-phosphate levels and cardiovascular disease in community-dwelling adults: The atherosclerosis risk in communities (ARIC) study. Am Heart J 2008; 156: 556 – 563.

[10] Muntner P, Hamm LL, Kusek JW, Chen J, Whelton PK, He J. The prevalence of nontraditional risk factors for coronary heart disease in patients with chronic kidney disease. Ann Intern Med 2004; 140: 9 – 17.

[11] Trimarchi H. The endothelium and hemodialysis. In: Goretti-Penido, M (ed.) Special Problems in hemodialysis patients. Riejka: InTech; 2011. P 167-192.

[12] Fouque D, Kalantar-Zadeh K, Kopple J, et al. A proposed nomenclature and diagnostic criteria for protein-energy wasting in acute and chronic kidney disease. Kidney Int. 2008;73:391–398.

[13] Muntner P, He J, Astor BC, Folsom AR, Coresh J. Traditional and nontraditional risk factors predict coronary heart disease in chronic kidney disease: results from the atherosclerosis risk in communities study. J Am Soc Nephrol. 2005;16:529–538.

[14] Cheung AK, Sarnak MJ, Yan G, et al. Atherosclerotic cardiovascular disease risks in chronic hemodialysis patients. Kidney Int. 2000;58: 353–362.

[15] Himmelfarb J, Stenvinkel P, Ikizler TA, Hakim RM. The elephant of uremia: oxidative stress as a unifying concept of cardiovascular disease in uremia. Kidney Int. 2002; 62:1524–1538.

[16] Wang TJ, Gona P, Larson MG, et al. Multiple biomarkers for the prediction of first major cardiovascular events and death. N Engl J Med. 2006;21:2631–2639.

[17] Stenvinkel P, Carrero JJ, Axelsson J, Lindholm B, Heimbürger O, Massy Z. Emerging biomarkers for evaluating cardiovascular risk in the chronic disease patient: how do new pieces fit into the uremic puzzle? Clinl J Am Soc Nephrol. 2008;3:505–521.

[18] Caro J, Brown S, Miller O, Murray TG, Erslev AJ: Erythropoietin levels in uremic nephric and anephric patients. J Lab Clin Med 1979; 93: 449–454.

[19] Jonger M, VanDerVijgh W, Lip P, Netclenbos J: Measurement of vitamin D metabolites in anephrotic subjects. Nephron 1984; 36: 230–236.

[20] Morduchowicz G, Winkler J, Zabludowski J, Boner G: The effect of residual renal function in hemodialysis patients. Intern Urol Nephrol 1994; 1: 125–131.

[21] Milutinovic J, Cutler R, Hoover P, Meijsen B, Scribner B: Measurement of residual glomerular filtration rate in the patient receiving repetitive hemodialysis. Kidney Int 1975; 8: 185–190.

[22] Weber MH, Reetze P, Norman F, Worneke G, Scheler F: Influence of CAPD and residual diuresis on the serum level of alpha 1 aminoglobulin in ESRD. Nephron 1985; 51: 367–374.

[23] Tattersall JE, Doyle S, Greenwood RN, Farrington K: Kinetic modeling and under dialysis in CAPD patients. Nephrol Dial Transplant 1993; 8: 535–538.

[24] Blake PG: Targets in CAPD and APD prescription. Perit Dial Int 1996; 16[Suppl 1]: S143–S146.

[25] Canada-USA (CANUSA) Peritoneal Dialysis Study Group: Adequacy of dialysis and nutrition in continuous peritoneal dialysis associated with clinical outcomes. J Am Soc Nephrol 1996; 7: 198– 207.

[26] Bargman J, Thorpe K, Churchill D: The importance of residual renal function for survival in patients on peritoneal dialysis [Abstract]. J Am Soc Nephrol 1997; 8: 185A.

[27] Ravid M, Lang R, Rolson M: The importance of daily urine volume and residual renal function in patients treated with chronic hemodialysis. Dial Transplant 1985; 9: 763–765.

[28] Bonomini V, Albertazzi A, Vangelistu A, Bortolotti G, Stefoni S, Scolari M: Residual renal function and effective rehabilitation in chronic dialysis. Nephron 1976; 16: 89– 99.

[29] Hunsicker LG, Adler S, Cagsiulla A, England B, Greene T, Kusek JW, Rogers NL, Teschen PE: Modification of Diet in Renal Disease Study Group. Predictors of progression of renal disease. Kidney Int 1997; 51: 1908–1919.

[30] Lysaght M, Vonesh E, Gotch F, Ibels L, Keen M, Lindholm B, Nolph K, Pollock C, Prowant B, Farrell, P: The influence of dialysis treatment modality on the decline in remaining renal function. ASAIO Trans 1991; 37: 598–604.

[31] Rottembourg J, Issad B, Gallego J, Degoulet P, Aime F, Gueffaf B, Legrain M: Evolution of residual renal function in patients undergoing maintenance hemodialysis or continuous ambulatory peritoneal dialysis. Proc Eur Dial Transplant Assoc 1982; 19: 397– 409.

[32] Cancarini G, Bunori G, Camererini C, Brasa S, Manili L, Maiorca R: Renal function recovery and maintenance of residual diuresis in CAPD and hemodialysis. Perit Dial Bull 1986; 6: 77–79.

[33] Hiroshige K, Yuu K, Masasake S, Takasugi M, Kuroiwa A: Rapid decline of residual renal function on automated peritoneal dialysis. Perit Dial Int 1996; 16: 307–315.

[34] VanStone J: The effect of dialyzer membrane and etiology of kidney disease on the preservation of residual renal function in chronic hemodialysis patients. ASAIO J 1995; 41: M713–M716.

[35] Hartmann J, Fricke H, Schittle H: Biocompatible membranes preserve renal function in patients undergoing hemodialysis. Am J Kidney Dis 1997; 30: 366–373.

[36] McCarthy JT, Jenson BM, Squillace DP, Williams AW: Improved preservation of residual renal function in chronic hemodialysis patients using polysulfone dialyzers. Am J Kidney Dis 1997; 29: 576–583.

[37] Maschio G: Protecting the RRF: How do ACE inhibitors and calcium channel blockers compare? Nephron 1994; 67: 257–262.

[38] Dworkin AD, Bernstein JA, Parker M, Tolbert E, Feiner E: Calcium antagonist and converting enzyme inhibitors reduce renal injury by different mechanisms. Kidney Int 1993; 43: 808–814.

[39] Rutherford W, Blondin J, Grunwalt A, Vavra J: Chronic progressive renal disease: Rate of change of serum creatinine concentration. Kidney Int 1997; 11: 62–70.

[40] Moist L, Port FK, Orzol SM, Young EW, Ostbye I, Wolfe RA, Hulbert-Shearon T, Jones CA, Bloembergen WE. Predictors of Loss of Residual Renal Function among New Dialysis Patients. J Am Soc Nephrol 2000; 11: 556–564.

[41] Coggins CH, Lewis JB, Caggiula AW, Castaldo LS, Klahr S, Wang S: Differences between women and men with chronic renal disease. Nephrol Dial Transplant 1998; 13: 1430–1437.

[42] Silbiger SR, Neugarten J: The impact of gender on the progression of chronic renal disease. Am J Kidney Dis 1995; 25: 515–533

[43] Hannedouche T, Chauveau P, Kalou F, Albouze G, Lacour B: Factors affecting progression in advanced chronic renal failure. Clin Nephrol 1993; 39: 312–320

[44] Hunt C, Short C, Mallick N: Prognostic indicators in patients presenting with the nephrotic syndrome. Kidney Int 1988; 34: 382–388

[45] Lopes AA, Hornbuckle K, Sherman AJ, Port FK: The joint effects of race and age on the risk of end-stage renal disease attributed to hypertension. Am J Kidney Dis 1994; 24: 554–560

[46] Bloembergen WE, Port FK, Mauger EA, Wolfe RA: A comparison of mortality between patients treated with hemodialysis and peritoneal dialysis. J Am Soc Nephrol 1995; 6: 177–191

[47] Held PJ, Port FK, Turenne MN, Gaylin DS, Hamburger RJ, Wolfe RA: Continuous ambulatory peritoneal dialysis and hemodialysis: Comparison of patient mortality with adjustment for comorbid conditions. Kidney Int 1994; 45: 1163–1169.

[48] Fenton SSA, Schaubel DE, Morrison HI, Mayo Y, Copleston P, Jeffery JR, Kjellstrand CM: Hemodialysis vs peritoneal dialysis: A comparison of adjusted mortality rates. Am J Kidney Dis 1997; 30: 334–342.

[49] Foley RN, Parfrey PS, Harnett JD, Kent GM, O'Dea R, Murray DC, Barre' PE: Mode of dialysis and mortality in end stage renal disease. J Am Soc Nephrol 1998; 9: 267–276.

[50]   Salem M, Bower J: Hypertension in the hemodialysis population: Any relation to one year survival? Am J Kidney Dis 1996; 28: 737–740.

[51]   Zager PG, Nikolic J, Brown RH, Campbell MA, Hunt WC, Peterson D, Van Stone J, Levey A, Meyer KB, Klag MJ, Johnson HK, Clark E, Sadler JH, Teredesai P, for the Medical Directors of Dialysis Clinic, Inc.: "U" curve association of blood pressure and mortality in hemodialysis patients. Kidney Int 1998; 54: 561–569.

[52]   Port FK, Hulbert-Shearon TE, Wolfe RA, Bloembergen WE, Golper T, Agodoa LY, Young E: Pre-dialysis blood pressure and mortality risk in a national sample of maintenance hemodialysis patients. Am J Kidney Dis 1999; 33: 507–517.

[53]   Hakim R, Breillat J, Lazarus J, Port F: Complement activation and hypersensitivity reactions to dialysis membranes. N Engl J Med 1984; 311: 878-882.

[54]   Chatoth DK, Golper TA, Gokal R. Morbidity and mortality in redefining adequacy of peritoneal dialysis: a step beyond the National Kidney Foundation Dialysis Outcomes Quality Initiative. Am J Kidney Dis 1999; 33:617–32.

[55]   Maiorca R, Brunori G, Zubani R, Cancarini CG, Manili L, Camerini C, et al. Predictive value of dialysis adequacy and nutritional indices for mortality and morbidity in CAPD and HD patients. A longitudinal study. Nephrol Dial Transplant 1995; 10:2295–305.

[56]   Churchill DN, Wayne T, Keshaviah PR, for CANADAUSA Peritoneal Dialysis Study Group. Adequacy of dialysis and nutrition in continuous peritoneal dialysis: association with clinical outcomes. J Am Soc Nephrol 1996; 7:198–207.

[57]   Lameire N, Van Biesen W. The impact of residual renal function on the adequacy of peritoneal dialysis. Perit Dial Int 1997; 17(Suppl 2):S102–10.

[58]   Tatterstall JE, Doyle S, Greenwood RN, Farrington K. Maintaining adequacy in CAPD by individualizing the dialysis prescription. Nephrol Dial Transplant 1994; 9:749–52.

[59]   Harty J, Boulton H, Venning M, Gokal R. Impact of increasing dialysis volume on adequacy targets: a prospective study. J Am Soc Nephrol 1997; 8:1304–10.

[60]   Bargman JM, Thorpe KE, Churchill DN, for CANUSA Peritoneal Dialysis Study Group. The importance of residual renal function for survival in patients on peritoneal dialysis (Abstract). J Am Soc Nephrol 1997; 8 (Suppl):185A.

[61]   Diaz-Buxo JA, Lowrie EG, Lew NL, Zhang SM, Zhu X, Lazarus JM. Associates of mortality among peritoneal dialysis patients with special reference to peritoneal transport rates and solute clearance. Am J Kidney Dis 1999; 33:523–34.

[62]   Lameire N. Cardiovascular risk factors and blood pressure control in continuous ambulatory peritoneal dialysis. Perit Dial Int 1993; 13(Suppl 2):S394–5.

[63] Bergström J, Furst P, Alvestrand A, Lindholm B. Protein and energy intake, nitrogen balance and nitrogen losses in patients treated with continuous ambulatory peritoneal dialysis. Kidney Int 1993; 44:1048–57.

[64] Jones MR. Etiology of severe malnutrition: results of an international cross-sectional study in continuous ambulatory peritoneal dialysis patients. Am J Kidney Dis 1994; 23:412–20.

[65] McCusker FX, Teehan BP, Thorpe KE, Keshaviah PR, Churchill DN, for CANUSA Peritoneal Dialysis Study Group. How much peritoneal dialysis is required for the maintenance of a good nutritional state? Kidney Int 1996; 50 (Suppl 56):S56–61.

[66] Rottembourg J. Residual renal function and recovery of renal function in patients treated by CAPD. Kidney Int 1993; 43(Suppl 40): S106–10.

[67] Cancarini GC, Brunori G, Camerini G, Brassa A, Manili L, Maiorca R. Renal function recovery and maintenance of residual diuresis in CAPD and hemodialysis. Perit Dial Bull 1986; 6:77–9.

[68] Lysaght MJ, Vonesh EF, Gotch F, Ibels L, Keen M, Lindholm B, et al. The influence of dialysis treatment modality on the decline of remaining renal function. Trans Am Soc Artif Intern Organs 1991; 37:598–604.

[69] Feber J, Scharer K, Schaefer F, Mikova M, Janda J. Residual renal function in children on hemodialysis and peritoneal dialysis therapy. Pediatr Nephrol 1994; 8:579–83.

[70] Lutes R, Perlmutter J, Holley JL, Bernardini J, Piraino B. Loss of residual renal function in patients on peritoneal dialysis. Adv Perit Dial 1993; 9:165–8.

[71] Hiroshige K, Yuu K, Soejima M, Takasugi M, Kuroiwa A. Rapid decline of residual renal function in patients on automated peritoneal dialysis. Perit Dial Int 1996; 16:307–15.

[72] Hufnagel G, Michel C, Queffeulou G, Skhiri H, Damieri H, Mignon F. The influence of automated peritoneal dialysis on the decrease in residual renal function. Nephrol Dial Transplant 1999; 14:1224–8.

[73] Shin SK, Noh H, Kang SW, Seo BJ, Lee IH, Song HY, et al. Risk factors influencing the decline of residual renal function in continuous ambulatory peritoneal dialysis patients. Perit Dial Int 1999; 19:138–42.

[74] Shemin D, Maaz D, St. Pierre D, Kahn SI, Chazan JA. Effect of aminoglycoside use on residual renal function in peritoneal dialysis patients. Am J Kidney Dis 1999; 34:14–20.

[75] Singal MK, Bashkaran S, Vidgen E, Bargman JE, Vas SI, Oreopoulos DG. Rate of decline of residual renal function in patients on continuous peritoneal dialysis and factors affecting it. Peritoneal Dialysis International, 2000; 20:429–438.

[76] Tzamaloukas AH, Murata GH, Malhotra D, Fox L, Goldman RS. An analysis of determinants of urinary urea and creatinine clearance in patients on continuous peritoneal dialysis. Adv Perit Dial 1997; 13:38–41.

[77] Misra M, Vonesh EF, Churchill DN, Moore H, Van Stone JC, Nolph KD. Preservation of glomerular filtration rate on dialysis when adjusted for patient drop out. Kidney Int 2000; 57:691–6.

[78] Iest CG, Vanholder RC, Ringoir SM. Loss of residual renal function in patients on regular hemodialysis. Int J Artif Organs 1989; 12:159–64.

[79] Davies SJ, Phillips L, Naish PF, Russell GI. Influence of primary diagnosis on the evolution of residual renal function and peritoneal solute transport in PD patients (Abstract). J Am Soc Nephrol 1997; 8:205A.

[80] Bommer J. Prevalence and socio-economic aspects of chronic kidney disease. Nephrol Dial Transplant. 2002; 17 (suppl 11): 8 – 12.

[81] Chadban SJ, Briganti EM, Kerr PG, Dunstan DW, Welborn TA, Zimmet PZ, et al. Prevalence of kidney damage in Australian adults the AusDiab Kidney Study. J Am Soc Nephrol. 2003; 14 (suppl 2): S131– S138.

[82] Stewart JH , McCredie MR, Williams SM, Jager KJ, Trpeski L, Mc-Donald SP. Trends in incidence of treated end-stage renal disease, overall and by primary renal disease, in persons aged 20-64 years in Europe, Canada and the Asia-Paci_c region, 1998–2002. Nephrology (Carlton). 2007; 12: 520 – 527.

[83] Wakai K, Nakai S, Kikuchi K, Iseki K, Miwa N, Masakane I, et al. Trends in incidence of end-stage renal disease in Japan, 1983–2000: age-adjusted and age-speci_c rates by gender and cause. Nephrol Dial Transplant. 2004; 19: 2044 – 2052.

[84] Najafi I, Shakeri R, Islami F, Malekzadeh F, Salahi R, Yapan-Gharavi M, Hosseini M, Hakemi M, Alatab S, Rahmati A, Broumand B, Malekzadeh R. Prevalence of Chronic Kidney Disease and its Associated Risk Factors: The First Report from Iran Using Both Microalbuminuria and Urine Sediment. Archives of Iranian Medicine, 2012; 15: 70-75.

[85] Bakris GL. Slowing nephropathy progression: Focus on proteinuria reduction. Clin J Am Soc Nephrol 2008; 3 Suppl 1: S3-S10.

[86] Peterson JC, Adler S, Burkart JM, Greene T, Hebert LA, Hunsicker LG, King AJ, Klahr S, Massry SG, Sefter JL. Blood pressure control, proteinuria, and the progression of renal disease. The Modification of Diet in Renal Disease Study. Ann Int Med 1995; 123: 754-762.

[87] De Zeew D, Remuzzi G, Parving HH, Keane WF, Zhang Z, Shahinfar S, Snapping S, Cooper ME, Mitch WE, Brenner BM. Proteinuria, a target for renoprotection in patients with type 2 diabetic nephropathy: Lessons from RENAAL. Kidney Int 2004; 65: 2309-2320.

[88] de Zeeuw, D. Albuminuria: A Target for Treatment of Type 2 Diabetic Nephropathy. Seminars in Nephrology 2007; 27: 70-74.

[89] Lattanzio MR, Weir MR. Have we fallen off target with concerns surrounding dual RAAS blockade?. Kidney Int 2010; 78: 539-545.

[90] Irie F, Iso H, Sairenchi T, Fukasawa N, Yamagishi K, Ikehara S, Kanashiki M, Saito Y, Ota H, Nose T: The relationships of proteinuria, serum creatinine, glomerular filtration rate with cardiovascular disease mortality in Japanese general population. Kidney Int 2006; 69: 1264–1271.

[91] Abbate M, Zoja C, Remuzzi G. How does proteinuria cause progressive renal damage? J Am Soc Nephrol 2006; 17: 2974-2984.

[92] GISEN: Randomized placebo-controlled trial effect of ramipril on decline in glomerular filtration rate and risk of terminal renal failure in proteinuric, non-diabetic nephropathy. Lancet 1997; 349: 1857–1863.

[93] Wapstra FH, Navis G, de Jong PE, de Zeeuw D. Prognostic value of the short-term antiproteinuric response to ACE inhibition for prediction of GFR decline in patients with nondiabetic renal disease. Exp Nephrol 1996; 4 (S 1): S47–S52.

[94] Lewis EJ, Hunsicker LG, Bain RP, Rohde RD. The effect of angiotensin-converting-enzyme inhibition on diabetic nephropathy. The Collaborative Study Group. N Engl J Med 1993; 329: 1456–1462.

[95] de Zeeuw D, Remuzzi G, Parving HH, et al. Albuminuria a therapeutic target for cardiovascular protection in type 2 diabetic patients with nephropathy. Circulation 2004; 110: 921–927.

[96] Chobanian AV, Bakris GL, Black HR. Seventh Report of the Joint National Committee on prevention, detection, evaluation, and treatment of high blood pressure. Hypertension 2003; 42: 1206-1252.

[97] Bakris GL, Williams M, Dworkin L. Preserving renal function in adults with Hypertension and Diabetes: a consensus approach. National Kidney Foundation Hypertension and Diabetes Executive Committees Working Group. Am J Kidney Dis 2000; 36: 646-661.

[98] De Zeew D, Remuzzi G, Parving HH, Keane WF, Zhang Z, Shaninfar S, Snappin S, Cooper ME, Mitch WE, Brenner BM. Albuminuria, a therapeutic target for cardiovascular protection in type 2 diabetic patients with nephropathy. Circulation 2004; 110: 921-927.

[99] KDOQI clinical practice guidelines and clinical practice recommendations for diabetes and chronic kidney disease. Am J Kidney Dis 2007; 49 Suppl 2: S1-S179.

[100] Garg JP, Bakris GL. Microalbuminuria: marker of vascular dysfunction, risk factor for cardiovascular disease. Vasc Med 2002; 7: 35-43.

[101] Mancia G, De Backer G, Dominiczak A. 2007 Guidelines for the management of arterial hypertension: The Task Force for the management of arterial hypertension of the European Society of Hypertension (ESH) and of the European Society of Cardiology (ESC). J Hypertens 2007; 25: 1105-1187.

[102] Trimarchi H. Role of aliskiren in blood pressure control and renoprotection. International Journal of Nephrology and Renovascular Disease 2011; 4: 1-8.

[103] Stenvinkel, P. Endothelial Dysfunction and Inflammation—Is There a Link?. Nephrol Dial Transplant 2001: 16: 1968-1971.

[104] Festa A, D'Agostino R, Howard G, Mykkanen L, Tracy RP, Haffner SM. Inflammation and Microalbuminuria in Non-Diabetic and Type 2 Diabetic Subjects: The Insulin Resistance Atherosclerosis Study. Kidney Int 2000; 58: 1703-1710.

[105] Breyer JA, Bain RP, Evans JK, Nahman NS Jr, Lewis EJ, Cooper M, McGill J, Berl T: Predictors of the progression of renal insufficiency in patients with insulin-dependent diabetes and overt diabetic nephropathy. The Collaborative Study Group. Kidney Int 1996; 50: 1651–1658.

[106] Tarver-Carr M, Brancati F, Eberhardt MS, Powe N: Proteinuria and the risk of chronic kidney disease (CKD) in the United States. J Am Soc Nephrol 2000; 11: 168A.

[107] Irie F, Iso H, Sairenchi T, Fukasawa N, Yamagishi K, Ikehara S, Kanashiki M, Saito Y, Ota H, Nose T: The relationships of proteinuria, serum creatinine, glomerular filtration rate with cardiovascular disease mortality in Japanese general population. Kidney Int 2006; 69: 1264–1271.

[108] Wapstra FH, Navis G, de Jong PE, de Zeeuw D: Prognostic value of the short-term antiproteinuric response to ACE inhibition for prediction of GFR decline in patients with nondiabetic renal disease. Exp Nephrol 4[Suppl 1]: 47–52, 1996

[109] Ruggenenti P, Perna A, Remuzzi G: Retarding progression of chronic renal disease: The neglected issue of residual proteinuria. Kidney Int 2003; 63: 2254–2261.

[110] Bjorck S, Mulec H, Johnsen SA, Norden G, Aurell M: Renal protective effect of enalapril in diabetic nephropathy. BMJ 1992; 304: 339–343.

[111] Brenner BM, Cooper ME, de Zeeuw D, Keane WF, Mitch WE, Parving H-H, Remuzzi G, Snapinn SM, Zhang Z, Shahinfar S: Effects of losartan on renal and cardiovascular outcomes in patients with type 2 diabetes and nephropathy. N Engl J Med 2001; 345: 861–869.

[112] Lewis EJ, Hunsicker LG, Clarke WR, Berl T, Pohl MA, Lewis JB, Ritz E, Atkins RC, Rohde R, Raz I: Renoprotective effect of the angiotensin-receptor antagonist irbesartan in patients with nephropathy due to type 2 diabetes. N Engl J Med 2001; 345: 851–860.

[113] Jafar TH, Stark PC, Schmid CH, Landa M, Maschio G, Marcantoni C, de Jong PE, de Zeeuw D, Shahinfar S, Ruggenenti P, Remuzzi G, Levey AS: Proteinuria as a modifi-

able risk factor for the progression of non-diabetic renal disease. Kidney Int 2001; 60: 1131–1140.

[114] Jafar TH, Schmid CH, Landa M, Giatras I, Toto R, Remuzzi G, Maschio G, Brenner BM, Kamper A, Zucchelli P, Becker G, Himmelmann A, Bannister K, Landais P, Shahinfar S, de Jong PE, de Zeeuw D, Lau J, Levey AS: Angiotensinconverting enzyme inhibitors and progression of nondiabetic renal disease. A meta-analysis of patient-level data. Ann Intern Med 2001; 135: 73–87.

[115] Ruggenenti P, Schieppati A, Remuzzi G: Progression, remission, regression of chronic renal diseases. Lancet 2001; 357: 1601–1608.

[116] Abbate M, Zoja C, Morigi M, Rottoli D, Angioletti S, Tomasoni S, Zanchi C, Longaretti L, Donadelli R, Remuzzi G: Transforming growth factor-beta1 is up-regulated by podocytes in response to excess intraglomerular passage of proteins. Am J Pathol 2002; 161: 2179–2193.

[117] Abbate M, Zoja C, Remuzzi G. How Does Proteinuria Cause Progressive Renal Damage? J Am Soc Nephrol 2006; 17: 2974–2984.

[118] Anavekar NS, Pfeffer MA. Cardiovascular Risk in Chronic Kidney Disease. Kidney Int 2004; 92: (S92): S11- S15.

[119] Tonelli M, Pfeffer MA. Kidney Disease and Cardiovascular Risk. Ann Rev Med 2007; 58: 123-139.

[120] Trimarchi H, Muryan A, Dicugno M, Young P, Forrester M, Lombi F, Pomeranz V, Iriarte R, Raña MS, Alonso M. Proteinuria: An ignored marker of inflammation and cardiovascular disease in chronic hemodialysis International Journal of Nephrology and Renovascular Disease 2012; 5: 1-7.

[121] Goldwasser P, Kaldas AI, Barth RH. Rise in serum albumin and creatinine in the first half year on hemodialysis. Kidney Int 1999; 56: 2260-2268.

[122] Trimarchi H, Muryan A, Martino D, Toscano A, Iriarte R, Campolo-Girard V, Forrester M, Pomeranz V, Fitzsimons C, Lombi F, Young P, Raña M, Alonso M· Creatinine-vs cystatin c-based equations compared with ^{99m}TcDTPA scyntigraphy to assess glomerular filtration rate in chronic kidney disease. Journal of Nephrology 2012; doi: 10.5301/jn.5000083 (Accessed 17 August 2012)

[123] Yeun JY, Levine RA, Mantadilok V, Kaysen GA. C-reactive protein predicts all-cause and cardiovascular mortality in hemodialysis patients. Am J Kidney Dis 2000; 35: 469-476.

[124] Li D, Keffer J, Corry K. Nonspecific elevation of troponin T levels in patients with chronic kidney failure. Clin Biochem 1995; 28: 474-477.

[125] Francis GS, Tang WH. Cardiac troponins in renal insufficiency and other non-ischemic cardiac conditions. Prog Cardiovasc Dis 2004; 47: 196-206.

[126] Fernandez-Reyes MJ, Mon C, Heras M. Predictive value of troponin T levels for is-
       chemic heart disease and mortality in patients on hemodialysis. J Nephrol 2004; 17:
       721-727.

[127] Kanderian AS, Francis GS. Cardiac troponins and chronic kidney disease. Kidney Int
       2006; 69: 1112-1114.

[128] Mallamaci F, Zoccali C, Parlongo S. Troponin is related to left ventricular mass and
       predicts all-cause and cardiovascular mortality in hemodialysis patients. Am J Kid-
       ney Dis 2002; 40: 68-75.

[129] de Filippi C, Wasserman S, Rosanio S. Cardiac troponin T and C-reactive protein for
       predicting prognosis, coronary atherosclerosis, and cardiomyopathy in patients un-
       dergoing long-term hemodialysis. JAMA 2003; 290: 353-359.

[130] Wong CK, Szeto CC, Chan MHM, Leung CB, LI PKT, Lam WK. Elevation of Pro-In-
       flammatory cytokines, C-Reactive Protein and cardiac Troponin T in chronic renal
       failure patients on dialysis. Immunol Invest 2007; 36: 47-57.

[131] Kuo HK, Al Snih S, Kuo YF, Raji MA. Cross-sectional associations of albuminuria
       and C-reactive protein with functional disability in older adults with diabetes. Diabe-
       tes Care 2011; 34:710-717.

[132] Salmon AHJ, Ferguson JK, Burford JL, Gevorgyan H, Nakano D, Harper SJ, Bates
       DO, Peti-Peterdi J. Loss of the Endothelial Glycocalyx Links Albuminuria and Vascu-
       lar Dysfunction. J Am Soc Nephrol 2012; 23: 1339-1350.

Chapter 8

Glycemic Control in Diabetic Patients on Long-Term Maintenance Dialysis

Pornanong Aramwit and Bancha Satirapoj

Additional information is available at the end of the chapter

1. Introduction

The epidemiology of end-stage renal disease (ESRD) varies considerably worldwide. In Thailand, the incidence of ESRD on renal replacement therapy (RRT) increased from 78.9 per million populations in 1999 to 552.8 per million populations in 2009. The yearly incidence of all RRT modalities increased by an average of 34.8% from 2007 to 2009 [1]. According to the estimation by the International Diabetes Foundation, by the year 2025 the frequency of diabetes is expected to increase threefold worldwide [2]. Diabetic nephropathy is the most common cause of ESRD [3], representing 30-47% of the United States and Asian populations undergoing long-term maintenance hemodialysis [4, 5]. Disparities in the incidence of ESRD due to diabetes among ethnic groups have existed for many years, but the magnitude may be increasing.

In the United States, from 1990 to 1996, the age-adjusted diabetes-related ESRD incidence increased from 299.0 to 343.2 per 100,000 diabetic patients. However, from 1996 to 2006, the age-adjusted diabetes-related ESRD incidence decreased by 3.9% per year from 343.2 to 197.7 per 100,000 diabetic patients [6]. Diabetes-related ESRD incidence in the diabetic population has declined in all age-groups, probably because of a reduction in the prevalence of ESRD risk factors, improved treatment and care, and other factors. An alternative explanation for the decline in diabetes-related ESRD incidence in the diabetic population might be that the patients are not surviving long enough to develop ESRD, which occurs typically between 10 and 15 years after the onset of the disease. Premature mortality among ESRD patients with diabetes as a result of the increasing prevalence of coronary heart disease and stroke by tenfold could reduce the number of people who ultimately develop ESRD [7, 8]. Even though diabetes-related ESRD incidence in the population with diabetes has decreased since 1996, diabetes-related ESRD incidence in the general population and the number of persons initiating treatment for kidney failure each year who have diabetes listed as a primary cause continue to increase [5, 9]. In Europe, data from the European Renal Association-European Dialysis and Transplant Association (ERA-EDTA) Registry shows an 11.9% annual increase in patients with type 2 diabetes entering RRT [10]. The most recent report of the Thailand RRT Registry shows a prevalence of diabetes among patients with ESRD of 47.6% and an incidence of 47.7%. The majority of patients with ESRD secondary to diabetes (51.0%) are treated by hemodialysis, 45.1% by peritoneal dialysis, and 3.9% have functioning renal transplants [1].

Diabetes-related ESRD is a costly and disabling condition with a high mortality rate. These patients are at a higher risk of mortality, mostly from cardiovascular complications, than other patients with diabetes. Apart from cardiac complications, the patients are subject to a wide range of vascular (e.g., peripheral vascular disease, stroke) and infectious complications. Patients with ESRD due to diabetes challenge the nephrologists because they have the greatest number of comorbid conditions, and the greatest dependency during daily activities. The goal of therapy is to improve quality of life, as well as reduce mortality. Attention to several basic principles helps to guide therapy: control of hypertension, control of hyperglycemia, control of lipid abnormalities, treatment of malnutrition, and attention to the effects of erythropoietin. Current cardio- and renoprotective treatment for diabetic nephropathy without ESRD includes optimization of glycemic control. Early intensive glycemic interventions reduce cardiovascular events as well as nephropathy by about half when compared with a conventional glycemic treatment. However, hypoglycemia is common because of impaired renal gluconeogenesis, malnutrition, chronic inflammation, decrease renal insulin clearance and the increased half-life of hypoglycemic agents [11]. Therefore, data are scarce on how diabetes should best be treated in patients in ESRD. In this chapter, we summarize the current evidence for glucose metabolism and glycemic control in diabetic patients on dialysis.

2. Glucose metabolism in dialysis

Hyperglycemia is an important factor in the progression of diabetic nephropathy. Early functional changes in diabetic nephropathy include glomerular hyperfiltration, glomerular and tubular epithelial hypertrophy, and the development of microalbuminuria, followed by the development of glomerular basement membrane (GBM) thickening, accumulation of mesangial matrix, and overt proteinuria, eventually leading to glomerulosclerosis and ESRD. Hyperglycemia-induced metabolic and hemodynamic pathways are recognized to be mediators of kidney injury [4].

Glucose transport activity is an important modulator of extracellular matrix formation by mesangial cells. Glucose transporter-1 (GLUT-1) regulates glucose entry into renal cells. Glucose and its metabolites subsequently activate metabolic pathways, and these pathways contribute to mesangial expansion and mesangial cell matrix-production, mesangial cell apoptosis and structural changes [12]. This may result from a similar increase in the mesangial cell glucose concentration, since similar changes in mesangial function can be induced in a normal glucose milieu by over-expression of GLUT1 [13]. Multiple biochemical pathways have been postulated that explain how hyperglycemia causes tissue damage including: non-enzymatic glycosylation that generates advanced glycosylation end products (AGE); activation of protein kinase C (PKC); and acceleration of the polyol pathway. Oxidative stress also seems to be a common theme. These pathways ultimately lead to increased renal albumin permeability and extracellular matrix accumulation, resulting in increasing proteinuria, glomerulosclerosis and ultimately renal fibrosis.

In ESRD, both uremia and dialysis can complicate blood glucose control by affecting the secretion, clearance, and peripheral tissue sensitivity of insulin. The abnormal glucose homeostasis in patients with dialysis is postulated to be multifactorial issues as Figure 1.

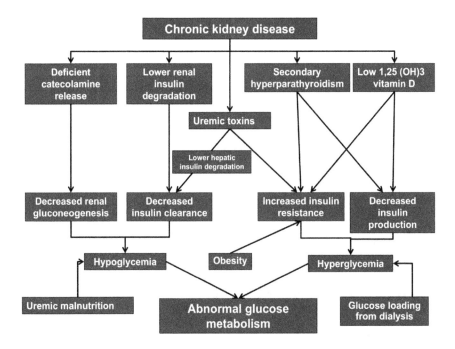

Figure 1. Contribution factors for the abnormal glucose metabolism in dialysis patients.

2.1. Hyperglycemia: Increased insulin resistance and decrease insulin production in dialysis

Advanced-stage chronic kidney disease (CKD) or ESRD can show mild fasting hyperglycemia and abnormal glucose tolerance, suggesting that the uremic state alters glucose homeostasis [14]. Insulin resistance is also frequently recognized in uremic patients and is a predictor of cardiovascular mortality in ESRD patients [15]. Impaired insulin sensitivity in the absence of overt diabetes play a central role in the development of atherosclerotic vascular disease [16]. Several clinical studies have noted impaired tissue sensitivity to insulin in diabetic nephropathy [17], and non-diabetic patients exhibit only mild to moderate reductions in renal function [18-20] and in ESRD [21, 22]. However, impaired insulin sensitivity in both dialysis groups after long-term dialysis was still higher than that of the non-dialysis ESRD group while no significant differences were noted between peritoneal dialysis and hemodialysis treatments [23]. The mechanism of increased insulin resistance in patients with kidney disease is not fully understood. Several factors, including uremic toxins, may increase insulin resistance in ESRD, leading to a blunted ability to suppress hepatic gluconeogenesis and regulate peripheral glucose utilization. In addition, in non-diabetic CKD patients, an independent factor for insulin resistance was the amount of total body fat and body mass index [20]. This change occurs in ESRD because of concomitant metabolic acidosis, deficiency of 1,25 dihydroxy-vitamin D, and secondary hyperparathyroidism. In addition, in uremic patients, previous studies have reported that treatment with hemodialysis, active vitamin D, erythropoietin and angiotensin receptor blocker can improve insulin insensitivity [21, 24-26].

Further complicating the effect of dialysis is the glucose load provided by both dialysis modalities. The dextrose concentration in the dialysate can also affect glucose control. In hemodialysis population, dialysates with lower dextrose concentrations are used and may be associated with hypoglycemia. Conversely, dialysates with higher dextrose concentrations are occasionally used in hypoglycemic patients on hemodialysis and low ultrafiltration patients on peritoneal dialysis (PD), but this can lead to hyperglycemia and insulin resistance [27].

2.2. Hypoglycemia: Decreased insulin clearance and renal gluconeogenesis in dialysis

Decreasing insulin requirements and frequent hypoglycemia also occur in diabetic patients on dialysis. Renal insulin clearance decreases as glomerular filtration rate decreases to less than 15 to 20 mL/min/1.73 m^2 [14]. Hepatic clearance of insulin is also decreased in patients with uremia. In addition, deficient gluconeogenesis along with malnutrition, deficient catecholamine release, and impaired renal insulin degradation and clearance, can contribute to frequent hypoglycemia in patients with CKD [28, 29].

Thus, advanced CKD and ESRD on dialysis exert opposing forces on insulin secretion, action, and metabolism, often creating unpredictable serum glucose values. Some patients who have insulin resistance would need more supplemental insulin. In contrast, the reduced renal gluconeogenesis and insulin clearance seen in ESRD may result in less requirement for insulin treatment. Together, all of these factors contribute to wide fluctuations in plasma glucose levels and increase the risk of both hyperglycemic and hypoglycemic events. Both of these abnormalities are at least partially reversed with the institution of dialysis. As a result, the insulin requirement in any given patient will depend upon the net balance between improving insulin secretion and insulin sensitivity, and restoring normal hepatic insulin metabolism.

3. Glycemic control in dialysis

Glycemic therapy in patients with diabetes has been shown to improve outcomes, especially microvascular complications in patients without kidney disease [30, 31]. The efficacy of glycemic control depends in part upon the stage at which it is begun and the degree of normalization of glucose metabolism. Glycemic control can partially reverse the glomerular hypertrophy and hyperfiltration that are thought to be important pathogenic pathways for diabetic nephropathy, and decrease the incidence of new-onset microalbuminuria in retrospective [32] and prospective studies of patients with diabetes [31, 33]. Progression of established overt nephropathy can also be stabilized or retarded through strict glycemic control. However, proving the efficacy of this treatment is difficult, and previous studies examining outcomes of glycemic control in dialysis patients gave conflicting results [34]. The benefit of glucose control on progression in patients with CKD who have advanced kidney disease is less well studied.

Interestingly, benefits of glycemic control after pancreas transplantation in patients with type 1 diabetes were observed: mesangial matrix volume, thickening of glomerular and tubular basement membranes, and nodular glomerular lesions were significantly decreased and/or returned to normal compared to the same measurements at zero and ten years [35, 36].

Effects of intensive glycemic control on prevention of macrovascular complications (e.g., coronary artery disease, peripheral artery disease, cerebrovascular disease) are less certain, particularly in type 2 diabetes. The 10-year follow-up study of patients with type 2 diabetes in the United Kingdom Prospective Diabetes Study (UKPDS) demonstrated risk reduction for myocardial infarction and death from any cause [37]. More recent studies, including the Action to Control Cardiovascular Risk in Diabetes (ACCORD), Action in Diabetes and Vascular Disease: Preterax and Diamicron MR Controlled Evaluation (ADVANCE), and the Veterans Affairs Diabetes Trial (VA-DT) that targeted even lower hemoglobin A_{1c} (HbA_{1c}) goals (<6–6.5%), failed to show cardiovascular disease risk reduction with more intensive glycemic control regimens [38-40].

Several observational studies showed that higher levels of hemoglobin A_{1c} were associated with higher mortality rates in patients with diabetes on long-term dialysis and CKD [41-44]. A previous study demonstrated that a paradoxically lower unadjusted mortality associated with greater hemoglobin A_{1c} levels were found in 23,618 dialysis patients with diabetes. However, after adjusting for markers of malnutrition and inflammation, hemodialysis patients with hemoglobin A_{1c} levels <5% or >7% became associated with greater mortality [45]. The data indicate that competing risk factors related to malnutrition, muscle wasting, and anemia may confound the association between glycemic control and survival in diabetic patients with long-term dialysis. In the study by Williams, hemoglobin A_{1c} levels >11.0% in type 1 diabetes on hemodialysis were required to observe a statistically significant higher mortality risk, but few subjects had hemoglobin A_{1c} levels in this category [46]. In a recent cohort of 54,757 diabetic hemodialysis patients, poor glycemic control (hemoglobin A_{1c} ≥8% or serum glucose ≥200 mg/dL) appears to be associated with high all-cause and cardiovascular death and very low glycemic levels (hemoglobin A_{1c} <7%) are also associated with high mortality risk [47]. In a single interventional study in 83 dialysis patients, patients in the intensive intervention group experienced improved quality of life and a decreased need for amputations and hospitalizations [48]. Larger clinical trials are needed to conclusively prove the concept that better glycemic control is beneficial in patients with advanced CKD. To date, there are no data available from randomized clinical trials targeting different hemoglobin A_{1c} levels and powered for cardiovascular events or mortality in ESRD populations. Careful evaluation of the relationship of hemoglobin A_{1c} with these outcomes in ESRD patients should be a high priority for future research to determine the risks and benefits of different hemoglobin A_{1c} targets.

The Kidney Disease Outcomes Quality Initiative (KDOQI) foundation state that target hemoglobin A_{1c} for people with diabetes should be <7%, irrespective of presence or absence of CKD. This recommendation is in line with diabetes management in the general population [11]. However, very few studies have addressed the benefits and risks of intensive glycemic control in late stages of CKD and ESRD. Recent evidence from randomized studies has highlighted the potential risks of aggressive glycemic control in non-ESRD diabetic populations [38, 39]. Moreover, because many dialysis patients are wasting, malnourished, and non-ambulatory, they may be less able to respond appropriately to hypoglycemia. Current evidence suggests that aggressive glycemic control cannot be routinely recommended for all diabetic hemodialysis patients on the basis of reducing mortality risk. Physicians are encouraged to individualize glycemic targets based on potential risks and benefits in diabetic ESRD patients.

The guidelines of the 2012 American Diabetes Association recommend lowering hemoglobin A_{1c} to below or around 7% for many adults, and to implement this soon after the diagnosis of diabetes that is associated with long-term reduction in macrovascular disease [49]. Providers might reasonably suggest more stringent hemoglobin A_{1c} goals (such as <6.5%) for selected individual patients, if this can be achieved without significant hypoglycemia or other adverse effects of treatment. Appropriate patients might include those with short duration of diabetes, long life-expectancy, and no significant cardiovascular disease. Less stringent hemoglobin A_{1c} goals (such as <8%) may be appropriate for patients with a history of severe hypoglycemia, limited life- expectancy, advanced microvascular or macrovascular complications, extensive comorbid conditions, and those with longstanding diabetes in whom the general goal is difficult to attain [49]. Therefore, providers should be vigilant in preventing severe hypoglycemia in patients with advanced kidney disease or ESRD and should not aggressively attempt to achieve near-normal hemoglobin A_{1c} levels in patients in whom such a target cannot be reasonably easily and safely achieved.

4. Monitoring of glycemia in dialysis

Glucose homeostasis is altered significantly in patients with uremia. Glycated hemoglobin (expressed as a percentage of total hemoglobin) or hemoglobin A_{1c} measurement is used as an indicator of integrated glucose control. Glycated hemoglobin is formed by the non-enzymatic reaction between glucose and the N-terminal amino group on the beta chain of hemoglobin. The good correlation between hemoglobin A_{1c} and blood glucose in non-CKD type 1 diabetic patients has been documented in the Diabetes Control and Complications Trial (DCCT) [50]. At present, this test is the most accurate method to assess chronic glycemic control based on clinical outcomes associated with certain hemoglobin A_{1c} levels in diabetic patients with normal kidney function [31]. The validity of glycated hemoglobin and hemoglobin A_{1c} has not been rigorously studied in patients with ESRD. These tests may be unreliable in dialysis patients because of assay interference due to the elevated blood urea nitrogen. Glycated hemoglobin tests, such as column- and ion-exchange chromatography and agar gel electrophoresis, are affected by uremia. This is due in part to analytical interference from carbamylated hemoglobin formed in the presence of elevated concentrations of urea, leading to false elevations in the hemoglobin A_{1c} level. Use of agarose affinity chromatography or the thiobarbituric acid method for analyzing hemoglobin A_{1c} can be used reliably in patients with ESRD. Other factors such as shorter life span of red blood cells, iron deficiency anemia, and recent transfusion may also cause underestimation of glucose control in diabetic hemodialysis patients (Table 1). In addition, patients treated with erythropoietin could lead to underestimation of glycemic control by using hemoglobin A_{1c} level, because of the greater proportion of young erythrocytes in the circulation of patients [51]. Therefore, hemoglobin A_{1c} levels tend to underestimate glycemic control in diabetic patients undergoing long-term maintenance hemodialysis [52, 53].

Falsely increased hemoglobin A_{1c}	Falsely decreased hemoglobin A_{1c}
Carbamylated hemoglobin for charge-dependent chromatography assays	Erythropoiesis supplement
Increased glycosylation rate	Shortened life span of red blood cells
Uremia	Blood transfusions
Metabolic acidosis	Hemoglobinopathy

Table 1. Glycated hemoglobin levels in dialysis patients

Despite anemia and shortened RBC lifespan in ESRD patients, hemoglobin A_{1c} in the range of 6% to 7% estimates glycemic control similarly to patients without severe renal impairment. Hemoglobin A_{1c} above 7.5% may overestimate hyperglycemia in patients with ESRD [43]. It is important to be aware of the specific assay used and the other factors affecting the accuracy of hemoglobin A_{1c} measurements in ESRD on hemodialysis and peritoneal dialysis.

Another potential method to monitor glycemic control in patients with uremia is glycated albumin. Some studies suggest that glycated albumin more accurately reflects glycemic control in diabetic hemodialysis patients than hemoglobin A_{1c} [54, 55]. However, falsely increased glycated albumin values have been measured in the presence of lipemia, hemolysis, and high bilirubin and uric acid concentrations. In addition, use of glycated albumin is hampered by conditions that alter protein metabolism including ESRD, their lack of availability in routine practice and the lack of established reference levels [56].

Despite the limitations in using hemoglobin A_{1c} in the dialysis population, this test is considered a reasonable measure of chronic glycemic control in this group. Patient self-monitoring of blood glucose is also available for patients to assess the effectiveness of the management plan on glycemic control. It provides real-time assessments of glycemic control and results of self-monitoring of blood glucose can be useful in preventing hypoglycemia and adjusting medications (particularly prandial insulin doses), and physical activity. There are some limitations of this method, because it is subject to errors from poor technique, problems with the meters and strips, and lower sensitivity in measuring low blood glucose levels. However, hemoglobin A_{1c} does not provide a measure of glycemic variability or hypoglycemia. Thus, for patients prone to glycemic variability (especially type 1 patients, or type 2 patients with severe insulin deficiency), glycemic control is best judged by the combination of results of self-monitoring of blood glucose testing and the hemoglobin A_{1c} assay [49]. Hemoglobin A_{1c} may also serve as a check for the accuracy of the patient's meter and the adequacy of the self-monitoring schedule of blood glucose testing.

5. Insulin therapy in dialysis

Insulin regulates glucose homeostasis at many sites, reducing hepatic glucose output by decreasing gluconeogenesis and glycogenolysis, and increasing the rate of glucose uptake, primarily into muscle and adipose tissue. Insulin affects cells through binding to its receptor on the surface of insulin-responsive cells. The stimulated insulin receptor phosphorylates itself, and several substrates including membranes of the insulin receptor substrate family and initiate downstream signaling events [27].

In healthy non-diabetic people, the pancreatic β-cells secrete half of the daily insulin requirement (approximately 0.5 units/kilogram/day) at a steady basal rate independent of glucose levels and the other half is secreted in response to prandial glucose stimulation [57]. Insulin is secreted into the portal system, it passes through the liver where approximately 75% is metabolized with the remaining 25% metabolized by the kidneys. About 60% of the insulin in the arterial bed is filtered by the glomerulus and 40% is actively secreted into the nephric tubules [58]. Most of the insulin in the tubules is metabolized into amino acids, and only 1% of insulin is secreted intact.

Interestingly, endogenous insulin is substantially degraded by the liver but exogenous insulin is eliminated mainly by the kidney. For diabetic patients receiving exogenous insulin, renal metabolism plays a more significant role since there is no first-pass metabolism in the liver. Insulin is freely filtered at the glomerulus and extensively reabsorbed in the proximal tubule after enzyme degradation into smaller peptides. As renal function starts to decline, insulin clearance does not change appreciably, due to compensatory peritubular insulin uptake [59]. However, once the glomerular filtration rate drops below 20 mL/min, insulin clearance decreases and the half-life of insulin increases, an effect compounded by a decrease in the hepatic metabolism of insulin that occurs in uremia [25]. Glucose and insulin homeostasis are altered in CKD patients even in the early stages of CKD, leading to insulin resistance by various pathways. Studies even in the 1980s showed that, although insulin secretion in CKD is normal, a decreased tissue sensitivity to insulin is responsible for the abnormal glucose uptake [60]. In advanced CKD, particularly in stages 4 and 5, significant metabolic derangements in insulin metabolism occur. Several factors have been implicated in the pathogenesis of insulin resistance including anemia, dyslipidemia, uremia, malnutrition, excess of parathyroid hormone, vitamin D deficiency, metabolic acidosis, and increase in plasma free fatty acids and proinflammatory cytokines. Thus, despite the increase in insulin resistance caused by renal failure, the net effect is a reduced requirement for exogenous insulin in ESRD patients [61]. Despite similar duration of disease and clinical characteristics, patients with type 2 diabetes with ESRD often show marked heterogeneity in terms of insulin requirement and dosages [62]. However, predictors for exogenous insulin requirement in patients with type 2 diabetes undergoing continuous ambulatory peritoneal dialysis (CAPD) have not been defined. Possible factors include β-cell function, endogenous metabolism and elimination of insulin, insulin resistance, body size, carbohydrate intake, and extra glucose absorbed from dialysate fluid [27].

Recent evidence showed that insulin is a anti-inflammatory hormone that suppresses several proinflammatory transcription factors such as nuclear factor κB (NF-κB), early growth response protein 1 and activating protein 1, which all mediate inflammation. An impairment of the action of insulin because of insulin resistance would therefore result in the activation of these proinflammatory transcription factors and in an increase of the expression of the corresponding genes. Derangements in other biologic effects of insulin could be associated with certain pathologic states in CKD such as hypertension and insulin resistance [63, 64].

Previous studies have shown that uremia was associated with an insulin-resistant state, mainly because of decreased insulin-stimulated uptake of glucose by muscle [65]. However, in clinical practice, with progressive renal failure, the insulin requirements of patients with diabetes for glycemic control often tend to decrease [66]. The determinants of insulin requirements in patients with diabetes with ESRD remain uncertain. This can be influenced by factors such as insulin resistance, production and metabolism of endogenous insulin, oral intake, extra carbohydrate absorbed from dialysis solution, and reduction of body weight in uremic patients [27, 67]. Possible factors for this reduction in insulin requirement include reduced renal clearance of both endogenous and exogenous insulin and progressive loss of appetite and body weight in uremic patients. However, several studies have shown similar fasting insulin levels between patients with renal failure and those with normal renal function [27, 68].

In PD patients, the development of insulin resistance after a initial improvement is generally attributed to a high glucose load absorbed from dialysis fluid, contributing to a wide spectrum of metabolic abnormalities including hypertriglyceridemia, poor glycemic control, new-onset diabetes, hypertension and central obesity. An amplifying loop in the process of glucose absorption appears to be a consequence of the modifications in the peritoneum associated with a loss of ultrafiltration capacity [69]. Disturbances of carbohydrate metabolism seem to be even more intense in non-diabetic PD patients than in hemodialysis patients. After PD initiation, a large number of patients developed new-onset hyperglycemia because of their exposure to hypertonic glucose solutions [27, 70, 71]. In fact, glucose absorption through the peritoneum results in significantly higher serum glucose levels than are produced by an equivalent dose of oral dextrose. Wong et al. show considerable variations in the need for insulin treatment and dosages in patients with type 2 diabetes undergoing CAPD despite similar disease duration, dialysis regimens, renal function, and glycemic control [67]. Duration of diabetes, hemoglobin A_{1c} level, and body weight were independent determinants of insulin requirement of patients with type 2 diabetes with ESRD patients undergoing CAPD. Dialysis regimen with estimated amount of glucose absorbed and Kt/V did not predict insulin requirement in these patients. Insulin resistance, insulin requirement, and fasting C-peptide levels, a crude measurement of basal pancreatic β-cell function in patients with diabetes with normal renal function, were not affected by dialysis dosage, reflected by a similar value of Kt/V [67]. Insulin-treated patients had lower C peptide concentrations than non-insulin-treated patients, and insulin dosage required was correlated with duration of diabetes mellitus, implying the significance of β-cell function in determination of insulin requirement in patients with type 2 diabetes with ESRD.

Insulin injection therapy remains the mainstay treatment to achieve good glycemic control in diabetic patients receiving hemodialysis therapy [72]. In hemodialysis patients, the insulin sensitivity normally improves on both an acute and chronic basis [66], mainly by clearing circulating urea, and also insulin clearance. The concentration of glucose and insulin is frequently affected by the dialysis procedure itself. Changes in glucose will vary with the concentration of glucose (dextrose) in the dialysis fluid, to which the patient's blood is indirectly exposed. Because glucose transfers to the dialysate according to its concentration gradient, dialysate lacking glucose is associated with significant decreases in plasma glucose levels in poorly and well-controlled diabetic patients as well as in some non-diabetic patients, and is no longer used. Plasma insulin levels also are decreased during the hemodialysis treatment, due to clearance by dialysis which varies among membranes and with the fall in glucose. Additional metabolic effects of dialysis include improvement in sensitivity to insulin and decrease in some cases of counter-regulatory hormones (e.g., growth hormone). In poorly controlled patients, hemodialysis-induced clearance of plasma immunoreactive insulin levels may result in hyperglycemia in the post-dialysis period [63].

Various insulin preparations are available in the market. In ESRD patients, insulin doses will need to be reduced, especially after dialysis has been initiated [63]. Sobngwi et al. show that the daily insulin needs on the day after hemodialysis should be decreased approximately 15% compared with the daily insulin needs before hemodialysis, with a significant reduction of basal hourly insulin requirement by 25%, unchanged boluses, and unchanged body weight-indexed total insulin dose in a group of type 2 diabetic patients on maintenance hemodialysis [73]. However, no evidence for the benefit of neutral protamine hagedorn (NPH) insulin or other long-acting insulin in patients with ESRD is available. On the other hand, insulin lispro which has a short onset of action and a short duration of action shows the benefit not only facilitate the correction of hyperglycemia but may also decrease the risk of late hypoglycemic episodes, which is of increased relevance in hemodialysis patients [64] because its pharmacokinetics is less affected in renal failure [74]. Long-acting insulin such as insulin glargine or NPH insulin can be widely used as basal requirements, along with a rapid-acting insulin analogue such as lispro or insulin aspart before meals two or three times daily [57]. When the glomerular filtration rate drops between 10 and 50 mL/min, the total insulin dose should be reduced by 25%. Once the filtration rate is below 10 mL/min, as in ESRD patients, the insulin dose should be decreased by 50% from the previous amount [75].

Unexpected hypoglycemia often occurs in dialysis patients during basal-bolus insulin therapy despite careful adjustment of their insulin dose which may due to 3 main factors: (1) prolongation of the elimination half-life of insulin associated with decreased renal degradation and excretion [68]; (2) impairment of gluconeogenesis by the kidneys and (3) weak gastric peristalsis in diabetic patients on dialysis, with prolongation of stomach food retention, resulting in delays in glucose absorption [76]. It is important to note that the signs and symptoms of hyperglycemia are modified in patients with ESRD [63]. Signs and symptoms of hyperglycemia may involve thirst, fluid overload, and hyperkalemia rather than polyuria. Lacking polyuria, patients experience volume expansion, not contraction; excessive thirst will result in large weight gains, which correlate with poor glycemic control between dialysis treatments. Severe hyperglycemia may result in hyperkalemia and complicate management further. Other findings may be pulmonary edema, hypertension, anorexia, altered mental status, nausea, vomiting, and gastroparesis, although symptoms are frequently nonspecific or lacking.

6. Oral antihyperglycemic drugs in dialysis

Therapeutic options for patients with diabetes with CKD and ESRD are limited because a reduced glomerular filtration rate results in the accumulation of certain drugs and/or their metabolism [77]. Most of oral antihyperglycemic drugs include the insulin secretagogues such as sulfonylureas and meglitinides, biguanides, thiazolidinediones, and alpha-glucosidase inhibitors are contraindicated in ESRD patients. However, some agents have been used in patients with CKD and were found to be effective and safe even in those on dialysis. Therefore, some medications may be useful therapeutic options for the management of diabetes in CKD.

As shown in Table 2, insulin secretagogues can be classified as sulfonylureas and meglitinides while alpha-glucosidase inhibitors are modifiers of glucose absorption and thiazolidinediones are insulin sensitizers. Incretin-related therapies include dipeptidylpeptidase-4 (DPP-4) inhibitors and incretin mimetics. DPP-4 inhibitors are oral antidiabetic agents, whereas incretin mimetics are used by subcutaneous injection.

Since many drugs bind to serum protein, primarily albumin and plasma concentration of albumin in patients with renal impairment is commonly decreased, the concentrations of unbound drugs are increased.

Sulfonylureas

Insulin secretagogues increase endogenous insulin levels. These agents work by binding to sulfonylurea receptors or nearby sites, resulting in closure of ATP-sensitive potassium channels of the pancreatic β-cell, depolarization of the cell membranes, calcium influx, and subsequently insulin release [72]. They have a wide volume of distribution and are highly protein-bound. However, only the unbound drug exerts a clinical effect. Because of high protein binding property, dialysis cannot effectively clear elevated levels of sulfonylurea drugs. As these agents increase endogenous insulin levels, they are associated with an increased risk of hypoglycemia. This risk is mitigated when shorter-acting agents are used. Furthermore, many ESRD patients take drugs such as sulfonamides, vitamin K antagonists, beta-blocker, salicylates and fibric acid derivatives which may displace sulfonylureas from albumin, thus increasing the risk of severe hypoglycemia.

Category	Action	Group	Medication	Medication	Medication	Dosing recommendation CKD stage 3, 4 or kidney transplant	Dialysis dose recommendation
Insulin	Sensitizers	Biguanides	Metformin			Contraindicated with kidney dysfunction defined as sCr ≥1.5 mg/dL in men or ≥1.4 mg/dL in women	Avoid
Insulin	Sensitizers	TZDs (PPAR)	Pioglitazone			No dose adjustment needed	No dose adjustment needed
Insulin	Sensitizers	TZDs (PPAR)	Rivoglitazone			No dose adjustment needed	No dose adjustment needed
Insulin	Sensitizers	TZDs (PPAR)	Rosiglitazone			No dose adjustment needed	No dose adjustment needed
Insulin	Sensitizers	Dual PPAR agonist	Aleglitazar			Use with caution	Use with caution
Insulin	Sensitizers	Dual PPAR agonist	Muraglitazar			Use with caution	Use with caution
Insulin	Sensitizers	Dual PPAR agonist	Tesaglitazar			Use with caution	Use with caution
Insulin	Secretagogues	K+ ATP	Sulfonylureas	1st generation	Acetohexamide	Avoid	Avoid
Insulin	Secretagogues	K+ ATP	Sulfonylureas	1st generation	Carbutamide	Avoid	Avoid
Insulin	Secretagogues	K+ ATP	Sulfonylureas	1st generation	Chlorpropamide	Reduce dose by 50% when GFR<70 and 50%mL/min/1.73m² and avoid when GFR<50 mL/min/1.73 m²	Avoid
Insulin	Secretagogues	K+ ATP	Sulfonylureas	1st generation	Metahexamide	Avoid	Avoid
Insulin	Secretagogues	K+ ATP	Sulfonylureas	1st generation	Tolbutamide	Avoid	Avoid
Insulin	Secretagogues	K+ ATP	Sulfonylureas	1st generation	Tolazamide	Avoid	Avoid
Insulin	Secretagogues	K+ ATP	Sulfonylureas	2nd generation	Glipizide	Preferred, no dose adjustment needed	Preferred, no dose adjustment needed
Insulin	Secretagogues	K+ ATP	Sulfonylureas	2nd generation	Gliclazide	Preferred, no dose adjustment needed	Preferred, no dose adjustment needed
Insulin	Secretagogues	K+ ATP	Sulfonylureas	2nd generation	Glyburide	Avoid	Avoid
Insulin	Secretagogues	K+ ATP	Sulfonylureas	2nd generation	Glimepiride	Initiate at low dose, 1 mg daily	Avoid
Insulin	Secretagogues	K+ ATP	Meglitinides	Nateglinide		Initiate at low dose, 60 mg before each meal	No dose adjustment needed
Insulin	Secretagogues	K+ ATP	Meglitinides	Repaglinide		No dose adjustment needed, initiate at 0.5 mg dose when GFR<40 mL/min/1.73 m²	No dose adjustment needed
Insulin	Secretagogues	K+ ATP	Meglitinides	Mitiglinide		No dose adjustment needed	
Insulin	Secretagogues	GLP-1 analogs (Incretin Mimetics)	Exenatide			Not recommended in patients with GFR<30 mL/min/1.73 m² and caution should be applied when GFR<30 and< 50 mL/min/1.73 m²; No dose adjustment needed when GFR<50 and <80 mL/min/1.73 m²	Avoid
Insulin	Secretagogues	GLP-1 analogs (Incretin Mimetics)	Liraglutide			No dose adjustment needed	No dose adjustment needed
Insulin	Secretagogues	DPP-4 inhibitors	Alogliptin			Reduce dose by 50% (12.5 mg/day) when GFR<50 and 30 mL/min/1.73 m² and by 75% (6.25 mg/day) when GFR<30 mL/min/1.73 m²	Reduce dose by 75% (6.25 mg/day)
Insulin	Secretagogues	DPP-4 inhibitors	Linagliptin			No dose adjustment needed	No dose adjustment needed
Insulin	Secretagogues	DPP-4 inhibitors	Sexagliptin			Moderate to severe kidney impairment should receive<2.5 mg/d	Moderate to severe kidney impairment should receive<2.5 mg/d
Insulin	Secretagogues	DPP-4 inhibitors	Sitagliptin			Reduce dose by 50% (50 mg/day) when GFR<50 and 30%mL/min/1.73 m² and by 75% (25 mg/day) when GFR<30 mL/min/1.73 m²	Reduce dose by 75% (25 mg/d)
Insulin	Secretagogues	DPP-4 inhibitors	Vildagliptin			Initiate at low dose	Initiate at low dose

Category	Action	Group	Medication	Medication	Medication	Dosing recommendation CKD stage 3, 4 or kidney transplant	Dialysis dose recommendation
Insulin	Analogs/other insulins	Rapid-acting	Regular			Preferred, normally no dose adjustment needed	Preferred, normally no dose adjustment needed but depends on dialysis factors as well
Insulin	Analogs/other insulins	Rapid-acting	Lispro			Preferred, normally no dose adjustment needed	Preferred, normally no dose adjustment needed but depends on dialysis factors as well
Insulin	Analogs/other insulins	Rapid-acting	Aspart			Preferred, normally no dose adjustment needed	Preferred, normally no dose adjustment needed but depends on dialysis factors as well
Insulin	Analogs/other insulins	Long-acting	NPH			Dose adjustment needed depends on individual factors	Reduce dose by 25% when GFR 10-50 mL/min and by 50% when GFR<10 mL/min
Insulin	Analogs/other insulins	Long-acting	Glargine			Dose adjustment needed depends on individual factors	Reduce dose by 25% when GFR 10-50 mL/min and by 50% when GFR<10 mL/min
Insulin	Analogs/other insulins	Long-acting	Determir			Dose adjustment needed depends on individual factors	Reduce dose by 25% when GFR 10-50 mL/min and by 50% when GFR<10 mL/min
Insulin	Analogs/other insulins	Premixed	70/30 human mix			Dose adjustment needed depends on individual factors	Dose adjustment needed depends on individual factors
Insulin	Analogs/other insulins	Premixed	70/30 aspart mix			Dose adjustment needed depends on individual factors	Dose adjustment needed depends on individual factors
Insulin	Analogs/other insulins	Premixed	75/25 lispro mix			Dose adjustment needed depends on individual factors	Dose adjustment needed depends on individual factors
Others	Alpha-glucosidase inhibitor		Acarbose			Not recommended in patients with sCr>2 mg/dL	Avoid
Others	Alpha-glucosidase inhibitor		Miglitol			Not recommended in patients with sCr>2 mg/dL	Avoid
Others	Alpha-glucosidase inhibitor		Vogibose			Not recommended in patients with sCr>2 mg/dL	Avoid
Others	Amylin analog		Pramlintide			No dose adjustment needed for GFR 20-50 mL/min/1.73 m^2	No data available
Others	SGLT2 inhibitor		Canagliflozin			No data available	No data available

* Modify from Masanori Abe, Kazuyoshi Okada and Masayoshi Soma "Antidiabetic agents in patients with chronic kidney disease and end-stage renal disease on dialysis: metabolism and clinical practice" Current Drug Metabolsim Volume 12, January 2011, with permission.

Table 2. Oral anti-diabetic drugs and insulin analogs

The first-generation sulfonylureas-chlorpropamide, acetohexamide, tolbutamide, and tolaza-mide are almost exclusively excreted by the kidney and are therefore contraindicated in ESRD patients [78]. Second-generation agents include glimepiride and glyburide which are metab-olized in the liver. However, their active metabolites are excreted in the urine and so these medications should be avoided in ESRD patients as well [72] but low-dose initiation can be used in patients with CKD [79]. Glipizide and gliclazide are the preferred agents and no dose adjustment has been necessary in a dialysis population [11].

Most sulfonylureas are not suitable for ESRD patients due to the risk of prolonged hypogly-cemic; furthermore, metformin is contraindicated [80]. From all medications in this group, the only sulfonylurea recommended in ESRD patients are glipizide and gliclazide which are also metabolized in the liver but has inactive or weakly active metabolites excreted in the urine [57]. Glipizide is eliminated primarily by hepatic biotransformation; < 10% of a dose is excreted as unchanged drug in urine or feces while approximately 90% is excreted as biotransformation products in urine (80%) and feces (10%). The major metabolites of glipizide are products of aromatic hydroxylation that have no hypoglycemic activity. A minor metabolite which accounts for < 2% of a dose, an acetylamino-ethyl benzene derivative, is reported to have 1/10 to 1/3 of the hypoglycemic activity compared to the parent compound. The suggested dose of glipizide is 2.5 to 10 mg/day. In ESRD patients, sustained-release forms should be avoids due to the concerns of hypoglycemia [81].

Meglitinides

Repaglinide, nateglinide and mitiglinide are insulin secretagogues that stimulate pancreat-ic β-cells. They are currently in clinical use because of their rapid onset of action result-ing in improvement in hyperglycemia. Like sulfonylureas, nateglinide is hepatically metabolized, with renal excretion of active metabolites. On the other hand, repaglinide is almost completely converted to inactive metabolites in the liver, and less than 10% is excreted by the kidneys [82, 83]. Nateglinide still pose a risk of hypoglycemia especially in ESRD patients. Because of that, this drug is not recommended to use in patients on hemodialysis [82, 83]. However, mitiglinide shows selective action on the ATP-sensitive potassium channel of pancreatic β-cells and the order of affinity is mitiglinide > repagli-nide > nateglinide [84]. This result suggests that mitiglinide induces insulin secretion by specifically acting on pancreatic β-cells and has few unwanted effects on the cardiovascu-lar system. Because mitiglinide is rarely accompanied by hypoglycemia, it may be an attractive therapeutic option for patients undergoing dialysis [85]. However, the optimal daily dose of mitiglinide is suggested to be lower in the diabetic hemodialysis patients than that in the diabetic patients with normal kidney function. Mitiglinide has the potential to reduce the number of type 2 diabetics on hemodialysis who ultimately require insulin injection therapy. The daily dose of mitiglinide (23 mg) was adequate, as evidenced by the fact that it was able to induce significant reductions in glycemic parameters such as fasting plasma glucose, hemoglobin A_{1c}, glycated albumin, and homeostasis model assessment for insulin resistance (HOMA-IR) levels [86]. This suggests that appropriate blood glucose levels can be maintained even at a low dose of mitiglinide, not only during the postprandial period but also before meals, due to the prolonged half-life of mitiglinide in patients on dialysis compared with the half-life in those with normal renal function. Abe et al. reported that mitiglinide significantly improved glycemic control, triglyceride levels and interdialytic weight gain even when administered for only a short duration [87]. Thus, mitiglinide not only improved hemoglobin A_{1c} and glycated albumin, the overall index of glycemic control in type 2 diabetes, but also effectively improved fasting plasma glucose in dialysis patients [72, 85].

Biguanides

Metformin, the drug of choice for many patients with type 2 diabetics, is a biguanide that reduces hepatic gluconeogenesis and glucose output. Metformin does not cause increase insulin levels, but rather decreases hepatic glucose output by suppressing fasting gluconeogenesis. It is absorbed via the small intestine and the absolute bioavailability is approximately 50-60%. Intravenous single-dose studies in normal subjects demonstrate that metformin is excreted unchanged in the urine and does not undergo hepatic metabolism or biliary excretion [88]. Renal clearance of metformin is approximately 3.5-fold greater than creatinine clearance, which indicates that tubular secretion via human organic cation transporter 2 is the major route of metformin elimination [89]. Single-dose and steady-state pharmacokinetics of metformin were compared between patients with normal renal function (CrCl > 90 mL/min), mild impaired renal function (CrCl 61-90 mL/min) as well as moderate (CrCl 31-60 mL/min) and severe impaired renal function (CrCl 10-30 mL/min). The results show that in patients with moderate to severe impaired renal function, C_{max} and AUC are increased 173% and 390%, respectively, compared to the patients with normal renal function [89]. In patients with decreased renal function, based on the measurement of CrCl, the plasma half-life of metformin is prolonged and renal clearance is decreased in proportion to the decrease in CrCl [89]. Therefore, metformin should be avoided in patients with moderate to severe CKD including those on dialysis since the risk of metformin accumulation and lactic acidosis increases in line with the degree of impairment of renal function [90].

Thiazolidinediones

Rosiglitazone and pioglitazone are highly potent, selective agonists that work by binding to and activating a nuclear transcription factor, specifically, peroxisome proliferator-activated receptor gamma (PPAR-gamma) which improves insulin resistance in type 2 diabetic patients [91, 92] as well as increase glucose uptake in muscles and adipose tissue, and decrease hepatic glucose production [92, 93]. Both rosiglitazone and pioglitazone have an adequate oral bioavailability and are extensively metabolized by the liver. Rosiglitazone is mainly metabolized by CYP2C8 into inactive metabolites and < 1% of the parent drug appears in the urine in unchanged form [80, 94]. The half-life of rosiglitazone is similar in patients with ESRD and in healthy individuals, and can therefore be administered to ESRD patients without dose adjustment or risk of causing hypoglycemia [95-97]. Pioglitazone is metabolized by CYP3A4 and CYP2C8/9 [98]. Metabolites of pioglitazone are more active than those of rosiglitazone and are excreted predominantly in bile. The pioglitazone metabolites do not accumulate in CKD. The pharmacokinetics profile of pioglitazone was found to be similar in healthy subjects and patients with moderately or severely impaired renal function who did not require dialysis [98]. Moreover, in patients who did require dialysis, pioglitazone was found to have a T_{max} of 1.8 h and a half-life of 5.4 h [98]. Therefore, a post-dialysis supplementary dose is not required, and pioglitazone can be administered irrespective of the time of dialysis. Due to the high molecular weight (392 Da), high protein-binding capacity (> 98%) and predominant hepatic metabolism of pioglitazone, its pharmacokinetics is similar in patients with normal renal function and CKD, and in those undergoing dialysis therapy. The main adverse reaction of these agents is edema, especially when they are used in combination with insulin. Because of that, a joint statement of the American Diabetes Association and the American Heart Association recommends avoiding thiazolidinediones in patients in New York Heart Association class III or IV heart failure [99]. Moreover, caution is required in patients in compensated heart failure (New York Heart Association class I or II) or in those at risk of heart failure such as patients with history of myocardial infarction or angina, hypertension, left ventricular hypertrophy, significant aortic or mitral value disease, age greater than 70 years, or diabetes for more than 10 years [99].

Thiazolidinediones have been reported to (1) reduce insulin requirements, (2) ameliorate albuminuria (3) have various roles in lipid metabolism, fibrinolysis, platelet aggregation and coagulation, (4) protect against impairment of endothelial function and (5) have an anti-inflammatory effect [100-103]. When used for the clinical management of type 2 diabetes and ESRD, thiazolidinediones are primarily metabolized in the liver and will not accumulate in patients with CKD. They might also improve uremia-associated insulin resistance and confer benefits at the metabolic, inflammatory, vascular, and hemodynamic levels [100]. The efficacy of this drug in patients with normal renal function is similar to the efficacy in those with mild to moderate renal impairment [104]. Administration of pioglitazone is also associated with mean decreases in triglyceride levels and mean increases in high-density lipoprotein (HDL)-cholesterol without consistent changes in the mean levels of total cholesterol or low-density lipoprotein (LDL)-cholesterol in non-uremic patients [105].

Thiazolidinediones are known to reduce HOMA-IR and levels of high-sensitivity C-reactive protein (hs-CRP) and tumor necrosis factor-alpha (TNF-α), and increase adiponectin levels in patients not undergoing dialysis [72]. In patients undergoing PD, thiazolidinediones have been reported to reduce hs-CRP levels, but levels of interleukin-6 (IL-6) and TNF-α were not reduced [91, 102]. In a short-term study of dialysis patients, thiazolidinediones are reported to reduce the levels of hs-CRP but not adiponectin [106]. It has been reported that pioglitazone treatment reduced the levels of hs-CRP, IL-6 and TNF-α and increased the high-molecular weight adiponectin level even in hemodialysis patients [107]. Moreover, the dosage of erythropoiesis-stimulating agents was significantly reduced during pioglitazone treatment with improvement in insulin resistance and a decrease in the levels of inflammatory cytokines [107].

It can be concluded that even though ESRD and dialysis do not affect the metabolism of thiazolidinediones, the medications in this group are not recommended in ESRD patients due to the associated risk of fluid accumulation and precipitation of heart failure.

Alpha-glucosidase inhibitors

Enzyme alpha-glucosidase is located in the gut and hydrolyzed oligosaccharides, trisaccharides and disaccharides into glucose in the brush border of the small intestine. The antihyperglycemic action of alpha-glucosidase inhibitors results from the reversible inhibition of membrane-bound intestinal alpha-glucoside hydrolase enzymes. Alpha-glucosidase inhibitors decrease the rate of breakdown of complex carbohydrates so that less glucose is absorbed and postprandial hyperglycemia is lowered but they do not enhance insulin secretion. The main side effects are gastrointestinal including flatulence and diarrhea.

Acarbose and miglitol slow carbohydrate absorption from the intestine. The levels of these drugs and their active metabolites are higher in patients with renal failure [80], and since data are scarce on the use of these drugs in ESRD, they are contraindicated in ESRD patients [11].

Acarbose is metabolized by intestinal bacteria and digestive enzymes exclusively within the gastrointestinal tract. Within 96 h of ingestion, 51% of an oral dose was excreted in the faces and unabsorbed drug-related radioactivity. Because acarbose acts locally within the gastrointestinal tract, low systemic bioavailability of the parent compound is therapeutically desirable. A fraction of these metabolites (about 34% of the dose) was absorbed and subsequently excreted in urine. The major metabolites have been identified as 4-methylpyrogallol derivatives (such as sulfate, methyl, and glucuronide conjugates). Moreover, one metabolite (formed by cleavage of a glucose molecule from acarbose) also has alpha-glucosidase inhibitory activity. This metabolite, together with the parent compound, recovered from the urine, accounts for < 2% of the total administered dose. Although < 2% of an oral dose of acarbose was absorbed as active drug, patients with severe renal impairment (CrCl < 25 mL/min) attained increases about 5-fold higher for peak plasma concentration of acarbose and 6-fold higher for AUC values than subjects with normal renal function [108]. Because long-term clinical trials in diabetic patients with significant renal dysfunction have not been conducted, treatment of these patients with acarbose is not recommended [108].

Miglitol is not metabolized in humans or other animal species [109]. No metabolites have been detected in plasma, urine, or feces indicating a lack of either systemic or presystemic metabolism. Miglitol is eliminated by renal excretion as unchanged drug [109]. Patients with CrCl < 25 mL/min taking the miglitol 25 mg 3 times daily exhibited a greater than 2-fold increase in miglitol plasma levels when compared to subjects with CrCl > 60 mL/min [109]. Dose adjustment to correct for the increased plasma concentrations is not feasible because miglitol acts locally. However, treatment of patients with CrCl < 25 mL/min with miglitol is not recommended because the safety of miglitol in these patients has not yet been elucidated [109].

Glucagon-like peptide-1 analogues

The intestinal hormone glucagon-like peptide-1 (GLP-1) stimulates glucose-dependent insulin release from pancreatic β-cells in a glucose-dependent manner and inhibits inappropriate postprandial glucagon release. It also shows gastric emptying and reduces food intake. However, its meal-induced secretion is generally decreased in patients with type 2 diabetes, and this may contribute to the amplification of postprandial hyperglycemia [72]. GLP-1 is rapidly inactivated by the enzyme dipeptidylpeptidase-4 (DPP-4) [110].

Therefore, an effective way to potentiate postprandial GLP-1 response is the use of selective DPP-4 inhibitors [111, 112].

Table 2 shows some of the medications in this group.

Sitagliptin is a highly selective, oral, once-daily administration DPP-4 inhibitor approved for the treatment of patients with type 2 diabetes [113]. DPP-4 inhibitors slow the degradation and the inactivation of the incretins, GLP-1 and glucose-dependent insulinotropic polypeptide [110]. These two incretins regulate glucose homeostasis by stimulating insulin release, while GLP-1 also suppresses glucagon release [72]. Sitagliptin can be used as initial pharmacologic therapy for type 2 diabetes, as a second agent in those who do not respond to a single agent such as a sulfonylurea [114], metformin [115-117], or a thiazolidinedione [118] and as an additional agent when dual therapy with metformin and a sulfonylurea does not provide adequate glycemic control [114]. CYP3A4 is the major CYP isozyme responsible for the limited oxidative metabolism of sitagliptin, with some minor contribution from CYP2C8. Sitagliptin is primarily renally eliminated with approximately 80% of the oral dose excreted unchanged in the urine [119, 120]. Excretion is thought to be via active secretion and glomerular filtration [119, 121]. Following single oral doses of sitagliptin, plasma level increases with decreasing renal function, as determined by 24 h CrCl. Relative to subjects with normal or mildly impaired renal function, patients with moderate renal insufficiency (CrCl 30-50 mL/min), severe renal insufficiency (CrCl < 30 mL/min, not on dialysis) or ESRD on dialysis have approximately 2.3-fold, 3.8-fold, or 4.5-fold higher plasma sitagliptin exposures, respectively, and the C_{max} increased by 1.4-fold to 1.8-fold [122]. T_{max} is significantly increased in patients with ESRD, and the terminal half-life increased with decreasing renal function [72]. Compared with values in subjects with normal renal function, the terminal half-life values of sitagliptin in those with mild, moderate, and severe renal impairment, and ESRD were raised to 16.1, 19.1, 22.5 and 28.4 h, respectively, compared to 13.1 h in normal renal function patients [122]. The fraction of dose removed by dialysis was low with 13.5% and 3.5% for dialysis initiated at 4 and 48 h post dose, respectively. Plasma protein binding of 38% was not altered in uremic plasma from patients with renal impairment. Based on these data, in order to achieve plasma sitagliptin concentrations comparable to those in patients with normal renal function, sitagliptin dose adjustments are recommended for patients with type 2 diabetes and moderate to severe renal insufficiency, as well as for those with ESRD requiring dialysis [123]. The usual dose of sitagliptin is 100 mg orally once daily, with reduction to 50 mg for patients with a glomerular filtration rate of 30-50 mL/min, and 25 mg for patients with a glomerular filtration rate less than 30 mL/min [122]. Sitagliptin may be used at does of 25 mg daily in ESRD patients, irrespective of dialysis timing. However, some side effects have been found after administration of sitagliptin such as anaphylaxis, angioedema and Steven-Johnson syndrome. Moreover, the risk of hypoglycemia increases when sitagliptin is used with sulfonylureas.

Vildagliptin is not a CYP enzyme substrate and does not inhibit or induce CYP enzymes, it is unlikely to interact with co-medications that are substrates, inhibitors, or inducers of these enzymes [124, 125]. The efficacy of vildagliptin in humans against the DPP-4 enzyme also shows a low *in vivo* IC_{50} (4.5 nM), which suggests a higher potency than that reported for sitaliptin (IC_{50} 26 nM) [119, 126]. Elimination of vildagliptin mainly involves renal excretion of unchanged parent drug and cyano group hydrolysis with little CYP involvement, suggesting a low potential for drug-drug interaction when co-administered with CYP inhibitors/inducers.

In patients with mild, moderate and severe renal impairment and ESRD patients on hemodialysis, systemic exposure to vildagliptin was increased (C_{max} 8-66%; AUC 32-134%) compared to subjects with normal renal function [72]. However, changes in exposure to vildagliptin did not correlate with the severity of renal function. In contrast, exposure of the main metabolite increased with increasing severity of renal function (AUC 1.6- to 6.7-fold), but this effect has no clinically relevant consequences because the metabolite is pharmacologically inactive. The elimination half-life of vildagliptin is not affected by renal function and it is well-tolerated in this population [127]. According to the label, no dosage adjustment of vildagliptin is required in patients with mild renal impairment. In clinical practice, special precautions are advised for the use of this drug in patients with moderate to severe renal impairment, including those on dialysis [72].

Alogliptin was rapidly absorbed and slowly eliminated primarily via urinary excretion in healthy subjects. In patients with type 2 diabetes, alogliptin is also primarily excreted renally with a renal clearance rate of 165-254 mL/min which is slightly higher than the normal glomerular filtration rate, suggesting the occurrence of some active renal secretion. The results of a single-dose (50 mg) pharmacokinetics study in patients with renal impairment showed an increase in alogliptin exposure compared with healthy volunteers; approximately 1.7-, 2.1-, 3.2- and 3.8-fold increase in patients with mild, moderate, and severe renal impairment, and in patients with ESRD, respectively [127, 128]. According to this data, to achieve plasma alogliptin concentrations comparable to those in patients with normal renal function, alogliptin dose adjustments are recommended for patients with type 2 diabetes and moderate to severe renal insufficiency, including those with ESRD requiring dialysis [72].

Saxagliptin is another DPP-4 inhibitor and its metabolite is pharmacologically active which makes saxagliptin difference from other medications in this group. The metabolism of saxagliptin is primarily mediated by CYP3A4/5 and its major metabolite is also a selective, reversible, competitive DPP-4 inhibitor which is 50% less potent than saxagliptin [129]. Saxagliptin is cleared by both metabolism and renal excretion. However, the degree of renal impairment does not affect the C_{max} of saxagliptin or its major metabolite [127]. In subjects with mild renal impairment, AUC from time 0 to infinity (AUC_∞) values of saxagliptin and its major metabolite are 1.2- and 1.7-fold higher than mean AUC_∞ in controls, respectively, while they are 1.4- and 2.9-fold higher in subjects with moderate renal impairment. Corresponding value are 2.1- and 4.5-fold higher in those with severe impairment [127]. A 4-h dialysis section removes approximately 23% of saxagliptin dose, AUC_∞ values for saxagliptin and its major metabolite are correlated with the degree of renal impairment, whereas C_{max} values are not well correlated. Renal function should be assessed before initiating saxagliptin therapy and patients with moderate to severe kidney impairment should receive less than 2.5 mg of saxagliptin/day and this drug can still be taken after dialysis in patients with ESRD.

Linagliptin is extensively protein bound (> 80% at the therapeutic dose) which is unlike other DPP-4 inhibitors. Because DPP-4 is expressed in various tissues but soluble DPP-4 is also present in plasma, binding to soluble DPP-4 may influence the pharmacokinetics of linagliptin. High-affinity but readily saturable binding of linagliptin to its target DPP-4 primarily accounted for the concentration-dependent plasma-protein binding at therapeutic plasma concentrations of linagliptin [130]. Fecal elimination is the dominant excretion pathway of linagliptin with 84.7 and 58.2% of the dose whereas renal excretion accounted for 5.4 and 30.8% of the dose administered orally or intravenously, respectively [131]. Renal excretion of unchanged linagliptin is < 1% after administration of 5 mg [132]. As absolute bioavailability is determined to be around 30%, renal excretion is a minor elimination pathway of linagliptin at therapeutic dose levels (compared to other DPP-4 inhibitors) and accordingly, a dose adjustment in patients with renal impairment is not anticipated for linagliptin [72].

Incretin mimetics

GLP-1 belongs to the incretin class of hormones which exert an influence over multiple physiologic functions, including a rapid blood glucose-lowering effect in response to enteral nutrient absorption [72]. Native GLP-1 is rapidly metabolized by DPP-4 which is found in many tissues and cell types, as well as in the circulation [133]. Clearance of native GLP-1 and its metabolites is largely mediated by the kidneys [133]. Incretins, such as GLP-1, enhance glucose-dependent insulin secretion and exhibit other antihyperglycemic actions following their release into the circulation from the gut. Exenatide and liraglutide are GLP-1 receptor agonists that enhance glucose-dependent insulin secretion by pancreatic β-cells, suppress inappropriately elevated glucagon secretion and slow gastric emptying [72].

Exenatide is one of the drugs in this group. The amino acid sequence of exenatide is partially homologous to that of human GLP-1. Exenatide binds and activates the human GLP-1 receptor which leads to an increase in both glucose-dependent synthesis of insulin and secretion of insulin from pancreatic β-cells. Exenatide is a naturally occurring GLP-1 analogue that is resistant to degradation by DPP-4 and has a longer half-life. The kidney provides the primary route for elimination and degradation of exenatide [134]. Given subcutaneously, exenatide undergoes minimal systemic metabolism. In subjects with mild to moderate renal impairment (CrCl 30-80 mL/min), exenatide exposure is similar to that of subjects with normal renal function and no dose adjustment is required. However, in subjects with ESRD receiving dialysis, mean exenatide exposure increased by 3.4-fold compared to that of subjects with normal renal function. Exenatide is contraindicated in patients undergoing hemodialysis, ESRD or in patients who have glomerular filtration rate less than 30 mL/min and it should be used with caution in patients undergone renal transplantation [135]. In patients with ESRD receiving dialysis, single dose of 5 μg exenatide are not well tolerated due to gastrointestinal side effects. Due to the side effects of exenatide such as nausea and vomiting with transient hypovolemia, treatment may worsen renal function. Caution is required when initiating or escalating doses of exenatide from 5 μg to 10 μg in patients with moderate renal impairment (CrCl 30-50 mL/min) [72].

Liraglutide is a once-daily human GLP-1 analog and has a high degree of sequence identity to human GLP-1 [136, 137]. The half-life of liraglutide is approximately 13 h after subcutaneous injection [138] and its metabolism is similar to that of large peptides which is fully degraded in the body [137]. There is no evidence that kidney is a major organ for elimination. Its pharmacokinetics parameters are essentially independent of renal function [139]. Renal dysfunction is not found to increase exposure of liraglutide and patients with type 2 diabetes and renal impairment can be treated with standard regimens of liraglutide [72].

Amylin analogs

Currently, pramlintide is the only drug in this group which is administered by subcutaneous injection and it is a naturally occurring neuroendocrine hormone co-secreted with insulin by pancreatic β-cells [140]. Amylin regulates gastric emptying [141], suppresses inappropriate postprandial glucagon secretion [142] and reduces food intake [143]. Through the mechanism similar to those of amylin, pramlintide reduces postprandial glucose, improving overall glycemic control [144, 145] and increases satiety resulting in reduced food intake and weight loss [146-148]. The half-life of pramlintide in healthy subjects, which is metabolized primarily by the kidney, is approximately 48 min. Its primary metabolite has a similar half-life and is biologically active. Patients with moderate or severe renal impairment (CrCl > 20 to < 50 mL/min) do not show increased pramlintide exposure or reduced pramlintide clearance when compared with subjects with normal renal function. However, no data is available for dialysis patients and further clinical studies are warranted in this population.

Sodium glucose co-transporter 2 (SGLT2) inhibitors

The plasma glucose level below which nearly all filtered glucose is reabsorbed by the kidneys, and above which glucose is excreted in urine, is designated as the renal threshold for glucose (RT_G) [149]. In healthy individuals, virtually all filtered glucose is reabsorbed up to a plasma glucose level of approximately 10 mmol/L (180 mg/dL), thus defining RT_G [150, 151]. At plasma glucose levels higher than RT_G, the renal glucose reabsorptive capacity is saturated and the amount of glucose in urine increases proportionately to plasma glucose concentration [152]. By inhibiting the proximal renal tubule glucose transporter responsible for the majority of glucose reabsorption, sodium glucose co-transporter 2 (SGLT2) inhibitors are predicted to lower RT_G, thereby increasing urinary glucose excretion [149]. In patients with diabetes, reduction of RT_G is expected to increase urinary glucose excretion and lower plasma glucose concentrations. Unlike other antidiabetic agents which often cause weight gain, the glucose-lowering effect with SGLT2 inhibitors is accompanied by urinary loss of calories, potentially resulting in weight loss. Moreover, SGLT2 inhibitors do not target the major pathophysiological defects in type 2 diabetes mellitus-namely insulin resistance and impaired insulin secretion-they represent a potentially promising new option in the treatment of diabetes [153]. One of the drug in this category is canagliflozin. In preclinical studies, a single oral administration of 3 mg/kg of canagliflozin decreased plasma glucose levels independent of food intake in mice on a high-fat, hyperglycemic diet [153]. In normo-glycemic mice, canagliflozin administration led to a minimal change in plasma glucose levels. Sha et al. show that canagliflozin was well tolerated in healthy men across the range of single does studied up to 800 mg. By inhibiting SGLT2, canagliflozin treatment dose dependently decreased RT_G, leading to a dose-dependent increase in urinary glucose excretion [149]. However, no data on its safety and efficacy is available for CKD or dialysis patients and further clinical studies are warranted in this population.

7. Combination therapy

Saxagliptin plus metformin

In order to obtain the better control of plasma glucose level and decrease the side effect of some medications in renal patients, combination therapy has been used. Scheen reviewed the use of metformin plus saxagliptin in renal impairment patients [154]. Since saxagliptin's license was recently extended to include diabetic patients with moderate or severe renal impairment while metformin is still widely prescribed in patients with some degree of renal impairment in real life even though it is contraindicated, the pro and contra of using this combination in type 2 diabetic patients with renal impairment need to be reviewed. Some recent data suggested that both metformin and saxagliptin may be used safely in type 2 diabetic patients with mild-to-moderate renal impairment, provided that dose reduction is made appropriately according to individual CrCl [154]. Because of the absence of pharmacokinetics interactions between the two drugs, this should be also the case with the saxagliptin-metformin combination. In this population, DPP-4 inhibitors offer advantages compared with sulfonylureas, especially because of the absence of hypoglycemia [155, 156]. A retrospective subgroup analysis of data from five randomized, double-blind, placebo-controlled, multicenter, 24-week, Phase III trials showed that saxagliptin 5 mg once-daily monotherapy and as add-on therapy are associated with clinically relevant and significant efficacy for reducing hemoglobin A_{1c} in older patients ($\geq$ 65 years; CrCl: 80±20 mL/min) versus younger patients (< 65 years; CrCl: 119±40 mL/min) [157]. Furthermore, saxagliptin was well-tolerated in older patients with a low incidence of hypoglycemia and no weight gain. Normally, patients with type 2 diabetes and renal impairment are exposed to a higher risk of cardiovascular disease. Therefore, reducing cardiovascular risk in this population should be considered as a main objective and drugs that have proven their efficacy and safety in this regard should be preferred. Treatment with metformin in type 2 diabetic patients is associated with a lower cardiovascular morbidity and mortality, compared with alternative glucose-lowering drugs [158]. It has also been suggested that metformin might exert direct protective effects on the heart [159]. Since both metformin and saxagliptin are excreted via the kidney, dose adjustment is required in case of moderate-to-severe renal impairment (ca. half dose of saxagliptin). Due to major discrepancies exist between guidelines (metformin excluded in case of renal impairment because of the risk of lactic acidosis) and real life, physicians should weigh the benefit/risk ratio carefully before deciding to prescribe or withdraw this combination in renal patients.

DDP-4 inhibitor plus thiazolidinedione

Thiazolidinediones are currently considered as the most efficacious class of oral anti-diabetics [160]. However, they carry the burden of weight gain and hemodilution which may lead to cardiovascular complications. It has been considered that the use of a low dose thiazolidinedione in combination with DPP-4 inhibitor may reduce the risk of dose dependent side effects of thiazolidinediones such as weight gain and hemodilution while, simultaneously, this combination may be more effective owing to different mechanisms of action of thiazolidinediones and DPP-4 inhibitors. Roy et al. demonstrated that in aged *db/db* mice, a combination therapy of low dose rosiglitazone and vildagliptin is safer and equally efficacious when compared to the therapeutic dose of rosiglitazone [160]. The combination therapy (1 mg/kg/day of rosiglitazone plus 5 mg/kg/day of vildagliptin) showed similar efficacy as that of 10 mg/kg/day rosiglitazone in lowering random blood glucose. GLP-1 and insulin levels were found to be elevated significantly in both vildagliptin and combination treated groups following oral glucose load. Vildagliptin alone had no effect on random glucose and glucose excursion during oral glucose tolerance test in severely diabetic *db/db* mice. The combination treatment showed no significant increase in body weight as compared to the robust weight gain by therapeutic dose of rosiglitazone. Rosiglitazone at 10 mg/kg/day showed significant reduction in hematocrit, red blood cell count, hemoglobin pointing towards hemodilution associated with increased mRNA expression of Na^+, K^+-ATPase-α and epithelial sodium channel gamma in kidney. The combination therapy escaped these adverse effects. The results suggest that combination of DPP-4 inhibitor with low dose thiazolidinedione can interact synergistically to represent a therapeutic advantage for the clinical treatment of type 2 diabetes without the adverse effects of haemodilution and weight gain associated with thiazolidinediones.

DDP-4 plus metformin

The retrospective analysis by Banerji et al. found that the combination of vildagliptin and metformin in type 2 diabetic patients with mild renal impairment is safe and tolerable, similar to that in patients with normal renal function [161]. Furthermore these results were similar to those in patients receiving a combination of thiazolidinedione and metformin. Higher incidence of headache and rash was noted in both vildagliptin groups, whereas those with mild renal impairment receiving thiazolidinedione experienced a higher incidence of peripheral edema.

Mitiglinide plus voglibose

Unlike typical sulfonylurea agents, mitiglinide, a benzylsuccinic acid derivative, is a rapid- and short-acting insulinotropic sulfonylurea receptor ligand with rapid hypoglycemic action. It alleviates postprandial hyperglycemia and, as a result, improves overall glycemic control [162]. The blood concentration of mitiglinide rapidly increases after oral administration and the drug quickly disappears subsequently; therefore, it is unlikely to exert hypoglycemic effects early in the morning and between meals. Abe et al. demonstrated that add-on therapy of mitiglinide with voglibose may be a therapeutic option for achieving good glycemic control in type 2 diabetic hemodialysis patients with otherwise poor glycemic control [86]. The daily dose of mitiglinide is suggested to be lower in the diabetic hemodialysis patients than that in the diabetic patients with normal kidney function. At low dose (23 mg), mitiglinide was adequate to induce significant reductions in glycemic parameters such as fasting plasma glucose, hemoglobin A_{1c}, glycated albumin levels and HOMA-IR. Mitiglinide also significantly improved glycemic control, triglyceride level and interdialytic weight gain even when it was administered only for a short duration [86].

8. Effects of high-flux dialyzer membranes on plasma insulin

Nowadays, several types of high-flux dialyzer membranes are on the market. The normally used ones are made from polysulfone, polyethersulfone, cellulose triacetate, polymethylmethacrylate or polyester-polymer alloy. The mechanism of plasma insulin clearance by hemodialysis is mainly by adsorption rather than diffusion or convection since no insulin is not normally detected in either the dialysate or the ultrafiltrate fluid during hemodialysis [163]. Furthermore, the amount of insulin adsorbed differed depending on the dialyzer membrane used. The insulin levels during a dialysis session depend not only on insulin removal by dialysis but also on the secretion of insulin from the pancreatic β-cells; this in turn is determined by the changes in plasma glucose induced by dialysis and the ability of the β-cells to respond to these glucose changes [163]. Therefore, it was suggested that an increase in endogenous insulin secretion may occur in response to hemodialysis treatment, in particular with the polysulfone membrane. On the other hand, plasma glucose levels at the post-dialysis stage were mainly determined by the glucose concentration in the dialysate; this is because the molecular weight of glucose is very small, and glucose rapidly transmigrates across the membrane during hemodialysis treatment. Therefore, plasma glucose levels at the post-dialysis stage should be similar in the case of polysulfone, cellulose triacetate and polyester polymer alloy membranes, regardless of the type of high-flux membrane. However, in the insulin-dependent diabetes mellitus (IDDM) subjects, who lack endogenous insulin secretion, the insulin reduction rate was significantly higher when the polysulfone membrane was used compared with the cellulose triacetate and polyester-polymer alloy membranes. This is because these patients have no residual β-cell function, which is responsible for insulin secretion; therefore, if plasma insulin was removed by hemodialysis, these cells could not have maintained the patients' insulin levels. Hence, plasma insulin removal is highly significant in the case of diabetic hemodialysis patients with low C-peptide levels, particularly those with type 1 or 2 diabetes with a deteriorated β-cell function [164]. Higher doses of injected insulin or antidiabetic agents might be added in order to achieve good glycemic control in such patients, because the surplus insulin is removed by hemodialysis, particularly when the polysulfone dialyzer is used [163]. Therefore, patient monitoring of blood glucose on the day that hemodialysis is performed could be useful for self-assessment of glycemic state, and if hyperglycemia was recognized, and additional dose of injected insulin after hemodialysis should be considered.

Due to the development in dialyzer technology, it was found that the biocompatible dialyzer membrane used in hemodialysis patients not only causes less hemodialysis-induced inflammation but also achieves better clearance of uremic toxins and medium- to large-sized molecules [165]. Moreover, high-flux dialyzers have been shown to be superior in terms of attenuating hyperlipidemia and alleviating oxidative stress [166, 167]. There is a significant reduction in patients' plasma insulin at different time point with each type of membranes, because various biological reactions can occur in the course of contact between artificial materials and blood components in the extracorporeal circulation [163]. The clearance of plasma immunoreactive insulin (IRI), a biologically active molecule, is significantly higher in patients used polysulfone membrane than by other membranes such as polyethersulfone, cellulose triacetate, polymethylmethacrylate or polyester-polymer alloy [168]. Moreover, no clinical difference has been found in the reduction rate of IRI between hemodialysis treatments when using either polysulfone, polyethersulfone, cellulose triacetate or polymethylmethacrylate except for polyester-polymer alloy [168]. From these results, it suggests that hemodialysis patients with residual β-cell function, the course of treatment for diabetic control would be unaffected by the differences resulting from the type of membrane used. However, in diabetic hemodialysis patients, particularly in type 1 and type 2 with deteriorated β-cell function, these differences might be very significant. Higher doses of injected insulin might be required to achieve good glycemic control in hyperinsulinemic patients because the surplus insulin is removed by hemodialysis, specifically by polysulfone, polyethersulfone, cellulose triacetate or polymethylmethacrylate, excluding polyester-polymer alloy membrane dialyzer. Polysulfone membrane dialyzer may worsen glycemic control and switching to the polyester-polymer alloy membrane dialyzer which shows a lower IRI clearance rate might improve the glycemic control in hemodialysis patients.

9. Conclusion

Although diabetes is the most common cause of ESRD and diabetic control is considered as one of the most important factor to prolong patients' life and improve their quality of life, data are scarce on how diabetes should be best treated in patients with CKD or ESRD. Since the glycemic control and monitoring in CKD and ESRD patients is complex, patient education is also one of the key factors for successful treatment. Moreover, patients with diabetic nephropathy are especially susceptible to hypoglycemia and diabetic drug therapy requires special caution. Adjustment of the type of drugs used or dosage regimen should be individualized based on self-monitored blood glucose patterns.

Acknowledgements

We are grateful for the support from The Thailand Research Fund and Bentham Science Publishers for permission of copyrighted material (Table 2).

Author details

Pornanong Aramwit[1*] and Bancha Satirapoj[2]

*Address all correspondence to: aramwit@gmail.com

1 Bioactive Resources for Innovative Clinical Applications Research Unit and Department of Pharmacy Practice, Faculty of Pharmaceutical Sciences, Chulalongkorn University, Phaya-Thai Road, Phatumwan, Bangkok, Thailand

2 Division of Nephrology, Phramongkutklao Hospital and College of Medicine, Bangkok, Thailand

References

[1] Praditpornsilpa K, Lekhyananda S, Premasathian N, Kingwatanakul P, Lumpaopong A, Gojaseni P, et al. Prevalence trend of renal replacement therapy in Thailand: impact of health economics policy. J Med Assoc Thai. 2011;94 Suppl 4 S1-6.

[2] King H, Aubert RE, Herman WH. Global burden of diabetes, 1995-2025: prevalence, numerical estimates, and projections. Diabetes Care. 1998;21(9) 1414-1431.

[3] Coresh J, Selvin E, Stevens LA, Manzi J, Kusek JW, Eggers P, et al. Prevalence of chronic kidney disease in the United States. JAMA. 2007;298(17) 2038-2047.

[4] Satirapoj B. Review on pathophysiology and treatment of diabetic kidney disease. J Med Assoc Thai. 2010;93 Suppl 6 S228-241.

[5] Collins AJ, Foley RN, Chavers B, Gilbertson D, Herzog C, Johansen K, et al. 'United States Renal Data System 2011 Annual Data Report: Atlas of chronic kidney disease & end-stage renal disease in the United States. Am J Kidney Dis. 2012;59(1 Suppl 1) A7, e1-420.

[6] Burrows NR, Li Y, Geiss LS. Incidence of treatment for end-stage renal disease among individuals with diabetes in the U.S. continues to decline. Diabetes Care. 2010;33(1) 73-77.

[7] Tuomilehto J, Borch-Johnsen K, Molarius A, Forsen T, Rastenyte D, Sarti C, et al. Incidence of cardiovascular disease in Type 1 (insulin-dependent) diabetic subjects with and without diabetic nephropathy in Finland. Diabetologia. 1998;41(7) 784-790.

[8] Adler AI, Stevens RJ, Manley SE, Bilous RW, Cull CA, Holman RR. Development and progression of nephropathy in type 2 diabetes: the United Kingdom Prospective Diabetes Study (UKPDS 64). Kidney Int. 2003;63(1) 225-232.

[9] Incidence of end-stage renal disease attributed to diabetes among persons with diagnosed diabetes --- United States and Puerto Rico, 1996-2007. MMWR Morb Mortal Wkly Rep. 2010;59(42) 1361-1366.

[10] Van Dijk PC, Jager KJ, Stengel B, Gronhagen-Riska C, Feest TG, Briggs JD. Renal replacement therapy for diabetic end-stage renal disease: data from 10 registries in Europe (1991-2000). Kidney Int. 2005;67(4) 1489-1499.

[11] KDOQI Clinical Practice Guidelines and Clinical Practice Recommendations for Diabetes and Chronic Kidney Disease. Am J Kidney Dis. 2007;49(2 Suppl 2) S12-154.

[12] Mishra R, Emancipator SN, Kern T, Simonson MS. High glucose evokes an intrinsic proapoptotic signaling pathway in mesangial cells. Kidney Int. 2005;67(1) 82-93.

[13] Heilig CW, Concepcion LA, Riser BL, Freytag SO, Zhu M, Cortes P. Overexpression of glucose transporters in rat mesangial cells cultured in a normal glucose milieu mimics the diabetic phenotype. J Clin Invest. 1995;96(4) 1802-1814.

[14] Mak RH. Impact of end-stage renal disease and dialysis on glycemic control. Semin Dial. 2000;13(1) 4-8.

[15] Shinohara K, Shoji T, Emoto M, Tahara H, Koyama H, Ishimura E, et al. Insulin resistance as an independent predictor of cardiovascular mortality in patients with end-stage renal disease. J Am Soc Nephrol. 2002;13(7) 1894-1900.

[16] Ginsberg HN. Insulin resistance and cardiovascular disease. J Clin Invest. 2000;106(4) 453-458.

[17] Satirapoj B, Supasyndh O, Dispan R, Punpanich D, Tribanyatkul S, Choovichian P. Insulin Resistance and Type 2 Diabetes Patients in Difference Stage of Nephropathy. Royal Thai Army Medical Journal. 2009;62(3) 113-122.

[18] Vareesangthip K, Tong P, Wilkinson R, Thomas TH. Insulin resistance in adult polycystic kidney disease. Kidney Int. 1997;52(2) 503-508.

[19] Fliser D, Pacini G, Engelleiter R, Kautzky-Willer A, Prager R, Franek E, et al. Insulin resistance and hyperinsulinemia are already present in patients with incipient renal disease. Kidney Int. 1998;53(5) 1343-1347.

[20] Satirapoj B, Supasyndh O, Boonyavarakul A, Luesutthiviboon L, Choovichian P. The correlation of insulin resistance and renal function in non diabetic chronic kidney disease patients. J Med Assoc Thai. 2005;88 Suppl 3 S97-104.

[21] DeFronzo RA, Tobin JD, Rowe JW, Andres R. Glucose intolerance in uremia. Quanti-
      fication of pancreatic beta cell sensitivity to glucose and tissue sensitivity to insulin. J
      Clin Invest. 1978;62(2) 425-435.

[22] Hong SY, Yang DH. Insulin levels and fibrinolytic activity in patients with end-stage
      renal disease. Nephron. 1994;68(3) 329-333.

[23] Satirapoj B, Supasyndh O, Phantana-Angkul P, Ruangkanchanasetr P, Nata N, Chai-
      prasert A, et al. Insulin resistance in dialysis versus non dialysis end stage renal dis-
      ease patients without diabetes. J Med Assoc Thai. 2011;94 Suppl 4 S87-93.

[24] Mak RH. Correction of anemia by erythropoietin reverses insulin resistance and hy-
      perinsulinemia in uremia. Am J Physiol. 1996;270(5 Pt 2) F839-844.

[25] Mak RH, DeFronzo RA. Glucose and insulin metabolism in uremia. Nephron.
      1992;61(4) 377-382.

[26] Satirapoj B, Yingwatanadej P, Chaichayanon S, Patumanond J. Effect of angiotensin
      II receptor blockers on insulin resistance in maintenance haemodialysis patients.
      Nephrology (Carlton). 2007;12(4) 342-347.

[27] Fortes PC, de Moraes TP, Mendes JG, Stinghen AE, Ribeiro SC, Pecoits-Filho R. Insu-
      lin resistance and glucose homeostasis in peritoneal dialysis. Perit Dial Int. 2009;29
      Suppl 2 S145-148.

[28] Arem R. Hypoglycemia associated with renal failure. Endocrinol Metab Clin North
      Am. 1989;18(1) 103-121.

[29] Cano N. Bench-to-bedside review: glucose production from the kidney. Crit Care.
      2002;6(4) 317-321.

[30] Effect of intensive diabetes treatment on the development and progression of long-
      term complications in adolescents with insulin-dependent diabetes mellitus: Diabetes
      Control and Complications Trial. Diabetes Control and Complications Trial Research
      Group. J Pediatr. 1994;125(2) 177-188.

[31] Intensive blood-glucose control with sulphonylureas or insulin compared with con-
      ventional treatment and risk of complications in patients with type 2 diabetes
      (UKPDS 33). UK Prospective Diabetes Study (UKPDS) Group. Lancet. 1998;352(9131)
      837-853.

[32] Kawazu S, Tomono S, Shimizu M, Kato N, Ohno T, Ishii C, et al. The relationship be-
      tween early diabetic nephropathy and control of plasma glucose in non-insulin-de-
      pendent diabetes mellitus. The effect of glycemic control on the development and
      progression of diabetic nephropathy in an 8-year follow-up study. J Diabetes Com-
      plications. 1994;8(1) 13-17.

[33] The effect of intensive treatment of diabetes on the development and progression of long-term complications in insulin-dependent diabetes mellitus. The Diabetes Control and Complications Trial Research Group. N Engl J Med. 1993;329(14) 977-986.

[34] Mulec H, Blohme G, Grande B, Bjorck S. The effect of metabolic control on rate of decline in renal function in insulin-dependent diabetes mellitus with overt diabetic nephropathy. Nephrol Dial Transplant. 1998;13(3) 651-655.

[35] Fioretto P, Steffes MW, Sutherland DE, Goetz FC, Mauer M. Reversal of lesions of diabetic nephropathy after pancreas transplantation. N Engl J Med. 1998;339(2) 69-75.

[36] Fioretto P, Sutherland DE, Najafian B, Mauer M. Remodeling of renal interstitial and tubular lesions in pancreas transplant recipients. Kidney Int. 2006;69(5) 907-912.

[37] Holman RR, Paul SK, Bethel MA, Matthews DR, Neil HA. 10-year follow-up of intensive glucose control in type 2 diabetes. N Engl J Med. 2008;359(15) 1577-1589.

[38] Gerstein HC, Miller ME, Byington RP, Goff DC, Jr., Bigger JT, Buse JB, et al. Effects of intensive glucose lowering in type 2 diabetes. N Engl J Med. 2008;358(24) 2545-2559.

[39] Patel A, MacMahon S, Chalmers J, Neal B, Billot L, Woodward M, et al. Intensive blood glucose control and vascular outcomes in patients with type 2 diabetes. N Engl J Med. 2008;358(24) 2560-2572.

[40] Duckworth W, Abraira C, Moritz T, Reda D, Emanuele N, Reaven PD, et al. Glucose control and vascular complications in veterans with type 2 diabetes. N Engl J Med. 2009;360(2) 129-139.

[41] Drechsler C, Krane V, Ritz E, Marz W, Wanner C. Glycemic control and cardiovascular events in diabetic hemodialysis patients. Circulation. 2009;120(24) 2421-2428.

[42] Tsujimoto Y, Ishimura E, Tahara H, Kakiya R, Koyama H, Emoto M, et al. Poor glycemic control is a significant predictor of cardiovascular events in chronic hemodialysis patients with diabetes. Ther Apher Dial. 2009;13(4) 358-365.

[43] Joy MS, Cefalu WT, Hogan SL, Nachman PH. Long-term glycemic control measurements in diabetic patients receiving hemodialysis. Am J Kidney Dis. 2002;39(2) 297-307.

[44] Menon V, Greene T, Pereira AA, Wang X, Beck GJ, Kusek JW, et al. Glycosylated hemoglobin and mortality in patients with nondiabetic chronic kidney disease. J Am Soc Nephrol. 2005;16(11) 3411-3417.

[45] Kalantar-Zadeh K, Kopple JD, Regidor DL, Jing J, Shinaberger CS, Aronovitz J, et al. A1C and survival in maintenance hemodialysis patients. Diabetes Care. 2007;30(5) 1049-1055.

[46] Williams ME, Lacson E, Jr., Wang W, Lazarus JM, Hakim R. Glycemic control and extended hemodialysis survival in patients with diabetes mellitus: comparative re-

sults of traditional and time-dependent Cox model analyses. Clin J Am Soc Nephrol. 2010;5(9) 1595-1601.

[47] Ricks J, Molnar MZ, Kovesdy CP, Shah A, Nissenson AR, Williams M, et al. Glycemic control and cardiovascular mortality in hemodialysis patients with diabetes: a 6-year cohort study. Diabetes. 2012;61(3) 708-715.

[48] McMurray SD, Johnson G, Davis S, McDougall K. Diabetes education and care management significantly improve patient outcomes in the dialysis unit. Am J Kidney Dis. 2002;40(3) 566-575.

[49] Standards of medical care in diabetes--2012. Diabetes Care. 2012;35 Suppl 1 S11-63.

[50] Rohlfing CL, Wiedmeyer HM, Little RR, England JD, Tennill A, Goldstein DE. Defining the relationship between plasma glucose and HbA(1c): analysis of glucose profiles and HbA(1c) in the Diabetes Control and Complications Trial. Diabetes Care. 2002;25(2) 275-278.

[51] Inaba M, Okuno S, Kumeda Y, Yamada S, Imanishi Y, Tabata T, et al. Glycated albumin is a better glycemic indicator than glycated hemoglobin values in hemodialysis patients with diabetes: effect of anemia and erythropoietin injection. J Am Soc Nephrol. 2007;18(3) 896-903.

[52] Ansari A, Thomas S, Goldsmith D. Assessing glycemic control in patients with diabetes and end-stage renal failure. Am J Kidney Dis. 2003;41(3) 523-531.

[53] Freedman BI, Shenoy RN, Planer JA, Clay KD, Shihabi ZK, Burkart JM, et al. Comparison of glycated albumin and hemoglobin A1c concentrations in diabetic subjects on peritoneal and hemodialysis. Peritoneal dialysis international : journal of the International Society for Peritoneal Dialysis. 2010;30(1) 72-79.

[54] Peacock TP, Shihabi ZK, Bleyer AJ, Dolbare EL, Byers JR, Knovich MA, et al. Comparison of glycated albumin and hemoglobin A(1c) levels in diabetic subjects on hemodialysis. Kidney Int. 2008;73(9) 1062-1068.

[55] Freedman BI, Shihabi ZK, Andries L, Cardona CY, Peacock TP, Byers JR, et al. Relationship between assays of glycemia in diabetic subjects with advanced chronic kidney disease. Am J Nephrol. 2010;31(5) 375-379.

[56] Goldstein DE, Little RR, Lorenz RA, Malone JI, Nathan DM, Peterson CM. Tests of glycemia in diabetes. Diabetes Care. 2004;27 Suppl 1 S91-93.

[57] Shrishrimal K, Hart P, Michota F. Managing diabetes in hemodialysis patients: observations and recommendations. Cleve Clin J Med. 2009;76(11) 649-655.

[58] Carone FA, Peterson DR. Hydrolysis and transport of small peptides by the proximal tubule. Am J Physiol. 1980;238(3) F151-158.

[59] Rabkin R, Simon NM, Steiner S, Colwell JA. Effect of renal disease on renal uptake and excretion of insulin in man. N Engl J Med. 1970;282(4) 182-187.

[60] DeFronzo RA, Alvestrand A, Smith D, Hendler R, Hendler E, Wahren J. Insulin resistance in uremia. J Clin Invest. 1981;67(2) 563-568.

[61] Biesenbach G, Raml A, Schmekal B, Eichbauer-Sturm G. Decreased insulin requirement in relation to GFR in nephropathic Type 1 and insulin-treated Type 2 diabetic patients. Diabet Med. 2003;20(8) 642-645.

[62] Avram MM, Paik SK, Okanya D, Rajpal K. The natural history of diabetic nephropathy: unpredictable insulin requirements--a further clue. Clin Nephrol. 1984;21(1) 36-38.

[63] Williams ME. Management of diabetes in dialysis patients. Curr Diab Rep. 2009;9(6) 466-472.

[64] Aisenpreis U, Pfutzner A, Giehl M, Keller F, Jehle PM. Pharmacokinetics and pharmacodynamics of insulin Lispro compared with regular insulin in haemodialysis patients with diabetes mellitus. Nephrol Dial Transplant. 1999;14 Suppl 4 5-6.

[65] Smith D, DeFronzo RA. Insulin resistance in uremia mediated by postbinding defects. Kidney Int. 1982;22(1) 54-62.

[66] Schmitz O. Insulin-mediated glucose uptake in nondialyzed and dialyzed uremic insulin-dependent diabetic subjects. Diabetes. 1985;34(11) 1152-1159.

[67] Wong TY, Chan JC, Szeto CC, Leung CB, Li PK. Clinical and biochemical characteristics of type 2 diabetic patients on continuous ambulatory peritoneal dialysis: relationships with insulin requirement. Am J Kidney Dis. 1999;34(3) 514-520.

[68] Rubenstein AH, Mako ME, Horwitz DL. Insulin and the kidney. Nephron. 1975;15(3-5) 306-326.

[69] Fortes PC, de Moraes TP, Mendes JG, Stinghen AE, Ribeiro SC, Pecoits-Filho R. Insulin resistance and glucose homeostasis in peritoneal dialysis. Peritoneal dialysis international : journal of the International Society for Peritoneal Dialysis. 2009;29 Suppl 2 S145-148.

[70] Szeto CC, Chow KM, Kwan BC, Chung KY, Leung CB, Li PK. New-onset hyperglycemia in nondiabetic chinese patients started on peritoneal dialysis. Am J Kidney Dis. 2007;49(4) 524-532.

[71] Mistry CD, Gokal R, Peers E. A randomized multicenter clinical trial comparing isosmolar icodextrin with hyperosmolar glucose solutions in CAPD. MIDAS Study Group. Multicenter Investigation of Icodextrin in Ambulatory Peritoneal Dialysis. Kidney Int. 1994;46(2) 496-503.

[72] Abe M, Okada K, Soma M. Antidiabetic agents in patients with chronic kidney disease and end-stage renal disease on dialysis: metabolism and clinical practice. Curr Drug Metab. 2011;12(1) 57-69.

[73] Sobngwi E, Enoru S, Ashuntantang G, Azabji-Kenfack M, Dehayem M, Onana A, et al. Day-to-day variation of insulin requirements of patients with type 2 diabetes and

end-stage renal disease undergoing maintenance hemodialysis. Diabetes Care. 2010;33(7) 1409-1412.

[74] Ersoy A, Ersoy C, Altinay T. Insulin analogue usage in a haemodialysis patient with type 2 diabetes mellitus. Nephrol Dial Transplant. 2006;21(2) 553-554.

[75] Charpentier G, Riveline JP, Varroud-Vial M. Management of drugs affecting blood glucose in diabetic patients with renal failure. Diabetes Metab. 2000;26 Suppl 4 73-85.

[76] Toyoda M, Kimura M, Yamamoto N, Miyauchi M, Umezono T, Suzuki D. Insulin glargine improves glycemic control and quality of life in type 2 diabetic patients on hemodialysis. J Nephrol. 2012;25(6) 989-995.

[77] Yale JF. Oral antihyperglycemic agents and renal disease: new agents, new concepts. J Am Soc Nephrol. 2005;16 Suppl 1 S7-10.

[78] Krepinsky J, Ingram AJ, Clase CM. Prolonged sulfonylurea-induced hypoglycemia in diabetic patients with end-stage renal disease. Am J Kidney Dis. 2000;35(3) 500-505.

[79] Rosenkranz B, Profozic V, Metelko Z, Mrzljak V, Lange C, Malerczyk V. Pharmacokinetics and safety of glimepiride at clinically effective doses in diabetic patients with renal impairment. Diabetologia. 1996;39(12) 1617-1624.

[80] Snyder RW, Berns JS. Use of insulin and oral hypoglycemic medications in patients with diabetes mellitus and advanced kidney disease. Semin Dial. 2004;17(5) 365-370.

[81] United Kingdom Prospective Diabetes Study (UKPDS). 13: Relative efficacy of randomly allocated diet, sulphonylurea, insulin, or metformin in patients with newly diagnosed non-insulin dependent diabetes followed for three years. BMJ. 1995;310(6972) 83-88.

[82] Nagai T, Imamura M, Iizuka K, Mori M. Hypoglycemia due to nateglinide administration in diabetic patient with chronic renal failure. Diabetes Res Clin Pract. 2003;59(3) 191-194.

[83] Inoue T, Shibahara N, Miyagawa K, Itahana R, Izumi M, Nakanishi T, et al. Pharmacokinetics of nateglinide and its metabolites in subjects with type 2 diabetes mellitus and renal failure. Clin Nephrol. 2003;60(2) 90-95.

[84] Reimann F, Proks P, Ashcroft FM. Effects of mitiglinide (S 21403) on Kir6.2/SUR1, Kir6.2/SUR2A and Kir6.2/SUR2B types of ATP-sensitive potassium channel. Br J Pharmacol. 2001;132(7) 1542-1548.

[85] Kaku K, Tanaka S, Origasa H, Kikuchi M, Akanuma Y. Effect of mitiglinide on glycemic control over 52 weeks in Japanese type 2 diabetic patients insufficiently controlled with pioglitazone monotherapy. Endocr J. 2009;56(6) 739-746.

[86] Abe M, Okada K, Maruyama T, Maruyama N, Matsumoto K. Combination therapy with mitiglinide and voglibose improves glycemic control in type 2 diabetic patients on hemodialysis. Expert Opin Pharmacother. 2010;11(2) 169-176.

[87] Abe M, Okada K, Maruyama T, Maruyama N, Matsumoto K. Efficacy and safety of mitiglinide in diabetic patients on maintenance hemodialysis. Endocr J. 2010;57(7) 579-586.

[88] Sirtori CR, Franceschini G, Galli-Kienle M, Cighetti G, Galli G, Bondioli A, et al. Disposition of metformin (N,N-dimethylbiguanide) in man. Clin Pharmacol Ther. 1978;24(6) 683-693.

[89] http://www.sanofi-aventis.ca/products/en/glucophage.pdf, Accessed 5th August, 2012.

[90] Martin Gomez MA, Sanchez Martos MD, Garcia Marcos SA, Serrano Carrillo de Albornoz JL. Metformin-induced lactic acidosis: usefulness of measuring levels and therapy with high-flux haemodialysis. Nefrologia. 2011;31(5) 610-611.

[91] Wong TY, Szeto CC, Chow KM, Leung CB, Lam CW, Li PK. Rosiglitazone reduces insulin requirement and C-reactive protein levels in type 2 diabetic patients receiving peritoneal dialysis. Am J Kidney Dis. 2005;46(4) 713-719.

[92] Ciaraldi TP, Huber-Knudsen K, Hickman M, Olefsky JM. Regulation of glucose transport in cultured muscle cells by novel hypoglycemic agents. Metabolism. 1995;44(8) 976-981.

[93] Spiegelman BM. PPAR-gamma: adipogenic regulator and thiazolidinedione receptor. Diabetes. 1998;47(4) 507-514.

[94] Krentz AJ, Bailey CJ. Oral antidiabetic agents: current role in type 2 diabetes mellitus. Drugs. 2005;65(3) 385-411.

[95] Thompson-Culkin K, Zussman B, Miller AK, Freed MI. Pharmacokinetics of rosiglitazone in patients with end-stage renal disease. J Int Med Res. 2002;30(4) 391-399.

[96] Goldstein BJ. Rosiglitazone. Int J Clin Pract. 2000;54(5) 333-337.

[97] Cox PJ, Ryan DA, Hollis FJ, Harris AM, Miller AK, Vousden M, et al. Absorption, disposition, and metabolism of rosiglitazone, a potent thiazolidinedione insulin sensitizer, in humans. Drug Metab Dispos. 2000;28(7) 772-780.

[98] Budde K, Neumayer HH, Fritsche L, Sulowicz W, Stompor T, Eckland D. The pharmacokinetics of pioglitazone in patients with impaired renal function. Br J Clin Pharmacol. 2003;55(4) 368-374.

[99] Nesto RW, Bell D, Bonow RO, Fonseca V, Grundy SM, Horton ES, et al. Thiazolidinedione use, fluid retention, and congestive heart failure: a consensus statement from the American Heart Association and American Diabetes Association. Diabetes Care. 2004;27(1) 256-263.

[100] Iglesias P, Diez JJ. Peroxisome proliferator-activated receptor gamma agonists in renal disease. Eur J Endocrinol. 2006;154(5) 613-621.

[101] Sarafidis PA, Bakris GL. Protection of the kidney by thiazolidinediones: an assessment from bench to bedside. Kidney Int. 2006;70(7) 1223-1233.

[102] Lin SH, Lin YF, Kuo SW, Hsu YJ, Hung YJ. Rosiglitazone improves glucose metabolism in nondiabetic uremic patients on CAPD. Am J Kidney Dis. 2003;42(4) 774-780.

[103] Martens FM, Visseren FL, Lemay J, de Koning EJ, Rabelink TJ. Metabolic and additional vascular effects of thiazolidinediones. Drugs. 2002;62(10) 1463-1480.

[104] Agrawal A, Sautter MC, Jones NP. Effects of rosiglitazone maleate when added to a sulfonylurea regimen in patients with type 2 diabetes mellitus and mild to moderate renal impairment: a post hoc analysis. Clin Ther. 2003;25(11) 2754-2764.

[105] Ginsberg H, Plutzky J, Sobel BE. A review of metabolic and cardiovascular effects of oral antidiabetic agents: beyond glucose-level lowering. J Cardiovasc Risk. 1999;6(5) 337-346.

[106] Chiang CK, Ho TI, Peng YS, Hsu SP, Pai MF, Yang SY, et al. Rosiglitazone in diabetes control in hemodialysis patients with and without viral hepatitis infection: effectiveness and side effects. Diabetes Care. 2007;30(1) 3-7.

[107] Abe M, Okada K, Maruyama T, Maruyama N, Soma M, Matsumoto K. Clinical effectiveness and safety evaluation of long-term pioglitazone treatment for erythropoietin responsiveness and insulin resistance in type 2 diabetic patients on hemodialysis. Expert Opin Pharmacother. 2010;11(10) 1611-1620.

[108] http://www.accessdata.fda.gov/drugsatfda_docs/label/2008/020482s023lbl.pdf, Accessed 5th August, 2012.

[109] http://www.pfizer.com/files/products/uspi_glyset.pdf, Accessed 5th August, 2012.

[110] Drucker DJ, Nauck MA. The incretin system: glucagon-like peptide-1 receptor agonists and dipeptidyl peptidase-4 inhibitors in type 2 diabetes. Lancet. 2006;368(9548) 1696-1705.

[111] Richter B, Bandeira-Echtler E, Bergerhoff K, Lerch CL. Dipeptidyl peptidase-4 (DPP-4) inhibitors for type 2 diabetes mellitus. Cochrane Database Syst Rev. 2008(2) CD006739.

[112] Idris I, Donnelly R. Dipeptidyl peptidase-IV inhibitors: a major new class of oral antidiabetic drug. Diabetes Obes Metab. 2007;9(2) 153-165.

[113] Herman GA, Stein PP, Thornberry NA, Wagner JA. Dipeptidyl peptidase-4 inhibitors for the treatment of type 2 diabetes: focus on sitagliptin. Clin Pharmacol Ther. 2007;81(5) 761-767.

[114] Hermansen K, Kipnes M, Luo E, Fanurik D, Khatami H, Stein P. Efficacy and safety of the dipeptidyl peptidase-4 inhibitor, sitagliptin, in patients with type 2 diabetes mellitus inadequately controlled on glimepiride alone or on glimepiride and metformin. Diabetes Obes Metab. 2007;9(5) 733-745.

[115] Nauck MA, Meininger G, Sheng D, Terranella L, Stein PP. Efficacy and safety of the dipeptidyl peptidase-4 inhibitor, sitagliptin, compared with the sulfonylurea, glipizide, in patients with type 2 diabetes inadequately controlled on metformin alone: a randomized, double-blind, non-inferiority trial. Diabetes Obes Metab. 2007;9(2) 194-205.

[116] Goldstein BJ, Feinglos MN, Lunceford JK, Johnson J, Williams-Herman DE. Effect of initial combination therapy with sitagliptin, a dipeptidyl peptidase-4 inhibitor, and metformin on glycemic control in patients with type 2 diabetes. Diabetes Care. 2007;30(8) 1979-1987.

[117] Charbonnel B, Karasik A, Liu J, Wu M, Meininger G. Efficacy and safety of the dipeptidyl peptidase-4 inhibitor sitagliptin added to ongoing metformin therapy in patients with type 2 diabetes inadequately controlled with metformin alone. Diabetes Care. 2006;29(12) 2638-2643.

[118] Rosenstock J, Brazg R, Andryuk PJ, Lu K, Stein P. Efficacy and safety of the dipeptidyl peptidase-4 inhibitor sitagliptin added to ongoing pioglitazone therapy in patients with type 2 diabetes: a 24-week, multicenter, randomized, double-blind, placebo-controlled, parallel-group study. Clin Ther. 2006;28(10) 1556-1568.

[119] Herman GA, Stevens C, Van Dyck K, Bergman A, Yi B, De Smet M, et al. Pharmacokinetics and pharmacodynamics of sitagliptin, an inhibitor of dipeptidyl peptidase IV, in healthy subjects: results from two randomized, double-blind, placebo-controlled studies with single oral doses. Clin Pharmacol Ther. 2005;78(6) 675-688.

[120] Herman GA, Bergman A, Stevens C, Kotey P, Yi B, Zhao P, et al. Effect of single oral doses of sitagliptin, a dipeptidyl peptidase-4 inhibitor, on incretin and plasma glucose levels after an oral glucose tolerance test in patients with type 2 diabetes. J Clin Endocrinol Metab. 2006;91(11) 4612-4619.

[121] Chu XY, Bleasby K, Yabut J, Cai X, Chan GH, Hafey MJ, et al. Transport of the dipeptidyl peptidase-4 inhibitor sitagliptin by human organic anion transporter 3, organic anion transporting polypeptide 4C1, and multidrug resistance P-glycoprotein. J Pharmacol Exp Ther. 2007;321(2) 673-683.

[122] Bergman AJ, Cote J, Yi B, Marbury T, Swan SK, Smith W, et al. Effect of renal insufficiency on the pharmacokinetics of sitagliptin, a dipeptidyl peptidase-4 inhibitor. Diabetes Care. 2007;30(7) 1862-1864.

[123] Chan JC, Scott R, Arjona Ferreira JC, Sheng D, Gonzalez E, Davies MJ, et al. Safety and efficacy of sitagliptin in patients with type 2 diabetes and chronic renal insufficiency. Diabetes Obes Metab. 2008;10(7) 545-555.

[124] Croxtall JD, Keam SJ. Vildagliptin: a review of its use in the management of type 2 diabetes mellitus. Drugs. 2008;68(16) 2387-2409.

[125] Henness S, Keam SJ. Vildagliptin. Drugs. 2006;66(15) 1989-2001; discussion 2002-1984.

[126] He YL, Serra D, Wang Y, Campestrini J, Riviere GJ, Deacon CF, et al. Pharmacokinetics and pharmacodynamics of vildagliptin in patients with type 2 diabetes mellitus. Clin Pharmacokinet. 2007;46(7) 577-588.

[127] Scheen AJ. Pharmacokinetics of dipeptidylpeptidase-4 inhibitors. Diabetes Obes Metab. 2010;12(8) 648-658.

[128] Pratley RE. Alogliptin: a new, highly selective dipeptidyl peptidase-4 inhibitor for the treatment of type 2 diabetes. Expert Opin Pharmacother. 2009;10(3) 503-512.

[129] Fura A, Khanna A, Vyas V, Koplowitz B, Chang SY, Caporuscio C, et al. Pharmacokinetics of the dipeptidyl peptidase 4 inhibitor saxagliptin in rats, dogs, and monkeys and clinical projections. Drug Metab Dispos. 2009;37(6) 1164-1171.

[130] Fuchs H, Tillement JP, Urien S, Greischel A, Roth W. Concentration-dependent plasma protein binding of the novel dipeptidyl peptidase 4 inhibitor BI 1356 due to saturable binding to its target in plasma of mice, rats and humans. J Pharm Pharmacol. 2009;61(1) 55-62.

[131] Blech S, Ludwig-Schwellinger E, Grafe-Mody EU, Withopf B, Wagner K. The metabolism and disposition of the oral dipeptidyl peptidase-4 inhibitor, linagliptin, in humans. Drug Metab Dispos. 2010;38(4) 667-678.

[132] Huttner S, Graefe-Mody EU, Withopf B, Ring A, Dugi KA. Safety, tolerability, pharmacokinetics, and pharmacodynamics of single oral doses of BI 1356, an inhibitor of dipeptidyl peptidase 4, in healthy male volunteers. J Clin Pharmacol. 2008;48(10) 1171-1178.

[133] Baggio LL, Drucker DJ. Biology of incretins: GLP-1 and GIP. Gastroenterology. 2007;132(6) 2131-2157.

[134] Copley K, McCowen K, Hiles R, Nielsen LL, Young A, Parkes DG. Investigation of exenatide elimination and its in vivo and in vitro degradation. Curr Drug Metab. 2006;7(4) 367-374.

[135] Linnebjerg H, Kothare PA, Park S, Mace K, Reddy S, Mitchell M, et al. Effect of renal impairment on the pharmacokinetics of exenatide. Br J Clin Pharmacol. 2007;64(3) 317-327.

[136] Knudsen LB, Nielsen PF, Huusfeldt PO, Johansen NL, Madsen K, Pedersen FZ, et al. Potent derivatives of glucagon-like peptide-1 with pharmacokinetic properties suitable for once daily administration. J Med Chem. 2000;43(9) 1664-1669.

[137] Malm-Erjefalt M, Bjornsdottir I, Vanggaard J, Helleberg H, Larsen U, Oosterhuis B, et al. Metabolism and excretion of the once-daily human glucagon-like peptide-1 ana-

log liraglutide in healthy male subjects and its in vitro degradation by dipeptidyl peptidase IV and neutral endopeptidase. Drug Metab Dispos. 2010;38(11) 1944-1953.

[138] Agerso H, Jensen LB, Elbrond B, Rolan P, Zdravkovic M. The pharmacokinetics, pharmacodynamics, safety and tolerability of NN2211, a new long-acting GLP-1 derivative, in healthy men. Diabetologia. 2002;45(2) 195-202.

[139] Jacobsen LV, Hindsberger C, Robson R, Zdravkovic M. Effect of renal impairment on the pharmacokinetics of the GLP-1 analogue liraglutide. Br J Clin Pharmacol. 2009;68(6) 898-905.

[140] Young A. Inhibition of glucagon secretion. Adv Pharmacol. 2005;52 151-171.

[141] Young AA, Gedulin B, Vine W, Percy A, Rink TJ. Gastric emptying is accelerated in diabetic BB rats and is slowed by subcutaneous injections of amylin. Diabetologia. 1995;38(6) 642-648.

[142] Gedulin BR, Rink TJ, Young AA. Dose-response for glucagonostatic effect of amylin in rats. Metabolism. 1997;46(1) 67-70.

[143] Lutz TA, Mollet A, Rushing PA, Riediger T, Scharrer E. The anorectic effect of a chronic peripheral infusion of amylin is abolished in area postrema/nucleus of the solitary tract (AP/NTS) lesioned rats. Int J Obes Relat Metab Disord. 2001;25(7) 1005-1011.

[144] Ratner RE, Dickey R, Fineman M, Maggs DG, Shen L, Strobel SA, et al. Amylin replacement with pramlintide as an adjunct to insulin therapy improves long-term glycaemic and weight control in Type 1 diabetes mellitus: a 1-year, randomized controlled trial. Diabet Med. 2004;21(11) 1204-1212.

[145] Whitehouse F, Kruger DF, Fineman M, Shen L, Ruggles JA, Maggs DG, et al. A randomized study and open-label extension evaluating the long-term efficacy of pramlintide as an adjunct to insulin therapy in type 1 diabetes. Diabetes Care. 2002;25(4) 724-730.

[146] Riddle M, Frias J, Zhang B, Maier H, Brown C, Lutz K, et al. Pramlintide improved glycemic control and reduced weight in patients with type 2 diabetes using basal insulin. Diabetes Care. 2007;30(11) 2794-2799.

[147] Hollander PA, Levy P, Fineman MS, Maggs DG, Shen LZ, Strobel SA, et al. Pramlintide as an adjunct to insulin therapy improves long-term glycemic and weight control in patients with type 2 diabetes: a 1-year randomized controlled trial. Diabetes Care. 2003;26(3) 784-790.

[148] Chapman I, Parker B, Doran S, Feinle-Bisset C, Wishart J, Strobel S, et al. Effect of pramlintide on satiety and food intake in obese subjects and subjects with type 2 diabetes. Diabetologia. 2005;48(5) 838-848.

[149] Sha S, Devineni D, Ghosh A, Polidori D, Chien S, Wexler D, et al. Canagliflozin, a novel inhibitor of sodium glucose co-transporter 2, dose dependently reduces calcu-

lated renal threshold for glucose excretion and increases urinary glucose excretion in healthy subjects. Diabetes Obes Metab. 2011;13(7) 669-672.

[150] Rave K, Nosek L, Posner J, Heise T, Roggen K, van Hoogdalem EJ. Renal glucose excretion as a function of blood glucose concentration in subjects with type 2 diabetes--results of a hyperglycaemic glucose clamp study. Nephrol Dial Transplant. 2006;21(8) 2166-2171.

[151] Nair S, Wilding JP. Sodium glucose cotransporter 2 inhibitors as a new treatment for diabetes mellitus. J Clin Endocrinol Metab. 2010;95(1) 34-42.

[152] Ruhnau B, Faber OK, Borch-Johnsen K, Thorsteinsson B. Renal threshold for glucose in non-insulin-dependent diabetic patients. Diabetes Res Clin Pract. 1997;36(1) 27-33.

[153] Chao EC, Henry RR. SGLT2 inhibition--a novel strategy for diabetes treatment. Nat Rev Drug Discov. 2010;9(7) 551-559.

[154] Scheen AJ. Saxagliptin plus metformin combination in patients with type 2 diabetes and renal impairment. Expert Opin Drug Metab Toxicol. 2012;8(3) 383-394.

[155] Schwartz SL. Treatment of elderly patients with type 2 diabetes mellitus: a systematic review of the benefits and risks of dipeptidyl peptidase-4 inhibitors. Am J Geriatr Pharmacother. 2011;8(5) 405-418.

[156] Bourdel-Marchasson I, Schweizer A, Dejager S. Incretin therapies in the management of elderly patients with type 2 diabetes mellitus. Hosp Pract (Minneap). 2011;39(1) 7-21.

[157] Doucet J, Chacra A, Maheux P, Lu J, Harris S, Rosenstock J. Efficacy and safety of saxagliptin in older patients with type 2 diabetes mellitus. Curr Med Res Opin. 2011;27(4) 863-869.

[158] Effect of intensive blood-glucose control with metformin on complications in overweight patients with type 2 diabetes (UKPDS 34). UK Prospective Diabetes Study (UKPDS) Group. Lancet. 1998;352(9131) 854-865.

[159] El Messaoudi S, Rongen GA, de Boer RA, Riksen NP. The cardioprotective effects of metformin. Curr Opin Lipidol. 2011;22(6) 445-453.

[160] Roy S, Khanna V, Mittra S, Dhar A, Singh S, Mahajan DC, et al. Combination of dipeptidylpeptidase IV inhibitor and low dose thiazolidinedione: preclinical efficacy and safety in db/db mice. Life Sci. 2007;81(1) 72-79.

[161] Banerji MA, Purkayastha D, Francis BH. Safety and tolerability of vildagliptin vs. thiazolidinedione as add-on to metformin in type 2 diabetic patients with and without mild renal impairment: a retrospective analysis of the GALIANT study. Diabetes Res Clin Pract. 2010;90(2) 182-190.

[162] Sunaga Y, Gonoi T, Shibasaki T, Ichikawa K, Kusama H, Yano H, et al. The effects of mitiglinide (KAD-1229), a new anti-diabetic drug, on ATP-sensitive K+ channels and

insulin secretion: comparison with the sulfonylureas and nateglinide. Eur J Pharmacol. 2001;431(1) 119-125.

[163] Abe M, Okada K, Ikeda K, Matsumoto S, Soma M, Matsumoto K. Characterization of insulin adsorption behavior of dialyzer membranes used in hemodialysis. Artif Organs. 2011;35(4) 398-403.

[164] Abe M, Okada K, Maruyama T, Ikeda K, Kikuchi F, Kaizu K, et al. Comparison of the effects of polysulfone and polyester-polymer alloy dialyzers on glycemic control in diabetic patients undergoing hemodialysis. Clin Nephrol. 2009;71(5) 514-520.

[165] Unruh M, Benz R, Greene T, Yan G, Beddhu S, DeVita M, et al. Effects of hemodialysis dose and membrane flux on health-related quality of life in the HEMO Study. Kidney Int. 2004;66(1) 355-366.

[166] Blankestijn PJ, Vos PF, Rabelink TJ, van Rijn HJ, Jansen H, Koomans HA. High-flux dialysis membranes improve lipid profile in chronic hemodialysis patients. J Am Soc Nephrol. 1995;5(9) 1703-1708.

[167] Seres DS, Strain GW, Hashim SA, Goldberg IJ, Levin NW. Improvement of plasma lipoprotein profiles during high-flux dialysis. J Am Soc Nephrol. 1993;3(7) 1409-1415.

[168] Abe M, Okada K, Matsumoto K. Plasma insulin and C-peptide concentrations in diabetic patients undergoing hemodialysis: Comparison with five types of high-flux dialyzer membranes. Diabetes Res Clin Pract. 2008;82(1) e17-19.

Chapter 9

Epidemiology of Chronic Dialysis Patients in the Intensive Care Unit

Melanie Chan and Marlies Ostermann

Additional information is available at the end of the chapter

1. Introduction

The incidence and prevalence of end-stage renal disease (ESRD) is rising worldwide, in part due to increasing rates of diabetes, hypertension and an ageing population [1,2]. Incidence rates of patients commencing renal replacement therapy (RRT) are estimated at 109 and 354 per million population (pmp) per year in the UK and US respectively [1,2], with the highest incidence seen in patients over 75 years of age.

Shifting demographics over the past two decades have resulted in an older and sicker long-term dialysis population, burdened with multiple and significant co-morbid conditions. ESRD patients experience higher rates of hospitalisation, cardiovascular events and all cause mortality when compared to patients with normal renal function, and are more likely to require admission to the intensive care unit (ICU) [3,4]. It has been estimated that 2% of all dialysis patients will require admission to ICU every year [5]. The presence of pre-existing end-stage organ failure, and often numerous co-morbidities, can impact on medical decisions regarding appropriateness of escalation of care and ICU admission. For a long time, it was thought that patients requiring long-term dialysis would have similarly poor ICU outcomes to those with acute kidney injury (AKI), however emerging evidence suggests otherwise.

This chapter aims to review the epidemiology, patient characteristics and short and long-term outcomes of critically unwell chronic dialysis patients, who require admission to ICU. Risk factors for early mortality, ICU prognostic scoring systems and end of life care planning will also be discussed in relation to the critically ill hemodialysis patient.

2. Characteristics on admission to ICU

Chronic dialysis patients have higher critical care admission rates than the general population; however there is a significant variation in estimates between published studies. This may reflect differences in referral rates, ICU admission policy and resource availability on a national and local level as well as the demographics of the surrounding population.

The largest cohort of critically ill ESRD patients studied derives from the Intensive Care National Audit & Research Centre (ICNARC) Case Mix Programme Database which records data of patients admitted to more than 200 ICUs across England, Wales and Northern Ireland. Analysis of this database showed that from 1995 to 2004 there were 270,972 admissions to ICU, of whom 1.3% were chronic dialysis patients [4]. The authors of the study projected that this was equivalent to six ICU admissions or 32 ICU bed days per 100 dialysis patient-years. When compared to annual ICU admission rates of 2 per 1,000 of the general population, this represents a 30-fold difference in critical care requirements. A more recent study using the same UK ICNARC database with data from 1995-2008, similarly found that ESRD patients accounted for 1.4% of all ICU admissions [6].

Other studies have proposed much higher estimates for admission rates of chronic dialysis patients to the ICU; however these are mostly single centre and involve significantly smaller study cohorts than Hutchinson et al [4]. A French prospective observational single-centre study admitted 92 chronic dialysis patients over a 3 year period, which gives a calculated admission rate of 8.6%, significantly higher than the UK database study [7]. Of note, this study was based at a teaching hospital which served as the sole critical care unit able to provide RRT to its large surrounding population.

Strijack and colleagues [8] report that 3.4% of all admissions to 11 adult ICUs in Winnipeg, Canada over a 6 year period were chronic dialysis patients, with crude admission rates for the ESRD population significantly higher than for those without ESRD (15.6 admissions per 100 prevalent patients with ESRD per year vs. 0.58 per 100 prevalent patients without ESRD per year). An American single-centre study conducted in Pittsburgh, and involving medical, surgical, trauma, neurological/neurosurgical, coronary and cardiothoracic ICUs found a similar admission rate for chronic dialysis patients of 3.6% [9]. In contrast to the 30-fold increase in critical care admissions for ESRD patients reported by Hutchinson et al [4], a multi-centre Australian study based on 3 months of data demonstrated a significantly lower 4-fold annual risk of ICU admission in dialysis patients compared to the general population [5].

Although ICU admission rates for the ESRD population vary from 1.3% - 8.6%, it is evident that patients with chronic renal disease are at higher risk of requiring critical care than the general population. Whether this is related to the underlying renal disease or associated co-morbidities remains to be seen. The decision to admit a patient to critical care is based on multiple factors, including the patient's and relatives' wishes, local admission policy, judgement of the clinicians involved and capacity.

Epidemiological data has shown that ESRD patients admitted to ICU are younger and more likely to be male in comparison to the general population [4,6-8,10]. The proportion of male admissions to the ICU is in keeping with the male preponderance in the dialysis population; however the reason for the lower mean age seen in critically ill ESRD patients requires further analysis.

3. Characteristics of critically ill dialysis patients

3.1. Severity of illness scores

Chronic dialysis patients requiring intensive care admission are more critically unwell and have a greater number of co-morbidities than the general population. Strijack et al [8] found they had significantly higher rates of diabetes (52.3% vs. 21.7%, p<0.0001) and peripheral arterial disease (29.7% vs. 12.3%, p<0.0001) than those without ESRD on admission to the ICU. Rates of coronary artery disease, stroke and cancer were comparable between the two groups.

Several studies have used ICU mortality and prognostication models such as the Acute Physiology and Chronic Health Evaluation II (APACHE) score [11] to attempt to quantify the severity of illness of dialysis patients admitted to critical care. Hutchinson et al [4] reported that both the APACHE II (24.7 vs. 16.6, p < 0.001) and Simplified Acute Physiology Score (SAPS) (17.2 vs. 12.6, p < 0.001) were significantly higher in dialysis patients when compared to those not requiring long-term renal replacement. Both scoring systems include physiological variables assessing cardiovascular, respiratory, biochemical, haematological and neurological status, within the first 24 hours of admission to ICU; however the APACHE II score places more emphasis on age and medical history than the SAPS. Strijack and colleagues [8] found a similar trend in their Canadian historical cohort study where patients with ESRD had a higher APACHE II score than those without ESRD (24 vs. 15, p < 0.0001), a finding that persisted even after removal of the renal component (serum creatinine and presence of AKI) of the score (20 vs. 14, p < 0.0001).

The fact that ESRD patients are more critically unwell on admission to ICU than the general population is an interesting concept. Certainly, this cohort is not being denied treatment based on illness severity, and it may reflect the differing admission diagnoses between the groups. However it does raise the possibility of whether there exists a higher threshold for seeking intensive care intervention in chronic dialysis patients, resulting in delayed referral, or whether patients need to be more critically unwell before being accepted into the ICU. It is also possible, that the commonly used scoring systems to assess severity of illness are not valid in chronic dialysis patients.

3.2. Reasons for admission to ICU

Dialysis patients are more likely to be admitted to ICU with a medical diagnosis than the general population (66.7% vs. 56.2%) [4]. Data shows that whilst there is a significant difference in critical care admissions after elective surgery (7.4% vs. 19%, p< 0.0001) between the two groups, with ESRD patients much less commonly admitted post operatively, the figures for admission after emergency surgery are comparable [8].

Interestingly, among patients with ESRD, admission after cardiopulmonary resuscitation (CPR) is a more frequent reason for ICU admission compared to other patient populations (13.6% vs. 7.3%, p < 0.001) [4]. Senthuran and colleagues [12] similarly found that 12% of their cohort of chronic dialysis patients were admitted to a single Australian ICU having survived a cardiac arrest. Epidemiological data from the US suggests that hemodialysis patients have a 10-fold increased risk of dying from cardiac arrest than the general population [2]. The fluid and electrolyte shifts experienced during and in between dialysis sessions may contribute to this increased risk in conjunction with left ventricular hypertrophy/dysfunction, ischaemic heart disease, autonomic dysfunction, hypertension, diabetes, and being male [13]. The fact that dialysis patients are more likely to have had CPR in the 24 hours prior to ICU admission is consistent with the finding that these patients are more critically unwell when they arrive in the ICU. Again whether this is an indirect consequence of delayed referral or acceptance or a direct consequence of the unphysiological fluid and electrolyte shifts experienced during hemodialysis is uncertain.

Cardiovascular disease and sepsis are the leading causes of death in patients with ESRD [1,2], and it is therefore not unexpected that these constitute two of the most common reasons for admission to ICU. Dialysis patients are particularly susceptible to infections due to uraemia related immune deficiency, defective phagocytic function, older age, and co-morbidities including diabetes mellitus. In addition, repeated vascular access for the purpose of hemo-dialysis increases the risk of bacteraemia. The annual percentage mortality rates secondary to sepsis for dialysis patients have been estimated at 100- to 300-fold higher than rates seen in the general population [14]. Between 5.6%-46% of chronic dialysis patients are admitted to ICU with a diagnosis of sepsis [4,7,8,10,12,15-18]. Strijack et al [8] found that significantly more ESRD patients were admitted to ICU with a diagnosis of sepsis compared to those without renal failure (15.8% vs. 6.5%, p< 0.0001), however the source of sepsis was not detailed, and whether this was related to vascular access infections cannot be determined. A small Brazilian study reported that the lung was the most frequent source of sepsis in the critically ill dialysis population, followed by soft tissue, catheter related/blood-stream and abdominal sources [17].

As well as having traditional cardiovascular risk factors, chronic kidney disease patients have associated non-traditional risk factors such as increased levels of inflammatory markers, left ventricular hypertrophy, anaemia, endothelial dysfunction, increased arterial calcification and stiffness, abnormal apolipoprotein levels, high plasma homocysteine and enhanced coagula-bility [3]. These factors are thought to put patients with renal dysfunction at a higher risk of adverse cardiac events including myocardial ischaemia, pulmonary oedema, cardiogenic shock, arrhythmias and sudden cardiac death. Studies have estimated that the proportion of ESRD patients admitted to ICU with a cardiac diagnosis (including pulmonary oedema) ranges from 5.1%-31% [4,7,8,10,12,15-17].

A recent study conducted in a single French ICU specifically analysed chronic dialysis patients admitted to their unit with acute pulmonary oedema [19]. Out of 102 patients with ESRD and pulmonary oedema admitted to ICU over an eight year period, they reported 41% could be attributed to an underlying cardiac cause, 26% to bronchopneumonia, 25% to excessive interdialytic weight gain and 23% secondary to an inappropriate dialysis prescription and incorrect assessment of dry weight. Interestingly they noted a distinct pattern to the ICU admissions related to patients' dialysis schedules; those dialysed on Monday-Wednesday-Friday were commonly admitted on Sunday and those on a Tuesday-Thursday-Saturday timetable were more likely to be admitted on Monday. The authors speculated that this may reflect a reduced tolerance to fluid overload in patients' with cardiac dysfunction and/or poor compliance with salt and water restriction over the weekend.

Gastrointestinal bleeding is the third most common reason for chronic dialysis patients to require critical care. Dara et al [10] report that between 1997 – 2002, 20% of their ESRD cohort had an ICU admission and the most common ICU admission diagnosis was gastrointestinal haemorrhage. However other studies have slightly lower estimates of 2.7%-15% [7,16,17].

It is difficult to ascertain precisely how often ESRD patients require critical care intervention for hemodialysis related complications, including pulmonary oedema, arrhythmias, hyperkalaemia or vascular access related septicaemia. Hutchinson and colleagues [4] report from their large UK database analysis that the most common ICU admission diagnosis for long-term dialysis patients is 'chronic renal failure' (8.6%), which they define as volume overload or electrolyte disturbance. Hyperkalaemia was recorded as the admitting diagnosis for 4.3% [7] and 3% [12] of ESRD patients admitted to single ICUs in France and Australia respectively. Clearly, these statistics depend not only on patients' severity of illness but also ICU admission policy, capacity, patients' wishes and whether a renal unit is on-site or not.

In summary, patients admitted to critical care on long-term dialysis are more likely to have multiple co-morbidities and have a higher severity illness score on admission than the general population. They more frequently present having had a cardiac arrest and CPR prior to admission and are more commonly admitted for medical rather than surgical reasons [18].

4. Short term outcomes of chronic dialysis patients admitted to ICU

4.1. Mortality

During the last ten years, numerous studies have focussed on the outcomes of critically ill long-term dialysis patients admitted to ICU (Table 1). Prior to this, it was believed that ICU mortality in this population was high, and comparable to those admitted with AKI. Reliable data on prognosis are necessary to enable patients and clinicians looking after critically ill dialysis patients to make well-informed and timely decisions regarding escalation of care.

Clermont et al [9] were among the first to attempt to evaluate ICU outcomes in ESRD patients admitted to eight American ICUs over a 10 month period. They reported an observed ICU mortality of 11% for ESRD patients compared to 5% in patients without renal failure. Numerous other studies have reported ICU mortality rates of 9-44% for chronic dialysis patients [4,5, 7,9,10,12,15-18,20-22].

Study	Country	Type of RRT	No of patients (n)	Mean age (years)	Mean severity score	ICU mortality (%)	Hospital mortality (%)	30-day mortality (%)	ICU LOS (days) Mean±SD or Median [range]	ICU readmission rate (%)
Clermont [9] 2002	USA	IHD, CVVHD	57	58	64 (APACHE III)	11	14	-		-
Uchino [5] 2003	Australia	CRRT	38	45	22 (APACHE II)	22	38	-	6	-
Dara [10] 2004	USA	N/A	93	66	64 (APACHE III)	9	16	22	2	-
Manhes [7] 2005	France	IHD	92	63	49.4 (SAPS II)	28	38	-	6.2±9.9	-
Bagshaw [22] 2006	Canada	IHD, CRRT	92	66	29.7 (APACHE II)	16	34	-	-	-
Hutchinson [4] 2007	UK	N/A	3420	57	24.7 (APACHE II)	26	45	-	1.9 [0.9-4.2]	9
Ostermann [21] 2008	UK and Germany	IHD, CRRT, PD	797	55	8 (SOFA)	21	35	-	2 [1-64]	-
Senthuran [12] 2008	Australia	IHD, CVVHDF, CAPD	70	57	26.1 (APACHE II)	17	29	-	2 [1-27]	-
Strijack [8] 2009	Canada	IHD, CVVHDF	619	62	24 (APACHE II)	-	16	-	4.3	12
Chapman [20] 2009	UK	N/A	199	59	27.6 (APACHE II)	44	56	-	7.5±10.1	-
Rocha [17] 2009	Brazil	IHD, CRRT, SLED	54	66	43.9 (SAPS II)	20	24	-	5 [3-11]	-
Juneja [16] 2010	India	IHD, CRRT, SLED	73	54	27.1 (APACHE II)	27	-	41	2 [1-20]	-
Sood [18] 2011	Canada	N/A	578	61	19 (APACHE II, renal adjusted)	13	-	-	-	-

Study	Country	Type of RRT	No of patients (n)	Mean age (years)	Mean severity score	ICU mortality (%)	Hospital mortality (%)	30-day mortality (%)	ICU LOS (days) Mean±SD or Median [range]	ICU readmission rate (%)
Walcher [24] 2011	USA	CRRT	28	58	-	36	39	39	9±8	-
O'Brien [6] 2012	UK	N/A	8991	59	24.6 (APACHE II)	24	42	-	2 [0.9-4.7]	-
Bell [37] 2008	Sweden	CRRT, IHD	245	-	-	-	-	90 day mortality 42%	-	-

Abbreviations: APACHE, Acute Physiology Assessment and Chronic Health Evaluation; SOFA, sequential organ failure assessment; SAPS, Simplified Acute Physiology Score; ICU, intensive care unit; LOS, length of stay; RRT, renal replacement therapy; CRRT, continuous renal replacement therapy; IHD, intermittent hemodialysis; CVVHDF, continuous hemodiafiltration; CVVHD, continuous hemodialysis; SLED, slow extended dialysis; CAPD, continuous ambulatory peritoneal dialysis; PD, peritoneal dialysis

Table 1.

Analysis of the UK ICNARC database showed an ICU mortality rate of 26.3% in patients with ESRD compared to 20.8% in those without ESRD (p< 0.001) [4]. This significant increase in mortality is however not surprising, given the higher illness severity scores of ESRD patients on admission to ICU. In 199 dialysis-dependent patients requiring support of two or more organ systems (including RRT) in ICU between 1999 - 2004, ICU mortality was 44% [20], which is similar to ICU mortality for patients with multi-organ failure which can range from 20-95% depending on number of organs involved and underlying comorbitdity [23].

Factors that are commonly associated with ICU mortality in chronic dialysis patients are age, number of non-renal organ system failures, an abnormal serum phosphorus level (high or low), higher mean APACHE II or SAPS II score and duration of mechanical ventilation [7,9,12]. There is clearly some overlap between these factors as confirmed by multivariate analyses [7]. The importance of abnormal serum phosphorus levels is unclear. Manhes et al [7] hypothesise that a low phosphate level can signify malnutrition and be related to severity of illness, where as hyperphosphataemia may be an indicator of inadequate renal replacement and a risk factor for cardiovascular disease in long-term dialysis patients, although the relevance of this to acute illness is uncertain.

4.2. Length of stay

Epidemiological data consistently show that chronic dialysis patients have comparable lengths of stay in ICU to the general population [4,7-9]. Mean length of stay ranged from 1.9 to 9 days [4,6-9,12,17,20,24], with Manhes [7] reporting a trend towards longer admissions in patients without ESRD. Clearly, the decision to discharge patients from ICU is influenced by the capabilities and staffing of the receiving ward which may explain some of the discrepancies between different studies. In hospitals with renal units offering level two care, safe discharge of patients may be possible earlier compared to hospitals without dedicated step-down units.

4.3. Re-admission to ICU

Studies have shown that ESRD patients have a higher rate of readmission to ICU during the same hospital stay than patients with normal renal function [4,8], with quoted figures of 9-12% [4,8,12]. Strijack et al [8] found a significant difference in readmission rates (12% vs. 4.9%, p < 0.0001) between those on chronic dialysis and the general population and reported twice the frequency of readmissions to ICU within three days in the former. A recent Canadian study explored ICU readmission rates even further by evaluating the impact of dialysis modality and vascular access. They found a significant reduction in readmission rates to ICU for hemodialysis patients using arterio-venous (AV) fistulae as opposed to central venous catheters (4.7% vs. 16.4%, p < 0.05) [18], but acknowledged that this finding was open to confounding as central venous catheters may be simply a surrogate for poor performance status. The same group also reported that dialysis dependence was independently associated with two-fold higher odds for ICU readmission in the elderly (> 65 years) population even after adjustment for case mix and illness severity variables [25].

Therefore, the literature suggests that sicker chronic dialysis patients have shorter stays in ICU but experience almost twice the number of readmissions. Readmission to ICU is associated with poor outcomes and while many renal units have considerable experience in managing unwell dialysis patients, careful planning for a timely and safe discharge from ICU to a suitable destination is paramount.

5. Longer term outcomes of critically ill dialysis patients

Having been discharged from ICU it is essential to know how an episode of critical illness impacts on the medium and long-term outcomes of patients requiring chronic dialysis. Several studies have attempted to quantify hospital and 30-day mortality rates for this cohort and report figures of between 14-56% [4-10,12,16,17,20,24] and 32-41% [10,16,24] respectively. Hospital mortality rates were significantly higher in chronic dialysis patients compared to the non-ESRD population after ICU discharge (45.3% vs. 31.2%, p < 0.001) [4]. The wide range seen in these figures can in part be attributed to differences in case-mix as well as variations in illness severity between the studies.

Chapman et al [20] reported the highest hospital mortality rate of 56% for their 199 chronic dialysis patients after discharge from ICU, but emphasised that their patient cohort had a longer length of stay in ICU and higher APACHE II score than other studies, suggesting that they were a sicker group of patients. Two year survival was 29%. Interestingly they reported that a medical admission reason to ICU was associated with a relative risk of death of 2.1 when compared to patients with surgical diagnoses. 61% of medical patients died, in contrast to 19% of surgical admissions to ICU. The effect remained significant even after discharge. Age, dialysis vintage and APACHE II score did not appear to significantly affect mortality in this cohort. The majority of deaths in critically ill dialysis patients occurred within the first month, and Chapman calculated that if a patient survived to one month or hospital discharge, then long-term survival reverted back to that of chronic dialysis patients who had not been admitted to ICU.

A large Swedish nationwide cohort study involving 32 ICUs followed up 245 ESRD patients who had been admitted to critical care [15]. 90-day mortality of ESRD patients was 42%. Diabetes and heart failure were significant predictors of 90-day mortality in this population with age adjusted odds ratios of 1.9 and 2, respectively. The long-term mortality in critically unwell ESRD patients was 25 times higher than expected from mortality rates in the general population (Standardized mortality ratio 25; 95% Confidence Interval 20-31), with the highest number of deaths occurring in the first year after ICU discharge, as might be expected. This is in contrast to the work of Chapman and colleagues who reported that on leaving hospital, mortality rates for ESRD patients reverted back to normal [20]. This discrepancy may be explained by different statistical methods used, for instance, Bell and team [15] did not exclude patients who had died in ICU from their calculations.

Dialysis access and modality have been found to impact on long term mortality rates in ESRD patients admitted to critical care. Sood and colleagues [18] evaluated the 6 and 12 month outcomes of 619 ESRD patients admitted to 11 Canadian ICUs. More than 80% of admission diagnoses were medical, most commonly sepsis, and 6 and 12 month mortality were 38% and 48%, respectively. Interestingly they reported that hemodialysis patients with central venous catheter access had higher crude mortality rates at both 6 and 12 months than those who dialysed with AV fistulae. Central venous catheters remained independently associated with death even after adjustment for baseline and ICU admission characteristics as well as comorbidities. Again, this finding is open to confounding, given that tunnelled lines are more commonly used in patients with a poor performance status, and pose an increased risk of infection. Two additional cohort studies have reported similar 6 and 12 month survival rates for critically ill chronic dialysis patients [7,22]. Bagshaw et al [22] found that chronic dialysis patients had a similar 1-year mortality rate to those with no kidney dysfunction after adjustment for age, severity of illness and admission type, a finding confirmed by Strijack and co-workers [8]. These studies suggest that although ESRD identifies a cohort with a worse ICU outcome than the general population, the prognosis is related to illness severity and co-morbidities rather than lack of renal function itself.

In addition to a medical admission diagnosis [4,20], diabetes, heart failure [15], and central venous catheter use [18], there are further factors which are associated with an increased mortality risk after discharge from ICU. Studies showed that older age, admission after emergency surgery, chronic health problems, CPR in the 24 hours preceding admission to ICU, having been in hospital for at least 7 days prior to ICU and the number of non-renal organ failures significantly affect outcome of ESRD patients post ICU [4,9,10,17]. As expected physiological and biochemical disturbances including hypotension, bradycardia, tachypnoea, hypoxia, reduced GCS, hyponatraemia, leucopenia and sepsis within the first 24 hours of ICU admission exert a significant impact on hospital mortality, too [4]. Mechanical ventilation and need for inotropic support are also significantly associated with mortality at 30 days [16]. Whilst many of these variables are risk factors for mortality in ICU patients in general, their impact on the ESRD population appears to be greater, perhaps due to a lack of physiological reserve in this group.

An important long-term outcome after ICU admission is quality of life and functional status. Unfortunately, to date this area has not been explored in detail in chronic dialysis patients but certainly deserves attention.

6. ICU outcomes in AKI compared to ESRD

Acute kidney injury is extremely common in critically ill patients and a frequent reason for admission to the ICU. A significant proportion require RRT and have a high associated mortality rate which can vary from 25-90% depending on patient characteristics and defining AKI criteria. Several studies have compared outcomes in patients with AKI to outcomes in critically ill chronic dialysis patients.

Clermont and colleagues [9] were among the first to examine ICU mortality in patients with AKI, ESRD and those with normal renal function. In spite of similar illness severity scores in the AKI and ESRD populations, ICU mortality rates were five times higher in the dialysis-requiring AKI group than those on chronic dialysis and ten times higher when compared to those with normal renal function (57% vs. 11% vs. 5%, respectively). There was no reported difference between patients with AKI on admission to ICU and those who developed AKI during their stay in ICU.

Similarly a small case-control study conducted in Brazil compared the outcome of AKI patients on RRT with ESRD patients, two cohorts characterised by loss of renal function. They reported double the ICU and hospital mortality rates in AKI patients compared to ESRD patients when matched for age, severity of illness and number of organ dysfunctions (42% vs. 20% and 50% vs. 24%, respectively) [17]. Length of stay in both ICU and hospital was also significantly increased in the AKI group. Having excluded patients admitted to ICU for post-operative monitoring and fluid overload or electrolyte imbalance secondary to inadequate dialysis, sepsis was the main reason for admission in both cohorts. In this study however they reported that patients with AKI were more likely to require mechanical ventilation and vasopressors than those on chronic dialysis, even when matched for severity of illness.

The largest comparison of outcomes in these two groups has come from a retrospective analysis of the Riyadh Intensive Care Program database, which recorded over 40,000 ICU admissions to nineteen units in the UK and three units in Germany over a 10 year period [21]. 1847 patients with AKI on RRT were compared to 797 ESRD patients. ICU and hospital mortality in addition to ICU length of stay were significantly increased in the cohort with AKI requiring RRT. ESRD patients had approximately half the ICU and hospital mortality rates of AKI patients on RRT (20.8% vs. 54.1%, p < 0.0001 and 34.5% vs. 61.6%, p < 0.0001, respectively). As expected, increasing ICU mortality was seen with an increasing number of organ failures in both cohorts, however the group of AKI patients on RRT had a significantly higher proportion with more than two non-renal organ failures (75.4% vs. 25.6%) and needed mechanical ventilation more often (91.3% vs. 60.9%, p<0.0001). The strongest independent risk factors for ICU mortality were mechanical ventilation, maximum number of organ failures and non-surgical reason for admission.

Walcher et al [24] also reported that significantly more AKI patients were mechanically ventilated than critically ill dialysis patients, even when well matched for illness severity scores and controlled for mode of RRT (89% vs. 57%, p = 0.0003). Mechanical ventilation was the single factor associated with increased hospital mortality with an odds ratio of 3.1. ICU, hospital, 30- and 60-day mortality rates as well as length of stay in ICU were higher in the AKI cohort compared to ESRD patients, when both received continuous renal replacement therapy (CRRT).

Although the majority of published literature indicates that ICU and hospital outcomes are significantly worse for AKI patients requiring RRT than critically ill chronic dialysis patients, one small Australian study reported comparable ICU and hospital mortality rates for diagnosis and severity-score matched AKI and ESRD patients receiving CRRT [5].

Most outcome studies are hampered by the difficulty in assessing severity of illness correctly in patients with ESRD. The commonly used ICU prognostic scoring systems are often applied to patients with ESRD despite the fact that they are not fully validated in this patient population and may over-estimate mortality rates. What is evident from the literature is that the requirement for mechanical ventilation appears to be significantly increased in patients with AKI and that this is independently associated with an increased mortality rate.

7. Validity of ICU severity scores in ESRD

ICU illness severity and organ dysfunction scoring systems are primarily used within critical care as research and audit tools to enable comparison between observed and predicted mortality and controlled matching between study cohorts. Whilst these scoring systems have been validated in a wide variety of different subspecialties, their application and accuracy in the ESRD population remains controversial.

The Acute Physiology and Chronic Health Evaluation (APACHE II and III) [11,26], SAPS II [27] and Sequential Organ Failure Assessment (SOFA) [28] scores are commonly used in critical care literature. The first two scores assess up to 20 physiological variables within 24 hours of admission to ICU, while the SOFA score is used to track progress between subsequent 24 hour periods in ICU. As might be expected all scoring systems have a renal component, taking into account urine output, urea, serum creatinine, serum potassium and bicarbonate to varying degrees. Application of these tools to chronic dialysis patients and their accuracy in predicting mortality in this group is therefore uncertain.

Several studies have attempted to assess the validity of different scoring systems when used in the ESRD population, with differing results. Hutchinson and co-workers [4] used the

APACHE II score and reported an area under the receiver operating curve (ROC) of 0.721 for their ESRD cohort, compared to 0.805 in the non-ESRD group, indicating that it is less accurate in predicting mortality in chronic dialysis patients. When using a modified renal-adjusted APACHE II score especially for dialysis patients the ROC improved to 0.817. Uchino [5] and Juneja [16] also reported a ROC of 0.81 and 0.86 respectively for the APACHE II score, using a much smaller cohort of long-term dialysis patients. The APACHE III score is an extension of its predecessor and takes into account twenty physiological variables as well as major disease categories and treatment location prior to ICU admission to provide risk estimates for hospital mortality for individual ICU patients. Two small studies have demonstrated that this score over-estimates 30-day mortality in ESRD [9,10]. Similarly, Strijack [8] found that the APACHE II score over predicted mortality in dialysis patients by a factor of 2.5.

The SOFA score assesses degree of dysfunction of six organ systems, including respiratory, cardiovascular, renal, hepatic, neurological and coagulation system. Data on its validity in patients with ESRD are conflicting. One study reported a ROC of 0.92 (although not significantly different from the APACHE II score) [16] whereas Dara et al [10] found the SOFA score to be less accurate than the APACHE III with a ROC of 0.66. Notably the patients in the first study were sicker than those included in the latter with an increased number of organ failures and greater need for mechanical ventilation and inotropes.

Therefore at present there is limited and conflicting information regarding the validity of commonly used scoring systems in chronic dialysis patients. The majority of studies have used too small sample sizes to make any reliable claims. As mentioned previously ESRD patients have similar illness severity scores to patients with AKI on admission to ICU, but have significantly better outcomes indicating that these prognostic tools over-estimate mortality in dialysis patients. The application of these tools in their current form to a population of anuric patients with chronically deranged biochemistry on long-term RRT is at best limited.

A group in Belgium have developed a renal specific prognostic score to predict outcomes in patients with AKI [29]. The Stuivenberg Hospital Acute Renal Failure Scoring System (SHARF II) is based on eight parameters; age, serum albumin, bilirubin, prothrombin time, respiratory support, sepsis, hypotension and heart failure and consists of two scores at AKI diagnosis and 48 hours later. ROC was 0.82 at diagnosis and 0.83 at 48 hours in a cohort of 293 patients admitted to the ICU with AKI. As with other prognostic tools, this system has limited clinical application because of its complexity and remains a research and audit tool. It has yet to be assessed in critically ill long-term dialysis patients and it would be interesting to investigate whether it is a more accurate predictor of mortality than current scoring systems.

8. End of life planning in critically ill dialysis patients

Advance care planning varies widely between institutions, regions and countries. The study to understand prognoses and preferences for outcomes and risks of treatments (SUPPORT) was published in 1995 and highlighted the shortcomings in end-of-life decision making practices [30]. The authors described issues with communication, frequency of intensive interventions and the way in which patients died. Less than half of physicians knew whether their patients wanted to avoid CPR, 46% of do-not-resuscitate (DNR) orders were signed within 2 days of death, and 38% of those who died had spent at least 10 days in ICU. More recently significant efforts have been made to try and improve end-of-life care for patients with chronic and terminal disease.

Critically ill patients in the ICU frequently lack the capacity to make decisions regarding life-saving and life-prolonging interventions [31]. Instead the burden falls to the family to act as surrogate decision makers in conjunction with the multi-disciplinary team. Good communication between health professionals and relatives in this scenario is essential in order to ascertain the patient's values and beliefs, as well as impart key information regarding prognosis, probability of survival and future quality of life. Decisions to withdraw active life sustaining therapies in ICU appear to be comparable between dialysis and non-dialysis patients [4].

A large retrospective mortality study using the US Renal Data System found that chronic dialysis patients over the age of 65 years experienced very high rates of medical intervention in the last month of their lives; 76% were hospitalized, 48.9% were admitted to ICU and 29% underwent at least one intensive intervention (mechanical ventilation, CPR or feeding tube placement) [32]. Unfortunately patients' preferences related to ICU admission and interventions were not explored.

With an increasingly elderly and unwell hemodialysis population advance care planning before an episode of critical illness or ICU admission is key [33]. Nephrologists have frequent contact with their patients and are in an ideal position of trust to explore any religious or cultural beliefs and discuss limitations of treatment. Advance care planning is known to address fears, prepare patients for death, and allow them to exert some control over their life as well as strengthen interpersonal relationships. Many physicians are reluctant to initiate such important discussions either through lack of adequate training or belief that patients will initiate any discussion when they are ready. In fact qualitative research has shown that ESRD patients prefer earlier physician initiation of end-of-life discussions and would welcome more information on prognosis and potential outcomes of their disease than is currently delivered [34]. These discussions are infinitely better suited to an outpatient environment rather than on a critical care unit.

A group in Saudi Arabia carried out a survey of 100 primarily Muslim dialysis patients on their views regarding advance care planning [35]. More than 95% had little knowledge of CPR, intubation or ventilation, however interestingly more than half of those surveyed had been admitted to ICU within the last 2 years. It was generally believed that CPR was effective in 50-90% of cases and the majority of patients opted to have CPR in the event of cardiac arrest. When informed about the more realistic success rates of CPR and potential ventilator dependency, brain injury and coma, the proportion of respondents agreeing to CPR fell to 35%. This study emphasises the importance of effective doctor-patient communication regarding prognosis and quality of life, supporting patients to make informed decisions.

Similarly a British study found that 76% of hemodialysis patients surveyed wished to receive CPR in the event of an in-hospital cardiac arrest not related to dialysis [36]. The patients who opted to receive CPR were significantly younger (59 ± 16 vs. 74 ± 10 years, $p < 0.01$) and had a significantly higher albumin level than those who declined or who were undecided, perhaps indicating a better chronic health status. Gender, comorbidity, dialysis vintage, proportion of patients with adequate dialysis and mean haemoglobin level were not associated with the decision.

It is evident that a large proportion of chronic dialysis patients experience an admission to ICU before they die. End-of-life discussions often fall to the family and health professionals caring for the patient. Research indicates that dialysis patients want to be involved in advance care planning at the earliest opportunity and the onus rests on the physician to enable patients to make well informed and timely decisions regarding end-of-life care.

9. Conclusion

Critically ill patients with ESRD are frequently admitted to the ICU, and although they display worse outcomes than those with normal renal function, their prognosis is better than that of ICU patients with AKI. Mortality is related primarily to the severity of the underlying illness and their co-morbidities rather than to lack of renal function itself. Having survived an episode of critical illness, data on longer-term outcomes remains conflicting and little is currently known about quality of life and performance status after discharge from ICU. Prognostic scoring systems used in critical care appear to over-estimate mortality in the chronic dialysis population and should be used with caution. There is a need for ESRD-specific tools to score severity of illness and predict mortality in the critically ill and enabling accurate research and audit in this population. Current evidence suggests that long-term dependence on dialysis should not prejudice against prompt referral or admission to ICU.

Author details

Melanie Chan and Marlies Ostermann*

*Address all correspondence to: marlies.ostermann@gstt.nhs.uk

Department of Critical Care, Guy's & St Thomas' Hospital, London, UK

References

[1] UK Renal Registry 13th Annual Report (December 2010). The Renal Association.

[2] Collins, A. J, Foley, R. N, Herzog, C, et al. US Renal Data System (2010). Annual Data Report. Am J Kidney Dis 2011;57:A8,e, 1-526.

[3] Go, A. S, Chertow, G. M, Fan, D, Mcculloch, C. E, & Hsu, C. Y. Chronic kidney disease and the risks of death, cardiovascular events, and hospitalization. N Engl J Med (2004). , 351, 1296-1305.

[4] Hutchison, C. A, Crowe, A. V, Stevens, P. E, Harrison, D. A, & Lipkin, G. W. Case mix, outcome and activity for patients admitted to intensive care units requiring chronic renal dialysis: a secondary analysis of the ICNARC Case Mix Programme Database. Crit Care (2007). R50.

[5] Uchino, S, Morimatsu, H, Bellomo, R, Silvester, W, & Cole, L. End-stage renal failure patients requiring renal replacement therapy in the intensive care unit: incidence, clinical features, and outcome. Blood Purif (2003). , 21, 170-175.

[6] Brien, O, Welch, A. J, Singer, C. A, Harrison, M, & Prevalence, D. A. and outcome of cirrhosis patients admitted to UK intensive care: a comparison against dialysis-dependent chronic renal failure patients. Intensive Care Med (2012). , 38(6), 991-1000.

[7] Manhes, G, Heng, A. E, Aublet-cuvelier, B, Gazuy, N, Deteix, P, & Souweine, B. Clinical features and outcome of chronic dialysis patients admitted to an intensive care unit. Nephrol Dial Transplant (2005). , 20, 1127-1133.

[8] Strijack, B, Mojica, J, Sood, M, Komenda, P, Bueti, J, Reslerova, M, Roberts, D, & Rigatto, C. Outcomes of chronic dialysis patients admitted to the intensive care unit. J Am Soc Nephrol (2009). , 20, 2441-2447.

[9] Clermont, G, Acker, C. G, Angus, D. C, Sirio, C. A, Pinsky, M. R, & Johnson, J. P. Renal failure in the ICU: comparison of the impact of acute renal failure and end-stage renal disease on ICU outcomes. Kidney Int (2002). , 62, 986-996.

[10] Dara, S. I, Afessa, B, Bajwa, A. A, & Albright, R. C. Outcome of patients with end-stage renal disease admitted to the intensive care unit. Mayo Clin Proc (2004). , 79, 1385-1390.

[11] Knaus, W. A, Draper, E. A, Wagner, D. P, Zimmerman, J. E, & Apache, I. I. a severity of disease classification system. Crit Care Med (1985). , 13(10), 818-29.

[12] Senthuran, S, Bandeshe, H, Ranganathan, D, & Boots, R. Outcomes for dialysis patients with end-stage renal failure admitted to an intensive care unit or high dependency unit. Med J Aust (2008). , 188, 292-295.

[13] Herzog, C. A. Cardiac arrest in dialysis patients: approaches to alter an abysmal outcome. Kidney Int (2003). Suppl 84]:SS200., 197.

[14] Sarnak, M. J, & Jaber, B. L. Mortality caused by sepsis in patients with endstage renal disease compared with the general population. Kidney Int (2000). , 58, 1758-1764.

[15] Bell, M, Granath, F, Schon, S, Lofberg, E, Ekbom, A, & Martling, C. R. Endstage renal disease patients on renal replacement therapy in the intensive care unit: short- and long-term outcome. Crit Care Med (2008). , 36, 2773-2778.

[16] Juneja, D, Prabhu, M. V, Gopal, P. B, Mohan, S, Sridhar, G, & Nayak, K. S. Outcome of patients with end stage renal disease admitted to an intensive care unit in India. Ren Fail (2010). , 32, 69-73.

[17] Rocha, E, Soares, M, Valente, C, Nogueira, L, & Bonomo, H. Jr., Godinho M, Ismael M, Valenca RV, Machado JE, Maccariello E. Outcomes of critically ill patients with acute kidney injury and end-stage renal disease requiring renal replacement therapy: a case-control study. Nephrol Dial Transplant (2009). , 24, 1925-1930.

[18] Sood, M. M, Miller, L, Komenda, P, Reslerova, M, Bueti, J, Santhianathan, C, Roberts, D, Mojica, J, & Rigatto, C. Long-term outcomes of end-stage renal disease patients admitted to the ICU. Nephrol Dial Transplant (2011). , 26, 2965-2970.

[19] Halle, M. P, Hertig, A, Kengne, A. P, Ashuntantang, G, Rondeau, E, & Ridel, C. Acute pulmonary oedema in chronic dialysis patients admitted into an intensive care unit. Nephrol Dial Transplant (2012). , 27, 603-607.

[20] Chapman, R. J, Templeton, M, Ashworth, S, Broomhead, R, Mclean, A, & Brett, S. J. Long-term survival of chronic dialysis patients following survival from an episode of multiple-organ failure. Crit Care (2009). R65.

[21] Ostermann, M. E, & Chang, R. Renal failure in the intensive care unit: acute kidney injury compared to end-stage renal failure. Crit Care (2008).

[22] Bagshaw, S. M, Mortis, G, Doig, C. J, Godinez-luna, T, Fick, G. H, & Laupland, K. B. One-year mortality in critically ill patients by severity of kidney dysfunction: a population-based assessment. Am J Kidney Dis (2006). , 48, 402-409.

[23] Marshall, J. C, Cook, D. J, Christou, N. V, Bernard, G. R, Sprung, C. L, & Sibbald, W. J. Multiple organ dysfunction score: a reliable descriptor of a complex clinical outcome. Crit Care Med (1995). , 23(10), 1638-52.

[24] Walcher, A, Faubel, S, Keniston, A, & Dennen, P. In critically ill patients requiring CRRT, AKI is associated with increased respiratory failure and death versus ESRD. Renal Failure (2011). , 33(10), 935-942.

[25] Sood, M. M, Roberts, D, Komenda, P, Bueti, J, Reslerova, M, Mojica, J, & Rigatto, C. End-stage Renal Disease Status and Critical Illness in the Elderly. Clin J Am Soc Nephrol (2011). , 6, 613-619.

[26] Knaus, W. A, Wagner, D. P, Draper, E. A, Zimmerman, J. E, Bergner, M, Bastos, P. G, Sirio, C. A, Murphy, D. J, Lotring, T, Damiano, A, et al. The APACHE III prognostic system. Risk prediction of hospital mortality for critically ill hospitalized adults. Chest (1991). , 100(6), 1619-36.

[27] Le Gall JLemeshow S, Saulnier F. A new simplified acute physiology score (SAPS II) based on a European/North American multicenter study. JAMA (1993). , 270, 2957-2963.

[28] Vincent, J. L, De Mendonça, A, Cantraine, F, Moreno, R, Takala, J, Suter, P. M, Sprung, C. L, Colardyn, F, & Blecher, S. Use of the SOFA score to assess the incidence of organ dysfunction/failure in intensive care units: results of a multicenter, prospective study. Working group on "sepsis-related problems" of the European Society of Intensive Care Medicine. Crit Care Med (1998). , 26(11), 1793-800.

[29] Lins, R. L, Elseviers, M. M, Daelemans, R, Arnouts, P, Billiouw, J. M, Couttenye, M, Gheuens, E, Rogiers, P, Rutsaert, R, Van Der Niepen, P, & De Broe, M. E. Re-evaluation and modification of the Stuivenberg Hospital Acute Renal Failure (SHARF) scoring system for the prognosis of acute renal failure: an independent multicentre, prospective study. Nephrol Dial Transplant (2004). , 19(9), 2282-8.

[30] The SUPPORT Principal InvestigatorsA controlled trial to improve care for seriously ill hospitalized patients. The study to understand prognoses and preferences for outcomes and risks of treatments (SUPPORT). JAMA (1995). , 274(20), 1591-8.

[31] Curtis, J. R, & Vincent, J. L. Ethics and end-of-life care for adults in the intensive care unit. Lancet (2010). , 376, 1347-1353.

[32] Wong, S. P, Kreuter, W, & Hare, O. AM. Treatment intensity at the end of life in older adults receiving long-term dialysis. Arch Intern Med (2012). , 172(8), 661-3.

[33] Arulkumaran, N, Szawarski, P, & Phillips, B. J. End-of-life care in patients with endstage renal disease. Nephrol Dial Transplant (2012). , 27(3), 879-81.

[34] Davison, S. N. Facilitating advance care planning for patients with endstage renal disease: the patient perspective. Clin J Am Soc Nephrol (2006). , 1, 1023-1028.

[35] Al-jahdali, H. H, Bahroon, S, Babgi, Y, Tamim, H, Al-ghamdi, S. M, & Al-sayyari, A. A. Advance care planning preferences among dialysis patients and factors influencing their decisions. Saudi J Kidney Dis Transpl (2009). , 20(2), 232-239.

[36] Ostermann, M. E, & Nelson, S. R. Haemodialysis patients' views on their resuscitation status. Nephrol Dial Transplant (2003). , 18, 1644-1647.

[37] Bell, M, Granath, F, Schön, S, & Löfberg, E. SWING, Ekbom A, Martling CR. End-stage renal disease patients on renal replacement therapy in the intensive care unit: short- and long-term outcome. Crit Care Med (2008). , 36(10), 2773-2778.

Chapter 10

More than Half of Patients Receiving Hemodialysis with Leg Ulcer Require Amputation

Masaki Fujioka

Additional information is available at the end of the chapter

1. Introduction

Patients receiving hemodialysis (HD) often develop leg ulcers, which are difficult to heal because of complications of other diseases, including diabetes mellitus (DM), calciphylaxis, collagen disease, peripheral arterial disorder (PAD), chronic anemia, and weakness of the skin (Figure 1) [1-3]. Especially, infection of an ulcer is associated with the risk of sepsis, which may be fatal if the blood access shunt becomes infected [4]. Some surgical treatment is usually required in these cases.

This article focuses on the prognosis and results of treating these wounds in patients receiving HD.

2. Patients and methods

We evaluated 57 patients receiving HD (male: 37, female: 20, and 32 because of diabetes mellitus, 22 because of chronic glomerulonephritis, 2 because of polycystic kidney, and 1 because of systemic lupus erythematosus) who had leg ulcers and underwent surgical treatment in our unit from 2004 through 2011. Patients ranged in age from 43 to 95 years (median age: 69 years).

Ninety-four patients with leg ulcers due to DM (male: 53, female: 41) who underwent surgical treatment in our unit from 2004 through 2011, were also investigated as a control. They ranged in age from 26 to 93 years (median age: 59.5 years) (no significant difference, Wilcoxon rank sum test).

I investigated differences in the cause of wounds, type of surgery, and their mortality to evaluate the severity of the wounds in patients receiving HD.

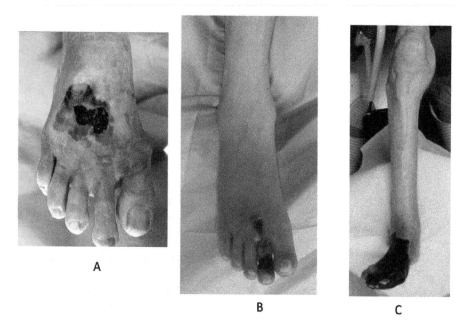

Figure 1. Patients receiving hemodialysis often develop leg ulcers due to several causes, including trauma (A: skin defect following developing a hematoma due to falling on a step), infection (B: diabetic gangrene), peripheral arterial disorder (C: leg dry necrosis due to arteriosclerosis obliterans).

3. Results

3.1. Causes of leg ulcers in patients with HD and DM

Leg ulcers in patients undergoing hemodialysis were originated due to ischemia in 34 cases (60%), infection in 13 cases (23%), and trauma in 10 cases (17%). Those in patients with DM were originally due to ischemia in 18 cases (19%), infection in 61 cases (65%), and trauma in 15 cases (16%) (Figure 2). HD-receiving patients were significantly more likely to develop leg ulcers due to PAD comparing to those with DM (p<0.001, Chi-square test).

3.2. Treatments for leg ulcers in patients with HD and DM

In the HD-receiving patient group, 30 patients (52%) underwent amputation surgery. Among them, 19 (33%) required major (below or above the knee) amputations, while 39 (42%) underwent amputation surgery, including 11 (12%) major amputations in the patients with leg ulcers due to DM (Figure 3). There was a significant differences between the groups in the frequency of amputation (p<0.05, Chi-square test) and that of major amputation (p<0.001, Chi-square test).

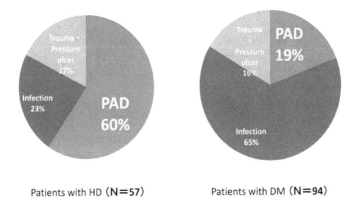

Patients with HD (N=57)   Patients with DM (N=94)

Figure 2. Causes of leg ulcers in patients with HD and DM (PAD: peripheral arterial disorder)

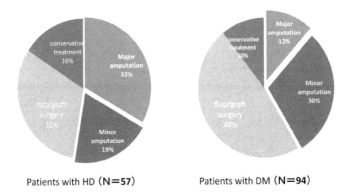

Patients with HD (N=57)   Patients with DM (N=94)

Figure 3. Treatments for leg ulcers in patients with HD and DM

3.3. Mortality of patients with leg ulcers

Three patients (5%) with HD died of contaminated foot ulcers, and 3 (3%) with DM (Figure 4). There were no significant differences in mortality between the 2 groups (p>0.05, Chi-square test).

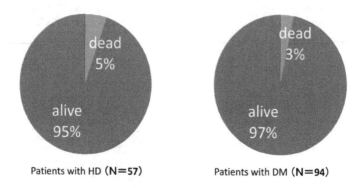

Patients with HD (N=57)   Patients with DM (N=94)

Figure 4. Mortality of patients with leg ulcers

4. Discussion

Chronic renal failure (CRF) affects all the systems of the body, causing neurological, gastrointestinal, cardiovascular, pulmonary, hematological, endocrine-metabolic, and dermatological
disorders [5]. Among them, cutaneous disorders are one of the common problems in patients
on long-term hemodialysis. The commonest skin disorders are xerosis and pruritus [6, 7]. The
skin of patients on hemodialysis is dry, and so the skin barrier structure and function are impaired [8]. Formerly, it was believed that the impaired skin resistance and stimuli caused by
scrunching because of itchy skin cause continuous inflammations, which contribute to local
skin ulcers [9]. Of course, these problems may be the causes of erosion or slight ulcers in HD-receiving patients. However, my study revealed that severe leg ulcers, which may require amputation, were mainly caused by some complications such as PAD and infection[10].

Difficulty healing wounds is a frequent problem in patients on HD because of their poor
general conditions, including malnutrition, inflammation, and PAD [1]. Mistrík et al. reported a significant decrease in skin blood flow during the HD procedure, and concluded that
the skin blood flow may be impaired in HD patients, which leads to the development of difficulty in healing skin wounds [3]. Regarding cutaneous infection, the incidence of fungal infection in patients undergoing hemodialysis was 67%, which suggested that adequate foot
care had not been performed for these patients [11]. CRF patients exhibit impaired cellular
immunity due to a decreased T-lymphocyte cell count; this could explain the increased
prevalence of infections [12]. Consequently, patients receiving HD were associated with
higher complication rates and mortality when they developed leg ulcers [13].

Patients with severely ischemic legs due to maintenance HD often require multiple surgeries
because arteriosclerosis obliterans usually progresses, which causes other ischemic ulcers
(Figure 5-8). Amputations of legs or fingers are sometimes performed for these complex ulcers, because patients receiving HD are thought to present with immunocompromised con-

ditions, and aggressive life-threatening infections such as sepsis require immediate surgical debridement in order to salvage the blood access line and save their lives (Figures 7, 9, 10). Administering antibiotics for a contaminated wound containing necrotic tissue is of no use because they cannot affect a non-vascularized or necrotic mass. Immediate surgical debridement is the only choice to improve these soft tissue infections [14, 15]. Surgical amputation is sometimes recommended to resurface these wounds, especially for some ischemic wounds including dry necrosis of toes and feet (Figure 9). My study revealed that more than half of patients underwent toe or leg amputation.

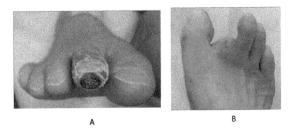

A   B

Figure 5. Case 1. Ischemic ulcer (A) The photograph shows a necrotic wound of right 2nd toe in a patient receiving HD at the initial examination. He was also diagnosed with peripheral arterial disorder. (B) He underwent amputation of the toe and the wound was healed.

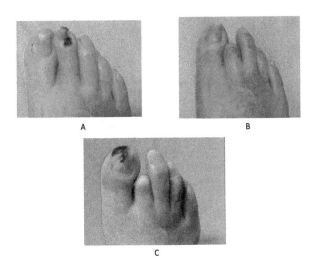

A   B

C

Figure 6. Case 2. Ischemic ulcer (PAD) (A) The photograph shows a necrotic wound of the right 2nd toe in a patient receiving HD at the initial examination. He was also diagnosed with peripheral arterial disorder. (B) He underwent amputation of the toe and the wound was healed. (C) However, he developed another ischemic ulcer 20 months later and required another amputation.

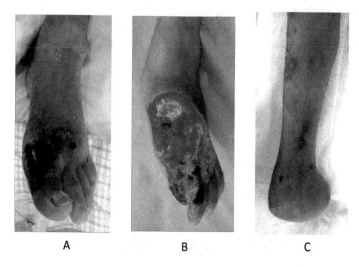

Figure 7. Case 3. Foot burn (trauma) (A) The patient was referred from an emergency unit for a complex necrotic ulcer caused by a burn to the left foot, with a high fever. As his blood access shunt in the right elbow also showed inflammation, amputation of the left big and 2nd toes was immediately performed. (B) As soft tissue necrosis progressed after debridement, and osteomyelitis occurred 1 month later, he underwent further amputation. (C) Finally, he underwent Chopart's joint amputation 2 months later.

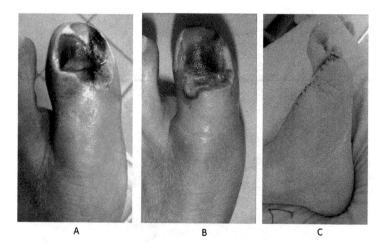

Figure 8. Case 4. Onychia periungualis (infection) (A) An HD-receiving patient developed onychia periungualis of the left 1st toe. (B) Although, he underwent the removal of the nail and antibiotic treatment, the ulcer and toe necrosis progressed. (C) The patient underwent amputation of the 1st and 2nd toes. (D) However, wound healing was unfavorable, because of the peripheral arterial disorder, thus, further amputation was required. (E) One month after the 3rd toe amputation, the wounds healed satisfactorily.

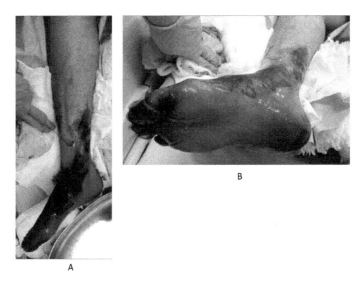

Figure 9. Case 5. Ischemic ulcer (PAD) (A) The photograph shows a necrotic wound of the right foot in a patient receiving HD at the initial examination. He was also diagnosed with peripheral arterial disorder. (B) As he developed sepsis and his blood access shunt in the right elbow also showed inflammation, he underwent below the knee amputation immediately, and the wound healed.

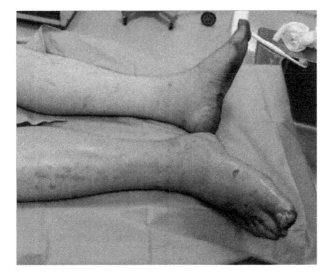

Figure 10. Case 6. Necrotizing fasciitis (infection) The photograph shows necrotizing fasciitis of the right foot in a patient receiving HD at the initial examination. He underwent below the knee amputation immediately.

I have investigated ulcers requiring surgical treatment, and the present study indicates that the development of severe leg ulcers in patients with HD is strongly influenced by ischemia due to PAD. Several investigators have reported incidences of peripheral arterial occlusive disease in patients receiving HD, ranging from 2.5 to 19.0% [16, 17].

These wounds usually develop infection, and often result in higher mortality rates because blood access shunts, especially when an artificial vessel is grafted, are easily infected. All my patients with infectious wounds (14 cases) required immediate debridement, including amputation to prevent such unfavorable general infections, because aggressive local inflammatory reactions had already developed.

On the other hand, the development of ulcers in patients with DM (control group) was mainly due to infection, which is so-called diabetic gangrene and is known to be life-threatening. My study revealed that there were no significant differences in mortality between the DM and HD groups. This suggested that the control of infection by aggressive debridement, including amputation, is the most important for the treatment of both local and general infection and saving the lives of patients. When initial debridement is insufficient and local infection recurs, further debridement should be performed. Wound infection cannot be controlled in the presence of necrotic tissue; therefore, amputation of fingers or legs is sometimes recommended, especially, when the patients show an septic status.

5. Conclusion

I conclude that patients receiving HD developed leg ulcers mainly due to PAD. They were likely to be more severe and progressive. Thus, they frequently require amputation before blood access shunts are infected.

Author details

Masaki Fujioka

Address all correspondence to: mfujioka@nmc.hosp.go.jp

Department of Plastic and Reconstructive Surgery, National Hospital Organization Nagasaki Medical Center, Ohmura City, Japan

References

[1] Mistrík E, Dusilová-Sulková S, Bláha V, Sobotka L.Plasma albumin levels correlate with decreased microcirculation and the development of skin defects in hemodialyzed patients.Nutrition. 2010 Sep;26(9):880-5.

[2] Stein, A. A. and Wiersum, J.: The Role of Renal Dysfunction in Abdominal Wound Dehiscence.J. Urol., 1959;82:271.

[3] Mistrík E, Dusilová-Sulková S, Bláha V, Sobotka L.Plasma albumin levels correlate with decreased microcirculation and the development of skin defects in hemodialyzed patients.Nutrition. 2010;26(9):880-885.

[4] Fujioka Masaki, Oka Kiyoshi, Kitamura Riko, Yakabe Aya.Complex wounds tend to develop more rapidly in patients receiving hemodialysis because of diabetes mellitus Hemodial Int. (2009). , 13(2), 168-171.

[5] Hajheydari Z, Makhlough A.Cutaneous and mucosal manifestations in patients on maintenance hemodialysis: a study of 101 patients in Sari, Iran.Iran J Kidney Dis. 2008;2(2):86-90.

[6] Robinson-Boston, L., & Di Giovanna, J. J. Cutaneous Manifestations of end-stage renal descase. J Am Acad Dermatol. (2000). , 43, 975-986.

[7] Udayakumar P, Balasubramanian S, Ramalingam KS, Lakshmi C, Srinivas CR, Mathew AC.Cutaneous manifestations in patients with chronic renal failure on hemodialysis.Indian J Dermatol Venereol Leprol. 2006;72(2):119-125.

[8] Yosipovitch G, Duque MI, Patel TS, Ishiuji Y, Guzman-Sanchez DA, Dawn AG, Freedman BI, Chan YH, Crumrine D, Elias PM.Skin barrier structure and function and their relationship to pruritus in end-stage renal disease.Nephrol Dial Transplant. 2007;22(11):3268-3272.

[9] Razeghi E, Omati H, Maziar S, Khashayar P, Mahdavi-Mazdeh M.Chronic inflammation increases risk in hemodialysis patients.Saudi J Kidney Dis Transpl. 2008;19(5): 785-789.

[10] Masaki Fujioka.Complex Wounds in Patients Receiving Hemodialysis.In:Maria GP. (ed.)Technical Problems in Patients on Hemodialysis., Rijeka:InTech; (2011). , 121-146.

[11] Bencini, P. L., Montagnino, G., Citterio, A., Graziani, G., Crosti, C., & Ponticelli, C. (1985). Cutaneous abnormalities in uremic patients. *Nephron*, 40, 316-321.

[12] Pico, M. R., & Lugo-Somolinos, A. Cutaneous alterations in patients with chronic renal failure. Int J Dermatol (1992). , 31, 860-863.

[13] Patel MS, Malinoski DJ, Nguyen XM, Hoyt DB.The impact of select chronic diseases on outcomes after trauma: a study from the National Trauma Data Bank.J Am Coll Surg. 2011;212(1):96-104.

[14] Schultz GS, Sibbald RG, Falanga V, Ayello EA, Dowsett C, Harding K, Romanelli M, Stacey MC, Teot L, Vanscheidt W.Wound bed preparation: a systematic approach to wound management.Wound Repair Regen. 2003;11 Suppl 1:S1-28.

[15] Attinger CE, Janis JE, Steinberg J, Schwartz J, Al-Attar A, Couch K.Clinical approach to wounds: débridement and wound bed preparation including the use of dressings and wound-healing adjuvants. Plast Reconstr Surg. 2006;117(7 Suppl):72S-109S.

[16] Ibels LS, Stewart JH, Mahony JF, Neale FC, SheilAG.Occlusive arterial disease in uraemic and haemodialysis patients and renal transplant recipients. A study of the incidence of arterial disease and of the prevalence of risk factors implicated in the pathogenesis of arteriosclerosis.Q J Med. (1977). , 46, 197-214.

[17] Bergesio F, Ciuti R, Salvadori M,et al.Are lipid abnormalities reliable cardiovascular risk factors in dialysis patients?Int J Artif Organs. 1989;12:677-682.

Chapter 11

Disturbances in Acid-Base Balance in Patients on Hemodialysis

Alexandre Braga Libório and Tacyano Tavares Leite

Additional information is available at the end of the chapter

1. Introduction

The prevalence of metabolic acidosis increases in Chronic Kidney Disease (CKD) patients according to the fall in glomerular filtration rate (GFR). In early stages of renal dysfunction acid retention is mainly due to the reduced tubular ammonium (NH^{4+}) secretion. As GFR declines retention of organic acids (HSO^{-s}_4, HPO^-_4) is also observed. The acid load resultant from diet and protein catabolism was believed to be the main responsible for acidosis in hemodialysis patients, however recent studies have shown an increasingly important role of hyperchloremia in the genesis of metabolic acidosis and pathophysiological disorders associated with it [1]. This finding was made possible through the use of Stewart's [2] physicochemical approach for diagnosis and classification of acid base disorders. This new approach not only enables the identification and classification of acid-base disorders and allows the quantification of the magnitude of each component to the disorder genesis [3,4].

The current K/DOQI recommendation for the treatment of metabolic acidosis in the patients on hemodialysis therapy is for maintaining a serum bicarbonate of at least 22 mEq/l [5]. Although consensus recommendation, the studies on metabolic acidosis in these patients showed that hemodialysis fail to raise the levels of serum bicarbonate to the desired value. Santos et al. [6] in a study of metabolic acidosis (HCO^-_3 < 22 mEq/L) in dialysis patients found a 90% prevalence of metabolic acidosis. Libório et al. found an average level of serum bicarbonate in dialysis patients of 18 to 19 mEq/L in their trials [1,7].

The deleterious effects of maintaining metabolic acidosis in this population of individuals are well known, endocrine disorders and anorexia leading to catabolism of endogenous proteins and changes in bone mineral metabolism all these contributing to increased morbidity and mortality in these patients [8].

CKD related acidosis is associated with several life-threatening conditions. Adequate treatment of this condition might be associated with better outcomes in the dialysis population as shown in some studies reporting improvement in nutritional status with oral bicarbonate supplementation or higher dialysis solution bicarbonate [6]. Data on involvement of chloride as cause of acidosis and its implication on acidosis complications are scarce.

In this chapter we intend to approach the importance of metabolic acidosis for dialysis patients, discuss the possible pathophysiological mechanisms involved in the genesis of the acidosis and the consequences that this disorder brings to these individuals, using quantitative physicochemical approach. We propose to conduct a literature review about the therapeutic alternatives as well as dialysis treatment modalities that could be used for the correction of this disorder.

2. The acid–base equilibrium: Henderson–Hasselbalch

The Henderson–Hasselbalch equation is still the standard method for interpreting acid–base equilibrium in clinical practice [9]. It is based in the following equation:

$$pH = pK1' + log\, HCO^{3-} / (Sx\, PCO_2) \tag{1}$$

This equation describes how plasma CO_2 tension, plasma bicarbonate (HCO^{3-}) concentration, the apparent dissociation constant for plasma carbonic acid (pK) and the solubility of CO2 in plasma interact to determine plasma pH. The magnitude of the metabolic acidosis is generally quantified by the base deficit or base excess, which is defined as the amount of base (or acid) that must be added to a liter of blood to return the pH to 7.4 at a partial pressure of carbon dioxide (PCO_2) of 40 mmHg [10].

3. Stewart model for acid base disorders

The traditional approach has been criticized as being descriptive rather than mechanistic in nature and limited in scope and therefore unable to make complete diagnosis in patients with complex disorders. In contrast, proponents of Stewart's approach believe it to be mechanistic in nature and comprehensive in scope, able to detect important hidden disorders [10,11]. The fundamental underpinning of Stewart's approach is the concept of independent and dependent variables in acid-base homeostasis. According to Stewart, "Independent variables in any system are those which can be directly altered from outside the system without affecting each other" and "...dependent variables in a system can be thought of as internal to the system. Their values represent the system's reaction to the externally imposed values of the independent variables." [12].

On the basis of Stewart's definition, H^+ and bicarbonate are dependent variables whose concentrations are determined by the three independent variables, Strong Ion Difference (SID),

PCO$_2$, and total concentration of weak acids (ATOT), mainly composed of albumin and phosphate [12]. In Stewart's approach, similar to the traditional approach, respiratory disorders are those that are due to a primary alteration in PCO$_2$. Metabolic disorders, however, are due to primary alterations in SID or ATOT and not bicarbonate. By the law of electroneutrality [4]:

$$([Na^+] + [K^+] + [Ca^{2+}] + [Mg^{2+}]) - ([Cl^-] + [lactate + other\ strong\ anions]) - ([HCO_3^-] + [A^-]) = 0 \qquad (2)$$

This formula can be rearranged as follows:

$$([Na^+] + [K^+] + [Ca^{2+}] + [Mg^{2+}]) - ([Cl^-] + [lactate + other\ strong\ anions]) = [HCO_3^-] + [A^-] \qquad (3)$$

Therefore,

$$SID = ([Na^+] + [K^+] + [Ca^{2+}] + [Mg^{2+}]) - ([Cl^-] + [lactate + other\ strong\ anions]) = [HCO_3^-] + [A^-] \qquad (4)$$

Under normal conditions, concentration of lactate and other strong ions is very low and can be ignored. The formula could therefore be simplified to

$$SID = ([Na^+] + [K^+] + [Ca^{2+}] + [Mg^{2+}]) - ([Cl^-]) = [HCO_3^-] + [A^-] \qquad (5)$$

SID therefore can be calculated as the difference between fully dissociated cations and anions or sum of bicarbonate and A$^-$ where A$^-$ represents total charges contributed by all nonbicarbonate buffers, primarily albumin, phosphate, and, in whole blood, hemoglobin. SID is therefore the same as buffer base concept introduced by Singer and Hasting more than five decades ago. When an abnormal anion is present, a gap will appear between SID calculated by the difference between strong ions (the so-called "apparent SID", SIDa) and calculated by the addition of bicarbonate and nonbicarbonate buffers (so called "effective SID" SIDe) (Figure 1). This difference, named strong ion gap (SIG), is a marker for the presence of an abnormal anion. Anion gap (AG) is also calculated on the basis of the principal of electroneutrality as shown as follows [4]:

$$([total\ cations] - [total\ anions]) = ([measured\ cations] + [unmeasured\ cations]) - ([measured\ anions] + [unmeasured\ anion]) = 0 \qquad (6)$$

This can be rearranged as:

$$([measured\ cations] - [measured\ anions]) = ([unmeasured\ anions] - [unmeasured\ cations]) = AG \qquad (7)$$

In normal state, plasma unmeasured anions reflect charges contributed by the nonbicarbonate anions (A$^-$), primarily albumin and phosphate. The unmeasured cations are primarily made up of calcium, magnesium, and, depending on the formula used, potassium. AG, the difference between the abnormal and normal (or baseline) AG, represents the amount of abnormal anion(s) present in plasma. SIG, as pointed out already, also represents the amount of abnormal anion(s) present in plasma and is expected to be mathematically equal to ΔAG (Figure 1) [4].

This relationship could have been even stronger if ΔAG were calculated in a more precise manner by using actual baseline values for AG in each patient rather than the mean value of 12 [13]. It should be clear that specific components of Stewart's formulas, such as SID and SIG, are conceptually and mathematically closely related to specific components of traditional formulas such as bicarbonate, AG, and ΔAG[4].

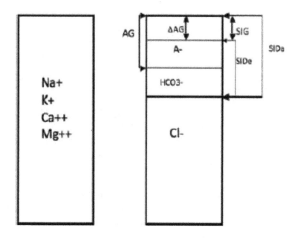

Figure 1. Relation between Strong Ion Gap (SIG) and ΔAG [4]

4. Classical X Stewart's approach

One important goal of any method used to analyze acid base disorders is to develop a clinically useful classification. The traditional approach, using a robust body of empirical observations, has developed a classification that contains six primary disorders: Metabolic acidosis, metabolic alkalosis, acute and chronic respiratory acidosis, and acute and chronic respiratory alkalosis. Metabolic acidosis can further be classified as anion gap or hyperchloremic acidosis. In addition, by using compensatory formulas as well as ΔAG, the traditional approach is capable of diagnosing complex acid-base disorders [14].

In Stewart's approach, classification of acid base disorders is based on changes in the three "independent" variables (Table 1) [15]. Respiratory disorders, as in the traditional approach, are due to a change in PCO_2, whereas metabolic disorders are due to alterations in either SID or ATOT. SID is decreased in metabolic acidosis and increased in metabolic alkalosis. By calculating SIG, one can further classify metabolic acidosis. In hyperchloremic metabolic acidosis, both effective and apparent SID decrease equally, as the increase in chloride is counterbalanced by an equal decrease in the bicarbonate concentration. SIG therefore remains at or near zero. In AG metabolic acidosis, apparent SID does not change (as chloride concentration is unchanged), but effective SID decreases (as a result of a decrease in bicarbonate concentration) and SIG therefore becomes positive [15]. One major departure from the traditional approach is classification of acid-base disorders as a result of alteration in ATOT. ATOT, representing all nonbicarbonate buffers pairs (HA + A-), is made up of charges contributed primarily by serum proteins (mainly albumin) with phosphate and other buffers playing a minor role. On the basis of this classification, an increase in serum protein would result in metabolic acidosis and a decrease, metabolic alkalosis [15,16].

Parameter	Acidosis	Alkalosis
Respiratory	$\uparrow$PCO2	$\downarrow$PCO2
Nonrespiratory (metabolic)		
Abnormal SID		
Water excess/deficit	$\downarrow$SID, $\downarrow$ [Na]	$\uparrow$SID, $\uparrow$[Na]
Imbalance of Strong anions		
Chloride excess/deficit	$\downarrow$SID, $\uparrow$[Cl]	$\uparrow$SID, $\downarrow$[Cl]
Unidentified anion excess	$\downarrow$SID, SIG "/> 0	
Nonvolatile weak acids		
Serum albumin	$\uparrow$[Alb]	$\downarrow$[Alb]
Inorganic phosphate	$\uparrow$[Pi]	$\downarrow$[Pi]

Table 1. Classification of acid-base disturbances according to Stewart´s approach [4]

5. Pathophysiology of acidosis in CKD

Classical uremic acidosis is characterized by a reduced rate of NH_4^+ production and excretion because of cumulative and significant loss of renal mass [17]. Usually, acidosis does not occur until a major portion of the total functional nephron population (>75%) has been destroyed, because of the ability of surviving nephrons to increase ammonia genesis. However, there is a decrease in total renal ammonia excretion as renal mass is reduced to a level at which the GFR is 20 mL/min or less. PO_4^{3-} balance is maintained as a result of both hyperparathyroidism, which decreases proximal PO_4^{3-}absorption, and an increase in plasma PO_4^{3-} as GFR declines. In advanced renal insufficiency, including hemodialysis patients, the hyperchloremic acidosis discussed earlier converts to a typical high AG acidosis. Poor filtration plus continued reabsorption of poorly identified uremic organic anions resulting from diet and body metabolism contributes to the pathogenesis of this metabolic disturbance [17].

Libórioet al. [1] showed when using Stewart's approach to acid–base disorders in maintenance hemodialysis that unmeasured anions are an important cause of acidosis in this population, contributing to more than 40% of reduction in serum bicarbonate. A surprising
finding was the role of hyperchloremia in acidosis etiology, which had a similar quantitative
effect in acidosis. Recently, a study carried out in nondialysis chronic renal failure patients
disclosed the main role of hyperchloremia in acidosis [18]; however, the acidosis composition in the dialysis population is still largely unknown.

The lack of quantitative analysis has led major textbooks to the assumption that the acidosis
in these patients is due to the accumulation of unmeasured anions only, leading to high
anion gap acidosis. Rocktaeschelet al. [19] showed in acute renal failure, acidosis also has
complex and multiple etiologies in maintenance hemodialysis.

Sevelamer hydrochloride is a known cause of acidosis in hemodialysis due to the load of hydrochloric acid (each 800 mg tablet of sevelamer hydrochloride leads to an acid load equivalent to 4 mEq hydrochloric acid) [20].Another potential culprit in the cause of
hyperchloremia is the chloride levels in the dialysate bath. In a literature review,15 considerable variations were found in dialysate chloride levels: from 90 to 125 mEq/l. The elevation
in chloride is accompanied by a reduction in dialysate SID. Considering this fact, the maximum level of dialysate chloride must be 105 mEq/l, allowing the dialysate SID to increase
up to 40 mEq/l, a value similar to that of plasma [7].

Acidosis in maintenance hemodialysis has multiple etiologies. Unmeasured anions and hyperchloremia are the main components, and hyperphosphatemia has a minor effect. Hyperchloremia cannot be attributed to sevelamer hydrochloride therapy alone, and we speculate
that high levels of chloride in dialysate constitute a potential culprit. Additional studies assessing the relationship between the nature of acidosis and its detrimental effects on bone,
inflammation, and nutrition are warranted [1].

6. Consequences of metabolic acidosis

6.1. Exacerbation of bone disease and impaired growth in children

Studies indicate that metabolic acidosis can be a contributory factor to the development or
exacerbation of bone disease in both adults and children and that it can impair growth in
children with or without CKD. Direct effects of an acidic milieu on bone and indirect effects
mediated by changes in PTH levels and/or its actions or vitamin D levels appear to contribute to these pathological effects [21].

Bone disease in CKD is mainly due to alterations in parathyroid hormone (PTH) and vitamin D levels. Certain toxins, such as aluminum may play a role [22]. However there is a substantial amount of data relating chronic metabolic acidosis as an additional important factor
[23,24]. In vitro and in vivo studies have demonstrated that prolonged metabolic acidosis

can directly stimulate osteoclast-mediated bone resorption and inhibit osteoblast mediated bone formation [24-27]. Some animal and human studies have shown that metabolic acidosis can reduce vitamin D levels and stimulate PTH secretion. Metabolic acidosis also attenuates the cellular response to PTH, as measured by cAMP accumulation in rat tissues. The actions of the calcium sensing receptor might also be attenuated by a decrease in extracellular pH, perhaps contributing to an increase in PTH levels [21]. Chloride might also be related to higher PTH levels and worsening bone disease. Using Stewart's physicochemical approach Liborio et al. [28] found a higher PTH levels in hemodialysis patients with higher chloride serum concentration and a significant relationship between chloride, PTH levels and serum markers of mineral bone disease.

In adult patients on chronic maintenance hemodialysis, amelioration of the acidosis by raising the dialysate base concentration was found to attenuate the rise in PTH, reduce bone resorption, and improve bone formation. In another study in dialysis patients, correction of the acidosis restored the normal suppression of PTH secretion in response to infused calcium [21]. Although controlled studies of the impact of correction of metabolic acidosis alone on the growth in children with CKD are not available, metabolic acidosis is considered to be a contributory factor to short stature in children with CKD prior to or after initiation of chronic maintenance dialysis. It's recommended that it be corrected prior to the initiation of growth hormone therapy [29].

Data about chloride and SID changing in dialysis bath and bone disease outcomes are still lacking. New studies in dialysis population assessing the long term effect this measure might influence in the amelioration of bone disease must emerge.

6.2. Increased muscle wasting

Muscle wasting is increased in CKD. This is not only due nutritional deprivation or exposure to a uremic milieu. Metabolic acidosis in CKD stimulates muscle wasting and may impair growth in children [30].

The increased protein degradation was due to the increased transcription of genes encoding proteins of the ATP-dependent ubiquitin–proteasome pathway, resulting in increased activity of the ATP-dependent ubiquitin–proteasome system (UPS) [30]. Of interest, activation of muscle protein degradation requires endogenous glucorticoids [21]. Recent studies have identified the dependency on glucocorticoids to increase muscle protein wasting as a nongenomic mechanism by which the glucocorticoid receptor sequesters phosphatidylinositol-3-kinase to interrupt insulin–IGF-1 signaling [31]. Several conditions including CKD and metabolic acidosis appear to be related to the activation of the UPS. In several studies, amelioration of metabolic acidosis by the provision of base to patients with CKD before or after initiation of maintenance dialysis decreased the rate of protein degradation and urea generation, resulting in improved protein balance and increased muscle mass [30].

Similar to bone disease, some evidence suggests that a detectable fall in serum [HCO_3^-] may not be necessary to stimulate muscle degradation. [21]

6.3. Reduced albumin synthesis

Hypoalbuminemia is the most common marker of protein-energy wasting in dialysis patients and has strong association with increased morbidity and mortality. Hypoalbuminemia is associated with development and recurrent cardiac failure in hemodialysis patients [32].

Experimental induction of metabolic acidosis in normal humans for at least 7 days has in some studies caused a reduction in albumin synthesis, thereby predisposing the individual to the development of hypoalbuminemia [33,34]. Indeed, analysis of more than 1500 patients > 20 years of age who participated in the NHANES III study revealed that the age-adjusted odds ratio of serum [HCO_3^-] for hypoalbuminemia rose from 1.0 for serum [HCO_3^-] > 28 mEq/l to 1.54 for serum [HCO_3^-] ≤22 mEq/l [35]. Furthermore, in two studies of adult patients with CKD either prior to or after initiation of chronic maintenance dialysis, improvement of the metabolic acidosis by the provision of base caused the serum albumin concentration to rise and protein catabolic rate to fall [36,37].

Reduced protein synthesis, increased protein breakdown, and enhanced amino acid oxidation have all been suggested as factors contributing to a reduced serum albumin concentration with metabolic acidosis. A decrease in protein intake might also play a role, although in one study in which dietary intake was examined, no difference in protein intake was found in patients with CKD before or after correction of the acidosis [21].

6.4. Accelerating the progression of CKD

Studies in humans have supported the potential role of metabolic acidosis in the progression of CKD. In a large cohort of patients with CKD followed at a single medical center, a serum [HCO_3^-] of <22 mEq/l was associated with a 54% increased hazard of progression of CKD when compared with a serum [HCO_3^-] of 25–26 mEq/L [38]. In two separate studies, one in patients with hypertensive renal disease [39]and another in patients with CKD of diverse etiology [40], the administration of base slowed the progression of CKD. In the latter study, the rate of decline in GFR in those given bicarbonate was less than half that in the control group. Moreover, the bicarbonate group was less likely to experience a rapid decline in GFR or develop end-stage renal disease [21].

Three mechanisms have been postulated to explain the acceleration of progression of CKD in response to metabolic acidosis. First, it has been suggested that the increase in renal medullary ammonia concentration resulting from the stimulation of ammonia production by metabolic acidosis activates the alternative complement pathway and causes progressive tubulointerstitial injury [41]. Second, it has been suggested that new bicarbonate synthesized by the kidney in response to acidosis alkalinizes the interstitium and encourages precipitation of calcium in the kidney [42]. Finally, evidence in both animals and humans has been accrued to suggest that increased endothelin production may mediate the tubulointerstitial injury and decline in GFR noted with the metabolic acidosis of CKD [43].

6.5. Impaired glucose homeostasis

Studies in patients with CKD demonstrated impaired glucose tolerance and insulin resistance, both prior to and after the initiation of chronic maintenance dialysis. The effect of uremia on insulin resistance appeared to be related, in part, to metabolic acidosis, because the administration of base to stable hemodialysis patients improved, although it did not normalize, insulin sensitivity. The insulin resistance and glucose intolerance of uremia per se are generally not severe, but it is possible that they contribute to the development of other clinical abnormalities [21].

6.6. Accumulation of β2-microglobulin

The accumulation of β2-microglobulin in individuals with CKD contributes to the development of amyloidosis. Amyloid infiltration can cause the carpal tunnel syndrome, bone cysts and, possibly, cardiomyopathy [44]. This accumulation of β2-microglobulin is primarily related to the number of years on dialysis, which has been interpreted as suggesting that the predilection to amyloidosis is due to reduced excretion of β2-microglobulin and, in the case of hemodialysis, also to chronic exposure of blood to the dialysis membrane [44].

Metabolic acidosis has been suggested as a possible additional factor in promoting β2-microglobulin accumulation. First, there is an inverse correlation between serum [HCO_3^-] and β2-microglobulin levels in patients with CKD. Furthermore, β2-microglobulin concentrations have been found to be higher in patients dialyzed with acetate who have a lower serum [HCO_3^-] than those dialyzed with bicarbonate [44].

6.7. Abnormal thyroid function

Individuals with uremia have low basal metabolic rates. This could be related in part to the associated metabolic acidosis affecting thyroid hormone levels, since ammonium chloride-induced metabolic acidosis has been found to be associated with reduced triiodothyronine (T3) and thyroxine (T4) and elevated thyroid-stimulating hormone levels [21]. Correction of metabolic acidosis in patients with CKD causes T3 levels to rise towards normal [45].

6.8. Stimulation of inflammation

Exposure of macrophages to an acidic environment leads to the increased production of tumor necrosis factor α (TNFα) [46]. In one study, the correction of metabolic acidosis in a small number of patients maintained on chronic ambulatory peritoneal dialysis was associated with a reduction in TNFα levels [21]. Thus, it has been suggested that metabolic acidosis is associated with the stimulation of inflammation and, therefore, that it represents a chronic inflammatory state. However, no significant difference was observed in the serum levels of C-reactive protein and interleukin-6 (two biomarkers of inflammation) among three separate groups of dialysis patients with a mean serum [HCO_3^-] of 19.2, 24.4, and 27.5 mEq/L, respectively [47].

6.9. Development or exacerbation of cardiac disease and increase in mortality

Low serum bicarbonate level is related to higher mortality in CKD patients both prior [48] to and after initiation of chronic maintenance dialysis [21]. A retrospective analysis of laboratory data obtained from more than 12,000 hemodialysis patients showed an increased risk of death in patients with a serum [HCO_3^-] <15–17 mEq/L [49]. Also, patients with CKD not on dialysis had a greater risk of death when their serum [HCO_3^-] was <22 mEq/L [50]. Navaneethanet al. [48]found a higher mortality rate in the group of patients with lower serum bicarbonate ([HCO_3^-] < 23 mEq/L) level in a trial of 41.445 stage 3 and 4 CKD patients. An interesting finding of this trial was that higher level ([HCO_3^-] > 32 mEq/L) was also associated with poor outcome and higher mortality rate. The DOPPS study [51] showed better outcomes in maintenance hemodialysis patients with midweek bicarbonate serum level of 21,1 to 22 mEq/L. In this study both low ([HCO_3^-] < 17 mEq/L) and higher (>24 mEq/L) were related to higher hospitalization and mortality rate. These data point to the importance of a strict control of metabolic acid base disturbances in CKD patients and the harmful effect of overcorrection of acidosis.

Cardiovascular disease is the most common cause of death in patients with CKD. There are strong evidence that inflammation plays an important role in the genesis and progression of atherosclerotic heart disease. As discussed earlier in this text acidosis is a chronic inflammatory state and it is reasonable to speculate that metabolic acidosis could be related to increased prevalence or severity of cardiovascular disease [21].

6.10. Renal replacement therapy and liver failure

Anticoagulation with heparin might be a problem in patients with increased bleeding risk specially critically ill patients and cirrhotic patients requiring continuous renal replacement therapy (CRRT). There is increasing evidence questioning the safety of heparin in such patients and there are accumulating data on a potential better alternative, regional anticoagulation with citrate. Sodium citrate administered before the filter inhibits the generation of thrombin. For anticoagulation the citrate dose is adjusted to blood flow to attain low ionized calcium (< 0,4 mmol/l) concentration in the filter, the lower the calcium concentration the higher the degree of anticoagulation. Citrate is partially removed by the filter and the remaining amount is metabolized in citric acid cycle predominantly in the liver. The chelated calcium is than released and the lost calcium is replaced after filter. The systemic coagulation is unaffected [52].

Buffer strength of citrate depends on the proportion of strong cations in the fluid counterbalancing citrate concentration. Assuming the citrate is completely metabolized, one micromole of trisodium citrate provides the buffer as 3 mmol sodium bicarbonate. The Stewart Concept provides an easier way to understand the buffering effect of citrate: after metabolized in the liver the remaining sodium increases serum SID. Increased SID produces alkalosis. Sodium citrate has a SID of zero until citrate is metabolized, so in conditions where citrate metabolism is grossly impaired, such as severe liver dysfunction the citrate alkalinizing effect might be compromised. Citrate accumulation decreases the SID leading to a metabolic acidosis [52]. For this reason anticoagulation free or low heparin regimens have been used for patients with severe liver dysfunction requiring continuous renal replacement therapy. This strategy reduces bleeding risk however lowers the procedure efficiency and thefilter patency.

Recent studies have emerged showing protocol using sodium citrate as a safe alternative for anticoagulation even in patients with liver dysfunction. In a prospective randomized open label crossover trial of regional citrate anticoagulation vs. anticoagulation free liver dialysis by the Molecular Adsorbents Recirculating System (MARS) Meijers et al. [53] demonstrated that citrate anticoagulation significantly increased the likelihood of completed MARS treatment (P = 0,04), higher bilirubin reduction ratio when citrate was applied and improvement in systemic ph levels. In this study, systemic ionized calcium concentrations were significantly reduced during citrate anticoagulation but remained within a safe range even using standard protocol for extracorporeal calcium levels. There were no major adverse events in the citrate group. Other study in early post liver transplantation patients requiring CRRT showed efficacy and safety of regional citrate anticoagulation without severe decrease in calcium concentration and acidosis [54]. Another study applied anticoagulation with sodium citrate in patients with severely impaired liver dysfunction (mean Child-Pugh score: 10,5) under renal replacement therapy with sustained low efficiency dialysis (SLED) after repeated filter clotting (filter lifetime < 2h) under heparin free or low dose heparin therapy. The dialysis time with citrate anticoagulation was 17,3 h, filter lifetime increased to 23,3 h. No major bleeding episodes related to dialysis therapy were observed, total calcium, ionized calcium, calcium gap, electrolytes and base excess were maintained at stable levels during therapy and thereafter. There were no significant hypotensive episodes and norepinephrine dose was reduced during therapy. This protocol used lower citrate infusion rate with higher post-filter ionized calcium levels and absence of routine calcium supplementation at venous line and the use of high-flux dialyser for reducing the risk of accumulating calcium citrate complexes [55].

These data show increasing evidence that citrate might be used for anticoagulation even in patients with impaired liver function. However clinicians should be alert when using this strategy, measuring the citrate levels and use of high-flux dialyser must be applied for warranting safety of maintaining low citrate concentrations. Data showing safety of citrate regional anticoagulation and recommendation of its use in patients with liver impairment under CRRT are scarce and don't warranty recommendation of its application for this modality of treatment.

7. Treatment of metabolic acidosis in hemodialysis patients

The standard recommendation for correction of metabolic acidosis in CKD patients is for reaching a bicarbonate level at least 22 mEq/L in dialytic and conservative management patients [5]. Reaching this level may be a challenging schedule [1,6,7]. Current dialysate base standards appear to be somewhat arbitrarily chosen. Standard concentrations of bicarbonate in dialysates (33–35 mEq/L) do not completely correct the acidosis [56].

Alkali therapy has been shown to retard the progression of CKD in patients with reduced GFR not in dialysis therapy [57]. Benefits of correcting this disturbance in hemodialysis patients have already been reported in this chapter.

Routine measuring bicarbonate serum levels and the application of one of the following strategies might be of utility for maintaining bicarbonate target concentration and improving outcomes.

7.1. Oral supplementation

In CKD patients in conservative management acidosis should be treated by administering base in the form of oral bicarbonate or organic anions that are metabolized to bicarbonate such as citrate. Once serum bicarbonate reaches the desired level, the amount of base administered can be reduced to the minimal necessary to maintain this level [21]. A Systematic review on treatment of metabolic acidosis in non-dialysis patients showed improvement in kidney function, which may afford a long term benefit in slowing the progression of CKD [57]. Papadoyannakis et al. [58]found that ingestion of sodium bicarbonate corrects metabolic acidosis and increases appetite and body mass of the end-stage renal failure patients.

In dialysis patients oral administration of calcium carbonate at a dosage of 3–6 g/daily raises pre-dialysis plasma bicarbonate [59]. Calcium carbonate induces positive nitrogen balance due to correction of metabolic acidosis. Furthermore, calcium carbonate serves as a phosphate binder [60]. Instead of ingestion of the bicarbonate, calcium salts of organic acids could also be used as phosphate binders, i.e. acetate, citrate, gluconate or ketogluterate, which all could be metabolized into bicarbonate [61].

7.2. Bicarbonate based dialysis solution

Whichever dialysis therapy is used, there is a similar need for correcting the acid-base balance. The most important tool for this aim is the buffer in the dialysis fluid. Bicarbonate dialysis achieves much better hemodialysis stability [62]. Based on clinical and experimental studies, different side effects of hemodialysis treatment have been attributed to acetate, such as nausea, vomiting, headache, muscle cramps, hypotension, hemodynamic instability and increased cytokine release [63,64]. In contrast to acetate dialysis, bicarbonate dialysis does not interfere with gluconeogenesis and lipid synthesis [65]. The buffer source in all modern versions of these therapies should be bicarbonate. Bicarbonate is a physiological buffer, therefore in bicarbonate dialysis, plasma bicarbonate concentration and blood pH progressively increase during the dialysis session[65].

7.3. Higher bicarbonate in dialysate

Rising bicarbonate level in dialysate is effective in correcting metabolic acidosis. This correction is associated with improvement in CKD related anorexia and influencing the nutritional status [6]. Choosing dialysate bicarbonate level might be challenging. Some observations confirmed that dialysate bicarbonate concentrations of 40 mEq/L appear safe and well tolerated [66,67]. Oettinger and Oliver [68] demonstrated that high-bicarbonate dialysate (42 mEq/L) corrects pre-dialysis acidosis in 75% of hemodialysis patients without causing progressive alkalemia, hypoxia, or hypercarbia and that pre-dialysis BUN, calcium, ionized calcium and phosphorus are unaffected by high-bicarbonate dialysate. Williams et al. [69] demonstrated that bicarbonate dialysate concentrations of 40 mEq/L were safe, well tolerated and produced better control of acidosis (significantly higher pre-dialysis arterial plasma pH values as pre-dialysis serum total CO_2), with an increase in triceps skinfold thickness, compared to a bicarbonate concentration of 30 mEq/L. The amount of base transferred to the patient during dialysis depends on the patient's needs. Agroyannis et al. [70] showed a significant correlation between interdialytic weight gain and the values of pre-hemodialysis blood pH and bicarbonate, suggesting an important role of the interdialytic weight gain on acid-base equilibrium of uremic patients undergoing hemodialysis.

There is no doubt that individualized bicarbonate concentration is necessary for hemodialysis patients. Therefore, the choice of dialysate bicarbonate concentration should also be predicted on the basis of the patient's determinants (hydrogen generation, bicarbonate distribution space) and technique-related factors (membrane permeability, ultrafiltration rate, blood and dialysate flow) [71]. This can be achieved by new dialysis machines and by bicarbonate profiling.

7.4. Changing SID – The physicochemical approach

The base supply by dialysis does not seem to represent the main mechanism for acid-base correction by dialysis. Using Stewart's physicochemical approach Liborio et al. [1], showed in that chloride might play a pivotal role in pathogenesis of metabolic acidosis in hemodialysis patients. Other study found a better correction in bicarbonate levels after dialysis with a chloride level of 107 mEq/L rather than 111 mEq/L [7]. Such correction in serum bicarbonate might be possible due to elevation in plasma SID by exposing plasma to higher SID in dialysis solution. However although not expected, correction of metabolic acidosis in this study was mainly due to reduction of unmeasured anions, represented in Stewart's model by SIG.

This unexpected reduction in unmeasured anions can be explained by Gibbs Donnan equilibrium. The reduction in serum chloride during the post-dialysis period can facilitate redistribution from the intracellular or interstitial compartment, this decrease in intracellular chloride can improve the intracellular capacity of buffering other negative charges, reducing plasma unmeasured anions. Another possible explanation may be found in the dialysate compartment. It has been suggested that a higher dialysate chloride concentration, through Gibbs-Donnan equilibrium across the dialyzer membrane, partially prevents an adequate clearance of unmeasured anions due to a charge effect, i.e., electric repulsion of a negative charge. Moreover, based on this principle, it is not possible to exclude that an improvement in bicarbonate diffusion might have been the result of using a lower dialysate chloride concentration [7].

Diet, intestine, bone and intermediate metabolism could play a pivotal role in the acid-base status of uremic patients. Probably, more attention needs to be paid to the possible noxious effect of overcorrection of acidosis. Rapid correction of acidosis by bicarbonate dialysis may cause drowsiness, unconsciousness, hypokalemia and cardiac arrhythmia [72].

8. Conclusion

Metabolic acidosis is a detrimental condition both for CKD patients on hemodialysis therapy or conservative management. Several adverse effects of maintenance of an acidic state
come with the falling in GFR and developing and worsing of acidosis. Several strategies
have been employed for correction of that disturbance as listed before, some need more researches for finding consistent results of the benefits of such strategies. Stewart's approach
brought new perspectives for understanding and treating this disturbance. Studies validat-
ing changing SID, chloride or other components of the dialysate bath are still need.

Attention must be paid for the metabolic alkalosis in this population as a result of overcorrection or overtreatment of acidosis. This one brings deleterious effects like metabolic acidosis. How metabolic alkalosis impairs survival in CKD is still unknow, new researches are
need in this field.

Author details

Alexandre Braga Libório and Tacyano Tavares Leite

General Hospital of Fortaleza, Fortaleza, Ceará, Brazil

References

[1] Libório AB, Daher EF, De Castro MCM. Characterization of acid-base status in maintenance hemodialysis: physicochemical approach. J Artif Organs 2008;11(3) 156-159.

[2] Stewart PA. How to Understand Acid-Base: A Quantitative Acid-Base Primer for Biology and Medicine. New York: Elsevier, 1981.

[3] Greenbaum J, Nirmalan M. Stewart's physicochemical approach. Current Anaesthe-
sia and Critical Care 2005;16(3) 74-80.

[4] Rastegar A, Clinical Utility of Stewart's Method in diagnosis and Management of
Acid-base disorders. Clin J Am SocNephrol 2009; 4 1267-1274.

[5] National Kidney Foundation. NKF-K/DOQI clinical practice guidelines for bone metabolism and disease in chronic kidney disease. Am J Kidney Dis 2003.

[6] Santos EMC, Petrubú MMV, Gueiros JEB, Cabral PC, et al. Efeitobenéfico da correção
da acidosemetabólicanaestadonutricional de pacientesemhemodiálise. J Bras Nefrol
2009;31(4) 244-251.

[7] Marques FO, Libório AB, Daher EF, Effect of chloride dialysate concentration on metabolic acidosis in maintenance hemodialysis patients. Brz J Med Biol Res 2010;43(10)
996-1000.

[8] Leal VO, Júnior ML, Mafra D, Acidosemetabólicanadoença renal crônica: abordagemnutricional. Rev Nutr, 2008.

[9] Hesselbalch KA. Die berechnungderwasserstoffzahldêsblutes auf der frejen und gebrndenenkohlensauredesselben, um die sauerstoffbindungdêsblutesalsfunktion der wasserstoffzahl. Biochem Z 1916; 78 112-144.

[10] Fencl V, Leith DE: Stewart's quantitative acid-base chemistry: Application in biology and medicine. RespirPhysiol 1993;9 11-16.

[11] Kellum J: Clinical Review: Reunification of acid-base Physiology. Crit Care 2005;9 500-507.

[12] Stewart PA: Independent a dependent variables of acid base conrol. RespPhysiol 1978;33 9-26.

[13] Rastegar A: Use of the AG/HCO3 ratio in the diagnosis of mixed acid-base disorders. J Am SocNephrol 2007;18 2429-2431.

[14] Rastegar A: Mixed acid-base disorders: Acid Base Disorders and Their Treatment, edited by Gennari FJ, Adrouge HJ, Galla JG, Madias NE, Boca Raton, Taylor & Francis, 2005, 681-696.

[15] Fencl V, Jabor A, Kazda A, Figge J: Diagnosis of metabolic acid-base disturbances in critically ill patients. Am J RespirCrit Care Med 2000;162 2246-2251.

[16] Fencl V. Acid base disorders in critical care medicine. Annu Rev Med 1989;40 17-29.

[17] Brenner & Rector's The Kidney edited by Maarten W. Taal et al. Elselvie, 9th edition, Elselvier Saunders, 2012.

[18] Story DA, Tosolini A, Bellomo R, et al. Plasma acid-base changes in chronic renal failure: a stewart analysis. IntArtif Organs 2005;28:961-965.

[19] Rocktaeschel J, Morimatsu H, Uchino S, et al. Acid-basestarus of critically ill patients with acute renal failure: analysis basid on Stewart-Figge Methodology. Crit Care 2003;7 60-66.

[20] Brezina B, QunibiWy, Nolan CR. Acid loading during treatment with sevelamer hydrochloride: mechanism and clinical implications. Kidney Int 2004;66 39-45.

[21] Kraut FA, Madias NE. Consequences and therapy of the metabolic acidosis of crhonic kidney disease. PediatrNephrol 2011;26 19-28.

[22] Bushinsky DA. Nephology forum: The contribution of acidosis to renal osteodystrophy. Kidney Int 1999;47 1816-1832.

[23] Kraut JA, Kurtz I. Metabolic acidosis of CKD: Diagnosis, clinical characteristics and treatment. Am J Kidney Dis 2005;45 978-993.

[24] Kraut JA. Disturbances of acid-base balance and bone disease in end stage renal disease. Semin Dial 2000;13 261-265.

[25] Lemann J Jr, Bushinsky DA, Hamm LL. Bone buffering of acid and base in humans. Am J Physiol 2003;285 811-832.

[26] Krieger NS, Sessler NE, Bushinsky DA. Acidosis inhibits osteoblastic and stimulates osteoclastic activity in vitro. Am J Physiol 1992;262 442-448.

[27] Kraut JA, Mishler DR, Singer, FR, Goodman WG. The effects of metabolic acidosis on bone formation and bone resorptioninrat. Kidney Int 1986;30 694-700.

[28] Libório AB, Noritomi DT, de Castro MCM. Chloride, but not unmeasured anions, is correlated with renal boné disease markers. Jnephrol 2007;20(4) 474-481.

[29] Mahan JD, Warady BA. Assesment and treatment of short stature in pediatric patients with chronic kidney disease: a consensus statement. PediatrNephrol 2006;21 917-930.

[30] Workeneh BT, Mitch WE. Review of muscle wasting associated with chronic kidney disease. Am J ClinNutr 2010;91 1128-1132.

[31] Hu ZY, Wang HL, Lee IH, DU J, Mitch WE. Endogenous glucocorticoids and impaired insulin signaling are both required to stimulate muscle wasting under pathophysiological conditions in mice. J. Clin Invest 119 3059-3069.

[32] Bonanni A, Mannucci I, Versola D, Sofia A, Saffioti S, Gianetta E, Garibotto G. Protein-Energy Wasting and Mortality in chronic Kidney disease. Int J Environ Res Public Health 2011;8 1631-1654.

[33] Ballmer PE, McNurlan MA, Hulter HN, Anderson SE, Garlick PJ, Krapf R. Chronic metabolic acidosis decreases albumin synthesis and induces negative nitrogen balance in humans. J Clin Invest 1995;95 39–45.

[34] Kleger GR, Turgay M, Imoberdorf R, McNurlan MA, Garlick PJ, Ballmer PE. Acute metabolic acidosis decreases muscle protein synthesis but not albumin synthesis in humans. Am J Kidney Dis 2001;38 1199–1207.

[35] Eustace JA, Astor B, Muntner PM, Ikizler TA, Coresh J. Prevalence of acidosis and inflammation and their association with low serum albumin in chronic kidney disease. Kidney Int 2004;65 1031–1040.

[36] Movilli E, Zani R, Carli O, Sangalli L, Pola A, Camerini C, Cancarini GC, Scolari F, Feller P, Maiorca R. Correction of metabolic acidosis increases serum albumin concentrations and decreases kinetically evaluated protein intake in haemodialysis patients: a prospective study. Nephrol Dial Transplant 1998;13 1719–1722.

[37] Verove C, Maisonneuve N, El Azouzi A, Boldron A, Azar R. Effect of the correction of metabolic acidosis on nutritional status in elderly patients with chronic renal failure. J RenNutr 2002;12 224–228.

[38] Shah SN, Abramowitz M, Hostetter TH, Melamed ML. Serum bicarbonate levels and the progression of kidney disease: a cohort study. Am J Kidney Dis 2009;54 270–277.

[39] Phisitkul S, Khanna A, Simoni A, Broglio K, Rajab MH, Wesson DE. Amelioration of metabolic acidosis in patients with low GFR reduced kidney endothelin production and kidney injury, and better preserved GFR. Kidney In 2010;77:617–623.

[40] Brito-Ashurst I, Varagunam M, Raftery MJ, Yaqoob MM. Bicarbonate supplementation slows progression of CKD and improves nutritional status. J Am SocNephrol 2009;20 2075–2084.

[41] Nath KA, Hostetter MK, Hostetter TH. Increased ammoniagenesis as a determinant of progressive renal injury. Am J Kidney Dis 1991;17:654–657.

[42] Halperin ML, Ethier JH, Kamel KS. Ammonium excretion in chronic metabolic acidosis: benefits and risks. Am J Kidney Dis 1989;14 267–271.

[43] Phisitkul S, Hacker C, Simoni J, Tran RM, Wesson DE. Dietary protein causes a decline in the glomerular filtration rate of the remnant kidney mediated by metabolic acidosis and endothelin receptors. Kidney Int 2008;73 192–199.

[44] Sonikian M, Gogusev J, Zingraff J, Loric S, Quednau B, Bessou G, Siffert W, Drueke TD, Reusch H, Luft FC. Potential effect of metabolic acidosis on beta2-microglobulin generation: In vivo and in vitro studies. J Am SocNephrol 1996;7 350–356.

[45] Wiederkehr MR, Kalogiros J, Krapf R. Correction of metabolic acidosis improves thyroid and growth hormone axes in haemodialysis patients. Nephrol Dial Transplant 2004;19 1190–1197.

[46] Bellocq A, Suberville S, Philippe C, Bertrand F, Perez J, Fouqueray B, Cherqui G, Baud L. Low environmental pH is responsible for the induction of nitric-oxide synthase in macrophages—evidence for involvement of nuclear factor-kappa B activation. J BiolChem 1998;273 5086–5092.

[47] Lin SH, Lin YF, Chin HM, Wu CC. Must metabolic acidosis be associated with malnutrition in haemodialysed patients? Nephrol Dial Transplant 2002;17 2006–2010.

[48] Navaneethan SD, Schold JD, Arrigain S, Jolly SE, Wehbe E, Raina R et al. Serum bicarbonate and mortality in stage 3 and stage 4 chronic kidney disease. Clin J Am SocNephrol 2011;6 2395-2402.

[49] Bommer J, Locatelli F, Satayathum S, Keen ML, Goodkin DA, Saito A, Akiba T, Port FK, Young EW. Association of pre-dialysis serum bicarbonate levels with risk of mortality and hospitalization in the Dialysis Outcomes and Practice Patterns Study (DOPPS) Am J Kidney Dis 2004;44 661–671.

[50] Kovesdy CP, Anderson JE, Kalantar-Zadeh K. Association of serum bicarbonate levels with mortality in patients with non-dialysis-dependent CKD. Nephrol Dial Transplant 2009;24 1232–1237.

[51] Bommer J, Locatelli F, Satyathum S, Keen M, Goodkin DA, Saito A et al. Association of pre-dialysis serum bicarbonate levels with risk of mortality and hospitalization in

the Dialysis Outcomes and Pactice Patterns Study (DOPPS). Am J Kid diseases 2004;44(4) 661-671.

[52] Straaten HMO, Kellum JA, Bellomo R. Clinical Review: Anticoagulation or continuous renal replacement therapy – heparin or citrate? Critcal Care 2011; 15 202-211

[53] Meijers B, Laleman W, Vermeersch P, Nevens F, Wilmer A, Evenepoel P. A prospective randomized open-label crossover trial of regional citrate anticoagulation vs. anticoagulation free liver dialysis by the Molecular Adsorbents Recirculating System. Critcal Care 2012; 16 R20-R28

[54] Saner FH, Treckmann JW, Geis A, Lösh C, Witzke O, CanbayA et al. Efficacy and safety of regional citrate anticoagulation in liver transplant patients requiring postoperative renal replacement therapy. Nephrol Dial Transplant 2012; 27 1651-1657

[55] Morath C, Miftari N, Dikow R, Heiner C, Zeier M, Morgera S et al. Sodium citrate anticoagulation during sustained low efficicency dialysis (SLED) in patients with acute renal failure and severely impaired liver function. Nephrol Dial Transplant 2007; 23 421-422

[56] Kraut JA, Madias NE: Treatment of metabolic acidosis in end-stage renal failure: Is dialysis with bicarbonate sufficient. Semin Dial 1996;9 378-383.

[57] Susantitaphong P, Sewaralthahab K, Balk EM, Jaber B, Madias NE. Short and long-term effects of alkali therapy in chronic kidney disease: a systematic review. Am J Nephrol 2012;35 540-547.

[58] Papadoyannakis NJ, Stefanidis CJ, McGeown M. The effect of the correction of metabolic acidosis on nitrogen and potassium balance of patients with chronic renal failure. Am J ClinNutr 1984;40 623–627.

[59] Anelli A, Brancaccio D, Damasso R, Padovese P, Gallieni M, Garella S. Substitution of calcium carbonate for aluminum hydroxide in patients on hemodialysis. Effects on acidosis, on parathyroid function, and on calcemia. Nephron 1989;52 125–132.

[60] Makoff R. The value of calcium carbonate in treating acidosis, phosphate retention and hypocalcemia. Nephrol News Issues 1991;5 1618–1632.

[61] Classen HG, Schutte K, Schimatschek HF. Different effects of three high-dose oral calcium salts on acid-base metabolism, plasma electrolytes and urine parameters of rats. Methods Find ExpClinPharmacol 1995;17 437–442.

[62] Mehta BR, Fischer D, Ahmad M, Dubose T. Effects of acetate and bicarbonate hemodialysis on cardiac function in chronic dialysis patients. Kidney Int 1983;24 782–787.

[63] Berland Y, Brunt R, Ragon A, Reynier JP. Dialysis fluid water: Their roles in biocompatibility. Nephrol Dial Transplant 1995;10 45–47.

[64] Velez RL, Woodard TD, HenrichWl. Acetate and bicarbonate hemodialysis in patients with and without autonomic dysfunction. Kidney Int 1984;26 59–65.

[65] Van Stone JC. Bicarbonate dialysis: Still more to learn. Semin Dial 1994;7 168–169.

[66] Ahmad S, Pagel M, Vizzo J, Scribner BH. Effect of the normalization of acid base balance on postdialysis plasma bicarbonate. Trans Am SocArtif Intern Organs 1980;26 318–321.

[67] Kobrin SM, Raja RM. Effect of varying dialysate bicarbonate concentration on serum phosphate. Trans Am SocArtif Intern Organs 1989;35 423–425.

[68] Oettinger CW, Oliver JC. Normalization of uremic acidosis in haemodialysis patients with a high bicarbonate dialysate. J Am SocNephrol 1993;3 1804–1807.

[69] Williams AJ, Dittmer ID, McArley A, Clarke J. High bicarbonate dialysate in haemodialysis patients. Effects on acidosis and nutritional status. Nephrol Dial Transplant 1997;12 2633–2637.

[70] Agroyannis B, Fourtounas C, Tzanatos H, Dalamangas A, Vlahakos DV: Relationship between interdialytic weight gain and acid-base status in hemodialysis by bicarbonate. Artif Organs 2002;26 385–387.

[71] Zucchelli P, Santoro A: Correction of acid-base balance by dialysis. Kidney IntSuppl 1993;41 179–183.

[72] Kovacic V, Roguljic L, Kovacic V. Metabolic Acidosis of Chronically Hemodialyzed Patients. Am J Nephrol 2003;23 158–164.

Chapter 12

Site and Size of Vascular Calcifications Are Different in Dialysis Patients with Various Underlying Diseases

H. Suzuki, T. Inoue, H. Okada, T. Takenaka, Kunihiko Hayashi, Jyunnichi Nishiyama, Takashi Yamazaki, Yuji Nishiyama and Keiko Kaneko

Additional information is available at the end of the chapter

1. Introduction

Computed tomography (CT) constitutes the gold standard for quantification of vascular calcification (VC) and, being the most effective and widely available with reproducible measurements, is also useful for monitoring progression as well as assessing the effect of therapeutic strategies to modify progression [1] [2]. VC has a significant effect in cardiovascular diseases on dialysis patients. Tanne et al. [3] focused on calcification of the thoracic aorta and found that it associated with coronary and valvular calcification in hypertensive patients. In the Calcification Outcome in Renal Disease (CORD) study, abdominal aortic calcification was found to have the predictive value for the occurrence of cardiovascular events and mortality in dialysis patients [4]. Coll et al. [5] reported that VC in large, conduit arteries was prevalent in patients on dialysis patients, and that age, dialysis vintage, past medical history of cardiovascular disease, atherosclerosis and inflammation were variable significantly influencing VC. From these studies, it is suggested that VC occurs in vessels of various diameters. However, no definitive studies have determined the significance of VC in different vessels in patients receiving dialysis therapy until the present time. Moreover, there have been few studies examining a relation between semi-quantitative measures of VC and their contributing factors. The aim of this work presented here is to examine a relation between semi quantitatively measured calcification of three major vessels, the thoracic aorta, the abdominal aorta and the iliac arteries and several known contributing factors to VC such as underlying diseases, age, gender, vintage of dialysis, values of serum calcium and phosphate, use of calcium-based phosphate binders and so on.

2. Methods

All HD patients received three dialysis sessions of at least 4 h duration per week. HD was performed using low flux polysalphose dialyhsers (1.5-2.0 m2 APS Asahi Medical R Tokyo, Japan). All HD patients were dialyzed using bicarbonate-bound 1.25 mmol/L, calcium and 134 mmol/sodium containing dialysate. Patients were all dialysed at the Dialysis Unit of Irumadai Hospital.

This was an observational and cross-sectional study that included 79 hemodialysis patients at the Dialysis Unit of Irumadai Hospital, who gave their informed consent to enroll in this study. The inclusion criteria were patient providing informed consent, age ≥ 40 years and duration of dialysis ≥ 1 year. Exclusion criteria were significant fetal diseases that were estimated to reduce life expectancy to < 6 months and patients in whom it was impossible to measure CT scan.

The recorded cardiovascular history and smoking status were obtained. The following baseline biochemical data were obtained; serum calcium, phosphorus, intact parathyroid hormone, albumin, total cholesterol, low-density lipoprotein cholesterol. Data on weight, height, body mass index and duration of dialysis and use of medications: phosphate binders, vitamin D, statins, erythropoietin and antihypertensive agents. Clinical characteristics and laboratory variables including dual-energy x-ray absorptiometry and pulse wave velocity. This study complies with the Declaration of Helsinki and was in agreement with the guidelines approved by the ethics committee at the institution.

2.1. Computed tomography

CT scan of the aorta and arteries was performed with a 16-detector CT scan {Prime Purpose MDCT (GE Healthcare, Milwaukee, WI USA)}. Scanning time was 0.5 s for two contiguous 1.25 mm sections and 20±5 seconds for the entire zone of interest. Examination was performed during a single, unforced, withheld inspiration. During scanning with the tube rotating at 2 rotation/second and the table moving at 55 mm/s with a 1:1.375 scanning pitch, images were obtained with an effective section thickness of 10 mm. Scanning was performed with 120 kVp and 350 mAs, standard resolution, and a 28-36 cm field of view. The total duration of the procedure was 5min. The range of CT scan was illustrated in Fig. 1.

2.2. Evaluation of thoracic and abdominal aorta and iliac artery

Volume acquisitions were analyzed using Volume Viewer software (GE Healthcare). The thoracic and abdominal aorta were segmented manually. In order to reduce errors due to noise, a cut-off of 130 Housefield Unit (HU) was applied. The total calcification volume was calculated as the sum of all voxels in the remaining volume.

2.3. Biochemistry

Blood samples were collected at monthly intervals. The results presented here were time-averaged results from the preceding 6 months prior to the CT scan.

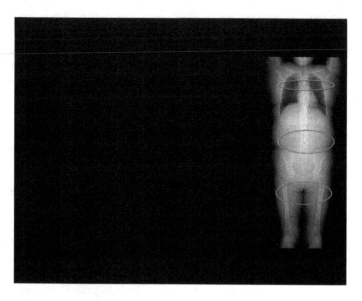

Figure 1. A range of computed tomography (CT) scan is illustrated.

2.4. Blood pressure

Three blood pressure (BP) recording were taken suing automated device.

2.5. Statistics

Data are expressed as means ± SD. Using variables found to be significant in the univariate analysis and potential confounders, we applied forward stepwise logistic regressions, in order to determine which of these variables were most significantly associated with calcification of the thoracic and abdominal aorta and the arteries of the lower limbs. F-to-Remove was set at 2.9. $P<0.05$ was considered as significance.

3. Results

3.1. Patients characteristics

The underlying kidney diseases were diabetic nephropathy [32], chronic glomerulonephritis (23), nephrosclerosis, polycystic kidney disease (3) and others (12).

Baseline demographics and laboratory and hemodynamic values of the study population are shown in Tables 1, 2 and 3 and current medications used are listed in Table 4.

Age (years)	62.3±12.8
Dialysis duration (months)	76.6±83.8
Gender (male/female)	52/27
Diabetes/non diabetes	32/47
Smoking/non smoking	36/43
Body mass index (kg/m²)	21.9±1.6

Table 1. Characteristics of patients

Systolic Blood Pressure (mmHg)	154±122
Diastolic Blood Pressure (mmHg)	79±13
Heart Rate (beats/min)	74±12

Table 2. Hemodynamic markers

Calcium (mg/dL)	8.9±0.8
Phosphate (mg/dL)	5.6±1.2
Intact PTH (ng/mL)	125.5±65.4
Creatinine (mg/dL)	12.5±1.1
Blood urea nitrogen (mg/dL)	98.4±12.2
Uric acid (mg/dL)	6.3±0.5
Hemoglobin (g/dL)	10.7±0.6
Low density lipoprotein (mg/dL)	84.2±27.0
Albumin (g/dL)	3.7±0.4

Table 3. Serum markers

Agent	Percentage of patients
Phosphate binders	
Calcium containing	86
Sevelamer	65
Vitamin D analogues	59
Cinacalcet	72
Statins	12
Antihypertensives	96
Erythropoiesis stimulating agents	98

Table 4. Current medications of the study population

3.2. Calcification of vessels

In Table 5, the average of calcification scores is shown.

All three lesions correlated significantly with each other. Stepwise regression was applied in which the independent variables were identified from the univariate analyses. Significant associations were seen for the following: the prevalence of calcification; the thoracic aorta with period of dialysis, elevations of both systolic and diastolic blood pressure and levels of serum albumin (Table 6); in the abdominal aorta with age, presence of diabetes, and calcium supplement (Table 7); arteries of the lower limbs with presence of diabetes mellitus, use of sevelamer and cinacalcet and serum levels of intact parathyroid hormone and albumin (Table 8).

Vessels	
Thoracic aorta	3.49 + 4.65
Abdominal aorta	5.21 + 7.21
Iliac artery	1.18 + 1.92

Table 5. Calcification scores of thoracic aorta, abdominal aorta and iliac artery

Constant	Coefficient	Standard Error	F	P
Dialysis vintage (months)	0.011	0.006	3.401	0.050
SBP (mmHg)	0.090	0.029	9.336	0.003
DBP (mmHg)	-0.210	0.054	15.071	0.001
Albumin (g/dL)	-2.181	1.206	3.270	0.045

SBP: systolic blood pressuer, DBP: diastolic blood pressure

Table 6. Significant correlations with calcification of thoracic aorta

Constant	Coefficient	Standard Error	F	P
Age (years)	0.2445	0.68	13.156	0.001
Presence of DM	3.997	1.715	5.431	0.002
$CaCO_3$	0.001		4.066	0.048
Vitamin D	-4.89	2.231	4.802	0.032
Ca (mg/dL)	2.32	1.224	3.595	0.043

DM: diabetes mellitus, $CaCO_3$: oral administration (g/day), Vitamin D: oral administration (µg/day)

Table 7. Significant correlations with calcification of abdominal aorta

Constant	Coefficient	Standard Error	F	P
Presence of DM	1.346	0.416	10.469	0.002
Savelamer	1.403	0.430	10.632	0.002
Cinacalcet	0.882	0.482	3.353	0.072
Intact PTH	-0.006	0.003	3.446	0.048
Albumin (g/dL)	-1.414	0.473	8.944	0.004

DM: diabetes mellitus, Savelamer: oral administration (g/day), Cinacalcet: oral administration (mg/day)

Table 8. Significant correlations with calcification of lower limb

4. Discussion

In the present study, we found that the contributing factors to VC were different in the different vessels. The development and progression of VC is a multifactorial process. Potentially differing factors may exert their maximum influence at either the predisposition, initiation and continuation phases of the process. The multivariate analysis performed on these data attempt to elucidate which factors might be most significant to the development of VC. In the present study, age, duration of HD, systolic and diastolic BP, presence of DM serum levels of Ca, intact PTH, calcium modulating drugs and albumin contributed differently in the different vessels. Albumin was negatively correlated with the severity of VC. This suggests that a characteristic state of low albumin as seen in malnutrition, inflammation or atherosclerosis complex is most important, as suggested by Wang et al. [6]. Factors shown to predict VC in the current study included older age, longer dialysis vintage, diabetes, higher concentrations of serum phosphorus and calcium are associated with more extensive VC among patients on HD and result partially consistent with those reported previously [7] [8] [9] [10].

Adler et al [11] demonstrated a strong association of coronary calcification and calcification of the thoracic aorta on spiral CT. The aortic calcification signifies a higher probability of coronary atherosclerosis and ischemic stroke (Cerebrovascular disease). Also, Tanne et al. [3] found that severe calcification in descending aorta is a predictor of ischemic cerebrovascular events. Calcification of the thoracic aorta is not a direct causative factor for embolic stroke, but rather a marker of increased burden of vascular (atherosclerotic disease) disease [12]. However, Honkanen et al. [4] reported that although the duration of HD correlates with calcification in coronary [1], carotid and peripheral arteries [7], the association is less clear in the thoracic arteries [8].

In the present study, calcification of the thoracic aorta had a strong association with dialysis vintage, systolic and diastolic BP and albumin, which are a major factors contributing to cardiovascular diseases. From these data, it is possible that severe calcification of the thoracic aorta is produced by hemodynamic, malnutrition and uremia in combination.

Abdominal aorta calcification has been well studied, has been associated with an increase risk of cardiovascular morbidity and mortality in patients with HD [13]. Hanada et al. [14] proposed that the section of the aorta chosen for measuring the semiquantitative calcification score is suitable for evaluation of the severity of VC because the site is associated with turbulent flow and is susceptible to development of atheroma. The chosen site is also simple to investigate radiologically since it is in a significant part of the aorta and is vertical to the transverse section. In the present study, VC of the abdominal aorta was correlated with the presence of diabetes, which is a well-known atherosclerotic risk factor. In addition, the factors relating with calcium-phsophate modulation, such as concentrations of calcium, PTH and so on are frequently evoked as the principal causes associated with vascular remodeling and/or arterial calcifications [15] [16]. Guerin et al. [17] reported that in HD patients, there is an association between the presence of aortic calcification and increased Ca x P products. In contrast, Arad et al. did not find the serum concentrations of calcium, 1,25-Vit D, and PTH to be associated with the presence of arterial calcifications [18]. Besides, the amount of CaO_3 prescribed as a phosphate binder was independently associated with the score of vascular calcifications. One of the adverse effects of calcium based phosphate binders is hypercalcemia, which may in turn result in arterial calcification. It is therefore likely that development of VC of the abdominal aorta is associated with calcium and phosphorus regulation in HD patients. Moreover, mineral bone disease-related factors such as serum calcium, phosphorus and PTH are thought to be strongly associated with the severity of VC in dialysis patients [19] [20].

Sigrist et al. [21] described a simple, sensitive low radiation dose technique as an alternative to coronary artery and aortic measurements to quantify a calcification score for the superficial femoral artery (SFA). The sector of artery chosen for this study is ideal as it avoids major bifurcations and arterial branching, and therefore, obvious site for turbulent flow and the development of atheroma. In the present study, factors contributing to VC of the iliac arteries are similar with those of the abdominal aorta.

In the Calcification Outcome in Renal Disease (CORD) study, 19% of patients had no visible calcification in their abdominal aorta [4]. These findings are partially in line with certain previous observations and it has been suggested that these individuals rarely develop calcification at follow-up [22] [8] [23]. In the present study, we did not find these individuals. Recently, further reports from CORD study provided a new evidence that no coronary [24] or thoracic aortic calcification at baseline, but their calcification developed during 2 years of observation and was most prevalent in those receiving calcium-containing binders. Besides, retrospective and cross-sectional data have given contradicting results with some publication showing a contribution of Vit D to VC [15], whereas others do not support this contention [25]. It is therefore unlikely that HD patients receiving calcium-containing binders and Vitamin D analogues have no VC of the vessels.

Recently Allison et al. [26] demonstrated that in terms of extent of calcification, the iliac arteries showed the strongest association for all mortality and end points, consistent with the well-known association between the severity of peripheral artery disease and both CVD and total mortality [27].

In addition, they concluded [26] that higher levels of calcium in different vascular beds are associated not only with CVD mortality but also with non-CVD and total mortality and that location of the arterial calcification appears to be relevant to the strength of the association with mortality, and the CVD risk factors appear to mediate some of this association.

4.1. Study limitations

First, the imaging methods used in this study did not distinguish the two types of VC (pathy calcification of the intima and calcification of the media). As is known, mineral metabolism disturbances link specifically with medial rather than intimal V and intima calcification associates with atherosclerosis. Second, our studies was cross-sectional, it does not directly show how detection of VC in various vessels predict incident cardiovascular events in the dialysis patients. Third, VC represents the result of long-standing atherosclerotic and calcification processes. It is unclear whether the steady-state of serum chemistry such as calcium, phosphate, intact PTH concentrations measured in this study accurately represents pathological process that occurred when VC was developing.

5. Conclusion

Presence and extension of VC in thoracic and abdominal aortas and lower limbs might be regulated in complex manner and caution should be needed to use these variables as a marker of the burden of vascular disease. The associations between calcified atherosclerosis and mortality differ by vascular bed, suggesting that the location and severity of calcification in different vascular beds provide unique information for mortality.

Author details

H. Suzuki[1], T. Inoue[1], H. Okada[1], T. Takenaka[1], Kunihiko Hayashi[2], Jyunnichi Nishiyama[2], Takashi Yamazaki[2], Yuji Nishiyama[2] and Keiko Kaneko[2]

1 Department of Nephrology, Saitama Medical University Saitama, Japan

2 Department of Internal Medicine, Irumadai Clinic, Saitama, Japan

References

[1] Moe SM, O'Neill KD, Fineberg N, Persohn S, Ahmed S, Garrett P, et al. Assessment of vascular calcification in ESRD patients using spiral CT. Nephrol Dial Transplant. 2003;18(6):1152-8.

[2] Raggi P, Giachelli C, Bellasi A. Interaction of vascular and bone disease in patients with normal renal function and patients undergoing dialysis. Nat Clin Pract Cardiovasc Med. 2007;4(1):26-33.

[3] Tanne D, Tenenbaum A, Shemesh J, Schwammenthal Y, Fisman EZ, Schwammenthal E, et al. Calcification of the thoracic aorta by spiral computed tomography among hypertensive patients: associations and risk of ischemic cerebrovascular events. Int J Cardiol. 2007;120(1):32-7.

[4] Honkanen E, Kauppila L, Wikstrom B, Rensma PL, Krzesinski JM, Aasarod K, et al. Abdominal aortic calcification in dialysis patients: results of the CORD study. Nephrol Dial Transplant. 2008;23(12):4009-15.

[5] Coll B, Betriu A, Martinez-Alonso M, Amoedo ML, Arcidiacono MV, Borras M, et al. Large artery calcification on dialysis patients is located in the intima and related to atherosclerosis. Clin J Am Soc Nephrol. 2011;6(2):303-10.

[6] Wang AY, Woo J, Lam CW, Wang M, Chan IH, Gao P, et al. Associations of serum fetuin-A with malnutrition, inflammation, atherosclerosis and valvular calcification syndrome and outcome in peritoneal dialysis patients. Nephrol Dial Transplant. 2005;20(8):1676-85.

[7] London GM, Guerin AP, Marchais SJ, Metivier F, Pannier B, Adda H. Arterial media calcification in end-stage renal disease: impact on all-cause and cardiovascular mortality. Nephrol Dial Transplant. 2003;18(9):1731-40.

[8] Hujairi NM, Afzali B, Goldsmith DJ. Cardiac calcification in renal patients: what we do and don't know. Am J Kidney Dis. 2004;43(2):234-43.

[9] Raggi P, Bellasi A. Clinical assessment of vascular calcification. Adv Chronic Kidney Dis. 2007;14(1):37-43.

[10] Floege J, Raggi P, Block GA, Torres PU, Csiky B, Naso A, et al. Study design and subject baseline characteristics in the ADVANCE Study: effects of cinacalcet on vascular calcification in haemodialysis patients. Nephrol Dial Transplant. 2010;25(6):1916-23.

[11] Adler Y, Fisman EZ, Shemesh J, Tanne D, Hovav B, Motro M, et al. Usefulness of helical computed tomography in detection of mitral annular calcification as a marker of coronary artery disease. Int J Cardiol. 2005;101(3):371-6.

[12] Jayalath RW, Mangan SH, Golledge J. Aortic Calcification. European Journal of Vascular and Endovascular Surgery. 2005;30(5):476-88.

[13] Okuno S, Ishimura E, Kitatani K, Fujino Y, Kohno K, Maeno Y, et al. Presence of abdominal aortic calcification is significantly associated with all-cause and cardiovascular mortality in maintenance hemodialysis patients. Am J Kidney Dis. 2007;49(3): 417-25.

[14] Hanada S, Ando R, Naito S, Kobayashi N, Wakabayashi M, Hata T, et al. Assessment and significance of abdominal aortic calcification in chronic kidney disease. Nephrol Dial Transplant. 2010;25(6):1888-95.

[15] Milliner DS, Zinsmeister AR, Lieberman E, Landing B. Soft tissue calcification in pediatric patients with end-stage renal disease. Kidney Int. 1990;38(5):931-6.

[16] Goldsmith DJ, Covic A, Sambrook PA, Ackrill P. Vascular calcification in long-term haemodialysis patients in a single unit: a retrospective analysis. Nephron. 1997;77(1): 37-43.

[17] Guerin AP, London GM, Marchais SJ, Metivier F. Arterial stiffening and vascular calcifications in end-stage renal disease. Nephrol Dial Transplant. 2000;15(7):1014-21.

[18] Arad Y, Spadaro LA, Roth M, Scordo J, Goodman K, Sherman S, et al. Serum concentration of calcium, 1,25 vitamin D and parathyroid hormone are not correlated with coronary calcifications. An electron beam computed tomography study. Coron Artery Dis. 1998;9(8):513-8.

[19] Cozzolino M, Dusso AS, Slatopolsky E. Role of calcium-phosphate product and bone-associated proteins on vascular calcification in renal failure. J Am Soc Nephrol. 2001;12(11):2511-6.

[20] Floege J, Ketteler M. Vascular calcification in patients with end-stage renal disease. Nephrol Dial Transplant. 2004;19 Suppl 5:V59-66.

[21] Spiegel DM, Raggi P, Mehta R, Lindberg JS, Chonchol M, Ehrlich J, et al. Coronary and aortic calcifications in patients new to dialysis. Hemodial Int. 2004;8(3):265-72.

[22] Goodman WG, London G, Amann K, Block GA, Giachelli C, Hruska KA, et al. Vascular calcification in chronic kidney disease. Am J Kidney Dis. 2004;43(3):572-9.

[23] Qunibi WY. Reducing the burden of cardiovascular calcification in patients with chronic kidney disease. J Am Soc Nephrol. 2005;16 Suppl 2:S95-102.

[24] Asmus HG, Braun J, Krause R, Brunkhorst R, Holzer H, Schulz W, et al. Two year comparison of sevelamer and calcium carbonate effects on cardiovascular calcification and bone density. Nephrol Dial Transplant. 2005;20(8):1653-61.

[25] London GM, Guerin AP, Verbeke FH, Pannier B, Boutouyrie P, Marchais SJ, et al. Mineral metabolism and arterial functions in end-stage renal disease: potential role of 25-hydroxyvitamin D deficiency. J Am Soc Nephrol. 2007;18(2):613-20.

[26] Allison MA, Hsi S, Wassel CL, Morgan C, Ix JH, Wright CM, et al. Calcified atherosclerosis in different vascular beds and the risk of mortality. Arterioscler Thromb Vasc Biol. 2012;32(1):140-6.

[27] Fowkes FG, Murray GD, Butcher I, Heald CL, Lee RJ, Chambless LE, et al. Ankle brachial index combined with Framingham Risk Score to predict cardiovascular events and mortality: a meta-analysis. JAMA. 2008;300(2):197-208.

Chapter 13

Helicobacterpylori Infection for Hemodialysis Patients

Yoshiaki Kawaguchi and Tetsuya Mine

Additional information is available at the end of the chapter

1. Introduction

Helicobacter pylori (*HP*) infection is reported to be closely associated with upper gastrointestinal disorders, such as gastroduodenal ulcers, chronic gastritis, and gastric cancer. Furthermore, patients with chronic renal failure receiving hemodialysis often complain of digestive symptoms. There are many possible factors causing these symptoms, including reduced gastrointestinal motility attributable to diabetes mellitus, uremia, intestinal ischemia associated with circulatory failure, and adverse reactions to many oral medications including non-steroidal anti-inflammatory drugs. Although *HP* infection is amongthe factors that may cause upper gastrointestinal disorders in patients with chronic renal failure, the association with*HP* infection has not as yet been elucidated. According to recent reports, the prevalence of *HP* infection is significantly lower in patients with chronic renal failure than in controls with normal renal function, and the prevalence is even reported to decrease with longer duration of hemodialysis. However, there are also previous reports presenting contrary findings. This chapter describes *HP* infection and eradication therapy in hemodialysis patients.

2. Is the prevalence of *HP* infection low in hemodialysis patients?

It is often reported that the prevalence of *HP* infection tends to be lower in patients with chronic renal failure receiving hemodialysis than in control groups with normal renal function [1-19]. In a study conducted in 539 hemodialysis patients, the prevalence of *HP* infection was 48.6%, whereas health check-up examinees with normal renal function showed a significantly higher prevalence of 69.4% ($P < 0.001$) [15]. Another report also showed that, compared to a 27.5% prevalence of *HP* infection in hemodialysis patients, the prevalence in patients with chronic renal failure not receiving hemodialysis was significantly higher at 56.0% [4]. Although there is a report showing the prevalence of *HP* infection to also be low in patients undergoing renal transplantation, it seems that most had received hemodialysis before transplantation [3]. Based on the above observations, the prevalence of *HP* infection would appear to be low in hemodialysis patients, suggesting that the hemodialysis proce- dure itself may be involved in the low prevalence of *HP* infection.

3. Are duration of hemodialysis and prevalence of *HP* infection inversely correlated?

How are duration of hemodialysis and prevalence of *HP* infection associated? There are re- ports that the prevalence of *HP* infection tends to be lower with longer duration of hemo- dialysis [9, 15, 20, 21]. Nakajima et al. report that the prevalence of *HP* infection gradually decreases with a 2-year or longer duration of hemodialysis, and Sugimoto et al reported that the prevalence gradually decreases within 4 years of hemodialysis [15]. Moriyama et al. re- port that such a tendency is revealed in patients receiving hemodialysis for 8 years or longer [20]. There is also a report that the prevalence of *HP* infection in health check-up examinees with normal renal function was similar to that in patients with chronic renal failure who had received hemodialysis for less than 1 year [15]. Meanwhile, other studies have shown that there is no such association [22, 23]. However, Sugimoto et al. conducted a 4-year follow-up study in hemodialysis patients with *HP* infection and found that the prevalence gradually decreased from 51.6% at the start to 38.3% at the end [15]. Given that the spontaneous elimi- nation rate of *HP* infection is generally reported to be 0.6% annually [24], it must be as- sumed from these results that the hemodialysis procedure itself contributes to the observed decrease in the prevalence of *HP* infection.

4. Is there variation in *HP* infection rates among different countries?

The gastricmucosa of approximately 50% of the world's populationis infected with *HP*, and the infectionlevels exceed 70% in some developing areas [25, 26].

There is variation in *HP* infection ratesamong different countries. It may, therefore, be impor- tant to evaluate the infection rate in various countries. In East Asian countries, the prevalence of *HP*infection in patients receiving chronic hemodialysis is44.5% (95% confidence interval (CI): 41.5–47.6%], 474/1065), which is significantly lower than in all patients with nor malrenal function [54.0% [95% CI: 50.9–57.1%], 560/1038,*P* <0.001] [27]. On the other hand, because the prevalenceof *HP*in other areas, such as Europe, Middle East, and South Asia has a wide varia- tion, it isdifficult to evaluate the prevalence of *HP*infectionin those areas.

5. Why does the hemodialysis procedure reduce the prevalence of *HP* infection?

One reason is eradication of *HP*by antibiotics that are administeredas therapy for other in- fections experienced by hemodialysis patients. Antibiotics are the most typically prescribed drugs in general. In hemodialysis patients, antibiotics may be used for the treatment of bacterial infections as often as or even more frequently than in the general population. It is assumed that patients with renal failure are often prescribed reduced doses of antibiotics. However, compared to the general population with normal renal function, blood levels of antibiotics are likely to be higher after administration in patients with renal failure, and the elimination time is expected to be longer. Thus, in hemodialysis patients with a long duration of renal failure, the spontaneous elimination rate of HP infection might be increased by repeated administration of antibiotics. Because blood urea levels are increased in hemodialysis patients, urea levels in gastric juice are also high. The increased urea levels are considered to suppress the growth of HP in the stomach [28]. Another possible explanation is that up-regulation of pro-inflammatory cytokines in hemodialysis patients triggers the infiltration of inflammatory cells activated by the gastric mucosa, resulting in progression of gastric mucosal atrophy, an increase in pH, and ultimately HP elimination [29, 30]. While there are as yet no data clearly supporting this explanation, the prevalence of HP infection may be decreased by a combination of various factors.

6. What are the harmful effects of a decreased prevalence of HP infection on hemodialysis patients?

In general, HP infection is considered to be a cause of gastroduodenal ulcers, and a decrease in the prevalence of HP infection is favorable in this regard. It is widely known that HP eradication suppresses gastric acid secretion, which causes gastric erosion [31]. The frequency of endoscopically detected gastric erosion is reported to be high in hemodialysis patients [20, 32, 33], which may be associated with a decrease in HP infection. Because gastric erosion may cause gastrointestinal bleeding, caution is required especially in hemodialysis patients [20]. They are often receiving anticoagulant or antiplatelet drugs, and gastrointestinal bleeding can thus be fatal.

Prophylactic administration of anti-acid secretory drugs, such as proton pump inhibitors (PPI), is recommended. While long-term hemodialysis is reported to carry a high risk for reflux esophagitis [32-34], this may also be attributable to suppressedgastric acid secretion due to a decrease in HP infection. In patients receiving long-term hemodialysis, administration of anti-acid secretory drugs is recommended to prevent reflux esophagitis.

7. Is HP eradication necessary for hemodialysis patients?

While the previous section described the harmful effects of a reduced prevalence of HP infection on hemodialysis patients, the harmful effects of HP infection include the aforementioned association with gastroduodenal ulcers, chronic gastritis and gastric cancer, as well as gastric mucosa associated-lymphoid tissue lymphoma, etc. Especially in hemodialysis patients, the frequency of gastroduodenal ulcers and gastric cancer is reported to be higher than in healthy people [3, 35]. Because hemodialysis patients are often receiving anticoagulant or antiplatelet drugs, bleeding from gastroduodenal ulcers may be fatal. Thus, *HP* eradication is considered to be an important treatment for hemodialysis patients in order to prevent gastroduodenal ulcers and gastric cancer. Although spontaneous elimination of *HP* infection can be expected in hemodialysis patients, the earliest possible *HP* eradication is recommended especially in those with a history of gastroduodenal ulcer and confirmed current *HP* infection.

8. How is *HP* eradication best achieved in hemodialysis patients?

According to recent reports, the major regimen is a combination of a PPI selected from among omeprazole, lansoprazole, and esomeprazole and 2 antibiotics selected from among clarithromycin, amoxicillin, and metronidazole, which are administered for 1 or 2 weeks [1, 6, 36-40]. Although the eradication rate fluctuates slightly from 72.7 to 96.0%, it averages around 90%. There seems to be no substantial difference in comparison with the eradication rate of *HP* infection in the general population. The factors contributing to eradication failure include a history of previous eradication therapy, suggesting that the presence or absence of resistant strains to antibiotics iskey to the success of eradication therapy [6].

9. What are the precautions for *HP* eradication therapy in hemodialysis patients?

Caution should be considered in performing eradication therapy for hemodialysis patients to avoidexcessive doses of drugs. Administration of low doses results in high blood levels. However, hemodialysis removes both PPI and antibiotics, lowering their blood levels. In consideration of this fact, without adjustment of the therapy by administering the drugs after the hemodialysis session on the day of hemodialysis, the eradication rate of *HP* infection may be decreased. Safe and effective optimal dosages and administration procedures should be established. In patients with chronic renal failure before the initiation of hemodialysis, attention should be paid to the nephrotoxicity of amoxicillin, and the eradication therapy needs to be adjusted by substituting amoxicillin with metronidazole [39, 41, 42].

Moreover, hemodialysis patients often receive oral antibiotics, and the duration of circulation of these antibiotics in the body is prolonged due to delayed metabolism. Thus, it seems that *HP* often acquires resistance to antibiotics. According to a report on resistance to clarithromycin, resistant *HP* strains were detected in 36.4% of patients with renal failure and 15.2% of healthy volunteers, showing the prevalence of resistant *HP* strains to be significantly lower in the latter [43].

10. Conclusion

This chapter has described *HP* infection in hemodialysis patients. Because the prevalence of *HP* infection is lower in these patients than in healthy people, attention should be paid to symptoms due to gastric hyperacidity. For those with *HP* infection, eradication therapy is recommended in order to prevent gastrointestinal ulcers and gastric cancer. Even after *HP* eradication, prophylaxis against gastric erosion and reflux esophagitis should be performed with anti-acid secretory drugs.

Author details

Yoshiaki Kawaguchi and Tetsuya Mine

Tokai University School of Medicine, Japan

References

[1] Sezer S, Ibis A, Ozdemir BH et al. Association of Helicobacterpylori infection with nutritional status in hemodialysispatients. Transplant Proc 2004;36:47–9.

[2] Sotoudehmanesh R, Ali Asgari A, Ansari R, Nouraie M.Endoscopic findings in end-stage renal disease. Endoscopy2003;35:502–5.

[3] Khedmat H, Ahmadzad-Asl M, Amini M et al. Gastroduodenallesions and Helico-bacter pylori infection in uremicpatients and renal transplant recipients. Transplant Proc2007;39:1003–7.

[4] Nakajima F, Sakaguchi M, Amemoto K et al. Helicobacterpylori in patients receiving long-term dialysis. Am J Nephrol2002;22:468–72.

[5] Fabbian F, Catalano C, Bordin V, Balbi T, Di Landro D.Esophagogastroduodenosco-py in chronic hemodialysispatients: 2-year clinical experience in a renal unit. Clin-Nephrol2002;58:54–9.

[6] Tsukada K, Miyazaki T, Katoh H et al. Seven-day tripletherapy with omeprazole, amoxycillin and clarithromycin forHelicobacter pylori infection in haemodialysis patients. ScandJ Gastroenterol2002;37:1265–8.

[7] Marsenic O, Peco-Antic A, Perisic V, Virijevic V, Kruscic D,Kostic M. Upper gastrointestinal lesions in children on chronichaemodialysis. Nephrol Dial Transplant 2003;18:2687–8.

[8] Lopez T, Quesada M, Almirall J, Sanfeliu I, Segura F, CalvetX. Usefulness of non-invasive tests for diagnosing Helicobacterpylori infection in patients undergoing dialysis forchronic renal failure. Helicobacter 2004;9:674–80.

[9] Nakajima F, Sakaguchi M, Oka H et al. Prevalence of Helicobacterpylori antibodies in long-term dialysis patients. Nephrology2004;9:73–6.

[10] Al-Mueilo SH. Gastroduodenal lesions and Helicobacterpylori infection in hemodialysis patients. Saudi Med J 2004;25:1010–14.

[11] Trimarchi H, Forrester M, Schropp J, Pereyra H, Freixas EA.Low initial vitamin B12 levels in Helicobacter pylori—positivepatients on chronic hemodialysis. Nephron ClinPract2004;96:c28–32.

[12] Blusiewicz K, Rydzewska G, Rydzewski A. Gastric juiceammonia and urea concentrations and their relation to gastricmucosa injury in patients maintained on chronic hemodialysis.RoczAkad Med Bialymst2005;50:188–92.

[13] Lentine KL, Parsonnet J, Taylor I,Wrone EM, Lafayette RA.Associations of serologic markers of infection and inflammationwith vascular disease events and mortality in Americandialysis patients. Clin ExpNephrol2006;10:55–62.

[14] Gioe FP, Cudia B, Romano G et al. Role and clinical importanceof Helicobacter pylori infection in hemodialysis patients.G Chir2008;29:81–4.

[15] Sugimoto M, Sakai K, Kita M, Imanishi J, Yamaoka Y. Prevalenceof Helicobacter pylori infection in long-term hemodialysispatients. Kidney Int2009;75:96–103.

[16] LuiSL,Wong WM, Ng SY, Chan TM, Lai KN, Lo WK. Seroprevalenceof Helicobacter pylori in Chinese patients on continuousambulatory peritoneal dialysis. Nephrology 2005;10:21–4.

[17] Altay M,Turgut F, Akay H et al. Dyspepsia inTurkish patientson continuous ambulatory peritoneal dialysis. IntUrolNephrol2008;40:211–17.

[18] Schoonjans R, Van VB, Vandamme W et al. Dyspepsia andgastroparesis in chronic renal failure: the role of Helicobacterpylori. ClinNephrol2002;57:201–7.

[19] Strid H, Simren M, StotzerPO, Abrahamsson H, BjornssonES. Delay in gastric emptying in patients with chronic renalfailure. Scand J Gastroenterol2004;39:516–20.

[20] Moriyama T, Matsumoto T, Hirakawa K, et al. Helicobacter pylori status and esophagogastroduodenal mucosallesions in patients with end-stage renal failure on maintenancehemodialysis. J Gastroenterol2010;45:515–522.

[21] Munoz de Bustillo E, Sanchez Tomero JA, Sanz JC, Moreno JA,Jimenez I, Lopez-Brea M, et al. Eradication and follow-up ofHelicobacter pylori infection in hemodialysis patients. Nephron.1998;79:55–60.

[22] O° zgur O, Boyacioglu S, Ozdogan M, Gur G, Telatar H, HaberalM. Helicobacter pylori infection in haemodialysis patients andreal transplant recipients. Nephrol Dial Transplant. 1997;12:289–91.

[23] Huang JJ, Huang CJ, Ruaan MK, Chen KW, Yen TS, Sheu BS.Diagnostic efficacy of (13) C-urea breath test for Helicobacterpylori infection in hemodialysis patients. Am J Kidney Dis.2000;36:124–9.

[24] Valle J, Kekki M, Sipponen P, Ihamaki T, Siurala M. Long-termcourse and consequence of Helicobacter pylori gastritis. Resultsof a 32-year follow-up study. Scand J Gastroenterol. 1996;31:546–50.

[25] Rocha GA, Queiroz DM, Mendes EN et al. Indirect immunofluorescencedetermination of the frequency of anti-H. pyloriantibodies in Brazilian blood donors. Braz J Med BiolRes1992;25:683–9.

[26] Perez-Perez GI, Taylor DN, Bodhidatta L et al. Seroprevalenceof Helicobacter pylori infections in Thailand. J Infect Dis1990; 161:1237–41.

[27] Sugimoto M, Yamaoka Y. Review of Helicobacter pylori infection and chronicalfailure. Therapeutic Apheresis and Dialysis 2011; 15:1–9.

[28] Gladziwa U, Haase G, Handt S et al. Prevalence of Helicobacterpylori in patients with chronic renal failure. NephrolDial Transplant 1993; 8:301–6.

[29] Hwang IR, Kodama T, Kikuchi S et al. Effect of interleukin 1polymorphisms on gastric mucosal interleukin 1beta productionin Helicobacter pylori infection. Gastroenterology 2002;123:1793–803.

[30] Wesdorp RI, Falcao HA, Banks PB, Martino J, Fischer JE.Gastrin and gastric acid secretion in renal failure. Am J Surg1981;141:334–8.

[31] Miyake K, Tsukui T, Futagami S, Tatsuguchi A, Shinoki A,Hiratsuka T, et al. Effect of acid suppression therapy on developmentof gastric erosions after cure of Helicobacter pyloriinfection. Aliment PhamacolTher. 2002;16[Suppl 2]:210–6.

[32] Kawaguchi Y, Mine T, Kawana I, et al. Gastroesophageal Reflux Disease in Hemodialysis Patients. Tokai J ExpClin Med. 2009; 34: 48-52.

[33] Kawaguchi Y, Mine T, Kawana I, et al. Gastroesophageal Reflux Disease in Chronic Renal Failure Patients: evaluation by endoscopic examination. Tokai J ExpClin Med. 2009; 34: 80-83.

[34] Doherty CC. Gastrointestinal bleeding in dialysis patients.Nephron. 1993;63:132–6.

[35] Ota K,Yamashita N, Suzuki T, AgishiT.Malignanttumours indialysis patients: a nationwidesurvey. Proc Eur Dial TransplantAssoc1981;18:724–30.

[36] Itatsu T, Miwa H, Nagahara A et al. Eradication of Helicobacterpylori in hemodialysis patients. Ren Fail 2007;29:97–102.

[37] Mak SK, Loo CK,Wong AM et al. Efficacy of a 1-week courseof proton-pump inhibitor-based triple therapy for eradicatingHelicobacter pylori in patients with and without chronic renalfailure. Am J Kidney Dis 2002;40:576–81.

[38] Mak SK, Loo CK, Wong PN et al. A retrospective study onefficacy of proton-pump inhibitor-based triple therapy foreradication of Helicobacter pylori in patients with chronicrenal failure. Singapore Med J 2003;44:74–8.

[39] Sheu BS, Huang JJ,YangHB,HuangAH,WuJJ.The selectionof triple therapy for Helicobacter pylori eradication in chronicrenal insufficiency. Aliment PharmacolTher2003;17:1283–90.

[40] Tseng GY,LinHJ,Fang CT et al. Recurrence of peptic ulcer inuraemic and non-uraemic patients after Helicobacter pylorieradication: a 2-year study. Aliment PharmacolTher2007;26:925–33.

[41] Arancibia A, Drouguett MT, Fuentes G et al. Pharmacokineticsof amoxicillin in subjects with normal and impaired renalfunction. Int J ClinPharmacolTherToxicol1982;20:447–53.

[42] Jones DP, Gaber L, Nilsson GR, Brewer ED, Stapleton FB.Acute renal failure following amoxicillin overdose. ClinPediatr1993;32:735–9.

[43] Aydemir S, Boyacioglu S, Gur G et al. Helicobacter pyloriinfection in hemodialysis patients: susceptibility to amoxicillinand clarithromycin. World J Gastroenterol2005;11:842–5.

Chapter 14

Colloids in Dialytic Refractory Hypotension

Guy Rostoker

Additional information is available at the end of the chapter

1.Introduction

1.1. Definition and epidemiology of dialytic hypotension

Intradialytic hypotension is the most common complication of hemodialysis,occurring in up to 33% of patients. There are two main clinical patterns of dialysis-associated hypotension : the first is episodic hypotension (defined by a sudden drop of systolic blood pressure below 100 mmHg or at least 30 mmHg with accompanying clinical symptoms), that typically oc- curs during the later stages of dialysis sessions and is generally favored by excessive weight gain ; the second is chronic persistent hypotension, which affects about 10% of long-term di- alysis patients [1, 2], most of whom experience frequent episodes of hypotension during di- alysis sessions, whereas some patients have permanent hypotension with low predialysis systolic pressure, often less than 100 mmHg [3, 4]. Intradialytic hypotension not only causes discomfort and has a negative impact on health-related quality of life but it may also ad- versely affect the outcome of chronic hemodialysis, reducing patients' life expectancy and favoring underdialysis [5-10]. According to recent data, low pre-dialytic systolic and diastol- ic pressures, like low post-dialytic systolic pressure and the occurrence of hypotensive epi- sodes during dialysis sessions, are associated with a significantly increased risk of death [5-9]. Moreover, a recent Japanese study has shown a link between dialysis-related hypoten- sion and the occurrence of progressive frontal lobe atrophy [10]. The incidence of intradia- lytic hypotension is expected to grow with the increasing number of elderly and diabetic patients and patients with cardiovascular disease who are now starting hemodialysis, to- gether with the use of long-term dialysis in an increasing number of hemodialyzed patients. In addition, dialysis treatment time has had a tendency to decrease over the last two deca- des and all these situations are known to be risk factors for this phenomenon [2,3].

1.2. Etiology and pathogenesis of dialytic hypotension

Several factors contribute to dialytic hypotension. These include too rapid fluid removal in an attempt to reach dry weight, a rapid reduction in plasma osmolality which causes extracellular water to move into cells, high interdialytic weight gain, anemia, poor nutritional status with hypoalbuminemia, autonomic neuropathy, anephric status, reduced pressor response to vasopressor agents, reduced cardiac reserve, increased arterial stiffness, impaired venous compliance, use of acetate rather than bicarbonate as a dialysate buffer, ingestion of a meal immediately before or during the dialysis session, use of low sodium or high magnesium concentrations in the dialysate, and intake before the dialysis session of anti-hypertensive medications that can impair cardiovascular stability (especially nitrate derivatives) [1-4, 11,12]. In a recent cross-sectionnal study of a cohort of 72 hemodialysis patients, 36 of whom suffered from dialysis-relatedchronic hypotension, cardiac diastolic dysfunction was found to be associated with dialysis hypotension [13]. The excessive release of several endogenous vasodilatators such as nitric oxide, adrenomedullin and adenosine, has been implicated in the pathogenesis of dialytic hypotension, together with an imbalance in the synthesis of the endogenous vasoconstrictors endothelin and vasopressin [14-17]. The immediate cause of intradialytic hypotension is acute central hypovolemia [2,4]. Frank hypotension occurs when cardiovascular mechanisms do not adequately compensate for the blood volume reduction resulting from the imbalance between the ultrafiltration rate and the plasma-refilling rate [12].

2. Management and prevention of dialytic hypotension

Management of intradialytic hypotension involves treating the acute episode and applying measures to prevent future episodes [4,11,18]. The acute management of intradialytic hypotension includes the following measures : reducing or halting ultrafiltration, use of the Trendelenburg position and often a reduction in the blood flow rate and use of volume expanders, regardless of the underlying mechanism [4,11,18]. Normal saline is the most widely used volume expander and has been advocated as first-line therapy for intradialytic hypotension [4,11,18]. Commonly used second and third-line fluids are hypertonic saline, dextran, hydroxyethyl starch (HES), mannitol, albumin and gelatin solutions [4,11,18,19]. Standard measures to prevent or alleviate intradialytic hypotension include accurate setting of the dry weight, avoidance of modifiable factors known to favor this phenomenon (e.g. excessively rapid fluid removal in an attempt to reach dry weight, anemia, poor nutritional status with hypoalbuminemia, ingestion of a meal immediately before or during the dialysis session, and intake before the dialysis session of anti-hypertensive medications) that can impair cardiovascular stability, adjustment of the dialysate sodium and/or calcium concentration and temperature, use of initial ultrafiltration followed by standard (or isovolemic) dialysis, use of sodium, and ultrafiltration modeling [1-4,14]. Among resistant patients, the most effective strategies to prevent intradialytic hypotension are to increase the dialysis time (for example by using either short daily hemodialysis sessions or frequent nocturnal hemo-dialysis) or to switch to peritoneal dialysis [1-4,14].

3. Use of colloids in refractory dialytic hypotension

Recent studies have shown that human albumin is safe in intensive care unitsand can also be useful in this setting in patients with acute renal failure secondary to sepsis or associated with profound hypoalbuminemia [20]. As central hypovolemia is the initiating factor in the pathogenesis of dialytic hypotension [2, 12], recent studies have hypothesized and analyzed the potential benefit of systematic infusion of colloids -- 20% albumin or 4% gelatin -- during dialysis sessions in hypotension-prone patients unresponsive to usual preventive measures [21, 22]. Until recently, few studies have evaluated colloids and especially albumin as a pri-ming fluid for hemodialysis in septic patients or as preventive or curative therapy for hypo-tension-prone dialysis patients. Jardin and coworkers showed that infusion of 300 ml of 17.5% albumin as a priming fluid at the start of the dialysis session resulted in better ultrafil-tration and hemodynamic stability than saline infusion in patients with sepsis-induced anuric acute renal failure ; these authors also showed that hypovolemia(as reflected indirect-ly by reduced left ventricular filling pressure), reduced cardiac output and the decline in mean arterial pressure were better corrected by 17.5% albumin than by saline [23]. McLi-geyo first reported an improvement in hemodynamic parameters in four hemodialysis pa-tients with chronic persistent hypotension receiving systematic infusions of 100 ml of 25% albumin [24]. More recently, Van der Sande and coworkers showed in nine cardiac-compro-mised hypotension-prone dialysis patients that 100 ml of 20% albumin and 100 ml of hy-droxyethyl starch preserved systolic blood pressure and relative blood volume better than 33 ml of 3% saline during a hypotensive episode [25]. However, the side effects of hydrox-yethyl starch (prolonged bleeding time, deposition of HES in various tissues and especially the liver) preclude its use in this setting and it is now forbidden in France and in numerous countries in dialysis patients [26, 27].

We recently conducted a single blind prospective cross-over study of systematic infusion of 200 ml of 20% albumin as compared to 200 ml of 4% gelatin in 10 patients on long-term bi-carbonate hemodialysis with refractory permanent hypotension (despite cool dialysate asso-ciated with sodium and ultrafiltration profiling, at an ideal dry weight assessed by echocardiography) ; the study lasted 20 weeks [21]. We analyzed the effect of albumin and gelatin infusions on systolic and diastolic pressure and the number of hypotensive episodes by using the n-of-1 trial methodology and the Wilcoxon matched-pairs signed-ranks test [21]. Statistical analysis of individual data showed that 20% albumin increased systolic pres-sure in 6 patients ($p < 0.05$ Wilcoxon test) whereas 4% gelatin improved systolic pressure in only 2 patients ($p < 0.05$ Wilcoxon test) [21].

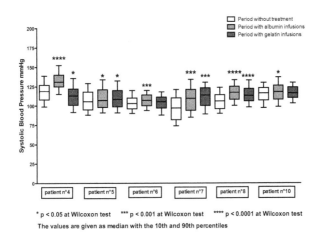

Figure 1. Evolution of systolic blood pressure with 20% albumin and 4% gelatin infusions in improved patients according toRostoker G,et al. A pilot study of routine colloid infusion in hypotension-prone dialysis patients unresponsive to preventive measures. J Nephrol 2011; 24(02) : 208-217; *p<0.5 at Wilcoxon test, ***p<0.001 at Wilcoxon test, ****p<0.0001 at Wilcoxon test; The values are given as median with the 10th and 90th percentiles

Albumin infusions increased diastolic pressure in 4 patients (p< 0.05 Wilcoxon test) whereas gelatin improved diastolic pressure in only 1 patient (p< 0.05 Wilcoxon test) [21].

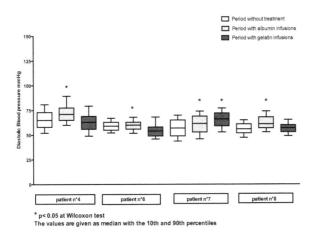

Figure 2. Evolution of diastolic blood pressure with 20% albumin and 4% gelatin infusions in improved patients accordingtoRostoker G,et al. A pilot study of routine colloid infusion in hypotension-prone dialysis patients unresponsive to preventive measures. J Nephrol 2011; 24(02): 208-217; *p<0.05 at Wilcoxon test; The values are given as median with the 10th and 90th percentiles

The median number of hypotensive episodes (systolic pressure < 100 mmHg) fell significantly in 3 patients during 20% albumin infusion and in 2 patients receiving 4% gelatin (p< 0.05, Wilcoxon test) [21]. Dialysis quality assessed by the Kt/V ratio and the relative blood volume reduction were also stable, whereas ionic dialysance at the end of the dialysis session was improved by albumin but not by gelatin (p< 0.05, repeated measure ANOVA) [21]. Thus,in this single blind cross-over pilot study using n-of-1 methodology, we found that systematic infusion of 20% albumin or 4% gelatin during hemodialysis sessions improved hemodynamic parameters (systolic blood pressure, diastolic blood pressure and the number of hypotensive episodes) and the ultrafiltration rate in most hypotension-prone patients unresponsive to usual preventive measures [21]. Albumin was proved to be superior to gelatin; however, both colloids were ineffective in some patients, suggesting the need for careful and objective evaluation of these expensive therapeutics on an individual level [21].

4. Hemodynamic mechanisms of action of colloids in refractory dialytic hypotension

In hemodialysis sessions, during ultrafiltration, the refilling rate is dependent on colloid osmotic pressure [28]. Therefore, systematic infusion of 20% albumin during the dialysis session and, to a lesser extent, 4% gelatin, would be expected to increase colloid osmotic pressure, enhance plasma refilling and thus prevent an abrupt reduction in blood volume and acute hypovolemia. Albumin has a water binding capacity of 18 ml per gram, and 200 ml of 20% albumin solution binds 720 ml of water for 6-8 hours, whereas 200 ml of 4% gelatin binds only 200 ml of water for 4-5 hours [29, 30]. It is also tempting to postulate that colloids counteract the reduced cardiac preload with both atrial and ventricular underfilling as recently shown by Graziani and coworkers at the end of the ultrafiltration session in the subset of patients with severe dialysis-related hypotension [31]. Finally, systematic infusion of colloids could improve cardiac output in patients with diastolic dysfunction: the German nephrologic school postulated in the late 1980s, and demonstrated in the early 1990s, that left-ventricular hypertrophy was a risk factor for dialysis-related hypotension due to diastolic dysfunction [32-35]. In contrast to German nephrologists, we found no relationship between diastolic dysfunction and left ventricular mass [13]. The latter finding might be related to changes in the epidemiology of dialysis over the last two decades: patients in the eighties had left ventricular hypertrophy related to both hypertension and uremic fibrosing cardiomyopathy, promoted by a long history of chronic dialysis with cuprophane membranes, while dialysis patients are now older and have diabetes or cardiovascular diseases (especially ischemic cardiopathy), which are known to cause left ventricular diastolic dysfunction and diastolic heart failure [13]. In patients with a very long dialysis vintage left ventricular enlargement is attributable to chronic volume and flow overload associated with anemia, presence of arteriovenous fistulas, sodium, water and uremic toxins retention [36]. Several mechanisms are involved in the pathophysiology of dialytic hypotension secondary to cardiac diastolic dysfunction: first, diastolic dysfunction in hemodialysis patients induces filling disturbances in diastole leading to systolic dysfunction especially a fall in stroke volume during hypohydratation induced by rapid ultrafiltration or when plasma refilling compensatory mechanisms are deficient resulting in central hypovolemia and abrupt hypotension: central hypovolemia in such cases could be counteracted by infusions of colloids [37,38]. Second, these hearts have a limited ability to utilize the Franck-Starling mechanism during exercise or its counterpart such as a dialysis session. Such limited preload reserve especially if coupled with chronotropic incompetence seen with advancing age limits cardiac output during exercise and dialysis sessions ; this leads to lactate accumulation and functional abnormalities of the myocardium [37,38]. Third, a substantial number of patients who have left ventricular hypertrophy with high wall thickness and a small end diastolic volume exhibit a low stroke volume and depressed cardiac output [35].

5. Modulation of oxidative stress and microinflammatory status by colloids in refractory dialytic hypotension

Data on the association between inflammatory status and dialysis hypotension are scarce: Tomita and coworkers have shown in nine patients with a history of intradialytic hypotension when compared with eight patients without dialysis associated hypotension a correlation between the levels of CRP and IL6 and the maximum percent change in mean arterial pressure over multiple dialysis sessions suggesting that dialysis hypotension may trigger inflammation [39]. This is consistent with the finding of Bergamini et al who found a significant release of TNF-alpha during hypotension episodes [40]. We recently hypothesized that frequent hypotension episodes may induce a noxious inflammatory response mediated by oxidative stress induced by ischemia-reperfusion phenomenon [22]. In a prospective cross-over study (lasting 20 weeks) of routine infusion of 200 ml of 20% albumin versus 200 ml of 4% gelatin in 10 patients with refractory intradialytic hypotension, we analyzed the effect of 20% albumin and 4% gelatin on microinflammatory status, oxidative stress, serum nitrite and nitrate levels by analysis of variance [22]. A significant decrease in serum ceruloplasmin and serum C3 was observed during the albumin period ($p < 0.05$, repeated measure ANOVA) [22]. A significant decrease in serum hydrogen peroxide was seen during albumin and gelatin administration ($p < 0.01$, repeated measure ANOVA) and a dramatic decrease in serum lipid peroxides was observed during the albumin period only ($p < 0.01$, Friedman test) [22].

Serum lactoferrin, serum proinflammatory cytokines and serum nitrite and nitrate levels remained stable during the different periods of this pilot trial [22]. These results strongly suggest that the improvement in microinflammatory status observed in hypotension prone dialysis patients may be related to the decrease in ischemia-reperfusion of noble organs by infusions of colloids together with a specific reduction of oxidative stress by 20% albumin.

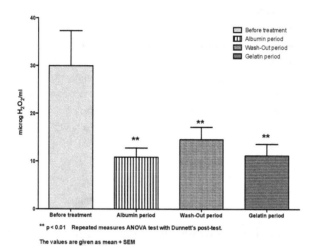

Figure 3. Concentration of serum hydrogen peroxide in patients with refractory dialytic hypotension treated by systematic infusion of colloids during dialysis sessions, according to Rostoker G et al Modulation of oxydative stress and microinflammatory status by colloids in refractory dialytic hypotension. BMC Nephrol 2011; oct 20; 12 (1): 58; **p<0.01 Repeated measures ANOVA test with Dunnett's post-test

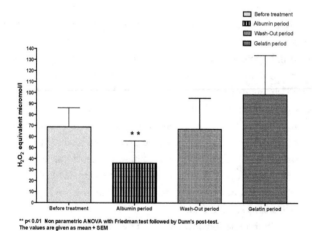

Figure 4. Concentration of serum lipid peroxides in patients with refractory dialytic hypotension treated by systematic infusion of colloids during dialysis sessions, according to Rostoker G et al Modulation of oxydative stress and microinflammatory status by colloids in refractory dialytic hypotension. BMC Nephrol 2011; Oct 20; 12 (1): 58 ; **p<0.01 Non parametric ANOVA with Friedman test followed by Dunn's post-test.; The values are given as mean + SEM

6. Anti-inflammatory mechanisms of action of colloids in refractory dialytic hypotension

In the aforementioned pilot study, C3 and ceruloplasmin were significantly lowered during the albumin period but not during the gelatin period [22]. This is consistent with recent studies using experimental models of hemorrhagic shock, which indicated that the type of resuscitation fluid greatly influences proinflammatory responses and especially neutrophil activation and nuclear factor-Kappa B gene transcription; albumin was found to be the least proinflammatory fluid [41, 42]. Conversely, ex-vivo data suggest that uremia may also increase vascular permeability [43] which may be acutely raised during dialysis–associated hypotension via released mediators such as adenosine aimed to preserve perfusion of the noble organs [17]; in this setting, albumin may itself influence vascular integrity by binding to the interstitial matrix and sub-endothelium and by altering the permeability of these layers to large molecules and solutes; these effects may be mediated by the binding of arachidonic acid to albumin and by polynitroxylated albumin, which inhibits xanthine-oxidase-mediated adhesion of human neutophils to endothelial cells [44].

In this trial, serum hydrogen peroxide levels were significantly lowered during both the albumin and the gelatin periods, suggesting that the improvement in hemodynamic parameters by colloids reduces oxidative stress related to the ischemia-reperfusion of noble organs that occurs during dialytic hypotension [22,45]. Besides this classical ischemia-reperfusion mechanism, by analogy with heart failure, it was hypothesized that entry of bacterial endotoxin during dialysis sessions might be the result of intermittent underperfusion of the intestine during dialysis-associated hypotension episodes leading to cardiac stunning and oxydative stress [46,47,48]; thus in this setting, colloids may improve both systemic and intestinal perfusion and reduce gut ischemia [22,46,47,48]. In the latter pilot study, serum lipid peroxide levels were also significantly reduced only during the albumin period. This is consistent with data showing that human serum albumin and bovine serum albumin provide protection from lipid peroxidation propagated by inorganic reactive oxygen species generated from xanthine oxidase/hypoxanthine in artificial systems [49] and that persistent hypoalbuminemia in hemodialysis patients is associated with peroxidation of erythrocyte membranes [50]. Moreover, albumin is the major extracellular source of reduced sulphydryl groups, termed thiols which are avid scavengers of reactive oxygen and nitrogen species;in this way albumin influences redox balance [51, 52]. All these data also strongly suggest that dialytic hypotension may contribute by different ways to the overproduction of reactive oxygen species seen in end-stage renal failure patients, a multifactorial process mainly related to uremia per-se, the hemoincompatibility of the dialysis system and trace amounts of endotoxin in the dialysate, gut ischemia and that colloids may indifferent mechanisms counteract it [22, 53].

7. Conclusions

Recent studies have shown that systematic infusions of 20% albumin and 4% gelatin during hemodialysis sessions improve hemodynamic parameters and ultrafiltration rate in most hypotension prone dialysis patients unresponsive to the usual preventive manoeuvers. An improvement in microinflammatory status was observed in parallel, which might be related to the decrease in both ischemia-reperfusion of noble organs, gut ischemia and oxidative stress. Hyperoncotic 20% albumin was found to have greater anti-inflammatory and anti-oxidative properties than 4% gelatin. Moreover, in the case of a new and expensive therapy such as 20% albumin (cost of 200 ml 20% albumin : 80 Euros as compared to 4 Euros for 200 ml 4% gelatin, in France), n-of-1 trials can furnish powerful evidence for provision on an individual basis, allaying managerial and medical fears as to the cost of frequently ineffective therapies being applied to an expanding at-risk population. From a pragmatic point of view, we advise practitioners to initiate first gelatin which is much less expensive when a treatment of systematic infusion of colloids is scheduled during dialysis sessions. Owing to its high cost, hyperoncontic albumin should be considered as a second-line therapy.Further well-designed controlled trials with a sufficient number of patients, of hyperoncotic 20% albumin and 4% gelatin in hypotension-prone dialysis patients are warranted to assess the benefit of colloids infusions in dialytic refractory hypotension.

Author details

Guy Rostoker*

Address all correspondence to: rostotom@orange.fr

Service de Néphrologie et de Dialyse, Hôpital Privé Claude Galien, Quincy Sous Sénart, France

References

[1] Leunissen KM, Kooman JP, Van Kuijk W, et al. Preventing haemodynamic instability in patients at risk for intra-dialytic hypotension. Nephrol Dial Transplant 1996; 11(Suppl 2): 11-15

[2] Sulowicz W, Radziszewski A. Pathogenesis and treatment of dialysis hypotension. Kidney Int 2006; 70: S36-S39

[3] Tislér A, Akócsi K, Hárshegi I, et al. Comparison of dialysis and clinical characteristics of patients with frequent and occasional hemodialysis associated hypotension. Kidney Blood Press Res 2002; 25: 97-102

[4] Zucchelli P, Santoro A. The management of hypotension in dialyzed patients. Miner Electrolyte Metab 1999; 25: 105-108

[5] Iseki K, Miyasato F, Tokuyama K, et al. Low diastolic blood pressure, hypoalbuminemia and risk of death in a cohort of chronic hemodialysis patients. Kidney Int 1997; 51: 1212-1217

[6] Zager P, Nikolic J, Brown R, et al. "U" curve association of blood pressure and mortality in hemodialysis patients. Kidney Int 1998; 54: 561-569

[7] Port FK, Hulbert-Shearon TE, Wolfe RA, et al. Predialysis blood pressure and mortality risk in a national sample of maintenance hemodialysis patients. Am J Kidney Dis 1999; 33: 507-517

[8] Shoji T, Tsubakihara Y, Fujii M, Imai E. Hemodialysis-associated hypotension as an independent risk factor for two-year mortality in hemodialysis patients. Kidney Int 2004; 66: 1212-1220

[9] Tislér A, Akócsi K, Borbás B, et al. The effect of frequent or occasional dialysis-associated hypotension on survival of patients on maintenance hemodialysis. Nephrol Dial Transplant 2003; 18: 2601-2605

[10] Mizumasa T, Hirakata H, Yoshimitsu T, et al. Dialysis-related hypotension as a cause of progressive frontal lobe atrophy in chronic hemodialysis patients: a 3-year prospective study. Nephron ClinPract 2004; 97: c23-c30

[11] Kooman J, Basci A, Pizzarelli F, et al. European Best Practice Guidelines: guideline on hemodynamic instability. Nephrol Dial Transplant 2007; 22 (Suppl 2) ii22-ii44

[12] Daugirdas JT. Pathophysiology of dialysis hypotension: an update. Am J Kidney Diseases 2001; 38 (Suppl 4): S11-S17

[13] Rostoker G,Griuncelli M, Loridon C, Benmaadi A, Illouz E. Left-ventricular diastolic dysfunction as a risk factor for dialytic hypotension. Cardiology 2009; 114(2): 142-149

[14] Nishimura M, Takahashi H, Maruyama K, Ohtsuka K, Nanbu A, Hara K, Yoshimura M. Enhanced production of nitric oxide may be involved in acute hypotension during maintenace hemodialysis. Am J Kidney Diseases 1998; 31: 809-817

[15] Cases A, Esforzado N, Lario S, Vera M, Lopez-Pedret J, Rivera-Fillat F, Jimenez W. Increased plasma adrenomedullin levels in hemodialysis patients with sustained hypotension. Kidney Int 2000; 57: 664-670

[16] Raj DS, Vincent B, Simpson K, Sato E, Jones KL, Welbourne TC, Levi M, Shah V, Blandon P, Zager P, Robbins RA. Hemodynamic changes in hemodialysis: role of nitric oxide and endothelin. Kidney Int 2002; 61: 697-704

[17] Franssen CFM. Adenosine and dialysis hypotension. Kidney Int 2006; 69: 789-791

[18] Schreiber MJ. Clinical case-based approach to understanding intradialytic hypotension. Am J Kidney Dis 2001; 38 (Suppl 4)S37-S47

[19] Emili S, Black NA, Paul RV, et al. A protocol-based treatment for intradialytic hypotension in hospitalized hemodialysis patients. Am J Kidney Dis 1999; 33: 1107-1114

[20] The SAFE study investigators. A comparison of albumin and saline for fluid resuscitation in the intensive care unit. New Engl J Med 2004; 350: 2247-2256

[21] Rostoker G,Griuncelli M, Loridon C, Bourlet T, IllouzE, Benmaadi A. A pilot study of routine colloid infusion in hypotension-prone dialysis patients unresponsive to preventive measures. J Nephrol 2011; 24(02): 208-217

[22] Rostoker G,Griuncelli M, Loridon C, Bourlet T, Illouz E, Benmaadi A. Modulation of oxidative stress and microinflammatory status by colloids in refractory dialytic hypotension. BMC Nephrol 2011; oct 20; 12 (1): 58

[23] Jardin F, Prost JF, Ozier Y, Margairaz A. Hemodialysis in septic patients: improvements in tolerance of fluid removal with concentrated albumin as the priming fluid. Crit Care Med 1982; 10: 650-652

[24] McLigeyo SO. Experience with the use of human albumin in renal patients at the Kenyatta National Hospital. East Afr Med J 1993; 70: 15-17

[25] Van Der Sande FM, Luik AJ, Kooman JP, et al. Effect of intravenous fluids on blood pressure course during hemodialysis in hypotension-prone patients. J Am SocNephrol 2000; 11: 550-555

[26] Sirtl C, Laubenthal H, Zumtobel V, Kraft D, Jurecka W. Tissue deposits of hydroxyethylstarch (HES) dose-dependent ant time-related. Br J Anaesth 1999; 82: 510-515

[27] www.afssaps.sante.fr: Hydroxyethylamidons: Enquêtenationale de Pharmacovigilance et décisions; 21 avril 1999

[28] Rodriguez M, Llach F, Pederson JA, Palma A. Changes in plasma oncotic pressure during isolated ultrafiltration.Kidney Int 1982; 21: 519-523

[29] Grocott MP, Hamilton MA. Resuscitation fluids. Vox Sang 2002; 82: 1-8

[30] Van Der Sande F, Kooman JP, Barendregt J, et al. Effect of intravenous saline, albumin or hydroxyethyl starch on blood volume during combined ultrafiltration and hemodialysis. J Am SocNephrol 1999; 10: 1303-1308

[31] Graziani G, Finazzi S, Mangiarotti R, Como G, Fedeli C, Oldani S, Morganti A, Badalamenti S. Different cardiovascular responses to hemodialysis-induced fluid depletion and blood pressure compliance. J Nephrol 2010; 23(01): 55-61

[32] Ritz E, Ruffmann K, Rambausek M, Mall G, Schmidli M. Dialysis hypotension - is it related to diastolic left ventricular malfunction?Nephrol Dial Transplant 1987; 2: 293-297

[33] Ritz E, Rambausek M, Mall G, Ruffmann K, Mandelbaum A. Cardiac changes in uremia and their possible relation to cardiovascular instability on dialysis. In Terminal

renal failure: therapeutic problems, possibilities and potentials. ContribNephrol. Klinkmann H, Smeby LC (eds). Basel, Karger 1990; vol 78pp 221-229

[34] Punzengruber C, Wallner M. Doppler echocardiographic analysis of diastolic left ventricular function in dialysis patients and its relation to intradialytic hypotension. J of Mol Med 1989; 67: 826-832

[35] Kramer W, Wizemann V, Lämmlein G, Thormann J, Kindler M, Schlepper M, Schütterle G. Cardiac dysfunction in patients on maintenance hemodialysis: II Systolic and diastolic properties of the left ventricle assessed by invasive methods. ContrNephrol (Karger, Basel) 1986; 52: 110-124

[36] London G. Left ventricular alterations and end-stage renal disease. Nephrol Dial Transplant 2002; 17 (Suppl 1): 29-36

[37] Gaash WH, Zile MR. Left ventricular diastolic dysfunction and diastolic heart failure. Annu Rev Med 2004; 55: 373-394

[38] Arias M, Alonso A, Garcia-Rio F. Diastolic heart failure. N Engl J Med 2005; 352: 307-308

[39] Tomita M, Malhotra D, Dheenan S, Shapiro JI, Henrich WL, Santoro TJ. A potential role for immune activation in hemodialysis hypotension. Renal Failure 2001; 23: 637-649

[40] Bergamini S, Vandelli L, Bellei E et Al. Relationship of asymmetric dimethylarginine to haemodialysis hypotension. Nitric Oxide 2004; 11: 273-278

[41] CantinAM, Paquette B, Richter M, Larivée P. Albumin-mediated regulation of cellular glutathione and nuclear factor kappa B activation. Am J RespCrit Care Med 2000; 162: 1539-1546

[42] Alam HB, Stanton K, Koustova E, Burris D, Rich N, Rhee P. Effects of different resuscitation strategies on neutrophil activation in a swine model of hemorrhagic shock. Resuscitation 2004; 60: 91-99.

[43] Harper SJ, Tomson CRV, Bates DO. Human uremic plasma increases microvascular permeability to water and proteins in vivo. Kidney Int 2002; 61: 1416-1422

[44] Evans TW. Albumin as a drug: biological effects on albumin unrelated to oncotic pressure. Aliment PharmacolTher 2002; 16(Suppl 5): 6-11

[45] Halliwell B. Free radicals, antioxidants and human disease: curiosity, cause or consequence? Lancet 1994; 344: 721-724

[46] Sandek A, Bjarnason I, Volkd HD, Crane R, Meddings JB, Niebauer J, Kaira PR, Buhner S, Herrmann R, Springer J, Doehner W, Von Haehling S, Anker SD, Rauchhaus M. Studies on bacterial endotoxin and intestinal absorption function in patients with chronic heart failure. Int J Cardiol 2012; 80-85

[47] Ritz E. Intestinal–renal syndrome: mirage or reality? Blood Purif 2011; 31: 70-76

[48] McIntyre CW, Harrison LE, Eldehni MT, Jefferies HJ, Szeto CC, John SG, Sigrist MK, Burton JO, Hothi D, Korsheed S, Owen PJ, Lai KB, Li PK. Circulating endotoxemia: a novel factor in systemic inflammation and cardiovascular disease in chronic kidney disease. Clin J Am SocNephrol 2011; 6: 133-141

[49] Radi R, Bush KM, Cosgrove TP, Freeman BA. Reaction of xanthine oxidase-derived oxidants with lipid and protein of human plasma. Arch BiochemBiophys 1991: 286: 117-125

[50] Soejima A, Matsuzawa N, Miyake N et Al. Hypoalbuminemia accelerates erythrocyte membrane lipid peroxidation in chronic hemodialysis patients. ClinNephrol 1999; 51: 92-97

[51] Hu ML, Louie S, Cross CE, Motchnik P, Halliwell B. Antioxidant protection against hypochlorous acid in human plasma. J Lab Clin Med 1993; 121: 257-262

[52] Quinlan GJ, Mumby S, Martin GS, Bernard GR, Gutteridge JM, Evans TW. Albumin influences total plasma antioxidant capacity favorably in patients with acute lung injury. Crit Care Med 2004; 32: 755-759

[53] Morena M, Delbosc S, Dupuy AM, Canaud B, Cristol JP. Overproduction of reactive oxygen species in end-stage renal disease patients: a potential component of hemodialysis-associated inflammation. Hemodialysis Int 2005; 9: 37-46

Permissions

The contributors of this book come from diverse backgrounds, making this book a truly international effort. This book will bring forth new frontiers with its revolutionizing research information and detailed analysis of the nascent developments around the world.

We would like to thank Professor Hiromichi Suzuki, for lending his expertise to make the book truly unique. He has played a crucial role in the development of this book. Without his invaluable contribution this book wouldn't have been possible. He has made vital efforts to compile up to date information on the varied aspects of this subject to make this book a valuable addition to the collection of many professionals and students.

This book was conceptualized with the vision of imparting up-to-date information and advanced data in this field. To ensure the same, a matchless editorial board was set up. Every individual on the board went through rigorous rounds of assessment to prove their worth. After which they invested a large part of their time researching and compiling the most relevant data for our readers. Conferences and sessions were held from time to time between the editorial board and the contributing authors to present the data in the most comprehensible form. The editorial team has worked tirelessly to provide valuable and valid information to help people across the globe.

Every chapter published in this book has been scrutinized by our experts. Their significance has been extensively debated. The topics covered herein carry significant findings which will fuel the growth of the discipline. They may even be implemented as practical applications or may be referred to as a beginning point for another development. Chapters in this book were first published by InTech; hereby published with permission under the Creative Commons Attribution License or equivalent.

The editorial board has been involved in producing this book since its inception. They have spent rigorous hours researching and exploring the diverse topics which have resulted in the successful publishing of this book. They have passed on their knowledge of decades through this book. To expedite this challenging task, the publisher supported the team at every step. A small team of assistant editors was also appointed to further simplify the editing procedure and attain best results for the readers.

Our editorial team has been hand-picked from every corner of the world. Their multi-ethnicity adds dynamic inputs to the discussions which result in innovative outcomes. These outcomes are then further discussed with the researchers and contributors who give their valuable feedback and opinion regarding the same. The feedback is then collaborated with the researches and they are edited in a comprehensive manner to aid the understanding of the subject.

Apart from the editorial board, the designing team has also invested a significant amount of their time in understanding the subject and creating the most relevant covers. They scrutinized every image to scout for the most suitable representation of the subject and create an appropriate cover for the book.

The publishing team has been involved in this book since its early stages. They were actively engaged in every process, be it collecting the data, connecting with the contributors or procuring relevant information. The team has been an ardent support to the editorial, designing and production team. Their endless efforts to recruit the best for this project, has resulted in the accomplishment of this book. They are a veteran in the field of academics and their pool of knowledge is as vast as their experience in printing. Their expertise and guidance has proved useful at every step. Their uncompromising quality standards have made this book an exceptional effort. Their encouragement from time to time has been an inspiration for everyone.

The publisher and the editorial board hope that this book will prove to be a valuable piece of knowledge for researchers, students, practitioners and scholars across the globe.

List of Contributors

Ane Cláudia Fernandes Nunes
Laboratory of Cellular, Genetic and Molecular Nephrology (LIM-29), Division of Ne-phrology, São Paulo University Medical School, University of São Paulo, São Paulo, Brazil
Developmental and Cell Biology Department, University of California, Irvine, CA, USA

Fernanda de Souza Messias
Laboratory of Cellular, Genetic and Molecular Nephrology (LIM-29), Division of Ne-phrology, São Paulo University Medical School, University of São Paulo, São Paulo, Brazil

Elvino José Guardão Barros
Service of Nephrology, Clinical Hospital of Porto Alegre, Federal University of Rio Grande do Sul. Porto Alegre, RS, Brazil

Han Li and Shixiang Wang
Blood Purification Center, Beijing Chaoyang Hospital, Capital Medical University, Beijing, China

F. Esra Güneş
Marmara University, Health Science Faculty, Department of Nutrition and Dietetic, Turkey

Gülsüm Özkan and Şükrü Ulusoy
Karadeniz Technical University, School of Medicine, Department of Nephrology, Turkey

Şükrü Ulusoy and Gülsüm Özkan
Karadeniz Technical University, School of Medicine, Department of Nephrology, Turkey

Yasuo Imanishi
Department of Metabolism, Endocrinology and Molecular Medicine, Osaka City University Graduate School of Medicine, Osaka, Japan

Masaaki Inaba
Department of Metabolism, Endocrinology and Molecular Medicine, Osaka City University Graduate School of Medicine, Osaka, Japan

Yoshiki Nishizawa
Osaka City University, Osaka, Japan

Hernán Trimarchi
Chief Nephrology Service, Hospital Británico de Buenos Aires, Buenos Aires, Argentina

Pornanong Aramwit
Bioactive Resources for Innovative Clinical Applications Research Unit and Department of Pharmacy Practice, Faculty of Pharmaceutical Sciences, Chulalongkorn University, Phaya- Thai Road, Phatumwan, Bangkok, Thailand

Bancha Satirapoj
Division of Nephrology, Phramongkutklao Hospital and College of Medicine, Bangkok, Thailand

Melanie Chan and Marlies Ostermann
Department of Critical Care, Guy's & St Thomas' Hospital, London, UK

Masaki Fujioka
Department of Plastic and Reconstructive Surgery, National Hospital Organization Na-gasaki Medical Center, Ohmura City, Japan

Alexandre Braga Libório and Tacyano Tavares Leite
General Hospital of Fortaleza, Fortaleza, Ceará, Brazil

H. Suzuki
Department of Nephrology, Saitama Medical University Saitama, Japan

T. Inoue
Department of Nephrology, Saitama Medical University Saitama, Japan

H. Okada
Department of Nephrology, Saitama Medical University Saitama, Japan

T. Takenaka
Department of Nephrology, Saitama Medical University Saitama, Japan

Kunihiko Hayashi
Department of Internal Medicine, Irumadai Clinic, Saitama, Japan

Jyunnichi Nishiyama
Department of Internal Medicine, Irumadai Clinic, Saitama, Japan

Takashi Yamazaki
Department of Internal Medicine, Irumadai Clinic, Saitama, Japan

Yuji Nishiyama
Department of Internal Medicine, Irumadai Clinic, Saitama, Japan

Keiko Kaneko
Department of Internal Medicine, Irumadai Clinic, Saitama, Japan

Yoshiaki Kawaguchi and Tetsuya Mine
Tokai University School of Medicine, Japan

Guy Rostoker
Service de Néphrologie ET de Dialyse, Hôpital Privé Claude Galien, Quincy Sous Sénart,
France

Embryonic Stem Cells: Differentiation Processes and Alternatives

Edited by **Jack Collins**

FOSTER
ACADEMICS

New Jersey

Published by Foster Academics,
61 Van Reypen Street,
Jersey City, NJ 07306, USA
www.fosteracademics.com

Embryonic Stem Cells: Differentiation Processes
and Alternatives
Edited by Jack Collins

International Standard Book Number: 978-1-63242-123-4 (Hardback)

Contents

Preface

This book provides elaborative information on embryonic cells. Embryonic stem cells require methods and protocols to turn these unspecialized cells into fully functioning cell types found in a wide variety of tissues and organs. This book presents an overview of contemporary research on differentiation of embryonic stem cells to a wide variety of cell types, including endothelial, osteogenic, and hepatic cells. Also, induced pluripotent stem cells and other pluripotent stem cell sources have been described. The book will prove to be a valuable resource for engineers, scientists, and clinicians as well as students in a wide range of disciplines.

Significant researches are present in this book. Intensive efforts have been employed by authors to make this book an outstanding discourse. This book contains the enlightening chapters which have been written on the basis of significant researches done by the experts.

Finally, I would also like to thank all the members involved in this book for being a team and meeting all the deadlines for the submission of their respective works. I would also like to thank my friends and family for being supportive in my efforts.

Editor

Part 1

General Differentiation

Bioactive Lipids in Stem Cell Differentiation

Erhard Bieberich and Guanghu Wang
Georgia Health Sciences University
U.S.A.

1. Introduction

Bioactive lipids are lipids with cell signaling functions. In the last two decades, they have become increasingly important in many fields of biology. They are the main diffusible mediators of inflammatory responses in tissues and regulate the polarity of cellular membranes. They are also critical for cell fate decisions during stem cell differentiation by inducing apoptosis or sustaining cell survival and polarity. The bioactive lipids discussed here belong to the classes of phospho- and sphingolipids. Mainly three different types of lipids and their function in stem cell differentiation will be reviewed in detail: phophatidylinositols (PIPs), lysophospholipids and eicosanoids, and the sphingolipid ceramide and its derivative sphingosine-1-phosphate (S1P).

2. Biological Function of bioactive lipids in stem cell differentiation

2.1 Phosphatidylinositols

The phosphatidylinositols PI(3,4)P2 and PI(3,4,5)P3 generated by class I phosphatidyinositol-3-kinase (PI3K) upon induction of tyrosine receptor kinases or G-protein coupled receptors (GPCRs) are known to be the major activators of the Akt/PKB cell signaling pathway for cell survival and differentiation (Callihan et al., 2011; Frebel &Wiese, 2006; Layden et al., 2010; Paling et al., 2004; Storm et al., 2007; Umehara et al., 2007). The phosphatase and tensin homolog deleted on chromosome 10 (PTEN) is a lipid phosphatase that catalyzes the hydrolysis of PIP3 to PIP2, which leads to inactivation of the Akt/PKB cell signaling pathway and loss of pluripotency in stem cells (Groszer et al., 2001; Korkaya et al., 2009; Otaegi et al., 2006). PTEN is a tumor suppressor mutated in many types of cancer and it is critical for the controlled growth of embryonic tissue and ES cells.

PTEN converts PIP3 into PIP2 (Fig. 1). Since PIP3 activates the Akt/PKB cell signaling pathway, thus PTEN catalyzing PIP3 hydrolysis is a negative regulator of Akt/PKB. Consistent with this function, deletion of PTEN activates Akt/PKB-dependent cell signaling pathways (Groszer et al., 2001). PTEN mutations are often found in human cancers such as glioblastoma, prostate cancer, and breast cancer. Loss of function of this tumor suppressor gene results in the up-regulation of the Akt/PKB-to-β-catenin pathway (Fig. 2A) (Korkaya et al., 2009). Akt/PKB phosphorylates and therefore, inactivates glycogen synthase-3β (GSK-3β), a protein kinase in the Wnt signaling pathway that phosphorylates β-catenin (Doble &Woodgett, 2003; Ikeda et al., 2000; van Noort et al., 2002). The oncogene β-catenin is an important adhesion protein and transcription factor for genes involved in proliferation. When phosphorylated by GSK-3β, β-catenin (in a protein complex with adenomatous polyposis coli or APC) is proteolytically degraded and thus, adhesion lost and proliferation reduced. Consistent with this function, deletion of β-catenin results in loss of pluripotency and early embryonic death of the respective knockout mouse (Haegel et al., 1995). Likewise, deletion of PTEN results in increased β-catenin levels and increased pluripotency or malignancy (Groszer et al., 2001). Therefore, the PTEN vs. PI3K-to-Akt/PKB antagonism is interesting in two biological contexts with respect to stem cell differentiation: maintenance of pluripotent stem cells and tumorigenesis of cancer stem cells. In the first context, inhibition of PTEN, activation of PI3K and Akt/PKB, or inhibition of GSK-3β will be useful to maintain pluripotent ES cells. In the second context, activation of PTEN, inhibition of PI3K and Akt/PKB, or activation of GSK-3β may be a useful strategy to eliminate cancer stem cells.

In the cultivation process of ES cells, elevated expression of the transcription factors Oct-4 and Nanog is essential for maintenance of pluripotency (Bhattacharya et al., 2003; Sato et al., 2004). It has been shown that two cell signaling pathways are critical for this regulation: the janus kinase/signal transducer and activator of transcription 3 (Jak/Stat3) and the Akt/PKB signaling pathways (Fig. 2A) (Kelly et al., 2011; Paling et al., 2004). In the cultivation of mouse ES cells, the most important growth factor activating Stat3 and Akt/PKB is LIF (leukemia inhibitory factor), an interleukin 6 class cytokine binding to LIF receptor α (LIFRα) (Cartwright et al., 2005; Niwa et al., 1998; Okita &Yamanaka, 2006; Schuringa et al., 2002; Takao et al., 2007). In vitro, LIF is added to the medium when cultivating undifferentiated mouse ES cells on feeder fibroblasts and in feeder-free culture. In vivo, LIF is generated by the trophoectoderm from where it penetrates the inner cell mass, the source of pluripotent ES cells in the pre-implantation embryo. In human ES cells, the role of LIF as "guardian" of pluripotency is taken over by fibroblast growth factor (FGF) (Lanner &Rossant, 2010; Li et al., 2007) (Fig. 2A). Binding of FGF-2 to the FGF receptor 2 (FGFR2) activates similar cell signaling pathways in human ES cells as stimulated by LIF in mouse ES cells: Jak/Stat3, mitogen-activated protein kinase (MAPK), and Akt/PKB (Lanner &Rossant, 2010; Li et al., 2007). However, FGFR-dependent signaling is very diverse and it depends on individual receptor protein complexes which specific response is elicited by FGF. For example, in mouse ES cells, FGF-2 is used to maintain the multipotent neuroprogenitor stage and to prevent further neuronal differentiation. In human ES cells, supplementation of the serum-free cell culture medium with FGF-2 is critical to prevent apoptosis and to maintain pluripotency.

The role of lipids as the key factors in the PI3K-to-Akt/PKB-to-β-catenin cell signaling pathway is obvious since phosphatidylinositols (PIPs) are lipids by provenance. Unfortunately, PIPs are not applicable as exogenous factors that can be simply added to stem cell media since these lipids are part of an intracellular cell signaling cascade not easily accessible to the outside of the cell. However, there are other lipid-regulated pathways that are dependent on the activation of cell surface receptors, which is of tremendous advantage if one attempts to use lipids as exogenously added growth or differentiation factors (see section 2.2). The two receptors involved in maintenance of pluripotency, LIFRα and FGFR2 are both tyrosine receptor kinases which are not directly activated by lipids, although indirect regulation by so-called "lipid rafts" has been discussed (see section 2.4) (Lee et al., 2010b; Yanagisawa et al., 2004b, 2005).

In addition to using natural lipids as ligands, stem cell differentiation can also be modulated by pharmacologic reagents that are either lipid analogs, inhibitors of enzymes in lipid

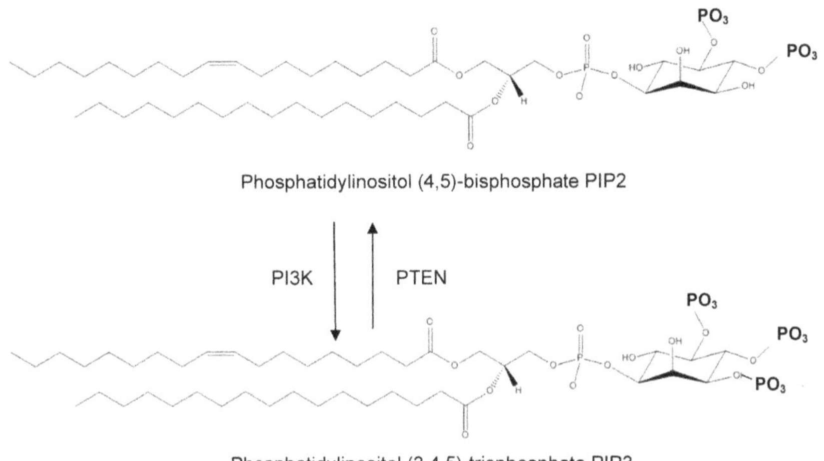

Phosphatidylinositol (4,5)-bisphosphate PIP2

Phosphatidylinositol (3,4,5)-trisphosphate PIP3

Fig. 1. Metabolism of phosphatidylinositols in the PI3K-to-Akt/PKB cells signaling pathway for ES cell pluripotency. PI3K, phosphatidylinositol 3-kinase; PTEN, phosphatase and tensin homolog deleted on chromosome 10

metabolism, or drugs targeting downstream effectors of lipid-regulated cell signaling pathways. Two drugs that are inhibitors of protein kinases in the LIFRα and FGFR2 pathways have been tested on their effect on pluripotency: LY294002 and indirubin-3-monoxime, two inhibitors specific for PI3K and GSK-3β, respectively (Chen et al., 2006; Chen et al., 2000; Ding &Schultz, 2004; Ding et al., 2003; Lyssiotis et al., 2011; Otaegi et al., 2006; Paling et al., 2004; Sato et al., 2004). The PI3K inhibitor LY294002 has been shown to reduce the capacity of mouse and human ES cells to self-renew and to undergo subsequent steps of lineage specification and differentiation (Paling et al., 2004). These effects are likely to involve differentiation stage-specific (contextual) other cell signaling pathways downstream (or parallel) to the PI3K-to-Akt/PKB signaling axis. While it may not be desired to interfere with ES cell pluripotency, LY294002 and other PI3K and Akt/PKB inhibitors are currently tested for cancer treatment, in particular for targeting cancer stem cells (Bleau et al., 2009; Plo et al., 1999). If one desires to sustain self-renewal of ES cells, GSK-3β inhibitors such as indirubin-3-monoxime or BIO are attractive candidates. BIO has been successfully used to maintain pluripotency in human ES cells (Sato et al., 2004). Additional effectors targeting GSK-3β are synthetic agonists of the Wnt receptor Frizzled, however, their use in stem cell differentiation is not yet sufficiently investigated (Lyssiotis et al., 2011).

Interestingly, inhibitors of the mitogen activated protein kinase (MAPK) pathway such as the MAPK kinase (MEK) inhibitor PD98059 have been used with mouse ES cells to promote self-renewal or pluripotency (Buehr &Smith, 2003; Li et al., 2007). This appears paradoxical since LIFRα as well as FGFR2 are known to activate MAPK, which suggests that activation of MAPK is involved in pluripotency. However, only transient MAPK activation to promote G1 re-entry is useful for self-renewal while prolonged activation will promote differentiation (Fig. 2B). Therefore, a combination of LIF with the MAPK-kinase (MEK) inhibitor PD95059 activating PI3K-to-Akt/PKB while inhibiting MAPK signaling has been successfully used to promote pluripotency in mouse ES cells, but also to enhance the

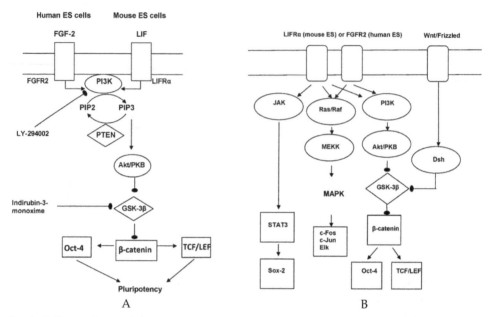

Fig. 2. Cell signaling pathways for ES cell pluripotency. Elliptic circles label enzymes that promote pluripotency, while diamonds label enzymes that reduce pluripotency and promote differentiation. MAPK shows both, pro-pluripotency or pro-differentiation activity in human or mouse ES cells, respectively.

generation of induced pluripotent stem (iPS) cells (Li et al., 2007; Lyssiotis et al., 2011). The situation in human ES cells, however, is different. In contrast to mouse ES cells, inhibition of the MAPK cell signaling pathway reduces the potential of undifferentiated human ES cells to self-renew, indicating that FGFR2-mediated activation of Ras/Raf-to-MEK-to MAPK is critical for human ES cell pluripotency (Ding et al., 2010). A similar role has been found for Bmp4, which promotes pluripotency in mouse and differentiation in human ES cells (Bouhon et al., 2005; Zeng et al., 2004; Zhang et al., 2010). It is quite possible that this difference depends on which other pathways for pluripotency are co-activated such as Jak/Stat3 in mouse or Activin in human ES cells. Bioactive lipids are important in that they co-regulate several cell signaling pathways critical for pluripotency and differentiation of ES cells, in particular MAPK and PI3K downstream of ClassA/Rhodopsin-like GPCRs, which will be discussed in the next section.

2.2 Lysophospholipids and eicosanoids

Lysophospholipids (LPLs) are lipids generated by hydrolytic cleavage of fatty acid from glycerophospholipids, which is catalyzed by phospholipases. Distinct phospholipases cleave off either one of the two (PLA1 and PLA2) or both (PLB) fatty acid residues, or they cleave off the phosphate-containing head group (PLC) or the alcohol (PLD) (Gardell et al., 2006; Hla et al., 2001; Hla et al., 2000; Lin et al., 2010; Meyer zu Heringdorf &Jakobs, 2007; Okudaira et al., 2010; Radeff-Huang et al., 2004; Tigyi &Parrill, 2003; Ye et al., 2002). PLA2 generates arachidonic acid, the precursor for the generation of eicosanoids, a group of inflammatory mediators including prostaglandins and leukotrienes (Funk, 2001; Jenkins et al., 2009; Khanapure et al., 2007; Lambeau &Gelb, 2008; Szefel et al., 2011; Wymann &Schneiter, 2008). Similar to the PLD reaction, lysophospholipase D or autotaxin generates lysophosphatidic acid (LPA) from lysophosphatidylcholine (Nakanaga et al., 2010; Okudaira et al., 2010; Samadi et al., 2011). LPA receptors are critical in cell proliferation and tumorigenesis and have recently been shown to promote proliferation of human neural precursor cells (Callihan et al., 2011; Hurst et al., 2008; Lin et al., 2010; Pebay et al., 2007; Pebay et al., 2005; Pitson &Pebay, 2009).

Arachidonic acid, generated by PLA2 from phospholipids such as phosphatidylcholine (Fig. 3A) is converted to a variety of pro-inflammotory eicosanoids among which prostaglandins, thromboxanes, and leukotrienes are the most important signaling lipids (Fig. 3B). The effect of eicosanoids on ES cells is not well understood and research is mostly limited to results with mouse ES cells. Interestingly, lysophospholipids such as LPA and eicosanoids such as prostaglandin E2 (PGE2) appear to activate similar downstream cell signaling pathways, mainly the PI3K-to-Akt/PKB, MAPK, and Wnt/GSK-3β pathways (Callihan et al., 2011; Goessling et al., 2009; Logan et al., 2007; North et al., 2007; Pebay et al., 2007; Pitson &Pebay, 2009; Yun et al., 2009). In contrast to LIFRα or FGFR2, however, stimulation of Akt/PKB by PGE2 has not been reported to sustain pluripotency, but is rather anti-apoptotic/cell protective and promotes stem cell proliferation. This may not be surprising since generation and conversion of arachidonic acid is often a response to hypoxic insults, which can damage mitochondria and induce apoptosis. Notably, inhibition of eicosanoid biosynthesis reduces the potential of mouse and human ES cells to self-renew, indicating a role of eicosanoids in stem cell maintenance or pluripotency (Yanes et al., 2010). Thromboxane has not been described to play a role in stem cell differentiation, maybe because its main function is rather confined to platelet aggregation. In contrast, prostacyclin, a similar eicosanoid in platelet aggregation has been shown to promote cardiogenic differentiation from human ES

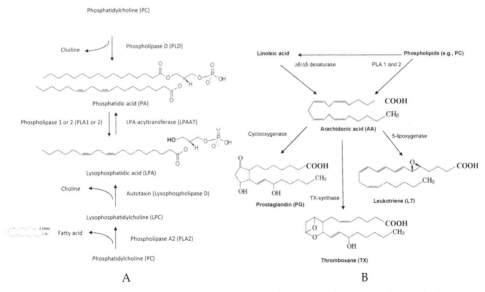

Fig. 3. Biosynthesis pathways in lysoposphatidic acid (LPA) and eicosanoid metabolism

cells (Chillar et al., 2010; Xu et al., 2008). In addition to prostacyclin, leukotriene of the LTD4 type has been used in several studies to promote proliferation and cardiovascular differentiation of mouse ES cells (Finkensieper et al., 2010; Funk, 2001; Kim et al., 2010).

The effect of prostaglandins and other eicosanoids on ES cells is worth discussing in an important aspect of human health care. Inhibitors of cyclooxygenase 2 (Cox-2), the enzyme critical for PGE2 production, are taken by nearly everyone to ease up head ache, back pain, and inflammation. The Cox-2 inhibitor aspirin is one of the most successfully administered drugs world-wide. A recent study on the negative effect of non-steroidal anti-inflammatory drugs (NSAIDs) such as aspirin on the differentiation of human ES cells suggests that one has to be careful with the use of NSAIDs when human ES cells are to be transplanted for heart tissue repair (Chillar et al., 2010). These observations suggest that eicosanoids are important in cardiogenic/cardiovascular differentiation of ES cells.

The eicosanoid as well as lysophospholipid receptors belong to the family of Class A Rhodopsin-like GPCRs (Callihan et al., 2011; Hla et al., 2001; Kostenis, 2004; Lin et al., 2010; Pitson &Pebay, 2009; Radeff-Huang et al., 2004). They mediate the activation of downstream cell signaling pathways through different types of GTPases, mainly Gi, Gq, and G12/13,

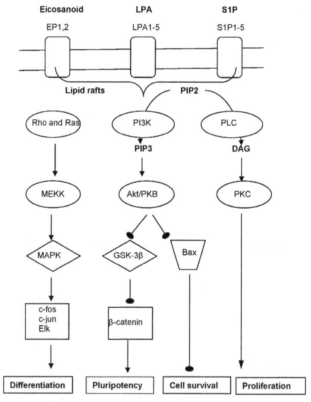

Fig. 4. GPCR-dependent cell signaling pathways with similar function for ES cell pluripotency and differentiation. DAG, diacylglycerol; PLC, phospholipase C; EP, eicosanoid receptor.

acting upon PI3K-to-Akt/PKB (Gi), Ras-to-ERK (Gi, Gq) Rho (G12/13), and PLC-to-PKC (Gq) cell signaling pathways for pluripotency and cell survival (Akt/PKB), proliferation (Rho and PKC), and differentiation/specification (MAPK) pathways (Fig. 4). Hence, combinations of particular cell signaling lipids with cytokines or growth factors such as LIF or FGF-2 activating similar effectors have been found to be useful in directing stem cell fate toward pluripotency, proliferation, or differentiation, respectively (Hurst et al., 2008; Kilkenny et al., 2003; Layden et al., 2010; Pebay et al., 2007; Radeff-Huang et al., 2004). There are five GPCRs for each LPA and sphingosine-1-phosphate (S1P) expressed in mouse and human ES cells.

2.3 Ceramide and sphingosine-1-phosphate
Sphingolipids are acyl (fatty acid) derivatives of the amino alcohol sphingosine. They encompass sphingosine, ceramide, and ceramide derivatives such as sphingomyelin, ceramide-1-phosphate, S1P, and glycosphingolipids (Fig. 5A for structures) (Bartke &Hannun, 2009; Chalfant &Spiegel, 2005; Chen et al., 2010; Futerman &Hannun, 2004; Hannun et al., 2001; Hannun &Obeid, 2002, 2008; Lebman &Spiegel, 2008; Merrill et al., 1997; Spiegel &Milstien, 2003; Strub et al., 2010; Takabe et al., 2008). Important biological functions of sphingolipids are cell signaling for inflammation, apoptosis, cell cycle regulation, and autophagy (Bartke &Hannun, 2009; Basu &Kolesnick, 1998; Bieberich, 2004, 2008a; Futerman &Hannun, 2004; Gulbins &Kolesnick, 2003; Haimovitz-Friedman et al., 1997; Hannun &Obeid, 2008; Morales et al., 2007). Most recently, particular sphingolipids have also been implicated in ES cell differentiation and cell polarity (Bieberich, 2004, 2008a, b, 2010; Bieberich et al., 2003; Bieberich et al., 2001; Bieberich et al., 2004; Gardell et al., 2006; Goldman et al., 1984; Harada et al., 2004; Hurst et al., 2008; Jung et al., 2009; Pebay et al., 2007; Pebay et al., 2005; Pitson &Pebay, 2009; Salli et al., 2009; Walter et al., 2007; Wang et al., 2008a; Wong et al., 2007; Yanagisawa et al., 2004a). Ceramide has been shown to induce apoptosis specifically in residual pluripotent stem (rPS) cells that cause teratomas (stem cell-derived tumors) after stem cell transplantation. S1P has been found to promote oligodendrocyte differentiation (see section 3.2. for discussion).
Ceramide is the precursor of all bioactive sphingolipids. It is synthesized in three different metabolic pathways. Figure 5B shows that sphingolipid metabolism is integrated into phospholipid (i.e., PC), one carbon unit (i.e., choline), fatty acid (i.e., palmitoyl CoA for de novo biosynthesis and other fatty acids in the salvage pathway), and amino acid (i.e., serine in de novo biosynthesis) metabolism (Bartke &Hannun, 2009; Bieberich, 2004, 2008a; Chen et al., 2010; Futerman &Hannun, 2004; Futerman &Riezman, 2005; Gault et al., 2010; Hannun et al., 2001; Luberto &Hannun, 1999). In cell cultures, plenty of these precursors are provided in the medium, which may not necessarily reproduce the metabolic situation of stem cells or other cell types in vivo. Recently, our group has found that neural crest-derived stem or progenitor cells are sensitive to alcohol due to ethanol-induced elevation of ceramide and induction of apoptosis (Wang &Bieberich, 2010). Apoptosis can be prevented by supplementing the medium with CDP-choline, This effect can be explained by providing excess of substrate required to drive conversion of ceramide to SM using the interconnection of the Kennedy pathway for phospholipid biosynthesis and the SM cycle (Fig. 5B). Choline can also be replenished from the one carbon unit metabolism, which establishes the interconnection of sphingolipid metabolism with this metabolic pathway.
The fatty acid metabolism interconnects with sphingolipid biosynthesis twice, in the de novo and salvage pathways. The de novo pathway uses palmitoyl CoA and serine for a

condensation reaction that is the first step in ceramide biosynthesis. Since serine is used as the second substrate, de novo biosynthesis ties into the amino acid metabolism as well. The salvage pathway uses a variety of activated fatty acids for re-attachment to sphingosine (Fig. 5B). While supply with precursors for lipid metabolism may not be critical in vitro, specialized tissues or cells such as astrocytes providing nutrients and metabolic precursors to neurons or neural stem cells in vivo maybe more sensitive toward lipid imbalances as observed in fetal alcohol syndrome and Alzheimer's disease (Adibhatla &Hatcher, 2008; Cutler et al., 2004; De Vito et al., 2000; Hirabayashi &Furuya, 2008; Jana et al., 2009; Jana &Pahan, 2010; Muscoli et al., 2010; Riboni et al., 2002; Satoi et al., 2005; Wang et al., 2008b). In particular, neural stem cells are confined to distinct morphological cell complexes which tightly control the interaction with other cells and therefore, comprise "metabolic niches" that may control supply with metabolic precursors and lipid cell signaling factors.

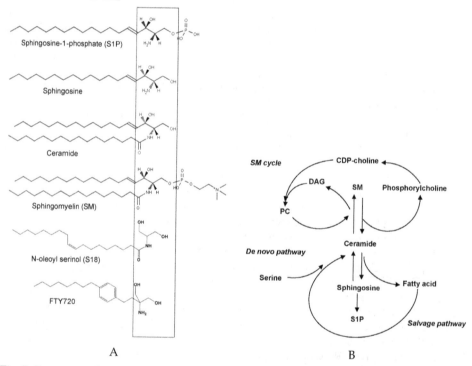

A   B

Fig. 5. Structures of ceramide precursors and derivatives with cell signaling function and interconnection of ceramide metabolism with other lipid and amino acid metabolism. N-oleoyl serinol (S18) or FTY720 are analogues of ceramide or S1P, respectively. Box shows common structural motif.

Regulation of sphingolipid metabolism by its interconnection with other lipid metabolic pathways has a direct impact on lipid-dependent cell signaling. Ceramide is the precursor of S1P, which is a ligand for five distinct S1P receptors (S1P1-5) on the cell surface and also binding partner/co-factor for at least three intracellular proteins, histone deacetylase 1 and 2

(HDAC 1 and 2) in the nucleus, the E3 ubiquitin ligase TRAF2, and prohibitin in the mitochondria (Alvarez et al., 2010; Callihan et al., 2011; Hait et al., 2009; Hait et al., 2006; Hurst et al., 2008; Pitson &Pebay, 2009; Radeff-Huang et al., 2004; Sanchez &Hla, 2004; Spiegel &Kolesnick, 2002; Strub et al., 2011) . The effect of intracellular S1P on stem cell differentiation is not known. However, there is solid experimental evidence that S1P has profound effects on ES cells and ES cell-derived neural progenitors via S1P receptors, which will be discussed in section 3.2.

2.4 Terpenoids, sterols, glycosphingolipids, and lipid rafts

The previous sections discussed bioactive lipids that are known to act through lipid receptors or binding proteins. There are many more lipids that regulate cell signaling pathways through a mechanism known as "lipid rafts" or "lipid microdomains" (Bieberich, 2008a; Lee et al., 2010b; Lingwood &Simons, 2010; Miljan &Bremer, 2002; Ohanian &Ohanian, 2001; Yanagisawa et al., 2005). Lipid rafts are areas in the cell membrane (or intracellular membranes) that emerge from the self-assembly of lipids in an ordered structure. They are believed to show high affinity to specific cell signaling proteins such as growth factor or cytokine receptors, which leads to clustering and activation of these receptors. Therefore, bioactive lipids can affect stem cell differentiation in two different ways: direct interaction with lipid receptors such as GPCRs and lipid raft-dependent activation of growth factor or cytokine receptors such as LIFRα or FGFR2 (Bieberich, 2008a; Bryant et al., 2009; Gutierrez &Brandan, 2010; Lee et al., 2010b; Yanagisawa et al., 2005). Lipids that form rafts are sphingomyelin, cholesterol, and glycosphingolipids. In addition, signal transduction proteins such as Ras can be modified with fatty acids (palmitoylation) or terpenoids (farnesylation, geranylation) and glycophosphatidylinositol (GPI anchor), which tremendously increases membrane binding and raft association (Levental et al., 2010; Lingwood &Simons, 2010; Resh, 2004; Roy et al., 2005). It has been shown that particular glycosphingolipids termed gangliosides can regulate ES cell differentiation by the activation of FGFR2 and other receptors in lipid rafts (Bieberich, 2004; Yanagisawa et al., 2005). An example for this mechanism is the corrective activity of the ganglioside GM1 on the effect of the fungus toxin fumonisin B1, which causes neural tube defects by inhibiting sphingolipid biosynthesis (Gelineau-van Waes et al., 2005; Marasas et al., 2004). It has also been demonstrated that the activity of sonic hedgehog, a morphogen critical for germ layer formation is functionally dependent on palmitoylation and modification with cholesterol (Gofflot et al., 2003; Guy, 2000; Incardona &Roelink, 2000; Karpen et al., 2001; Kelley et al., 1996; Lewis et al., 2001; Li et al., 2006). Inhibition of cholesterol biosynthesis with statins leads to aberrant embryo development. Although these are impressive examples of the effect of lipid modification and lipid raft formation on stem cell differentiation and embryo development, it is presently not known how to specifically utilize this mechanism in controlling the differentiation of ES cells. It is also not clear, which differentiation potential cholesterol has besides being critical for lipid raft formation. There is a plethora of steroid hormones such as estrogen or progesterone that are bioactive lipids activating nuclear receptors critical for embryo development. Progesterone is a particularly curious case since it is added to most of the supplements (e.g., N2, B27) found in defined media used for the in vitro maintenance and differentiation of ES cells. The use of this and other bioactive and synthetic lipids for the in vitro differentiation of ES cells will be discussed in the following section.

3. Bioactive lipids and their use for in vitro differentiation of embryonic stem cells

3.1 Induction of apoptosis in teratoma-forming stem cells by ceramide analogs

The reliability and safety of current stem cell differentiation protocols is still a matter of controversy. Many studies have shown that even when using similar protocols for the in vitro differentiation of ES cells, transplantation can lead to the formation of teratomas (Baker, 2009; Bieberich, 2008b; Blum &Benvenisty, 2008; Fong et al., 2010; Fujikawa et al., 2005; Lee et al., 2009; Vogel, 2005; Wang et al., 2010). Teratomas are stem cell-derived tumors that are fatal if they grow in the brain or heart. Teratomas may arise from any type of pluripotent cells, including induced pluripotent stem (iPS) cells. Therefore, they are a major safety concern, in particular when using larger numbers of ES or iPS cell-derived cells. Our studies have shown that teratomas arise from a particular type of residual pluripotent stem (rPS) cells that maintain the expression of the pluripotency transcription factor Oct-4 and fail to differentiate or undergo apoptosis (Bieberich, 2008a, b, 2010; Bieberich et al., 2003; Bieberich et al., 2004). However, we have also found that they co-express prostate apoptosis response 4 (PAR-4), a protein that sensitizes cells toward ceramide-induced apoptosis. Using a water-soluble ceramide analog termed N-oleoyl serinol or S18, which was for the first time synthesized in our laboratory, we were able to rid stem cells grafts of teratoma-forming rPS cells (Bieberich et al., 2002; Bieberich et al., 2000). We have shown that S18 promotes binding of atypical PKC (aPKC) to PAR-4, which inhibits the aPKC-activated NF-κB cell survival pathway and induces apoptosis in rPS cells (Bieberich, 2008a; Krishnamurthy et al., 2007; Wang et al., 2009; Wang et al., 2005). These cells are eliminated because they are sensitive to S18. Neural progenitor cells will survive and undergo further differentiation because they show no or only low level expression of PAR-4.

3.2 Induction of oligodendrocyte differentiation by S1P and S1P analogs

It has been shown that S1P and the S1P prodrug analog FTY720 promote cell survival and differentiation of primary cultures of oligodendroglial precursor cells (OPCs) (Bieberich, 2010; Coelho et al., 2010; Jung et al., 2007; Miron et al., 2008a; Saini et al., 2005). We have found that teratoma-forming rPS cells do not express the S1P receptor S1P1, which makes them vulnerable to ceramide or S18-induced apoptosis (Bieberich, 2008b, 2010; Bieberich et al., 2004). In contrast, ES cell-derived neural progenitor cells express S1P1. Our studies have shown that in the presence of S18 and FTY720, neural progenitor cells will survive and undergo oligodendroglial differentiation because they are insensitive to S18 (PAR-4 is not expressed). At the same time, OPC differentiation is promoted by FTY720 or S1P (S1P1 is expressed). Implantation of S18 and FTY720-treated neural progenitors does not result in teratoma formation and leads to integration of the grafted cells into highly myelinated areas of the brain such as the corpus callosum (Bieberich, 2010). Therefore, a combined treatment with ceramide analogs and S1P analogs or S1P receptor agonists is a promising strategy to control ES cell differentiation toward OPCs that are useful for treatment of de- or dysmelination diseases such as multiple sclerosis. Interestingly, the addition of S1P analogs to the ceramide analog S18 resulted in a shift of predominantly neuronal differentiation (as promoted by S18 alone) of ES cells toward oligodendroglial lineage, which is an impressive example for the impact of bioactive lipids on stem cell differentiation.

3.3 Synthetic lipids as small molecular effectors for ES cell differentiation

The use of defined media supplemented with small molecule effectors that control the in vitro differentiation of stem cells is a promising strategy to generate transplantable progenitor cells that have not been in contact with animal-derived products such as serum. Currently, there are more than twenty compounds available that specifically induce differentiation of ES cells toward progenitors of bone, heart, muscle, or brain tissue. Although most of these compounds are not considered bioactive lipids because they are synthetic drugs not found in biological organisms, almost all of them are lipids with respect to their chemical structure. One of the first synthetic lipids used a small molecule effector for ES cell differentiation is a bioactive lipid with critical function in brain development: retinoic acid (Dinsmore et al., 1996; Guan et al., 2001; Hu et al., 2009; Jiang et al., 2010; Lee et al., 2010a; Liour et al., 2006; Mayer-Proschel et al., 1997; Mummery et al., 1990; Murashov et al., 2005; Osakada &Takahashi, 2011; Plachta et al., 2004). Mouse and human ES cells respond to a brief exposure to retinoic acid by accelerating differentiation into motoneurons, interneurons, and even oligendendrocytes when combined with specific growth factors such as FGF-2 or platelet-derived growth factor (PDGF). Another bioactive lipid used for in vitro differentiation of mouse and human ES cells, in particular toward oligodendroglial lineage is thyroid hormone (T3) (Glaser et al., 2007; Kang et al., 2007).

In addition to these naturally occurring lipids, synthetic lipids have been isolated from chemical libraries using various bioassays for ES cell differentiation. Indirubin-3-oxime type compounds for maintenance of pluripotency have already been discussed in section 1. A more detailed discussion of these small molecule effectors can be found in the following articles (Ding et al., 2003; Lyssiotis et al., 2011; Zhu et al., 2010). The advantage of these compounds emerges from their lipid-like structure, which allows for penetration of the blood brain barrier. Provided that toxicity issues do not prevent the use of these compounds in vivo, bioactive and synthetic lipids are likely to develop into powerful pharmacologic drugs that can be used for in vitro differentiation of ES or iPS cells and then after transplantation, for further treatment of the patient to enhance the in vivo differentiation of the grafted cells. One of the first drugs with this dual potential of in vitro and in vivo use is FTY720 (Bieberich, 2010; Coelho et al., 2007; Lee et al., 2010a; Miron et al., 2008a; Miron et al., 2008b; Napoli, 2000). It is quite expectable that many of these "dual use" drugs will play an important role in the clinical application of ES and iPS cells.

4. Conclusions and perspectives

The goal of this chapter was to review current knowledge on bioactive lipids in embryonic stem cell differentiation. One of the important results of this analysis is the insight into the interconnection between lipid metabolism and signaling function. Unlike most proteins, lipids can be converted into derivatives that either complement or antagonize each other's cell signaling function. For example, conversion of PC to LPA and eisosanoids has similar effects on enhancing pluripotency. On the other hand, conversion of ceramide to S1P can have opposite functions, in particular with respect to apoptosis and survival of pluripotent stem cells. Another important insight is that most bioactive lipids cooperate with cytokine and growth factor receptors providing the possibility to combine these factors with the respective lipids in defined media for controlled stem cell differentiation. For example, FGF-2 can be combined with the ceramide analog S18 to promote neuronal differentiation, or with S18 and FTY720 to enhance specification to oligodendroglial lineage. This provides the opportunity to generate bioactive lipids or lipid analogs that can be applied for in vitro differentiation of stem cells and then for further treatment of the patient who has received the stem cell graft. These "dual use" bioactive lipids will be of tremendous value for the therapeutic application of stem cells.

5. Acknowledgment

The authors acknowledge support in part by the NIH (R01AG034389 to EB), March of Dimes Foundation (MOD 6-FY08-322 to EB), a Scientist Training Grant from the Georgia Health Sciences University (to GW), and a Scientist Development grant from the American Heart Association (to GW). We also thank the Institute of Molecular Medicine and Genetics (under directorship of Dr. Lin Mei) for institutional support.

6. References

Adibhatla, R.M. & Hatcher, J.F. (2008). Altered lipid metabolism in brain injury and disorders. *Subcell Biochem*, Vol.49241-268.

Alvarez, S.E.; Harikumar, K.B.; Hait, N.C.; Allegood, J.; Strub, G.M.; Kim, E.Y.; Maceyka, M.; Jiang, H.; Luo, C.; Kordula, T.; Milstien, S. & Spiegel, S. (2010). Sphingosine-1-phosphate is a missing cofactor for the E3 ubiquitin ligase TRAF2. *Nature*, Vol.465, No.7301, pp.1084-1088.

Baker, M. (2009). Stem cells: Fast and furious. *Nature*, Vol.458, No.7241, pp.962-965.

Bartke, N. & Hannun, Y.A. (2009). Bioactive sphingolipids: metabolism and function. *J Lipid Res*, Vol.50 SupplS91-96.

Basu, S. & Kolesnick, R. (1998). Stress signals for apoptosis: ceramide and c-Jun kinase. *Oncogene*, Vol.17, No.25, pp.3277-3285.

Bhattacharya, B.; Miura, T.; Brandenberg, R.; Mejido, J.; Luo, Y.; Yang, A.X.; Joshi, B.H.; Irene, G.; Thies, R.S.; Amit, M.; Lyons, I.; Condie, B.G.; Iskovitz-Eldor, J.; Rao, M.S. & Puri, R.K. (2003). Gene Expression in Human Embryonic Stem Cell Lines: Unique Molecular Signature. *Blood*.

Bieberich, E. (2004). Integration of glycosphingolipid metabolism and cell-fate decisions in cancer and stem cells: review and hypothesis. *Glycoconj J*, Vol.21, No.6, pp.315-327.

Bieberich, E. (2008a). Ceramide signaling in cancer and stem cells. *Future Lipidol*, Vol.3, No.3, pp.273-300.

Bieberich, E. (2008b). Smart drugs for smarter stem cells: making SENSe (sphingolipid-enhanced neural stem cells) of ceramide. *Neurosignals*, Vol.16, No.2-3, pp.124-139.

Bieberich, E. (2010). There is More to a Lipid than just Being a Fat: Sphingolipid-Guided Differentiation of Oligodendroglial Lineage from Embryonic Stem Cells. *Neurochem Res*.

Bieberich, E.; Hu, B.; Silva, J.; MacKinnon, S.; Yu, R.K.; Fillmore, H.; Broaddus, W.C. & Ottenbrite, R.M. (2002). Synthesis and characterization of novel ceramide analogs for induction of apoptosis in human cancer cells. *Cancer Lett*, Vol.181, No.1, pp.55-64.

Bieberich, E.; Kawaguchi, T. & Yu, R.K. (2000). N-acylated serinol is a novel ceramide mimic inducing apoptosis in neuroblastoma cells. *J Biol Chem*, Vol.275, No.1, pp.177-181.

Bieberich, E.; MacKinnon, S.; Silva, J.; Noggle, S. & Condie, B.G. (2003). Regulation of cell death in mitotic neural progenitor cells by asymmetric distribution of prostate apoptosis response 4 (PAR-4) and simultaneous elevation of endogenous ceramide. *J Cell Biol*, Vol.162, No.3, pp.469-479.

Bieberich, E.; MacKinnon, S.; Silva, J. & Yu, R.K. (2001). Regulation of apoptosis during neuronal differentiation by ceramide and b-series complex gangliosides. *J Biol Chem*, Vol.276, No.48, pp.44396-44404.

Bieberich, E.; Silva, J.; Wang, G.; Krishnamurthy, K. & Condie, B.G. (2004). Selective apoptosis of pluripotent mouse and human stem cells by novel ceramide analogues prevents teratoma formation and enriches for neural precursors in ES cell-derived neural transplants. *J Cell Biol*, Vol.167, No.4, pp.723-734.

Bleau, A.M.; Hambardzumyan, D.; Ozawa, T.; Fomchenko, E.I.; Huse, J.T.; Brennan, C.W. & Holland, E.C. (2009). PTEN/PI3K/Akt pathway regulates the side population phenotype and ABCG2 activity in glioma tumor stem-like cells. *Cell Stem Cell*, Vol.4, No.3, pp.226-235.

Blum, B. & Benvenisty, N. (2008). The tumorigenicity of human embryonic stem cells. *Adv Cancer Res*, Vol.100 133-158.

Bouhon, I.A.; Kato, H.; Chandran, S. & Allen, N.D. (2005). Neural differentiation of mouse embryonic stem cells in chemically defined medium. *Brain Res Bull*, Vol.68, No.1-2, pp.62-75.

Bryant, M.R.; Marta, C.B.; Kim, F.S. & Bansal, R. (2009). Phosphorylation and lipid raft association of fibroblast growth factor receptor-2 in oligodendrocytes. *Glia*, Vol.57, No.9, pp.935-946.

Buehr, M. & Smith, A. (2003). Genesis of embryonic stem cells. *Philos Trans R Soc Lond B Biol Sci*, Vol.358, No.1436, pp.1397-1402; discussion 1402.

Callihan, P.; Mumaw, J.; Machacek, D.W.; Stice, S.L. & Hooks, S.B. (2011). Regulation of stem cell pluripotency and differentiation by G protein coupled receptors. *Pharmacol Ther*, Vol.129, No.3, pp.290-306.

Cartwright, P.; McLean, C.; Sheppard, A.; Rivett, D.; Jones, K. & Dalton, S. (2005). LIF/STAT3 controls ES cell self-renewal and pluripotency by a Myc-dependent mechanism. *Development*, Vol.132, No.5, pp.885-896.

Chalfant, C.E. & Spiegel, S. (2005). Sphingosine 1-phosphate and ceramide 1-phosphate: expanding roles in cell signaling. *J Cell Sci*, Vol.118, No.Pt 20, pp.4605-4612.

Chen, S.; Do, J.T.; Zhang, Q.; Yao, S.; Yan, F.; Peters, E.C.; Scholer, H.R.; Schultz, P.G. & Ding, S. (2006). Self-renewal of embryonic stem cells by a small molecule. *Proc Natl Acad Sci U S A*, Vol.103, No.46, pp.17266-17271.

Chen, Y.; Li, X.; Eswarakumar, V.P.; Seger, R. & Lonai, P. (2000). Fibroblast growth factor (FGF) signaling through PI 3-kinase and Akt/PKB is required for embryoid body differentiation. *Oncogene*, Vol.19, No.33, pp.3750-3756.

Chen, Y.; Liu, Y.; Sullards, M.C. & Merrill, A.H., Jr. (2010). An introduction to sphingolipid metabolism and analysis by new technologies. *Neuromolecular Med*, Vol.12, No.4, pp.306-319.

Chillar, A.; So, S.P.; Ruan, C.H.; Shelat, H.; Geng, Y.J. & Ruan, K.H. (2010). A profile of NSAID-targeted arachidonic acid metabolisms in human embryonic stem cells (hESCs): Implication of the negative effects of NSAIDs on heart tissue regeneration. *Int J Cardiol*.

Coelho, R.P.; Payne, S.G.; Bittman, R.; Spiegel, S. & Sato-Bigbee, C. (2007). The immunomodulator FTY720 has a direct cytoprotective effect in oligodendrocyte progenitors. *J Pharmacol Exp Ther*, Vol.323, No.2, pp.626-635.

Coelho, R.P.; Saini, H.S. & Sato-Bigbee, C. (2010). Sphingosine-1-phosphate and oligodendrocytes: from cell development to the treatment of multiple sclerosis. *Prostaglandins Other Lipid Mediat*, Vol.91, No.3-4, pp.139-144.

Cutler, R.G.; Haughey, N.J.; Tammara, A.; McArthur, J.C.; Nath, A.; Reid, R.; Vargas, D.L.; Pardo, C.A. & Mattson, M.P. (2004). Dysregulation of sphingolipid and sterol metabolism by ApoE4 in HIV dementia. *Neurology*, Vol.63, No.4, pp.626-630.

De Vito, W.J.; Xhaja, K. & Stone, S. (2000). Prenatal alcohol exposure increases TNFalpha-induced cytotoxicity in primary astrocytes. *Alcohol*, Vol.21, No.1, pp.63-71.

Ding, S. & Schultz, P.G. (2004). A role for chemistry in stem cell biology. *Nat Biotechnol*, Vol.22, No.7, pp.833-840.

Ding, S.; Wu, T.Y.; Brinker, A.; Peters, E.C.; Hur, W.; Gray, N.S. & Schultz, P.G. (2003). Synthetic small molecules that control stem cell fate. *Proc Natl Acad Sci U S A*, Vol.100, No.13, pp.7632-7637.

Ding, V.M.; Ling, L.; Natarajan, S.; Yap, M.G.; Cool, S.M. & Choo, A.B. (2010). FGF-2 modulates Wnt signaling in undifferentiated hESC and iPS cells through activated PI3-K/GSK3beta signaling. *J Cell Physiol*, Vol.225, No.2, pp.417-428.

Dinsmore, J.; Ratliff, J.; Deacon, T.; Pakzaban, P.; Jacoby, D.; Galpern, W. & Isacson, O. (1996). Embryonic stem cells differentiated in vitro as a novel source of cells for transplantation. *Cell Transplant*, Vol.5, No.2, pp.131-143.

Doble, B.W. & Woodgett, J.R. (2003). GSK-3: tricks of the trade for a multi-tasking kinase. *J Cell Sci*, Vol.116, No.Pt 7, pp.1175-1186.

Finkensieper, A.; Kieser, S.; Bekhite, M.M.; Richter, M.; Mueller, J.P.; Graebner, R.; Figulla, H.R.; Sauer, H. & Wartenberg, M. (2010). The 5-lipoxygenase pathway regulates vasculogenesis in differentiating mouse embryonic stem cells. *Cardiovasc Res*, Vol.86, No.1, pp.37-44.

Fong, C.Y.; Gauthaman, K. & Bongso, A. (2010). Teratomas from pluripotent stem cells: A clinical hurdle. *J Cell Biochem*.

Frebel, K. & Wiese, S. (2006). Signalling molecules essential for neuronal survival and differentiation. *Biochem Soc Trans*, Vol.34, No.Pt 6, pp.1287-1290.

Fujikawa, T.; Oh, S.H.; Pi, L.; Hatch, H.M.; Shupe, T. & Petersen, B.E. (2005). Teratoma formation leads to failure of treatment for type I diabetes using embryonic stem cell-derived insulin-producing cells. *Am J Pathol*, Vol.166, No.6, pp.1781-1791.

Funk, C.D. (2001). Prostaglandins and leukotrienes: advances in eicosanoid biology. *Science*, Vol.294, No.5548, pp.1871-1875.

Futerman, A.H. & Hannun, Y.A. (2004). The complex life of simple sphingolipids. *EMBO Rep*, Vol.5, No.8, pp.777-782.

Futerman, A.H. & Riezman, H. (2005). The ins and outs of sphingolipid synthesis. *Trends Cell Biol*, Vol.15, No.6, pp.312-318.

Gardell, S.E.; Dubin, A.E. & Chun, J. (2006). Emerging medicinal roles for lysophospholipid signaling. *Trends Mol Med*, Vol.12, No.2, pp.65-75.

Gault, C.R.; Obeid, L.M. & Hannun, Y.A. (2010). An overview of sphingolipid metabolism: from synthesis to breakdown. *Adv Exp Med Biol*, Vol.6881-23.

Gelineau-van Waes, J.; Starr, L.; Maddox, J.; Aleman, F.; Voss, K.A.; Wilberding, J. & Riley, R.T. (2005). Maternal fumonisin exposure and risk for neural tube defects: mechanisms in an in vivo mouse model. *Birth Defects Res A Clin Mol Teratol*, Vol.73, No.7, pp.487-497.

Glaser, T.; Pollard, S.M.; Smith, A. & Brustle, O. (2007). Tripotential differentiation of adherently expandable neural stem (NS) cells. *PLoS One*, Vol.2, No.3, pp.e298.

Goessling, W.; North, T.E.; Loewer, S.; Lord, A.M.; Lee, S.; Stoick-Cooper, C.L.; Weidinger, G.; Puder, M.; Daley, G.Q.; Moon, R.T. & Zon, L.I. (2009). Genetic interaction of PGE2 and Wnt signaling regulates developmental specification of stem cells and regeneration. *Cell*, Vol.136, No.6, pp.1136-1147.

Gofflot, F.; Hars, C.; Illien, F.; Chevy, F.; Wolf, C.; Picard, J.J. & Roux, C. (2003). Molecular mechanisms underlying limb anomalies associated with cholesterol deficiency during gestation: implications of Hedgehog signaling. *Hum Mol Genet*, Vol.12, No.10, pp.1187-1198.

Goldman, J.E.; Hirano, M.; Yu, R.K. & Seyfried, T.N. (1984). GD3 ganglioside is a glycolipid characteristic of immature neuroectodermal cells. *J Neuroimmunol*, Vol.7, No.2-3, pp.179-192.

Groszer, M.; Erickson, R.; Scripture-Adams, D.D.; Lesche, R.; Trumpp, A.; Zack, J.A.; Kornblum, H.I.; Liu, X. & Wu, H. (2001). Negative regulation of neural stem/progenitor cell proliferation by the Pten tumor suppressor gene in vivo. *Science*, Vol.294, No.5549, pp.2186-2189.

Guan, K.; Chang, H.; Rolletschek, A. & Wobus, A.M. (2001). Embryonic stem cell-derived neurogenesis. Retinoic acid induction and lineage selection of neuronal cells. *Cell Tissue Res*, Vol.305, No.2, pp.171-176.

Gulbins, E. & Kolesnick, R. (2003). Raft ceramide in molecular medicine. *Oncogene*, Vol.22, No.45, pp.7070-7077.

Gutierrez, J. & Brandan, E. (2010). A novel mechanism of sequestering fibroblast growth factor 2 by glypican in lipid rafts, allowing skeletal muscle differentiation. *Mol Cell Biol*, Vol.30, No.7, pp.1634-1649.

Guy, R.K. (2000). Inhibition of sonic hedgehog autoprocessing in cultured mammalian cells by sterol deprivation. *Proc Natl Acad Sci U S A*, Vol.97, No.13, pp.7307-7312.

Haegel, H.; Larue, L.; Ohsugi, M.; Fedorov, L.; Herrenknecht, K. & Kemler, R. (1995). Lack of beta-catenin affects mouse development at gastrulation. *Development*, Vol.121, No.11, pp.3529-3537.

Haimovitz-Friedman, A.; Kolesnick, R.N. & Fuks, Z. (1997). Ceramide signaling in apoptosis. *Br Med Bull*, Vol.53, No.3, pp.539-553.

Hait, N.C.; Allegood, J.; Maceyka, M.; Strub, G.M.; Harikumar, K.B.; Singh, S.K.; Luo, C.; Marmorstein, R.; Kordula, T.; Milstien, S. & Spiegel, S. (2009). Regulation of histone acetylation in the nucleus by sphingosine-1-phosphate. *Science*, Vol.325, No.5945, pp.1254-1257.

Hait, N.C.; Oskeritzian, C.A.; Paugh, S.W.; Milstien, S. & Spiegel, S. (2006). Sphingosine kinases, sphingosine 1-phosphate, apoptosis and diseases. *Biochim Biophys Acta*, Vol.1758, No.12, pp.2016-2026.

Hannun, Y.A.; Luberto, C. & Argraves, K.M. (2001). Enzymes of sphingolipid metabolism: from modular to integrative signaling. *Biochemistry*, Vol.40, No.16, pp.4893-4903.

Hannun, Y.A. & Obeid, L.M. (2002). The Ceramide-centric universe of lipid-mediated cell regulation: stress encounters of the lipid kind. *J Biol Chem*, Vol.277, No.29, pp.25847-25850.

Hannun, Y.A. & Obeid, L.M. (2008). Principles of bioactive lipid signalling: lessons from sphingolipids. *Nat Rev Mol Cell Biol*, Vol.9, No.2, pp.139-150.

Harada, J.; Foley, M.; Moskowitz, M.A. & Waeber, C. (2004). Sphingosine-1-phosphate induces proliferation and morphological changes of neural progenitor cells. *J Neurochem*, Vol.88, No.4, pp.1026-1039.

Hirabayashi, Y. & Furuya, S. (2008). Roles of l-serine and sphingolipid synthesis in brain development and neuronal survival. *Prog Lipid Res*, Vol.47, No.3, pp.188-203.

Hla, T.; Lee, M.J.; Ancellin, N.; Paik, J.H. & Kluk, M.J. (2001). Lysophospholipids--receptor revelations. *Science*, Vol.294, No.5548, pp.1875-1878.

Hla, T.; Lee, M.J.; Ancellin, N.; Thangada, S.; Liu, C.H.; Kluk, M.; Chae, S.S. & Wu, M.T. (2000). Sphingosine-1-phosphate signaling via the EDG-1 family of G-protein-coupled receptors. *Ann N Y Acad Sci*, Vol.90516-24.

Hu, B.Y.; Du, Z.W. & Zhang, S.C. (2009). Differentiation of human oligodendrocytes from pluripotent stem cells. *Nat Protoc*, Vol.4, No.11, pp.1614-1622.

Hurst, J.H.; Mumaw, J.; Machacek, D.W.; Sturkie, C.; Callihan, P.; Stice, S.L. & Hooks, S.B. (2008). Human neural progenitors express functional lysophospholipid receptors that regulate cell growth and morphology. *BMC Neurosci*, Vol.9118.

Ikeda, S.; Kishida, M.; Matsuura, Y.; Usui, H. & Kikuchi, A. (2000). GSK-3beta-dependent phosphorylation of adenomatous polyposis coli gene product can be modulated by beta-catenin and protein phosphatase 2A complexed with Axin. *Oncogene*, Vol.19, No.4, pp.537-545.

Incardona, J.P. & Roelink, H. (2000). The role of cholesterol in Shh signaling and teratogen-induced holoprosencephaly. *Cell Mol Life Sci*, Vol.57, No.12, pp.1709-1719.

Jana, A.; Hogan, E.L. & Pahan, K. (2009). Ceramide and neurodegeneration: susceptibility of neurons and oligodendrocytes to cell damage and death. *J Neurol Sci*, Vol.278, No.1-2, pp.5-15.

Jana, A. & Pahan, K. (2010). Fibrillar amyloid-beta-activated human astroglia kill primary human neurons via neutral sphingomyelinase: implications for Alzheimer's disease. *J Neurosci*, Vol.30, No.38, pp.12676-12689.

Jenkins, C.M.; Cedars, A. & Gross, R.W. (2009). Eicosanoid signalling pathways in the heart. *Cardiovasc Res*, Vol.82, No.2, pp.240-249.

Jiang, P.; Selvaraj, V. & Deng, W. (2010). Differentiation of embryonic stem cells into oligodendrocyte precursors. *J Vis Exp*, No.39, pp.

Jung, C.G.; Kim, H.J.; Miron, V.E.; Cook, S.; Kennedy, T.E.; Foster, C.A.; Antel, J.P. & Soliven, B. (2007). Functional consequences of S1P receptor modulation in rat oligodendroglial lineage cells. *Glia*, Vol.55, No.16, pp.1656-1667.

Jung, J.U.; Ko, K.; Lee, D.H.; Chang, K.T. & Choo, Y.K. (2009). The roles of glycosphingolipids in the proliferation and neural differentiation of mouse embryonic stem cells. *Exp Mol Med*, Vol.41, No.12, pp.935-945.

Kang, S.M.; Cho, M.S.; Seo, H.; Yoon, C.J.; Oh, S.K.; Choi, Y.M. & Kim, D.W. (2007). Efficient induction of oligodendrocytes from human embryonic stem cells. *Stem Cells*, Vol.25, No.2, pp.419-424.

Karpen, H.E.; Bukowski, J.T.; Hughes, T.; Gratton, J.P.; Sessa, W.C. & Gailani, M.R. (2001). The sonic hedgehog receptor patched associates with caveolin-1 in cholesterol-rich microdomains of the plasma membrane. *J Biol Chem*, Vol.276, No.22, pp.19503-19511.

Kelley, R.L.; Roessler, E.; Hennekam, R.C.; Feldman, G.L.; Kosaki, K.; Jones, M.C.; Palumbos, J.C. & Muenke, M. (1996). Holoprosencephaly in RSH/Smith-Lemli-Opitz syndrome: does abnormal cholesterol metabolism affect the function of Sonic Hedgehog? *Am J Med Genet*, Vol.66, No.4, pp.478-484.

Kelly, K.F.; Ng, D.Y.; Jayakumaran, G.; Wood, G.A.; Koide, H. & Doble, B.W. (2011). beta-catenin enhances Oct-4 activity and reinforces pluripotency through a TCF-independent mechanism. *Cell Stem Cell*, Vol.8, No.2, pp.214-227.

Khanapure, S.P.; Garvey, D.S.; Janero, D.R. & Letts, L.G. (2007). Eicosanoids in inflammation: biosynthesis, pharmacology, and therapeutic frontiers. *Curr Top Med Chem*, Vol.7, No.3, pp.311-340.

Kilkenny, D.M.; Rocheleau, J.V.; Price, J.; Reich, M.B. & Miller, G.G. (2003). c-Src regulation of fibroblast growth factor-induced proliferation in murine embryonic fibroblasts. *J Biol Chem*, Vol.278, No.19, pp.17448-17454.

Kim, M.H.; Lee, Y.J.; Kim, M.O.; Kim, J.S. & Han, H.J. (2010). Effect of leukotriene D4 on mouse embryonic stem cell migration and proliferation: involvement of PI3K/Akt as well as GSK-3beta/beta-catenin signaling pathways. *J Cell Biochem*, Vol.111, No.3, pp.686-698.

Korkaya, H.; Paulson, A.; Charafe-Jauffret, E.; Ginestier, C.; Brown, M.; Dutcher, J.; Clouthier, S.G. & Wicha, M.S. (2009). Regulation of mammary stem/progenitor cells by PTEN/Akt/beta-catenin signaling. *PLoS Biol*, Vol.7, No.6, pp.e1000121.

Kostenis, E. (2004). A glance at G-protein-coupled receptors for lipid mediators: a growing receptor family with remarkably diverse ligands. *Pharmacol Ther*, Vol.102, No.3, pp.243-257.

Krishnamurthy, K.; Wang, G.; Silva, J.; Condie, B.G. & Bieberich, E. (2007). Ceramide Regulates Atypical PKC{zeta}/{lambda}-mediated Cell Polarity in Primitive Ectoderm Cells: A NOVEL FUNCTION OF SPHINGOLIPIDS IN MORPHOGENESIS. *J Biol Chem*, Vol.282, No.5, pp.3379-3390.

Lambeau, G. & Gelb, M.H. (2008). Biochemistry and physiology of mammalian secreted phospholipases A2. *Annu Rev Biochem*, Vol.77495-520.

Lanner, F. & Rossant, J. (2010). The role of FGF/Erk signaling in pluripotent cells. *Development*, Vol.137, No.20, pp.3351-3360.

Layden, B.T.; Newman, M.; Chen, F.; Fisher, A. & Lowe, W.L., Jr. (2010). G protein coupled receptors in embryonic stem cells: a role for Gs-alpha signaling. *PLoS One*, Vol.5, No.2, pp.e9105.

Lebman, D.A. & Spiegel, S. (2008). Cross-talk at the crossroads of sphingosine-1-phosphate, growth factors, and cytokine signaling. *J Lipid Res*, Vol.49, No.7, pp.1388-1394.

Lee, A.S.; Tang, C.; Cao, F.; Xie, X.; van der Bogt, K.; Hwang, A.; Connolly, A.J.; Robbins, R.C. & Wu, J.C. (2009). Effects of cell number on teratoma formation by human embryonic stem cells. *Cell Cycle*, Vol.8, No.16, pp.2608-2612.

Lee, C.W.; Choi, J.W. & Chun, J. (2010a). Neurological S1P signaling as an emerging mechanism of action of oral FTY720 (Fingolimod) in multiple sclerosis. *Arch Pharm Res*, Vol.33, No.10, pp.1567-1574.

Lee, M.Y.; Ryu, J.M.; Lee, S.H.; Park, J.H. & Han, H.J. (2010b). Lipid rafts play an important role for maintenance of embryonic stem cell self-renewal. *J Lipid Res*, Vol.51, No.8, pp.2082-2089.

Levental, I.; Grzybek, M. & Simons, K. (2010). Greasing their way: lipid modifications determine protein association with membrane rafts. *Biochemistry*, Vol.49, No.30, pp.6305-6316.

Lewis, P.M.; Dunn, M.P.; McMahon, J.A.; Logan, M.; Martin, J.F.; St-Jacques, B. & McMahon, A.P. (2001). Cholesterol modification of sonic hedgehog is required for long-range signaling activity and effective modulation of signaling by Ptc1. *Cell*, Vol.105, No.5, pp.599-612.

Li, J.; Wang, G.; Wang, C.; Zhao, Y.; Zhang, H.; Tan, Z.; Song, Z.; Ding, M. & Deng, H. (2007). MEK/ERK signaling contributes to the maintenance of human embryonic stem cell self-renewal. *Differentiation*, Vol.75, No.4, pp.299-307.

Li, Y.; Zhang, H.; Litingtung, Y. & Chiang, C. (2006). Cholesterol modification restricts the spread of Shh gradient in the limb bud. *Proc Natl Acad Sci U S A*, Vol.103, No.17, pp.6548-6553.

Lin, M.E.; Herr, D.R. & Chun, J. (2010). Lysophosphatidic acid (LPA) receptors: signaling properties and disease relevance. *Prostaglandins Other Lipid Mediat*, Vol.91, No.3-4, pp.130-138.

Lingwood, D. & Simons, K. (2010). Lipid rafts as a membrane-organizing principle. *Science*, Vol.327, No.5961, pp.46-50.

Liour, S.S.; Kraemer, S.A.; Dinkins, M.B.; Su, C.Y.; Yanagisawa, M. & Yu, R.K. (2006). Further characterization of embryonic stem cell-derived radial glial cells. *Glia*, Vol.53, No.1, pp.43-56.

Logan, C.M.; Giordano, A.; Puca, A. & Cassone, M. (2007). Prostaglandin E2: at the crossroads between stem cell development, inflammation and cancer. *Cancer Biol Ther*, Vol.6, No.10, pp.1517-1520.

Luberto, C. & Hannun, Y.A. (1999). Sphingolipid metabolism in the regulation of bioactive molecules. *Lipids*, Vol.34 SupplS5-11.

Lyssiotis, C.A.; Lairson, L.L.; Boitano, A.E.; Wurdak, H.; Zhu, S. & Schultz, P.G. (2011). Chemical control of stem cell fate and developmental potential. *Angew Chem Int Ed Engl*, Vol.50, No.1, pp.200-242.

Marasas, W.F.; Riley, R.T.; Hendricks, K.A.; Stevens, V.L.; Sadler, T.W.; Gelineau-van Waes, J.; Missmer, S.A.; Cabrera, J.; Torres, O.; Gelderblom, W.C.; Allegood, J.; Martinez, C.; Maddox, J.; Miller, J.D.; Starr, L.; Sullards, M.C.; Roman, A.V.; Voss, K.A.; Wang, E. & Merrill, A.H., Jr. (2004). Fumonisins disrupt sphingolipid metabolism, folate transport, and neural tube development in embryo culture and in vivo: a potential risk factor for human neural tube defects among populations consuming fumonisin-contaminated maize. *J Nutr*, Vol.134, No.4, pp.711-716.

Mayer-Proschel, M.; Kalyani, A.J.; Mujtaba, T. & Rao, M.S. (1997). Isolation of lineage-restricted neuronal precursors from multipotent neuroepithelial stem cells. *Neuron*, Vol.19, No.4, pp.773-785.

Merrill, A.H., Jr.; Schmelz, E.M.; Dillehay, D.L.; Spiegel, S.; Shayman, J.A.; Schroeder, J.J.; Riley, R.T.; Voss, K.A. & Wang, E. (1997). Sphingolipids--the enigmatic lipid class: biochemistry, physiology, and pathophysiology. *Toxicol Appl Pharmacol*, Vol.142, No.1, pp.208-225.

Meyer zu Heringdorf, D. & Jakobs, K.H. (2007). Lysophospholipid receptors: signalling, pharmacology and regulation by lysophospholipid metabolism. *Biochim Biophys Acta*, Vol.1768, No.4, pp.923-940.

Miljan, E.A. & Bremer, E.G. (2002). Regulation of growth factor receptors by gangliosides. *Sci STKE*, Vol.2002, No.160, pp.RE15.

Miron, V.E.; Jung, C.G.; Kim, H.J.; Kennedy, T.E.; Soliven, B. & Antel, J.P. (2008a). FTY720 modulates human oligodendrocyte progenitor process extension and survival. *Ann Neurol*, Vol.63, No.1, pp.61-71.

Miron, V.E.; Schubart, A. & Antel, J.P. (2008b). Central nervous system-directed effects of FTY720 (fingolimod). *J Neurol Sci*, Vol.274, No.1-2, pp.13-17.

Morales, A.; Lee, H.; Goni, F.M.; Kolesnick, R. & Fernandez-Checa, J.C. (2007). Sphingolipids and cell death. *Apoptosis*, Vol.12, No.5, pp.923-939.

Mummery, C.L.; Feyen, A.; Freund, E. & Shen, S. (1990). Characteristics of embryonic stem cell differentiation: a comparison with two embryonal carcinoma cell lines. *Cell Differ Dev*, Vol.30, No.3, pp.195-206.

Murashov, A.K.; Pak, E.S.; Hendricks, W.A.; Owensby, J.P.; Sierpinski, P.L.; Tatko, L.M. & Fletcher, P.L. (2005). Directed differentiation of embryonic stem cells into dorsal interneurons. *Faseb J*, Vol.19, No.2, pp.252-254.

Muscoli, C.; Doyle, T.; Dagostino, C.; Bryant, L.; Chen, Z.; Watkins, L.R.; Ryerse, J.; Bieberich, E.; Neumman, W. & Salvemini, D. (2010). Counter-regulation of opioid analgesia by glial-derived bioactive sphingolipids. *J Neurosci*, Vol.30, No.46, pp.15400-15408.

Nakanaga, K.; Hama, K. & Aoki, J. (2010). Autotaxin--an LPA producing enzyme with diverse functions. *J Biochem*, Vol.148, No.1, pp.13-24.

Napoli, K.L. (2000). The FTY720 story. *Ther Drug Monit*, Vol.22, No.1, pp.47-51.

Niwa, H.; Burdon, T.; Chambers, I. & Smith, A. (1998). Self-renewal of pluripotent embryonic stem cells is mediated via activation of STAT3. *Genes Dev*, Vol.12, No.13, pp.2048-2060.

North, T.E.; Goessling, W.; Walkley, C.R.; Lengerke, C.; Kopani, K.R.; Lord, A.M.; Weber, G.J.; Bowman, T.V.; Jang, I.H.; Grosser, T.; Fitzgerald, G.A.; Daley, G.Q.; Orkin, S.H. & Zon, L.I. (2007). Prostaglandin E2 regulates vertebrate haematopoietic stem cell homeostasis. *Nature*, Vol.447, No.7147, pp.1007-1011.

Ohanian, J. & Ohanian, V. (2001). Sphingolipids in mammalian cell signalling. *Cell Mol Life Sci*, Vol.58, No.14, pp.2053-2068.

Okita, K. & Yamanaka, S. (2006). Intracellular signaling pathways regulating pluripotency of embryonic stem cells. *Curr Stem Cell Res Ther*, Vol.1, No.1, pp.103-111.

Okudaira, S.; Yukiura, H. & Aoki, J. (2010). Biological roles of lysophosphatidic acid signaling through its production by autotaxin. *Biochimie*, Vol.92, No.6, pp.698-706.

Osakada, F. & Takahashi, M. (2011). Neural Induction and Patterning in Mammalian Pluripotent Stem Cells. *CNS Neurol Disord Drug Targets*.

Otaegi, G.; Yusta-Boyo, M.J.; Vergano-Vera, E.; Mendez-Gomez, H.R.; Carrera, A.C.; Abad, J.L.; Gonzalez, M.; de la Rosa, E.J.; Vicario-Abejon, C. & de Pablo, F. (2006). Modulation of the PI 3-kinase-Akt signalling pathway by IGF-I and PTEN regulates the differentiation of neural stem/precursor cells. *J Cell Sci*, Vol.119, No.Pt 13, pp.2739-2748.

Paling, N.R.; Wheadon, H.; Bone, H.K. & Welham, M.J. (2004). Regulation of embryonic stem cell self-renewal by phosphoinositide 3-kinase-dependent signaling. *J Biol Chem*, Vol.279, No.46, pp.48063-48070.

Pebay, A.; Bonder, C.S. & Pitson, S.M. (2007). Stem cell regulation by lysophospholipids. *Prostaglandins Other Lipid Mediat*, Vol.84, No.3-4, pp.83-97.

Pebay, A.; Wong, R.C.; Pitson, S.M.; Wolvetang, E.J.; Peh, G.S.; Filipczyk, A.; Koh, K.L.; Tellis, I.; Nguyen, L.T. & Pera, M.F. (2005). Essential roles of sphingosine-1-phosphate and platelet-derived growth factor in the maintenance of human embryonic stem cells. *Stem Cells*, Vol.23, No.10, pp.1541-1548.

Pitson, S.M. & Pebay, A. (2009). Regulation of stem cell pluripotency and neural differentiation by lysophospholipids. *Neurosignals*, Vol.17, No.4, pp.242-254.

Plachta, N.; Bibel, M.; Tucker, K.L. & Barde, Y.A. (2004). Developmental potential of defined neural progenitors derived from mouse embryonic stem cells. *Development*, Vol.131, No.21, pp.5449-5456.

Plo, I.; Bettaieb, A.; Payrastre, B.; Mansat-De Mas, V.; Bordier, C.; Rousse, A.; Kowalski-Chauvel, A.; Laurent, G. & Lautier, D. (1999). The phosphoinositide 3-kinase/Akt pathway is activated by daunorubicin in human acute myeloid leukemia cell lines. *FEBS Lett*, Vol.452, No.3, pp.150-154.

Radeff-Huang, J.; Seasholtz, T.M.; Matteo, R.G. & Brown, J.H. (2004). G protein mediated signaling pathways in lysophospholipid induced cell proliferation and survival. *J Cell Biochem*, Vol.92, No.5, pp.949-966.

Resh, M.D. (2004). Membrane targeting of lipid modified signal transduction proteins. *Subcell Biochem*, Vol.37217-232.

Riboni, L.; Tettamanti, G. & Viani, P. (2002). Ceramide in primary astrocytes from cerebellum: metabolism and role in cell proliferation. *Cerebellum*, Vol.1, No.2, pp.129-135.

Roy, S.; Plowman, S.; Rotblat, B.; Prior, I.A.; Muncke, C.; Grainger, S.; Parton, R.G.; Henis, Y.I.; Kloog, Y. & Hancock, J.F. (2005). Individual palmitoyl residues serve distinct roles in H-ras trafficking, microlocalization, and signaling. *Mol Cell Biol*, Vol.25, No.15, pp.6722-6733.

Saini, H.S.; Coelho, R.P.; Goparaju, S.K.; Jolly, P.S.; Maceyka, M.; Spiegel, S. & Sato-Bigbee, C. (2005). Novel role of sphingosine kinase 1 as a mediator of neurotrophin-3 action in oligodendrocyte progenitors. *J Neurochem*, Vol.95, No.5, pp.1298-1310.

Salli, U.; Fox, T.E.; Carkaci-Salli, N.; Sharma, A.; Robertson, G.P.; Kester, M. & Vrana, K.E. (2009). Propagation of undifferentiated human embryonic stem cells with nano-liposomal ceramide. *Stem Cells Dev*, Vol.18, No.1, pp.55-65.

Samadi, N.; Bekele, R.; Capatos, D.; Venkatraman, G.; Sariahmetoglu, M. & Brindley, D.N. (2011). Regulation of lysophosphatidate signaling by autotaxin and lipid phosphate phosphatases with respect to tumor progression, angiogenesis, metastasis and chemo-resistance. *Biochimie*, Vol.93, No.1, pp.61-70.

Sanchez, T. & Hla, T. (2004). Structural and functional characteristics of S1P receptors. *J Cell Biochem*, Vol.92, No.5, pp.913-922.

Sato, N.; Meijer, L.; Skaltsounis, L.; Greengard, P. & Brivanlou, A.H. (2004). Maintenance of pluripotency in human and mouse embryonic stem cells through activation of Wnt signaling by a pharmacological GSK-3-specific inhibitor. *Nat Med*, Vol.10, No.1, pp.55-63.

Satoi, H.; Tomimoto, H.; Ohtani, R.; Kitano, T.; Kondo, T.; Watanabe, M.; Oka, N.; Akiguchi, I.; Furuya, S.; Hirabayashi, Y. & Okazaki, T. (2005). Astroglial expression of ceramide in Alzheimer's disease brains: a role during neuronal apoptosis. *Neuroscience*, Vol.130, No.3, pp.657-666.

Schuringa, J.J.; van der Schaaf, S.; Vellenga, E.; Eggen, B.J. & Kruijer, W. (2002). LIF-induced STAT3 signaling in murine versus human embryonal carcinoma (EC) cells. *Exp Cell Res*, Vol.274, No.1, pp.119-129.

Spiegel, S. & Kolesnick, R. (2002). Sphingosine 1-phosphate as a therapeutic agent. *Leukemia*, Vol.16, No.9, pp.1596-1602.

Spiegel, S. & Milstien, S. (2003). Sphingosine-1-phosphate: an enigmatic signalling lipid. *Nat Rev Mol Cell Biol*, Vol.4, No.5, pp.397-407.

Storm, M.P.; Bone, H.K.; Beck, C.G.; Bourillot, P.Y.; Schreiber, V.; Damiano, T.; Nelson, A.; Savatier, P. & Welham, M.J. (2007). Regulation of Nanog expression by phosphoinositide 3-kinase-dependent signaling in murine embryonic stem cells. *J Biol Chem*, Vol.282, No.9, pp.6265-6273.

Strub, G.M.; Maceyka, M.; Hait, N.C.; Milstien, S. & Spiegel, S. (2010). Extracellular and intracellular actions of sphingosine-1-phosphate. *Adv Exp Med Biol*, Vol.688141-155.

Strub, G.M.; Paillard, M.; Liang, J.; Gomez, L.; Allegood, J.C.; Hait, N.C.; Maceyka, M.; Price, M.M.; Chen, Q.; Simpson, D.C.; Kordula, T.; Milstien, S.; Lesnefsky, E.J. & Spiegel, S. (2011). Sphingosine-1-phosphate produced by sphingosine kinase 2 in mitochondria interacts with prohibitin 2 to regulate complex IV assembly and respiration. *FASEB J*, Vol.25, No.2, pp.600-612.

Szefel, J.; Piotrowska, M.; Kruszewski, W.J.; Jankun, J.; Lysiak-Szydlowska, W. & Skrzypczak-Jankun, E. (2011). Eicosanoids in prevention and management of diseases. *Curr Mol Med*, Vol.11, No.1, pp.13-25.

Takabe, K.; Paugh, S.W.; Milstien, S. & Spiegel, S. (2008). "Inside-out" signaling of sphingosine-1-phosphate: therapeutic targets. *Pharmacol Rev*, Vol.60, No.2, pp.181-195.

Takao, Y.; Yokota, T. & Koide, H. (2007). Beta-catenin up-regulates Nanog expression through interaction with Oct-3/4 in embryonic stem cells. *Biochem Biophys Res Commun*, Vol.353, No.3, pp.699-705.

Tigyi, G. & Parrill, A.L. (2003). Molecular mechanisms of lysophosphatidic acid action. *Prog Lipid Res*, Vol.42, No.6, pp.498-526.

Umehara, H.; Kimura, T.; Ohtsuka, S.; Nakamura, T.; Kitajima, K.; Ikawa, M.; Okabe, M.; Niwa, H. & Nakano, T. (2007). Efficient derivation of embryonic stem cells by inhibition of glycogen synthase kinase-3. *Stem Cells*, Vol.25, No.11, pp.2705-2711.

van Noort, M.; Meeldijk, J.; van der Zee, R.; Destree, O. & Clevers, H. (2002). Wnt signaling controls the phosphorylation status of beta-catenin. *J Biol Chem*, Vol.277, No.20, pp.17901-17905.

Vogel, G. (2005). Cell biology. Ready or not? Human ES cells head toward the clinic. *Science*, Vol.308, No.5728, pp.1534-1538.

Walter, D.H.; Rochwalsky, U.; Reinhold, J.; Seeger, F.; Aicher, A.; Urbich, C.; Spyridopoulos, I.; Chun, J.; Brinkmann, V.; Keul, P.; Levkau, B.; Zeiher, A.M.; Dimmeler, S. & Haendeler, J. (2007). Sphingosine-1-phosphate stimulates the functional capacity of progenitor cells by activation of the CXCR4-dependent signaling pathway via the S1P3 receptor. *Arterioscler Thromb Vasc Biol*, Vol.27, No.2, pp.275-282.

Wang, G. & Bieberich, E. (2010). Prenatal alcohol exposure triggers ceramide-induced apoptosis in neural crest-derived tissues concurrent with defective cranial development. *Cell Death Dis*, Vol.1, No.5, pp.e46.

Wang, G.; Krishnamurthy, K.; Chiang, Y.W.; Dasgupta, S. & Bieberich, E. (2008a). Regulation of neural progenitor cell motility by ceramide and potential implications for mouse brain development. *J Neurochem*, Vol.106, No.2, pp.718-733.

Wang, G.; Krishnamurthy, K.; Umapathy, N.S.; Verin, A.D. & Bieberich, E. (2009). The carboxyl-terminal domain of atypical protein kinase Czeta binds to ceramide and regulates junction formation in epithelial cells. *J Biol Chem*, Vol.284, No.21, pp.14469-14475.

Wang, G.; Silva, J.; Dasgupta, S. & Bieberich, E. (2008b). Long-chain ceramide is elevated in presenilin 1 (PS1M146V) mouse brain and induces apoptosis in PS1 astrocytes. *Glia*, Vol.56, No.4, pp.449-456.

Wang, G.; Silva, J.; Krishnamurthy, K.; Tran, E.; Condie, B.G. & Bieberich, E. (2005). Direct binding to ceramide activates protein kinase Czeta before the formation of a pro-apoptotic complex with PAR-4 in differentiating stem cells. *J Biol Chem*, Vol.280, No.28, pp.26415-26424.

Wang, N.K.; Tosi, J.; Kasanuki, J.M.; Chou, C.L.; Kong, J.; Parmalee, N.; Wert, K.J.; Allikmets, R.; Lai, C.C.; Chien, C.L.; Nagasaki, T.; Lin, C.S. & Tsang, S.H. (2010). Transplantation of reprogrammed embryonic stem cells improves visual function in a mouse model for retinitis pigmentosa. *Transplantation*, Vol.89, No.8, pp.911-919.

Wong, R.C.; Tellis, I.; Jamshidi, P.; Pera, M. & Pebay, A. (2007). Anti-apoptotic effect of sphingosine-1-phosphate and platelet-derived growth factor in human embryonic stem cells. *Stem Cells Dev*, Vol.16, No.6, pp.989-1001.

Wymann, M.P. & Schneiter, R. (2008). Lipid signalling in disease. *Nat Rev Mol Cell Biol*, Vol.9, No.2, pp.162-176.

Xu, X.Q.; Graichen, R.; Soo, S.Y.; Balakrishnan, T.; Rahmat, S.N.; Sieh, S.; Tham, S.C.; Freund, C.; Moore, J.; Mummery, C.; Colman, A.; Zweigerdt, R. & Davidson, B.P. (2008). Chemically defined medium supporting cardiomyocyte differentiation of human embryonic stem cells. *Differentiation*, Vol.76, No.9, pp.958-970.

Yanagisawa, M.; Liour, S.S. & Yu, R.K. (2004a). Involvement of gangliosides in proliferation of immortalized neural progenitor cells. *J Neurochem*, Vol.91, No.4, pp.804-812.

Yanagisawa, M.; Nakamura, K. & Taga, T. (2004b). Roles of lipid rafts in integrin-dependent adhesion and gp130 signalling pathway in mouse embryonic neural precursor cells. *Genes Cells*, Vol.9, No.9, pp.801-809.

Yanagisawa, M.; Nakamura, K. & Taga, T. (2005). Glycosphingolipid synthesis inhibitor represses cytokine-induced activation of the Ras-MAPK pathway in embryonic neural precursor cells. *J Biochem*, Vol.138, No.3, pp.285-291.

Yanes, O.; Clark, J.; Wong, D.M.; Patti, G.J.; Sanchez-Ruiz, A.; Benton, H.P.; Trauger, S.A.; Desponts, C.; Ding, S. & Siuzdak, G. (2010). Metabolic oxidation regulates embryonic stem cell differentiation. *Nat Chem Biol*, Vol.6, No.6, pp.411-417.

Ye, X.; Ishii, I.; Kingsbury, M.A. & Chun, J. (2002). Lysophosphatidic acid as a novel cell survival/apoptotic factor. *Biochim Biophys Acta*, Vol.1585, No.2-3, pp.108-113.

Yun, S.P.; Lee, M.Y.; Ryu, J.M. & Han, H.J. (2009). Interaction between PGE2 and EGF receptor through MAPKs in mouse embryonic stem cell proliferation. *Cell Mol Life Sci*, Vol.66, No.9, pp.1603-1616.

Zeng, X.; Cai, J.; Chen, J.; Luo, Y.; You, Z.B.; Fotter, E.; Wang, Y.; Harvey, B.; Miura, T.; Backman, C.; Chen, G.J.; Rao, M.S. & Freed, W.J. (2004). Dopaminergic differentiation of human embryonic stem cells. *Stem Cells*, Vol.22, No.6, pp.925-940.

Zhang, P.; Andrianakos, R.; Yang, Y.; Liu, C. & Lu, W. (2010). Kruppel-like factor 4 (Klf4) prevents embryonic stem (ES) cell differentiation by regulating Nanog gene expression. *J Biol Chem*, Vol.285, No.12, pp.9180-9189.

Zhu, S.; Wurdak, H. & Schultz, P.G. (2010). Directed embryonic stem cell differentiation with small molecules. *Future Med Chem*, Vol.2, No.6, pp.965-973.

2

Role of Signaling Pathways and Epigenetic Factors in Lineage Determination During Human Embryonic Stem Cell Differentiation

Prasenjit Sarkar and Balaji M. Rao
Department of Chemical and Biomolecular Engineering,
North Carolina State University, Raleigh, NC,
USA

1. Introduction

Human embryonic stem cells (hESCs) are culture-adapted cells that were originally derived from the inner cell mass (ICM) of the blastocyst-stage embryo [1]. HESCs are pluripotent cells that can be propagated indefinitely in culture, while retaining the *in vivo* properties of ICM cells; they can give rise to all tissues of the three germ layers (ectoderm, mesoderm and endoderm). Due to their pluripotency, hESCs have been the subject of intense research since they were initially isolated in 1998. HESCs can serve as model systems to study early human development, in addition to providing a potentially unlimited source of functional tissues for use in drug evaluation and regenerative medicine. Nevertheless, despite major advances, the exact molecular mechanisms that govern the self-renewal and differentiation of hESCs remain unclear. Indeed, a mechanistic understanding of the molecular processes regulating hESC fate can elucidate early events in human development and enable the development of protocols for efficient generation of functional tissues. Here we review the molecular mechanisms that regulate hESC fate; specifically, we focus on the role of signaling pathways and factors regulating epigenetic changes, in hESC self-renewal and lineage-specific differentiation.

In hESCs, as in embryos, differentiation is triggered by developmental cues such as morphogens or cytokines that are present in the extracellular space. These morphogens or cytokines bind to their cognate plasma membrane-bound receptors and activate specific signaling pathways inside the cell. Activation of signaling pathways involves a sequence of phosphorylation events that eventually result in the regulation of specific transcription factors. These transcription factors, in turn, can recruit other co-factors and directly cause transcription of downstream genes. Furthermore, transcription factors can recruit histone modifying and chromatin remodeling enzymes to reshuffle the epigenetic structure, such that pluripotency genes become inaccessible for transcription and are repressed, whereas lineage-specific genes become accessible and are activated. This sequence of events finally leads to expression of lineage-specific proteins such as transcription factors and structural proteins, causing a morphological change in the cell. Also, pluripotency associated transcription factors and other pluripotency-associated genes are permanently repressed, thereby completing the process of differentiation. Thus, the process of differentiation is a rather complex cascade of events, controlled by signaling pathways, transcription factors, epigenetic factors and lineage-specific proteins. While significant understanding of each of these functional groups (i.e., signaling pathways, transcription factors, epigenetic factors and lineage-specific proteins) has been gathered in isolation, very little is known about the interactions amongst these groups, particularly in the context of hESC differentiation. In part, interactions amongst these groups confer lineage specificity to the process of differentiation and mediate the development of specific tissues upon exposure of hESCs to certain morphogens. In this review, we focus on the role of signaling pathways, transcription factors and epigenetic factors in the context of lineage-specific differentiation of hESCs and summarize the various links between these groups. Our goal is to present a mechanistic overview of the sequence of molecular events that regulate the differentiation of hESCs along various lineages.

2. The signaling pathways

As briefly described earlier, the self-renewal and differentiation of hESCs is governed by several developmental cues. The most well known among these are cytokines that trigger specific signaling pathways. These extracellular ligands initiate signaling through interactions with ligand-specific cell surface receptors. Receptor-binding typically results in association of multiple receptor subunits and activation of the kinase domains of receptors or other receptor-bound effector proteins. This triggers a sequence of phosphorylation events involving various other proteins, finally resulting in the activation or inhibition of transcription factors. These transcription factors in turn are directly responsible for activating or repressing their target genes. Thus, a group of signaling pathways is usually responsible for modulating gene expression in hESCs, leading to control of the transcriptome, the proteome and ultimately cellular physiology. In this section, we summarize key signaling pathways that have been implicated in the maintenance of undifferentiated hESCs and their lineage-specific differentiation.

2.1.1 The transforming growth factor-β pathway

The transforming growth factor β (TGF-β) pathway is well known for its involvement in embryonic development and patterning, as well as in epithelial-to-mesenchymal transformations and carcinogenesis [2-3]. This pathway (extensively reviewed elsewhere [2, 4-5]) is divided into two branches: the Activin/Nodal branch and the Bone Morphogenetic Protein (BMP) branch. The Activin/Nodal pathway is activated by ligands such as Activin, Nodal and TGFβ1. These ligands bind to their Type II receptor, which then recruits the Type I receptor. The Type II receptor phosphorylates the intracellular domain of the Type I receptor, creating a binding site for SMAD2 and SMAD3 transcription factors. Upon binding, SMAD2/3 is phosphorylated by the Type I receptor, leading to subsequent dissociation of SMAD2/3. Phosphorylated SMAD2/3 then associates with SMAD4 and can enter the nucleus to modulate gene expression. The BMP branch is activated by the BMP ligands; binding of BMP ligands results in phosphorylation of the type I receptor by the type II receptor, and subsequent intracellular binding and phosphorylation of SMAD1/5/8. Phosphorylated SMAD1/5/8 forms a complex with SMAD4 and subsequently enters the nucleus. Unlike ligands in the Activin/Nodal branch, the BMPs have high affinities for the type I receptor and bind weakly to the type II receptor; Activin/Nodal bind with high

Role of Signaling Pathways and Epigenetic Factors in Lineage Determination During
Human Embryonic Stem Cell Differentiation

27

affinity to their type II receptors and do not directly interact with their type I receptors. Numerous other proteins can modulate the localization and activity of SMADs (reviewed in [6-8]). Additionally, the activated TGFβ pathway receptors can also activate the Mitogen Activated Protein Kinase (MAPK) Pathway [9].

2.1.2 Role in lineage determination

The TGFβ pathway plays a significant role during embryogenesis across many species including flies, fishes, amphibians and mammals (reviewed in [10]). Specifically among vertebrates, Nodal is expressed throughout the epiblast [11] and is required for specification of mesoderm and endoderm from the epiblast [12]. Low levels of Nodal lead to mesoderm formation whereas high levels lead to endoderm formation [13]. Absence of Nodal signaling through active inhibition leads to ectoderm formation [12, 14]. Within the ectoderm, high levels of BMP cause formation of epidermis while low levels cause neural plate formation [15]. Intermediate levels of BMP lead to neural crest formation at the borders of the neural plate, although this a necessary but not a sufficient condition [16].

Not surprisingly, *in vitro* protocols for differentiating hESCs resemble *in vivo* conditions present during embryogenesis. Specifically, Activin causes endoderm differentiation from hESC cultures, while Activin and BMP simultaneously lead to mesoderm formation [17-21]. Inhibition of both Activin/Nodal and BMP causes neural differentiation [22] and this differentiation proceeds through an epiblast-like intermediate. Intriguingly, some amount of Activin/Nodal signaling is essential for hESC pluripotency; the pluripotency factor Nanog is a direct target of Smad2/3 [23-25] and inhibition of Activin/Nodal causes upregulation of BMP and subsequent trophectoderm differentiation [26]. Short term BMP treatment causes mesoderm formation [27] whereas long term BMP treatment leads to trophectoderm formation [28]. The disparity of BMP treatment leading to trophectoderm differentiation and not epidermal differentiation, as during embryogenesis, can in part be attributed to the fact that hESCs are derived from ICM cells and not epiblast cells. Thus, even though *in vivo* embryogenesis serves to provide guidelines for carrying out *in vitro* differentiation of hESCs, major challenges still remain. The biggest of these challenges is perhaps the heterogeneity in lineages of differentiated cells obtained through most *in vitro* protocols. This is primarily because most differentiation protocols rely on embryoid body (EB) formation which results in a heterogeneous environment for cells within the EB, and leads to heterogeneity in the lineages obtained after differentiation. Another challenge is the inability to form an absolute mechanistic link between the culture conditions used to differentiate hESCs, and the differentiation behavior seen in hESCs. This is mostly because the composition of serum, B27, serum replacer, conditioned medium and other components of media used for differentiation studies, are unknown [29].

2.2 The Fibroblast Growth Factor pathway

The Fibroblast Growth Factor (FGF) pathway is also known for its involvement in embryonic development and patterning, as well as in regulation of cell growth, proliferation and motility (extensively reviewed in [30-34]). The FGF pathway is activated when the FGF ligands, which have a strong affinity for Heparan Sulfate Proteoglycans (HSPGs), bind to FGF Receptors (FGFRs) forming a 2:2:2 combination of FGF: FGFR: HSPG on the cell surface. The ensuing receptor dimerization causes transphosphorylation of tyrosine residues in the intracellular domains of FGFRs through their tyrosine kinase domains. The phosphorylated tyrosines of FGFRs cause recruitment of the GRB2/SOS complex and its subsequent activation. SOS then activates RAS, which triggers the MAPK cascade, finally leading to the activation of extracellular-signal related kinases (ERKs). Activated Erk1/2 can phosphorylate and control the activity of a wide range of proteins [35]. Notably, Erk1/2 can phosphorylate the linker region of SMAD1 and inhibit BMP signaling [36-37]. Additionally, activated FGF receptors can also recruit FRS2/GRB2 and activate them, leading to recruitment of GAB1. GAB1 activates the Phosphatidylinositol 3-kinase (PI3K) pathway. Thus, FGF can also activate the PI3K pathway in a cell-specific context.

2.2.1 Role in lineage determination

The FGF pathway is needed for proper embryonic development in vertebrates. Experiments in mice have shown that FGF4 is required for ICM proliferation and maintenance [38-39], and for trophectoderm and primitive endoderm development [40]. FGF4 is secreted by the ICM and supports trophectoderm maintenance [41]. Interestingly, activation of HRas1 which is a component of the MAPK pathway, in mouse embryonic stem cells (mESCs) caused upregulation of Cdx2, a trophectoderm marker, and trophectoderm stem cells were derived from these mutants [42]. FGF4 secreted by ICM also causes primitive endoderm differentiation [43]. Further along the developmental timeline, FGF signaling is required for the induction of paraxial mesoderm and for maintenance (but not induction) of axial mesoderm [44-46]. FGF is required for primitive streak formation and cell migration during gastrulation [45, 47]. Inhibition of FGF is required for blood development [48-50], whereas activation of FGF signaling is required for neural differentiation [51]. However the mechanism by which FGF aids in embryonic neural differentiation is not fully understood [52-53]. *In vitro* studies have mimicked the role of FGF signaling in hESC maintenance and differentiation. FGF2 is required for maintaining hESCs in a pluripotent state [24, 54-55]. FGF signaling is also required for maintenance of mouse trophectoderm stem cells which are derived from the trophectoderm tissue of mouse embryos [56]. While there are no specific studies which delineate the inductive and maintenance/proliferative roles of FGF during hESC differentiation, work with mESCs have given ambiguous results, some showing that autocrine FGF2 is essential for neural differentiation [57] while others showing that FGF2 has a role in maintenance rather than induction of neural differentiation [58-59]. However, FGF signaling does seem to be necessary for inducing the posterior nervous system in vertebrate embryos [53, 60].

2.3 The Wnt pathway

The Wnt pathway is widely implicated during various stages of embryonic development, homeostasis as well as in cancer. This pathway (reviewed in [61-62]) has canonical and non-canonical branches. The canonical Wnt pathway is activated by binding of Wnt ligands to the Frizzled receptors and low-density lipoprotein receptor-related protein 5/6 (LRP5/6) co-receptors leading to the recruitment of Dishevelled to the Frizzled receptor. This causes recruitment of Axin to the receptor complex, causing the subsequent deactivation of Axin. In the absence of Wnt signaling, Axin associates with GSK3β, adenomatous polyposis coli (APC), casein kinase 1 (CK1) and β-catenin. CK1 and GSK3β phosphorylate β-catenin causing it to be degraded. Upon Wnt activation, Axin is inhibited and β-catenin becomes de-repressed, and subsequently enters the nucleus to function as a transcription factor. Various co-factors associate with β-catenin and control its promoter specificity, thus dictating the

Role of Signaling Pathways and Epigenetic Factors in Lineage Determination During
Human Embryonic Stem Cell Differentiation

29

target genes activated or repressed by β-catenin [63-64]. The non-canonical Wnt pathway acts independently of β-catenin and is also required during embryogenesis. The details of this Ca^{2+}-dependent pathway are reviewed in [62].

2.3.1 Role in lineage determination

The canonical Wnt pathway is activated during gastrulation [65] and mutation of Wnt3 blocks primitive streak formation resulting in lack of mesoderm and endoderm [66] (the primitive streak-specific transcription factor Brachyury is a direct target of Wnt3a signaling [67]). Similar defects are seen in Lrp5/6 double mutants and β-catenin loss-of-function mutants [68-69]. Interestingly, expression of Cripto, a co-receptor for Nodal signaling, is missing in β-catenin loss-of-function mutants [70]. Also, β-catenin is indispensable for endoderm formation and loss of β-catenin causes definitive endoderm to change into pre-cardiac mesoderm [71]. Although loss of Wnt signaling leads to loss of mesoderm formation, inhibition of Wnt signaling is required for a cardiac fate [65, 72], once pre-cardiac mesoderm has been induced. Remarkably, similar reports for the role of Wnt signaling have been obtained through *in vitro* differentiation studies in hESCs. Over-expression of β-catenin in hESC cultures lead to primitive streak formation [73]. Inputs form Activin/Nodal and BMP pathways are necessary for further lineage specification into mesoderm/endoderm. Blocking BMP signaling abolishes mesoderm and leads to endoderm formation, whereas Activin/Nodal is required for endoderm formation [73]. Wnt is required for mesoderm differentiation but must be inhibited thereafter for cardiac mesoderm formation [74].

2.4 The Phosphatidylinositol-3Kinase pathway

The Phosphatidylinositol-3Kinase (PI3K) pathway regulates cell survival, apoptosis and has been implicated in cancer. The pathway as well as its role in cancer is reviewed in [75-78]. It also has been, in select cases, implicated in lineage-specific hESC differentiation [79]. The pathway is activated when PI3K is phosphorylated; this can happen through binding of Insulin to the Insulin receptor or of Insulin-like growth Factor (IGF) to Insulin-like Growth Factor Receptor (IGFR), or as previously discussed, by recruitment and activation of GAB1 by FGFR. Activated PI3K phosphorylates Phosphatidylinositol (4, 5)-biphosphate to Phosphatidylinositol (3, 4, 5)-triphosphate and creates a docking site for proteins with a pleckstrin homology (PH) domain, such as Akt. Once Akt is properly docked, it is phosphorylated and activated by protein-dependent kinase 1 (PDK1). Akt can then dissociate and activate/repress numerous proteins by phosphorylating them [80]. The PI3K pathway has not received much attention during vertebrate embryogenesis, though some recent studies have emerged to show that it is necessary for normal embryo development [81-82]. Homozygous null mutations in the p110β subunit of PI3K cause embryonic lethality before formation of the blastocyst [83]. Thus, *in vivo* studies do not implicate PI3K signaling in differentiation of cells, but rather in maintenance of cell viability [82]. It has been hypothesized that growth factors maintain PI3K signaling during embryogenesis to guard against ectopic or metastatic growth of cells, since such ectopic/metastatic cells do not receive enough growth factors and enter the default apoptotic pathway [84]. In contrast, *in vitro* studies with hESCs have shown some supportive role for the PI3K pathway in definitive endoderm differentiation. Inhibition of PI3K signaling enhances definitive endoderm differentiation by Activin [85]. Other conflicting reports show that PI3K signaling stabilizes β-catenin during definitive endoderm formation [73]. A major challenge in elucidating the possible role of this pathway during differentiation is the inability to decouple its role in cell viability. Therefore, careful studies need to be designed to assess the extent of its role in causing differentiation.

2.5 The Hippo pathway

So far we have focused on developmental cues in the form of morphogens, i.e. protein ligands that physically diffuse through the embryonic tissue and pattern the embryo. Another developmental cue that has recently emerged to be of significant importance during embryogenesis is cell-cell contact. An increase in cell-cell contact is sensed by the cell through the activation of the Hippo pathway (reviewed in [86-87]). The Hippo pathway is important for organ size control, tumorigenesis, epithelial-to-mesenchymal transformation and cell-cell contact inhibition. Although the molecular mechanisms of cell-cell contact sensing are not fully understood, an increase in cell-cell contact is known to ultimately lead to phosphorylation of MST1/2 kinases. They then associate with SAV1 and phosphorylate the LATS1/2 kinases. Upon phosphorylation, LATS1/2 kinases recruit MOB1 and phosphorylate YAP and TAZ, both of which are homologues with non-redundant functions [86, 88]. Phosphorylation of TAZ and YAP leads to their association with 14-3-3 proteins and subsequent cytoplasmic retention [89-90]. YAP and TAZ act as co-factors for various transcription factors such as TEADs, RUNX, PAX3 and SMAD1/2/3/7 and modulate their nuclear localization and/or activity [91-96]. Additionally, TAZ can associate with DVL2 and inhibit its phosphorylation by CK1, thus possibly inhibiting β-catenin activation by Wnt factors [97]. Therefore, the nucleocytoplasmic shuttling of YAP and/or TAZ can lead to changes in the activity levels of associating transcription factors, leading to differentiation [93]. Indeed, low cell-cell contact at the periphery of the embryo leads to Yap activation, which in concert with Tead4, leads to trophoblast differentiation in mouse blastocysts [98]. The inner cell mass and epiblast tissues show predominantly cytoplasmic and weakly nuclear localization for Yap, Taz and phospho-Smad2 [98-99], in agreement with the fact that Taz controls Smad2 localization [93]. While cells of the mouse ICM continue to differentiate, in vitro cultures derived from ICM (i.e. mESCs) maintain high levels of Yap. Yap is downregulated during in vitro mESC differentiation and upregulated in mouse and human induced pluripotent stem (iPS) cells [100]. Ectopic Yap expression maintains mESC phenotype even under differentiation conditions. Though it remains to be seen whether downregulation of Yap/Taz is the cause of differentiation of ICM cells in vivo, experiments with hESCs show that downregulation of TAZ initiates neural differentiation [93]. Tead and Yap suppress terminal neuronal differentiation and maintain neural progenitor populations in the vertebrate neural tube [94]. Tead2 and Yap activate Pax3 expression during neural crest formation [101]. Tead1/2 and Yap also maintain the notochord which is formed from the axial mesoderm [102]. Thus the co-activators YAP and TAZ are important for the activity of many transcription factors during embryogenesis. However, further studies are needed to uncover the specific inductive/maintenance roles of these co-factors and their responsiveness to Hippo signaling in these tissues.

2.6 Crosstalk between signaling pathways

There is a vast amount of crosstalk between the various pathways described here, thus adding additional complexity in the regulation of downstream transcription factors [103]. As described earlier, the TGF-β pathway can activate the MAPK pathway directly

Role of Signaling Pathways and Epigenetic Factors in Lineage Determination During
Human Embryonic Stem Cell Differentiation

31

downstream of receptor activation [9]. Both TGF-β and FGF pathways can activate the PI3K pathways directly at the receptor level [9, 30]. However, the crosstalk between pathways is cell-specific, since the available pool of interacting proteins depends on the cell-type. Also, the promoter accessibility of downstream genes is dependent on cell-type. Therefore, here we restrict our discussion to crosstalk events identified specifically in hESCs. Activin/BMP signaling induces Wnt ligand expression in hESCs [74]. Also, Activin regulates FGF, Wnt and BMP pathways in hESCs [104]. Inhibition of Activin/Nodal signaling causes downregulation of Wnt3, FGF2, FGF4 and FGF8 expression [26] and upregulation of BMP signaling [26] while activation of Activin signaling causes upregulation of Wnt3 and FGF8 expression [104]. Interestingly, upregulation of Activin signaling also causes upregulation of Nodal and Lefty expression. Cerberus1, an inhibitor of Nodal signaling, is a downstream target of both Wnt and Nodal pathways in hESCs [105]. Expression of Cripto, a co-activator of Nodal signaling, is upregulated by FGF signaling in hESCs [24]. As described earlier, YAP, which is regulated by the Hippo pathway, controls the nuclear localization of Smad2 in hESCs [93]. Thus, it can be seen that hESCs exhibit considerable endogenous signaling wherein, signaling pathways not only control their own ligand expression but also the expression of ligands of other pathways.

3. Other regulators of differentiation

While morphogens and other developmental cues act as the environmental input to hESCs and trigger the process of differentiation, the molecular mechanisms responsible for carrying out differentiation inside the cell are complex and require many key factors. These factors are required for the following: 1) to bring about a change in gene expression which causes the cell to transition into the new lineage-specific physiology, 2) to reshuffle the epigenetic structure of the genome, and finally 3) to make the new epigenetic structure permanent, lending stability to the newly formed cellular physiology. We will now discuss these intracellular factors that mediate various aspects of the differentiation process.

3.1 MicroRNAs

MicroRNAs (miRNAs) have emerged as a new paradigm for regulating gene expression at the post-transcriptional level. The role of miRNAs in embryogenesis, stem cell fate and cancer is reviewed in [106-108]. Transcription factors regulate promoter regions of miRNAs, which upon synthesis can target many mRNAs and lead to downregulation of protein synthesis. MiRNAs, which upon transcription are called pri-miRNAs, fold into secondary structures with characteristic hairpin-loops. These are recognized by Drosha, which cleaves the hairpin-loop structures to generate pre-miRNAs. Pre-miRNAs are then exported to the cytoplasm and recognized by Dicer, which cleaves one of the strands and incorporates the other into the RNA-induced silencing complex (RISC). Once incorporated into RISC, the single-stranded miRNA recognizes target mRNAs (usually many different mRNA targets) through partial sequence complimentarily, and causes down-regulation of protein synthesis. It is now known that miRNAs play an important role in embryogenesis [109] and lineage-determination, and that many lineages have their characteristic miRNA expression patterns, akin to characteristic mRNA expression patterns [110]. The role of miRNAs in embryogenesis is evident from the fact that Dicer mutant mouse embryos die during gastrulation [111], while Dicer deficient zebrafish embryos do not develop beyond day8 [109]. The role of miRNAs in embryonic stem cell pluripotency and differentiation has also been demonstrated recently [107]. Dicer deficient mESCs fail to differentiate *in vitro* as well as *in vivo* [112]. Over-expression of miR-302 leads to reprogramming of human hair follicle cells and human skin cancer cells to form iPS cells [113-114]. During mESC differentiation, miR-134, miR-296 and miR-470 target and downregulate the transcription factors Nanog, Sox2 and Oct4 [115]. MiR-200c, miR-203 and miR-183 target and repress Sox2 and Klf4, both of which are involved in maintaining pluripotency in mESCs [116]. Similarly, during hESC differentiation, miR-145 targets and represses OCT4, SOX2 and KLF4 [117]. Sall4, another pluripotency-related transcription factor, is positively regulated by the ESC cell cycle regulating (ESCC) family of miRNAs and negatively regulated by the let7 family [118]. Additionally, miRNAs are also implicated during later stages of differentiation. The muscle-specific miR-1 controls cardiomyocyte differentiation and proliferation in mice by targeting the Hand2 transcription factor [119]. miR-181 controls hematopoietic differentiation in mice [120] and miR-143 regulates adipocyte differentiation [121]. MiR-196 is involved in HOX gene regulation [122-124] and the miR-200 family regulates olfactory neurogenesis [125]. MiRNAs have also been implicated in skin morphogenesis [126]. Most intriguingly, transfection of muscle-specific miR-1 or brain-specific miR-124 into human HeLa cells shifts the mRNA expression profile towards that of muscle or brain cells, respectively [127].

The expression of miRNAs is regulated by transcription factors which bind promoter regions of genes harboring miRNAs; more than half of known mammalian miRNA genes are within host gene introns and are spliced after transcription [128]. For example, Activin A signaling regulates the expression of ~12 miRNAs in hESC cultures [129]. OCT4, NANOG and SOX2 occupy the promoter regions of ~14 miRNAs in hESCs [130]. Additionally, miRNAs can be regulated directly by signaling pathways. In smooth muscle cells, BMP4 or TGF-β signaling causes increased processing of pri-miR-21 and pri-miR-199a [131] and regulates the processing of numerous other miRNAs [132]. The MAPK/ERK pathway can regulate miRNA maturation in the cytosol by controlling phosphorylation of TRBP, which functions with Dicer [133]. However, it is largely accepted that miRNAs do not trigger differentiation but rather, are required for carrying out the process of differentiation [107]. It is hypothesized that miRNAs are required to dampen the stochastic noise in mRNA transcription levels of genes during the process of differentiation. Thus, miRNAs add another layer of complexity to gene regulation during the process of differentiation, by fine-tuning active mRNA levels of a gene.

3.2 Epigenetic factors

Our discussion on signaling pathways focused on how a change in gene expression during differentiation is initiated; while miRNAs are most probably required to stabilize the mRNA levels against stochastic perturbations during differentiation. However, to provide long-term stability to the new gene expression pattern, the epigenetic structure of the genome needs to be changed. Epigenetic factors are responsible for modulating the epigenetic structure of hESCs, while it is pluripotent (reviewed in [134]) as well as while it goes through differentiation. The epigenetic structure of the genome dictates the promoter regions that would be accessible to transcription factors for initiating transcription; the heterochromatin, being densely packed, is inaccessible whereas the euchromatin is loosely packed and readily accessible. The epigenetic structure of hESCs is different from that of differentiated cells. The epigenetic structure also differs across various lineages of differentiation. Thus, epigenetic factors are involved in changing the epigenetic structure of the genome in a lineage-dependent fashion.

Role of Signaling Pathways and Epigenetic Factors in Lineage Determination During
Human Embryonic Stem Cell Differentiation

33

Epigenetic factors comprise broadly of histone modifying enzymes and chromatin remodeling complexes. The concerted action of both is needed to bring a stable change in the epigenetic landscape. Histone modifying enzymes are enzymes that modify histones post-translationally and create an epigenetic code of various acetylations, ubiquitinations and methylations throughout the genome (the histone code hypothesis [135-136]). This code is then recognized by chromatin remodeling enzymes, which alter the higher order structure of nucleosomes by creating heterochromatin and euchromatin. By controlling the formation of heterochromatin and euchromatin, these epigenetic factors control promoter accessibility and gene expression during differentiation. Differentiation is thought to proceed through activation of lineage-specific genes and repression of pluripotency genes [137]. This requires epigenetic factors to create repressive histone modifications on pluripotency genes (which were hitherto active) and reciprocally, to create activating histone modifications on lineage-specific genes (which were hitherto repressed). Permanent modification of histones also allows for epigenetic stability of the differentiated cell, which now becomes locked in this lineage. There is also some feedback from chromatin remodeling enzymes back to histone modifying enzymes. This means that certain chromatin remodeling enzymes can recruit back specific histone modifying enzymes for changing the histone code further. This is thought to provide more robustness to this system of epigenetic modification, thus lending further stability to the differentiated phenotype.

3.2.1 Histone Acetyltransferases

Of the various histone modifications, acetylation and methylation are critical for regulating the chromatin structure and gene expression [138]. These histone modifications, which create the genome-wide histone code, are regulated by Histone Acetyltransferases (HATs), Histone Deacetylases (HDACs), Histone Methyltransferases (HMTs) and Histone Demethylases. Histone Acetyltransferases are further classified into five families [139-140]: the Gcn5-related HATs (GNATs); the MYST (MOZ, Ybf2/Sas3, Sas2 and Tip60)-related HATs; p300/CBP HATs; general transcription factor HATs; and nuclear hormone-related HATs. In humans, the identified GNAT-related HAT complexes are PCAF, STAGA and TFTC. All three complexes have the chromatin-binding bromodomain which targets these complexes to chromatin. The bromodomain specifically recognizes and binds acetylated histones [141-142]. In mammals, the identified MYST-related HATs are Moz, Qkf, Mof, Tip60 (homologue of yeast NuA4 [143]) and Hbo1. The TIP60 complex contains the chromatin-binding chromodomain. The chromodomain of yeast SAGA HAT complex has been shown to recognize methylated histones [144] raising the possibility that TIP60 may also be recruited to methylated histones in humans. Together with the case of the bromodomain containing complexes, this implies that HATs may be recruited to specifically tagged histones and may function in a signaling cascade to modify the epigenetic map of the genome [145]. *Mof* homozygous null mice lack H4K16 acetylation and arrest at blastocyst stage [146]. Homozygous null *Tip60* mutant mice also die during blastocyst stage[147]. Tip60 has also been implicated in pluripotency of ESCs [148]. Qkf is required for normal development of neurons of the cerebral cortex [149], whereas Moz is required for normal hematopoietic stem cell development [150-152].

3.2.2 Histone Deacetylases

The family of Histone Deacetylases is classified into four groups [153-155]: the Class I HDACs (yeast Rpd3-like) comprising of HDAC1/2, HDAC3 and HDAC8; the Class II

HDACs (yeast Hda1-like) comprising of HDACs4-7, HDAC9 and HDAC10; the Class III HDACs (Sir2-like) comprising of SIRT1-7; and the Class IV HDACs (HDAC11-like) comprising of HDAC11. Of these, HDAC1 and HDAC2 have been identified in numerous complexes [156], namely: the SIN3 co-repressor complex, the nucleosome remodeling and deacetylase (NuRD) complex, the CoREST complex, the Nanog and Oct4 associated deacetylase (NODE) complex and the SHIP1 containing complex. HDACs complexes become associated with transcription factors through mediator proteins such as Sin3, NCoR, SMRT, CtBP and TLE [157]. Hdac1 and Hdac2 are important for embryonic development, especially during myogenesis, neurogenesis, haematopoiesis and epithelial cell differentiation [156]. The HDAC complexes NuRD and SIN3 are critical during different stages of embryonic development [158]. Mice embryos lacking Mbd3 or p66α, components of the NuRD complex, die during embryonic development [159-160]. *Mbd3* null mice show normal segregation of trophoblast and primitive endoderm, but fail to develop embryonic ectoderm and extraembryonic ectoderm [161]. ICM cells of these embryos continue expressing Oct4 and the primitive endoderm marker Gata4 and fail to expand in number. Further, even though the primitive endoderm is present, the visceral endoderm fails to form. Analogously, the ICM cells derived from *Mbd3* null mice did not expand ex-vivo and mESCs could not be formed [161]. *Mbd3* null mESCs could initiate differentiation but could not commit to the differentiated lineages [162]. Mbd3 was also shown to suppress trophoblast commitment of mESCs [163]. P66α, however, was not required for proper blastocyst formation and implantation, and *p66α* null mice died later during embryogenesis [160]. Mi-2β, another component of the NuRD complex, is important for haematopoiesis, lymphopoiesis and skin development [164-167]. Similar to *Mbd3* and *p66a*, *Sin3a* null mice embryos also die after implantation [168-169]. The ICM derived from these embryos shows severely retarded proliferation ex vivo [168]. *Sin3b* null embryos show defects in erythrocyte and granulocyte maturation and in skeletal development [170]. The Class III HDACs, known as Sirtuins (SirTs), are also implicated during differentiation and mammalian development [171]. SirT1 is highly expressed in ESCs and decreases during differentiation [172]. During late development, SirT2 modulates skeletal muscle and SirT1 modulates white adipose tissue differentiation [173-174]. Under oxidative stress, SirT1 causes astroglial differentiation in mouse neural progenitor cells [175]. SirtT2 controls gametogenesis in mice embryos [176].

3.2.3 Histone Methyltransferases
Various Histone Methyltransferases (HMTs) exist in the mammalian genome and many putative HMTs are yet to be discovered [177]. The major mammalian HMTs include Ash1l, Dot1l, Ezh1-2, G9a, GLP, Mll1-5, Nsd1, Prdm1-6, Prdm8-16, PrSet7, Setd1-7, Setdb1-2, Setmar, Smyd1-5, Suv39h1-2, Suv4-20h1-2 and Whsc1/1l. Their requirement during specific stages of mammalian development is comprehensively reviewed in [177]. These HMTs are associated with specific histone methylation activities on H3 and H4 histones. Although most of identified methylation marks are promiscuous and need further study, some histone methylation marks correlate well with gene activity. Transcriptionally active genes display H3K4me3 on their promoter region and H3K36me3 across the gene body, while repressed genes are enriched in H3K27me3 over the gene body, with some amount of H3K9me3 and H4K20me3 [178-180]. H3K4 methylation, which is associated with gene activation, is induced by Mll1-5, Setd1a/b and Ash1l. Therefore, these HMTs are critical during mammalian development. Mutations in *Mll1* lead to embryonic lethality in mice [181-182]

Role of Signaling Pathways and Epigenetic Factors in Lineage Determination During
Human Embryonic Stem Cell Differentiation

35

and cause aberrant regulation of Hox genes. Generation and/or expansion of hematopoietic stem cells, is abrogated in these embryos [183]. *Mll2* null mice are capable of blastocyst formation and normal implantation without any lineage-specific growth abnormalities, but die later during embryonic development [184]. Very few genes are misregulated in *Mll2* null mESCs, though *Mll2* is needed for spermatogenesis [185]. *Mll3* mutant mice show impaired differentiation towards the adipocyte lineage [186], while *Mll5* mutant mice show impaired hematopoietic development [187]. H3K27 methylation, which is associated with gene repression and is important for embryonic development, is caused by the Ezh1-2 HTMs. Again, *Ezh2* knockout causes early embryonic lethality in mouse embryos [188]. These embryos fail to complete gastrulation. Ezh2 is also shown to regulate epidermal and hematopoietic differentiation during embryogenesis [189-191]. H3K9 methylation is also associated with gene repression, and is induced by G9a, GLP, Prdm2, Setdb1 and Suv39h1-2. No gene targets for the Suv39h enzymes have been discovered though *Suv39h* double mutant mice display impaired viability as well as sterility [192]. In contrast, *Setdb1* knockout causes early embryonic lethality in mouse embryos due to aberrant blastocyst formation, and mESCs cannot be derived from these mutant blastocysts [193]. Setdb1 also controls the switch between osteoblastogenesis and adipogenesis from bone marrow mesenchymal progenitor cells [194]. Similar to *Setdb1*, both *G9a* and *GLP* null mice also show embryonic lethality, including aberrant somitogenesis and aberrant neural tube formation [195-196]. G9a inactivates ~120 genes during mESC differentiation including Oct4 and Nanog, in concert with DNA Methyltransferases Dnmt3a/b [197-198]. G9a is also implicated for genomic imprinting in the mouse placenta [199].

3.2.4 Histone Demethylases

In humans, the identified histone demethylases include the KDM (Lysine (K) Demethylase) families of demethylases (KDM1-6), the PHF family and the JMJD6 family (reviewed in [200-201]). As with histone methyltransferases, histone demethylases are critical for embryonic development. The KDM1 family comprises of KDM1A and KDM1B. Homozygous deletion mutants of *Kdm1a* are early embryonic lethal and do not gastrulate [202]. *Kdm1a* null ES cells are pluripotent but do not form embryoid bodies and do not differentiate [202]. *Kdm1b* mutant mice embryos are maternal embryonic lethal and defective in imprinting [203]. The KDM2 family comprises of KDM2A and KDM2B, of which, KDM2B is implicated in osteogenesis from mesenchymal stem cells [204]. The KDM3 family consists of KDM3A, KDM3B and JMJD1C. KDM3A is required for spermatogenesis [205-206]. KDM3A is positively regulated by Oct4 and depletion of KDM3A from ES cells leads to differentiation [207]. The KDM4 family consists of KDM4A, KDM4B, KDM4C and KDM4D, of which, KDM4C is also positively regulated by Oct4 [207]. Depletion of KDM4C causes differentiation in ES cells and KDM4C also positively regulates Nanog expression [207]. The KDM5 family comprises of KDM5A, KDM5B, KDM5C and KDM5D, of which, KDM5A has been implicated in differentiation [208]. The KDM6 family consists of KDM6A, UTY and KDM6B. KDM6A and KDM6B are shown to regulate HOX gene expression during development [209-210]. KDM6B also controls neuronal differentiation and epidermal differentiation [211-213]. The PHF family includes JHDM1D, PHF2 and PHF8, while the JMJD6 family includes only JMJD6. JHDM1D is required for neural differentiation in mESCs and knockdown of *Jhdm1d* blocks neural differentiation [214].

3.2.5 DNA Methyltransferases

The DNA Methyltransferases (DNMTs) in humans include DNMT1, DNMT2 and DNMT3 (reviewed in [215-216]). The identified isoforms of DNMT1 are DNMT1s, DNMT1o, DNMT1b and DNMT$^{\Delta E3-6}$. Members of DNMT3 are DNMT3a, DNMT3b and DNMT3L, of which, DNMT3a has isoforms DNMT3a1-4 and DNMT3b has isoforms DNMT3b1-8. *Dnmt1* null mice embryos die after gastrulation, before the 8-somite stage [217]. Double homozygous null mutations in *Dnmt3a* and *Dnmt3b* in mice embryos also caused similar phenotypes, with defects in neural tube closure and embryonic lethality at presomite stage [218-219]. During normal development, Dnmt3b is expressed in ICM, epiblast, embryonic ectoderm and spermatogonia of mouse embryo, whereas Dnmt3a is expressed throughout the embryo after E10.5 [220-221]. Dnmt3b is also expressed in progenitor population during hematopoiesis, spermatogenesis and neurogenesis [222]. During terminal neuronal differentiation, expression shifts to Dnmt3a [222]. Dnmt3l is required for genomic imprinting and female homozygous *Dnmt3l* null mice die during embryogenesis due to imprinting defects [223]. These mice show reduced spongiotrophoblast differentiation and excess trophoblast giant cell formation. Male homozygous *Dnmt3l* null mouse embryos show impaired spermatogenesis, but are viable [224]. Dnmt3a is also required for imprinting and spermatogenesis [225-226]. Curiously, triple homozygous knockout of *Dnmt1*, *Dnmt3a* and *Dnmt3b* causes no change in ESC self-renewal [227]. However, *Dnmt1* null ESCs with extremely low CpG methylation levels do not differentiate [228]. Similar blockage of differentiation is also observed in dual *Dnmt3a/Dnmt3b* homozygous null mutants [228].

3.2.6 Chromatin remodeling enzymes

Chromatin remodeling enzymes are involved in controlling the higher order structure of chromatin by creating heterochromatin and euchromatin, and utilize the energy of ATP to do so. Chromatin remodeling enzymes thereby control cell fate during differentiation of ESCs (reviewed in [229]). During *in vivo* development, chromatin remodeling enzymes have been shown to be important for myeloid differentiation, erythropoiesis, T-cell development, adipogenesis, neurogenesis and myogenesis (reviewed in [230]). Mammalian chromatin modeling enzymes are categorized into three families: SWI/SNF, ISWI and CHD. The SWI/SNF family is characterized by the presence of either Brg1 or Brm as the catalytic subunit, and is further categorized into two subfamilies: Baf and Pbaf [231]. *Brg1* homozygous null mice die at peri-implantation stage and their ICM as well as trophoblast tissues die [232]. Similar phenotypes are observed homozygous mice null for *Snf5*, another subunit of SWI/SNF complexes [233]. However, downregulation of Baf60c causes late embryonic lethality due to defects in cardiac and skeletal muscle development [234]. Similarly, ablation of *Baf180* leads to defects in heart development and placental trophectoderm development, and subsequent embryonic lethality [235] However, homozygous null mutations in *Baf155* caused early embryonic lethality due to failure of ICM cells, though trophoblast giant cells were found to be normal [236]. Heterozygotes null for *Baf155* showed defective brain development. In mESCs, knockdown of Brg1 leads to loss of self-renewal and impaired ability to differentiate to ectoderm and mesoderm [237]. Inactivation of *Baf250b* has been associated with reduced self-renewal and increased differentiation [238]. Interestingly, ablation of *Baf250a* caused failure of mesoderm formation in mouse embryos as well as in ESC-based embryoid body cultures [239]. However, primitive endoderm differentiation and neuronal differentiation could be established in these cells. Brg1, Baf47, Baf155 and Baf57 are

Role of Signaling Pathways and Epigenetic Factors in Lineage Determination During
Human Embryonic Stem Cell Differentiation

37

required to suppress Nanog expression during differentiation and knockdown of Baf155 or Baf57 lead to de-repression of Nanog levels during differentiation [240]. The ISWI family of chromatin remodelers is characterized by the presence of the Snf2h or Snf2l ATPase subunits that interact with unmodified histones. Snf2h is a part of the RSH, WICH, NoRC, CHRAC and ACF chromatin remodeling complexes. Snf2l is a part of the NURF and CERF complexes. Similar to *Brg1*, *Snf2h* homozygous null mice die at peri-implantation stage and both ICM and trophectoderm tissues degenerate [241]. Cecr2, a component of CERF, has been implicated in neural tube formation in mice [242]. Human NURF has also been implicated in neuronal development [243]. Interestingly, homozygous mice null for *Bptf*, a component of NURF, fail to form the visceral endoderm [244]. Bptf is required for ectoderm, mesoderm and both definitive and visceral endoderm development from ESCs in embryoid body cultures. Association between NURF complex and Smad transcription factors are necessary for endoderm formation [244]. The CHD family of chromatin remodelers is characterized by the presence of two chromodomains, with affinity for methylated histones. The CHD family is categorized into three subfamilies: family I with CHD1-2, family II with CHD3-4 and family III with CHD5-9. Downregulation of Chd1 in ESCs leads to impaired pluripotency, such that the cells are incapable of primitive endoderm and cardiac mesoderm differentiation and become prone to neural differentiation [245]. CHD3 and CHD4 are also found in NuRD histone deacetylase complexes described previously. Mutations in *Chd7* are embryonic lethal, showing that Chd7 is also important for embryonic development [246].

3.2.7 Regulation of epigenetic factors by transcription factors

Significant literature has been accumulated concerning the regulation of epigenetic factors by transcription factors. Transcription factors lie downstream of signaling pathways, raising the possibility that signaling pathways can control the recruitment of epigenetic factors to specific promoter regions. The vast number of interactions between the Smad transcription factors and epigenetic factors is extensively reviewed in [157]. Smads 1-4 can directly interact with HATs p300 and CBP [247] while Smads 2-3 can also interact with PCAF [248]. Smads 1, 2, 3 and 5 can interact with the HAT GCN5 [249] while Smad5 can also interact with the histone methyltransferases Suv39h2 [250]. Smad7 is acetylated and protected from degradation by p300 [251]. Smads 6 and 7 can also bind and recruit HDACs [252]. As discussed before, "bridging" proteins such as NCoR, Sin3, SMRT, CtBP and TLE can also help epigenetic factors to associate with transcription factors. Smad6 can directly bind CtBP [253]. Smads 3 and 4 can interact with NCoR and Sin3 through Dach1 [254]. Smad1 can also associate with Sin3a through Dach1 [255]. Smads 2, 3 and 4 can recruit NCoR as well as Sin3/HDAC through Ski [256-257]. Smad3 can associate with Hdac1 through TGIF2 [258]. Similarly, the transcription factor β-catenin can recruit epigenetic factors and influence the epigenetic state of cells (reviewed in [64]). β-catenin can associate with the HATs p300 and CBP [259-260] as well as TIP60 [261]. β-catenin can also associate with the chromatin remodeling factors Brg1 and ISWI [64]. Additionally, β-catenin can interact with the histone methyltransferases Mll1/Mll2 [261]. The Erk kinase, which is downstream of the MAPK pathway, can phosphorylate CBP [262], Smads 1-4 [263-265] as well as Brg1 and Brm [266]. Similarly, the Akt kinase, which is downstream of PI3K signaling, can associate with SWI/SNF components Ini1, Baf155 and Baf170, and can phosphorylate Baf155 [267]. Akt can interact with the histone methyltransferases Setdb1 [268] and Ezh2 and can phosphorylate and inhibit Ezh2 [269]. Akt can also phosphorylate and activate p300 [270]. Interestingly, the pluripotency factor Oct4 has also been shown to associate with numerous epigenetic factors including components of the NuRD HDAC complex (Chd4, p66α, p66β, Mbd3, Mta1-3 and Hdac1), chromatin remodeling proteins (Brg1, Baf155 and ISWI) and DNA methyltransferases (Dnmt3a and Dnmt3l) [271].

3.3 Cell polarity

Cell polarity is a feature of cellular physiology exhibited by epithelial cells. It refers to uneven spatial distribution of proteins across the cell, causing different parts of the cell to have different morphology and functions. Cell polarity can be classified as apical-basal polarity (epithelial cells), anterior-posterior polarity (neurons) and planar polarity (cochlea). In mammals, the apical-basal polarity of epithelial cells is regulated by three distinct protein complexes: the Crumbs/PALS1/PATJ complex, the Par3/Par6/aPKC complex and the Scribble/Dlg/Lgl complex. A detailed review of these complexes and their function in controlling epithelial architecture, cell migration and tumorigenesis can be found in [272]. The apical-basal polarity is lost during epithelial-to-mesenchymal transformation (EMT), a process that changes epithelial cells to mesenchymal cells with no apical-basal polarity and occurs during embryogenesis, fibrosis and cancer metastasis. Importantly, recent findings have indicated that epithelial cell polarity is required for early mouse embryogenesis and may be the driving factor for differentiation of certain early lineages. For example, the cell polarity regulator Par6 is required for proper trophectoderm formation in mouse embryos [273]. Downregulation of Par3 or aPKC drives blastomeres towards ICM instead of trophectoderm [274]. Interestingly, the Crumbs polarity complex has been found to interact with components of the Hippo signaling pathway [99], and the Hippo has been implicated in trophectoderm formation as discussed in the review. It will therefore be interesting to study whether cell polarity proteins indeed control trophectoderm differentiation during early stages of embryogenesis.

4. Conclusions

The development and morphogenesis of the embryo is under strict control by a rather small set of signaling pathways. However, the presence of multiple ligands and multiple receptors, numerous transcription factor-binding partners and significant crosstalk between pathways gives rise to vast complexity within this small set of signaling pathways. Further, lineage-specific differentiation is also controlled by complex regulation of various histone acetyltransferases, histone deacetylases, histone methyltransferases, histone demethylases, DNA methyltransferases and chromatin-remodeling enzymes. A detailed and molecular-level understanding of the determinants of lineage specificity of differentiation has only recently begun to emerge through studies of the signaling pathways and their downstream factors. We have summarized the signaling pathways and miRNAs associated with differentiation to various lineages in **Table 1**. Along similar lines, various histone modifying proteins and chromatin remodeling proteins associated with various lineages are summarized in **Table 2**. Even though these tables present a concise mechanistic linkage between various regulators of ESC differentiation, questions regarding how lineage-specific transcription factors are regulated and how a balance between opposing factors, such as HATs and HDACs, or HMTs and histone demethylases, is achieved in the cell remain largely unanswered. Further, the possible role of lineage-specific transcription factors in the recruitment of epigenetic factors also remains largely unknown. Thus, our understanding of the lineage-specificity of differentiation is still rudimentary and requires significant additional research.

Role of Signaling Pathways and Epigenetic Factors in Lineage Determination During
Human Embryonic Stem Cell Differentiation

39

Lineage	Signaling Pathways	Link with Lineage-specific Transcription Factors	Micro-RNAs
HESC	Activin/Nodal [23-24], FGF [24, 38-39, 54-55]	Smad2/3 activates Nanog promoter [25], Nanog binds and inhibits Smad1[275]	miR-302 [113-114], miR-145 [117]
Ectoderm	Block Activin/Nodal [12, 14]		
Mesoderm	Low Activin/Nodal [13, 18-19], Short-term BMP [18-19, 27], FGF [44-47], Wnt [66, 68-69, 73]	Smad1/5/8 binds Nanog promoter [25], Wnt3a activates Brachyury [67], β-catenin regulates Cripto promoter [70]	
Definitive Endoderm	High Activin/Nodal [13, 17, 20-21], Wnt [66, 68-69, 71, 73], Low PI3K [21, 85]	Wnt3a activates Brachyury [67]	
Epidermis	Block Activin/Nodal [12, 14], High BMP [15]	Smad1/5/8 binds Nanog promoter [25]	
Neural Plate / Neurogenesis	Block Activin/Nodal [12, 14, 22], Block BMP [15, 22], FGF [51, 53, 57, 60]		
Neural Crest	Block Activin/Nodal [12, 14], Low BMP [16], FGF [51, 57], Hippo [101] (?)	Smad1/5/8 binds Nanog promoter [25]d2 activates Pax3 promoter [101]	
Trophectoderm	Block Activin/Nodal [26], Long-term BMP[27-28], FGF[40-42, 56], Hippo [98]	Smad1/5/8 binds Nanog promoter [25], Ras/MAPK upregulates Cdx2 [42], Yap and Tead4 coactivate Cdx2 [98]	
Primitive Endoderm	FGF [40, 43]		
Hematopoietic Mesoderm	FGF [48-49]	FGF controls Runx1, Lmo2, Scl [50]	miR-181 [120]
Cardiac Mesoderm	Block Wnt [74]		miR-1 [119]
Adipocytic Mesoderm			miR-143 [121]

Table 1. Summary of signaling pathways, their link with lineage-specific transcription factors and micro-RNAs during embryogenesis and during hESC differentiation

Lineage	Epigenetic Factors					Chromatin Remodeling	Link with Lineage-specific Transcription factors
	HAT	HDAC	HMT	HDM	DNMT		
HESC	Tip60 [148]	NuRD [162]	Setdb1 [193]	KDM3A, KDM4C [207]		Brg1 [232] Baf155 [236] Baf250b [238] Snf2h [241]	Oct4 upregulates KDM3A and KDM4C. KDM4C upregulates Nanog [207], Oct4 associates with NuRD [271]
Ectoderm		NuRD [161]				Brg1 [237] NURF [244]	
Mesoderm						Brg1 [237] Baf250a [239] NURF [244]	Smad2 interacts with NURF [244], β-catenin can interact with Brg1 [64]
Definitive Endoderm						NURF [244]	Smad2 interacts with NURF [244]
Gametes		SirT2 [176]	Mll2 [185]	KDM3A [205-206]	Dnmt3l [224]		
Neural Plate/ Neurogenesis	Qkf [149]	HDAC1-2 [156], SirT1 [175]	G9a, GLP [195-196]	KDM6B [211-212] JHDM1D[214]	Dnmt3a, Dnmt3b [218-219]	Baf155 [236] Snf2l [242-243]	JHDM1D upregulates FGF4 [214]
Trophecto-derm		NuRD [163]			Dnmt3l [223]	Brg1 [232] Baf180 [235] Snf2h [241]	
Hematopoietic Mesoderm	Moz [150-152]	HDAC1-2 [156], NuRD [165-167]	Mll1 [183] Mll5 [187]				Smad2-4, 6-7 can interact with HDAC1-2 [252, 256-258], β-catenin can interact with Mll1 [261]
Cardiac Mesoderm		HDAC1-2 [156]				Baf60c [234] Baf180 [235] CHD1 [245]	Smad2-4, 6-7 can interact with HDAC1-2 [252, 256-258]
Adipocytic Mesoderm		SirT1 [174]	Mll3 [186]				
Myogenic Mesoderm		HDAC1-2 [156] SirT2 [173]				Baf60c [234]	Smad2-4, 6-7 can interact with HDAC1-2 [252, 256-258]
Primitive Endoderm		NuRD [161]				CHD1 [245]	

Table 2. Summary of epigenetic factors and their link with lineage-specific transcription factors during embryogenesis and during hESC differentiation. Abbreviations: HAT: Histone Acetyltransferase, HDAC: Histone Deacetylase, HDM: Histone Demethylase, DNMT: DNA Methyltransferase

Role of Signaling Pathways and Epigenetic Factors in Lineage Determination During
Human Embryonic Stem Cell Differentiation

41

5. Acknowledgments

The authors gratefully acknowledge funding support from the National Science Foundation
(NSF) Grant CBET-0966859.

6. References

[1] Thomson, J.A., et al., *Embryonic stem cell lines derived from human blastocysts*. Science, 1998. 282(5391): p. 1145-7.

[2] Gordon, K.J. and G.C. Blobe, *Role of transforming growth factor-beta superfamily signaling pathways in human disease*. Biochim Biophys Acta, 2008. 1782(4): p. 197-228.

[3] Blobe, G.C., W.P. Schiemann, and H.F. Lodish, *Role of transforming growth factor beta in human disease*. N Engl J Med, 2000. 342(18): p. 1350-8.

[4] Feng, X.H. and R. Derynck, *Specificity and versatility in tgf-beta signaling through Smads*. Annu Rev Cell Dev Biol, 2005. 21: p. 659-93.

[5] Shi, Y. and J. Massague, *Mechanisms of TGF-beta signaling from cell membrane to the nucleus*. Cell, 2003. 113(6): p. 685-700.

[6] Xu, L., *Regulation of Smad activities*. Biochim Biophys Acta, 2006. 1759(11-12): p. 503-13.

[7] Massague, J., J. Seoane, and D. Wotton, *Smad transcription factors*. Genes Dev, 2005. 19(23): p. 2783-810.

[8] Miyazawa, K., et al., *Two major Smad pathways in TGF-beta superfamily signalling*. Genes Cells, 2002. 7(12): p. 1191-204.

[9] Zhang, Y.E., *Non-Smad pathways in TGF-beta signaling*. Cell Res, 2009. 19(1): p. 128-39.

[10] Wu, M.Y. and C.S. Hill, *Tgf-beta superfamily signaling in embryonic development and homeostasis*. Dev Cell, 2009. 16(3): p. 329-43.

[11] Yamamoto, M., et al., *Nodal antagonists regulate formation of the anteroposterior axis of the mouse embryo*. Nature, 2004. 428(6981): p. 387-92.

[12] Schier, A.F., *Nodal signaling in vertebrate development*. Annu Rev Cell Dev Biol, 2003. 19: p. 589-621.

[13] Zorn, A.M. and J.M. Wells, *Molecular basis of vertebrate endoderm development*. Int Rev Cytol, 2007. 259: p. 49-111.

[14] Zhang, J., et al., *The role of maternal VegT in establishing the primary germ layers in Xenopus embryos*. Cell, 1998. 94(4): p. 515-24.

[15] Wilson, P.A., et al., *Concentration-dependent patterning of the Xenopus ectoderm by BMP4 and its signal transducer Smad1*. Development, 1997. 124(16): p. 3177-84.

[16] Sauka-Spengler, T. and M. Bronner-Fraser, *A gene regulatory network orchestrates neural crest formation*. Nat Rev Mol Cell Biol, 2008. 9(7): p. 557-68.

[17] D'Amour, K.A., et al., *Production of pancreatic hormone-expressing endocrine cells from human embryonic stem cells*. Nat Biotechnol, 2006. 24(11): p. 1392-401.

[18] Yao, S., et al., *Long-term self-renewal and directed differentiation of human embryonic stem cells in chemically defined conditions*. Proc Natl Acad Sci U S A, 2006. 103(18): p. 6907-12.

[19] Schuldiner, M., et al., *Effects of eight growth factors on the differentiation of cells derived from human embryonic stem cells*. Proc Natl Acad Sci U S A, 2000. 97(21): p. 11307-12.

[20] Kroon, E., et al., *Pancreatic endoderm derived from human embryonic stem cells generates glucose-responsive insulin-secreting cells in vivo*. Nat Biotechnol, 2008. 26(4): p. 443-52.

[21] D'Amour, K.A., et al., *Efficient differentiation of human embryonic stem cells to definitive endoderm*. Nat Biotechnol, 2005. 23(12): p. 1534-41.

[22] Chambers, S.M., et al., *Highly efficient neural conversion of human ES and iPS cells by dual inhibition of SMAD signaling*. Nat Biotechnol, 2009. 27(3): p. 275-80.

[23] James, D., et al., *TGFbeta/activin/nodal signaling is necessary for the maintenance of pluripotency in human embryonic stem cells*. Development, 2005. 132(6): p. 1273-82.

[24] Vallier, L., M. Alexander, and R.A. Pedersen, *Activin/Nodal and FGF pathways cooperate to maintain pluripotency of human embryonic stem cells*. J Cell Sci, 2005. 118(Pt 19): p. 4495-509.

[25] Xu, R.H., et al., *NANOG is a direct target of TGFbeta/activin-mediated SMAD signaling in human ESCs*. Cell Stem Cell, 2008. 3(2): p. 196-206.

[26] Wu, Z., et al., *Combinatorial signals of activin/nodal and bone morphogenic protein regulate the early lineage segregation of human embryonic stem cells*. J Biol Chem, 2008. 283(36): p. 24991-5002.

[27] Zhang, P., et al., *Short-term BMP-4 treatment initiates mesoderm induction in human embryonic stem cells*. Blood, 2008. 111(4): p. 1933-41.

[28] Xu, R.H., et al., *BMP4 initiates human embryonic stem cell differentiation to trophoblast*. Nat Biotechnol, 2002. 20(12): p. 1261-4.

[29] Suter, D.M. and K.H. Krause, *Neural commitment of embryonic stem cells: molecules, pathways and potential for cell therapy*. J Pathol, 2008. 215(4): p. 355-68.

[30] Villegas, S.N., M. Canham, and J.M. Brickman, *FGF signalling as a mediator of lineage transitions--evidence from embryonic stem cell differentiation*. J Cell Biochem, 2010. 110(1): p. 10-20.

[31] Dorey, K. and E. Amaya, *FGF signalling: diverse roles during early vertebrate embryogenesis*. Development, 2010. 137(22): p. 3731-42.

[32] Lanner, F. and J. Rossant, *The role of FGF/Erk signaling in pluripotent cells*. Development, 2010. 137(20): p. 3351-60.

[33] Kosaka, N., et al., *Pleiotropic function of FGF-4: its role in development and stem cells*. Dev Dyn, 2009. 238(2): p. 265-76.

[34] Ramos, J.W., *The regulation of extracellular signal-regulated kinase (ERK) in mammalian cells*. Int J Biochem Cell Biol, 2008. 40(12): p. 2707-19.

[35] Yoon, S. and R. Seger, *The extracellular signal-regulated kinase: multiple substrates regulate diverse cellular functions*. Growth Factors, 2006. 24(1): p. 21-44.

[36] Eivers, E., L.C. Fuentealba, and E.M. De Robertis, *Integrating positional information at the level of Smad1/5/8*. Curr Opin Genet Dev, 2008. 18(4): p. 304-10.

[37] Pera, E.M., et al., *Integration of IGF, FGF, and anti-BMP signals via Smad1 phosphorylation in neural induction*. Genes Dev, 2003. 17(24): p. 3023-8.

[38] Feldman, B., et al., *Requirement of FGF-4 for postimplantation mouse development*. Science, 1995. 267(5195): p. 246-9.

[39] Arman, E., et al., *Targeted disruption of fibroblast growth factor (FGF) receptor 2 suggests a role for FGF signaling in pregastrulation mammalian development*. Proc Natl Acad Sci U S A, 1998. 95(9): p. 5082-7.

[40] Goldin, S.N. and V.E. Papaioannou, *Paracrine action of FGF4 during periimplantation development maintains trophectoderm and primitive endoderm*. Genesis, 2003. 36(1): p. 40-7.

Role of Signaling Pathways and Epigenetic Factors in Lineage Determination During
Human Embryonic Stem Cell Differentiation

43

[41] Rappolee, D.A., et al., *Expression and function of FGF-4 in peri-implantation development in mouse embryos.* Development, 1994. 120(8): p. 2259-69.

[42] Lu, C.W., et al., *Ras-MAPK signaling promotes trophectoderm formation from embryonic stem cells and mouse embryos.* Nat Genet, 2008. 40(7): p. 921-6.

[43] Yamanaka, Y., F. Lanner, and J. Rossant, *FGF signal-dependent segregation of primitive endoderm and epiblast in the mouse blastocyst.* Development, 2010. 137(5): p. 715-24.

[44] Fletcher, R.B. and R.M. Harland, *The role of FGF signaling in the establishment and maintenance of mesodermal gene expression in Xenopus.* Dev Dyn, 2008. 237(5): p. 1243-54.

[45] Amaya, E., T.J. Musci, and M.W. Kirschner, *Expression of a dominant negative mutant of the FGF receptor disrupts mesoderm formation in Xenopus embryos.* Cell, 1991. 66(2): p. 257-70.

[46] Amaya, E., et al., *FGF signalling in the early specification of mesoderm in Xenopus.* Development, 1993. 118(2): p. 477-87.

[47] Ciruna, B. and J. Rossant, *FGF signaling regulates mesoderm cell fate specification and morphogenetic movement at the primitive streak.* Dev Cell, 2001. 1(1): p. 37-49.

[48] Isaacs, H.V., A.E. Deconinck, and M.E. Pownall, *FGF4 regulates blood and muscle specification in Xenopus laevis.* Biol Cell, 2007. 99(3): p. 165-73.

[49] Kumano, G. and W.C. Smith, *FGF signaling restricts the primary blood islands to ventral mesoderm.* Dev Biol, 2000. 228(2): p. 304-14.

[50] Walmsley, M., D. Cleaver, and R. Patient, *Fibroblast growth factor controls the timing of Scl, Lmo2, and Runx1 expression during embryonic blood development.* Blood, 2008. 111(3): p. 1157-66.

[51] Stern, C.D., *Neural induction: old problem, new findings, yet more questions.* Development, 2005. 132(9): p. 2007-21.

[52] Linker, C., et al., *Cell communication with the neural plate is required for induction of neural markers by BMP inhibition: evidence for homeogenetic induction and implications for Xenopus animal cap and chick explant assays.* Dev Biol, 2009. 327(2): p. 478-86.

[53] Wills, A.E., et al., *BMP antagonists and FGF signaling contribute to different domains of the neural plate in Xenopus.* Dev Biol, 2010. 337(2): p. 335-50.

[54] Chiao, E., et al., *Derivation of human embryonic stem cells in standard and chemically defined conditions.* Methods Cell Biol, 2008. 86: p. 1-14.

[55] Ludwig, T.E., et al., *Derivation of human embryonic stem cells in defined conditions.* Nat Biotechnol, 2006. 24(2): p. 185-7.

[56] Tanaka, S., et al., *Promotion of trophoblast stem cell proliferation by FGF4.* Science, 1998. 282(5396): p. 2072-5.

[57] Ying, Q.L., et al., *Conversion of embryonic stem cells into neuroectodermal precursors in adherent monoculture.* Nat Biotechnol, 2003. 21(2): p. 183-6.

[58] Smukler, S.R., et al., *Embryonic stem cells assume a primitive neural stem cell fate in the absence of extrinsic influences.* J Cell Biol, 2006. 172(1): p. 79-90.

[59] Holowacz, T. and S. Sokol, *FGF is required for posterior neural patterning but not for neural induction.* Dev Biol, 1999. 205(2): p. 296-308.

[60] Rentzsch, F., et al., *Fgf signaling induces posterior neuroectoderm independently of Bmp signaling inhibition.* Dev Dyn, 2004. 231(4): p. 750-7.

[61] MacDonald, B.T., K. Tamai, and X. He, *Wnt/beta-catenin signaling: components, mechanisms, and diseases.* Dev Cell, 2009. 17(1): p. 9-26.

[62] Sugimura, R. and L. Li, *Noncanonical Wnt signaling in vertebrate development, stem cells, and diseases*. Birth Defects Res C Embryo Today, 2010. 90(4): p. 243-56.

[63] Teo, J.L. and M. Kahn, *The Wnt signaling pathway in cellular proliferation and differentiation: A tale of two coactivators*. Adv Drug Deliv Rev, 2010. 62(12): p. 1149-55.

[64] Mosimann, C., G. Hausmann, and K. Basler, *Beta-catenin hits chromatin: regulation of Wnt target gene activation*. Nat Rev Mol Cell Biol, 2009. 10(4): p. 276-86.

[65] Yamaguchi, T.P., *Heads or tails: Wnts and anterior-posterior patterning*. Curr Biol, 2001. 11(17): p. R713-24.

[66] Liu, P., et al., *Requirement for Wnt3 in vertebrate axis formation*. Nat Genet, 1999. 22(4): p. 361-5.

[67] Yamaguchi, T.P., et al., *T (Brachyury) is a direct target of Wnt3a during paraxial mesoderm specification*. Genes Dev, 1999. 13(24): p. 3185-90.

[68] Huelsken, J., et al., *Requirement for beta-catenin in anterior-posterior axis formation in mice*. J Cell Biol, 2000. 148(3): p. 567-78.

[69] Kelly, O.G., K.I. Pinson, and W.C. Skarnes, *The Wnt co-receptors Lrp5 and Lrp6 are essential for gastrulation in mice*. Development, 2004. 131(12): p. 2803-15.

[70] Morkel, M., et al., *Beta-catenin regulates Cripto- and Wnt3-dependent gene expression programs in mouse axis and mesoderm formation*. Development, 2003. 130(25): p. 6283-94.

[71] Lickert, H., et al., *Formation of multiple hearts in mice following deletion of beta-catenin in the embryonic endoderm*. Dev Cell, 2002. 3(2): p. 171-81.

[72] Huelsken, J. and W. Birchmeier, *New aspects of Wnt signaling pathways in higher vertebrates*. Curr Opin Genet Dev, 2001. 11(5): p. 547-53.

[73] Sumi, T., et al., *Defining early lineage specification of human embryonic stem cells by the orchestrated balance of canonical Wnt/beta-catenin, Activin/Nodal and BMP signaling*. Development, 2008. 135(17): p. 2969-79.

[74] Paige, S.L., et al., *Endogenous Wnt/beta-catenin signaling is required for cardiac differentiation in human embryonic stem cells*. PLoS One, 2010. 5(6): p. e11134.

[75] Cantley, L.C., *The phosphoinositide 3-kinase pathway*. Science, 2002. 296(5573): p. 1655-7.

[76] Engelman, J.A., *Targeting PI3K signalling in cancer: opportunities, challenges and limitations*. Nat Rev Cancer, 2009. 9(8): p. 550-62.

[77] Engelman, J.A., J. Luo, and L.C. Cantley, *The evolution of phosphatidylinositol 3-kinases as regulators of growth and metabolism*. Nat Rev Genet, 2006. 7(8): p. 606-19.

[78] Wong, K.K., J.A. Engelman, and L.C. Cantley, *Targeting the PI3K signaling pathway in cancer*. Curr Opin Genet Dev, 2010. 20(1): p. 87-90.

[79] Ramasamy, T.S. and W. Cui, *Inhibition of phosphatidylinositol-3-kinase signalling promotes Activin A induced definitive endoderm differentiation of human embryonic stem cells*. Differentiation, 2010. 80: p. S25-S25.

[80] Franke, T.F., *PI3K/Akt: getting it right matters*. Oncogene, 2008. 27(50): p. 6473-88.

[81] Zheng, W. and K. Liu, *The emerging role of maternal phosphatidylinositol 3 kinase (PI3K) signaling in manipulating mammalian preimplantation embryogenesis*. Cell Cycle, 2011. 10(2): p. 178-9.

[82] O'Neill, C., *Phosphatidylinositol 3-kinase signaling in mammalian preimplantation embryo development*. Reproduction, 2008. 136(2): p. 147-56.

[83] Bi, L., et al., *Early embryonic lethality in mice deficient in the p110beta catalytic subunit of PI 3-kinase*. Mamm Genome, 2002. 13(3): p. 169-72.

Role of Signaling Pathways and Epigenetic Factors in Lineage Determination During
Human Embryonic Stem Cell Differentiation

45

[84]   Raff, M.C., et al., *Programmed cell death and the control of cell survival.* Philos Trans R Soc Lond B Biol Sci, 1994. 345(1313): p. 265-8.

[85]   McLean, A.B., et al., *Activin a efficiently specifies definitive endoderm from human embryonic stem cells only when phosphatidylinositol 3-kinase signaling is suppressed.* Stem Cells, 2007. 25(1): p. 29-38.

[86]   Zeng, Q. and W. Hong, *The emerging role of the hippo pathway in cell contact inhibition, organ size control, and cancer development in mammals.* Cancer Cell, 2008. 13(3): p. 188-92.

[87]   Oh, H. and K.D. Irvine, *Yorkie: the final destination of Hippo signaling.* Trends Cell Biol, 2010. 20(7): p. 410-7.

[88]   Lei, Q.Y., et al., *TAZ promotes cell proliferation and epithelial-mesenchymal transition and is inhibited by the hippo pathway.* Mol Cell Biol, 2008. 28(7): p. 2426-36.

[89]   Kanai, F., et al., *TAZ: a novel transcriptional co-activator regulated by interactions with 14-3-3 and PDZ domain proteins.* EMBO J, 2000. 19(24): p. 6778-91.

[90]   Oka, T. and M. Sudol, *Nuclear localization and pro-apoptotic signaling of YAP2 require intact PDZ-binding motif.* Genes Cells, 2009. 14(5): p. 607-15.

[91]   Ferrigno, O., et al., *Yes-associated protein (YAP65) interacts with Smad7 and potentiates its inhibitory activity against TGF-beta/Smad signaling.* Oncogene, 2002. 21(32): p. 4879-84.

[92]   Chan, S.W., et al., *TEADs mediate nuclear retention of TAZ to promote oncogenic transformation.* J Biol Chem, 2009. 284(21): p. 14347-58.

[93]   Varelas, X., et al., *TAZ controls Smad nucleocytoplasmic shuttling and regulates human embryonic stem-cell self-renewal.* Nat Cell Biol, 2008. 10(7): p. 837-48.

[94]   Cao, X., S.L. Pfaff, and F.H. Gage, *YAP regulates neural progenitor cell number via the TEA domain transcription factor.* Genes Dev, 2008. 22(23): p. 3320-34.

[95]   Wang, K., et al., *YAP, TAZ, and Yorkie: a conserved family of signal-responsive transcriptional coregulators in animal development and human disease.* Biochem Cell Biol, 2009. 87(1): p. 77-91.

[96]   Alarcon, C., et al., *Nuclear CDKs drive Smad transcriptional activation and turnover in BMP and TGF-beta pathways.* Cell, 2009. 139(4): p. 757-69.

[97]   Varelas, X., et al., *The Hippo pathway regulates Wnt/beta-catenin signaling.* Dev Cell, 2010. 18(4): p. 579-91.

[98]   Nishioka, N., et al., *The Hippo signaling pathway components Lats and Yap pattern Tead4 activity to distinguish mouse trophectoderm from inner cell mass.* Dev Cell, 2009. 16(3): p. 398-410.

[99]   Varelas, X., et al., *The Crumbs complex couples cell density sensing to Hippo-dependent control of the TGF-beta-SMAD pathway.* Dev Cell, 2010. 19(6): p. 831-44.

[100] Lian, I., et al., *The role of YAP transcription coactivator in regulating stem cell self-renewal and differentiation.* Genes Dev, 2010. 24(11): p. 1106-18.

[101] Milewski, R.C., et al., *Identification of minimal enhancer elements sufficient for Pax3 expression in neural crest and implication of Tead2 as a regulator of Pax3.* Development, 2004. 131(4): p. 829-37.

[102] Sawada, A., et al., *Redundant roles of Tead1 and Tead2 in notochord development and the regulation of cell proliferation and survival.* Mol Cell Biol, 2008. 28(10): p. 3177-89.

[103] Guo, X. and X.F. Wang, *Signaling cross-talk between TGF-beta/BMP and other pathways.* Cell Res, 2009. 19(1): p. 71-88.

[104] Xiao, L., X. Yuan, and S.J. Sharkis, *Activin A maintains self-renewal and regulates fibroblast growth factor, Wnt, and bone morphogenic protein pathways in human embryonic stem cells.* Stem Cells, 2006. 24(6): p. 1476-86.

[105] Katoh, M., *CER1 is a common target of WNT and NODAL signaling pathways in human embryonic stem cells.* Int J Mol Med, 2006. 17(5): p. 795-9.

[106] Wienholds, E. and R.H. Plasterk, *MicroRNA function in animal development.* FEBS Lett, 2005. 579(26): p. 5911-22.

[107] Tiscornia, G. and J.C. Izpisua Belmonte, *MicroRNAs in embryonic stem cell function and fate.* Genes Dev, 2010. 24(24): p. 2732-41.

[108] Navarro, A. and M. Monzo, *MicroRNAs in human embryonic and cancer stem cells.* Yonsei Med J, 2010. 51(5): p. 622-32.

[109] Wienholds, E., et al., *The microRNA-producing enzyme Dicer1 is essential for zebrafish development.* Nat Genet, 2003. 35(3): p. 217-8.

[110] Wienholds, E., et al., *MicroRNA expression in zebrafish embryonic development.* Science, 2005. 309(5732): p. 310-1.

[111] Bernstein, E., et al., *Dicer is essential for mouse development.* Nat Genet, 2003. 35(3): p. 215-7.

[112] Kanellopoulou, C., et al., *Dicer-deficient mouse embryonic stem cells are defective in differentiation and centromeric silencing.* Genes Dev, 2005. 19(4): p. 489-501.

[113] Lin, S.L., et al., *Regulation of somatic cell reprogramming through inducible mir-302 expression.* Nucleic Acids Res, 2011. 39(3): p. 1054-65.

[114] Lin, S.L., et al., *Mir-302 reprograms human skin cancer cells into a pluripotent ES-cell-like state.* RNA, 2008. 14(10): p. 2115-24.

[115] Tay, Y., et al., *MicroRNAs to Nanog, Oct4 and Sox2 coding regions modulate embryonic stem cell differentiation.* Nature, 2008. 455(7216): p. 1124-8.

[116] Wellner, U., et al., *The EMT-activator ZEB1 promotes tumorigenicity by repressing stemness-inhibiting microRNAs.* Nat Cell Biol, 2009. 11(12): p. 1487-95.

[117] Xu, N., et al., *MicroRNA-145 regulates OCT4, SOX2, and KLF4 and represses pluripotency in human embryonic stem cells.* Cell, 2009. 137(4): p. 647-58.

[118] Melton, C., R.L. Judson, and R. Blelloch, *Opposing microRNA families regulate self-renewal in mouse embryonic stem cells.* Nature, 2010. 463(7281): p. 621-6.

[119] Zhao, Y., E. Samal, and D. Srivastava, *Serum response factor regulates a muscle-specific microRNA that targets Hand2 during cardiogenesis.* Nature, 2005. 436(7048): p. 214-20.

[120] Chen, C.Z., et al., *MicroRNAs modulate hematopoietic lineage differentiation.* Science, 2004. 303(5654): p. 83-6.

[121] Esau, C., et al., *MicroRNA-143 regulates adipocyte differentiation.* J Biol Chem, 2004. 279(50): p. 52361-5.

[122] Kawasaki, H. and K. Taira, *MicroRNA-196 inhibits HOXB8 expression in myeloid differentiation of HL60 cells.* Nucleic Acids Symp Ser (Oxf), 2004(48): p. 211-2.

[123] Hornstein, E., et al., *The microRNA miR-196 acts upstream of Hoxb8 and Shh in limb development.* Nature, 2005. 438(7068): p. 671-4.

[124] Yekta, S., I.H. Shih, and D.P. Bartel, *MicroRNA-directed cleavage of HOXB8 mRNA.* Science, 2004. 304(5670): p. 594-6.

[125] Choi, P.S., et al., *Members of the miRNA-200 family regulate olfactory neurogenesis.* Neuron, 2008. 57(1): p. 41-55.

Role of Signaling Pathways and Epigenetic Factors in Lineage Determination During
Human Embryonic Stem Cell Differentiation

47

[126] Yi, R., et al., *Morphogenesis in skin is governed by discrete sets of differentially expressed microRNAs.* Nat Genet, 2006. 38(3): p. 356-62.

[127] Lim, L.P., et al., *Microarray analysis shows that some microRNAs downregulate large numbers of target mRNAs.* Nature, 2005. 433(7027): p. 769-73.

[128] Rodriguez, A., et al., *Identification of mammalian microRNA host genes and transcription units.* Genome Res, 2004. 14(10A): p. 1902-10.

[129] Tsai, Z.Y., et al., *Identification of microRNAs regulated by activin A in human embryonic stem cells.* J Cell Biochem, 2010. 109(1): p. 93-102.

[130] Boyer, L.A., et al., *Core transcriptional regulatory circuitry in human embryonic stem cells.* Cell, 2005. 122(6): p. 947-56.

[131] Davis, B.N., et al., *SMAD proteins control DROSHA-mediated microRNA maturation.* Nature, 2008. 454(7200): p. 56-61.

[132] Davis, B.N., et al., *Smad proteins bind a conserved RNA sequence to promote microRNA maturation by Drosha.* Mol Cell, 2010. 39(3): p. 373-84.

[133] Paroo, Z., et al., *Phosphorylation of the human microRNA-generating complex mediates MAPK/Erk signaling.* Cell, 2009. 139(1): p. 112-22.

[134] Lessard, J.A. and G.R. Crabtree, *Chromatin regulatory mechanisms in pluripotency.* Annu Rev Cell Dev Biol, 2010. 26: p. 503-32.

[135] Turner, B.M., *Histone acetylation and an epigenetic code.* Bioessays, 2000. 22(9): p. 836-45.

[136] Strahl, B.D. and C.D. Allis, *The language of covalent histone modifications.* Nature, 2000. 403(6765): p. 41-5.

[137] Hirabayashi, Y. and Y. Gotoh, *Epigenetic control of neural precursor cell fate during development.* Nat Rev Neurosci, 2010. 11(6): p. 377-88.

[138] Shahbazian, M.D. and M. Grunstein, *Functions of site-specific histone acetylation and deacetylation.* Annu Rev Biochem, 2007. 76: p. 75-100.

[139] Carrozza, M.J., et al., *The diverse functions of histone acetyltransferase complexes.* Trends Genet, 2003. 19(6): p. 321-9.

[140] Lee, K.K. and J.L. Workman, *Histone acetyltransferase complexes: one size doesn't fit all.* Nat Rev Mol Cell Biol, 2007. 8(4): p. 284-95.

[141] Dhalluin, C., et al., *Structure and ligand of a histone acetyltransferase bromodomain.* Nature, 1999. 399(6735): p. 491-6.

[142] Hassan, A.H., et al., *Function and selectivity of bromodomains in anchoring chromatin-modifying complexes to promoter nucleosomes.* Cell, 2002. 111(3): p. 369-79.

[143] Doyon, Y., et al., *Structural and functional conservation of the NuA4 histone acetyltransferase complex from yeast to humans.* Mol Cell Biol, 2004. 24(5): p. 1884-96.

[144] Pray-Grant, M.G., et al., *Chd1 chromodomain links histone H3 methylation with SAGA- and SLIK-dependent acetylation.* Nature, 2005. 433(7024): p. 434-8.

[145] Schreiber, S.L. and B.E. Bernstein, *Signaling network model of chromatin.* Cell, 2002. 111(6): p. 771-8.

[146] Gupta, A., et al., *The mammalian ortholog of Drosophila MOF that acetylates histone H4 lysine 16 is essential for embryogenesis and oncogenesis.* Mol Cell Biol, 2008. 28(1): p. 397-409.

[147] Hu, Y., et al., *Homozygous disruption of the Tip60 gene causes early embryonic lethality.* Dev Dyn, 2009. 238(11): p. 2912-21.

[148] Fazzio, T.G., J.T. Huff, and B. Panning, *An RNAi screen of chromatin proteins identifies Tip60-p400 as a regulator of embryonic stem cell identity.* Cell, 2008. 134(1): p. 162-74.

[149] Thomas, T., et al., *Querkopf, a MYST family histone acetyltransferase, is required for normal cerebral cortex development.* Development, 2000. 127(12): p. 2537-48.

[150] Perez-Campo, F.M., et al., *The histone acetyl transferase activity of monocytic leukemia zinc finger is critical for the proliferation of hematopoietic precursors.* Blood, 2009. 113(20): p. 4866-74.

[151] Thomas, T., et al., *Monocytic leukemia zinc finger protein is essential for the development of long-term reconstituting hematopoietic stem cells.* Genes Dev, 2006. 20(9): p. 1175-86.

[152] Katsumoto, T., et al., *MOZ is essential for maintenance of hematopoietic stem cells.* Genes Dev, 2006. 20(10): p. 1321-30.

[153] Dokmanovic, M., C. Clarke, and P.A. Marks, *Histone deacetylase inhibitors: overview and perspectives.* Mol Cancer Res, 2007. 5(10): p. 981-9.

[154] Gray, S.G. and T.J. Ekstrom, *The human histone deacetylase family.* Exp Cell Res, 2001. 262(2): p. 75-83.

[155] Khochbin, S., et al., *Functional significance of histone deacetylase diversity.* Curr Opin Genet Dev, 2001. 11(2): p. 162-6.

[156] Brunmeir, R., S. Lagger, and C. Seiser, *Histone deacetylase HDAC1/HDAC2-controlled embryonic development and cell differentiation.* Int J Dev Biol, 2009. 53(2-3): p. 275-89.

[157] van Grunsven, L.A., et al., *Smads and chromatin modulation.* Cytokine Growth Factor Rev, 2005. 16(4-5): p. 495-512.

[158] McDonel, P., I. Costello, and B. Hendrich, *Keeping things quiet: roles of NuRD and Sin3 co-repressor complexes during mammalian development.* Int J Biochem Cell Biol, 2009. 41(1): p. 108-16.

[159] Hendrich, B., et al., *Closely related proteins MBD2 and MBD3 play distinctive but interacting roles in mouse development.* Genes Dev, 2001. 15(6): p. 710-23.

[160] Marino, S. and R. Nusse, *Mutants in the mouse NuRD/Mi2 component P66alpha are embryonic lethal.* PLoS One, 2007. 2(6): p. e519.

[161] Kaji, K., J. Nichols, and B. Hendrich, *Mbd3, a component of the NuRD co-repressor complex, is required for development of pluripotent cells.* Development, 2007. 134(6): p. 1123-32.

[162] Kaji, K., et al., *The NuRD component Mbd3 is required for pluripotency of embryonic stem cells.* Nat Cell Biol, 2006. 8(3): p. 285-92.

[163] Zhu, D., et al., *Mbd3, a component of NuRD/Mi-2 complex, helps maintain pluripotency of mouse embryonic stem cells by repressing trophectoderm differentiation.* PLoS One, 2009. 4(11): p. e7684.

[164] Kashiwagi, M., B.A. Morgan, and K. Georgopoulos, *The chromatin remodeler Mi-2beta is required for establishment of the basal epidermis and normal differentiation of its progeny.* Development, 2007. 134(8): p. 1571-82.

[165] Naito, T., et al., *Antagonistic interactions between Ikaros and the chromatin remodeler Mi-2beta determine silencer activity and Cd4 gene expression.* Immunity, 2007. 27(5): p. 723-34.

[166] Williams, C.J., et al., *The chromatin remodeler Mi-2beta is required for CD4 expression and T cell development.* Immunity, 2004. 20(6): p. 719-33.

[167] Yoshida, T., et al., *The role of the chromatin remodeler Mi-2beta in hematopoietic stem cell self-renewal and multilineage differentiation.* Genes Dev, 2008. 22(9): p. 1174-89.

[168] Cowley, S.M., et al., *The mSin3A chromatin-modifying complex is essential for embryogenesis and T-cell development.* Mol Cell Biol, 2005. 25(16): p. 6990-7004.

Role of Signaling Pathways and Epigenetic Factors in Lineage Determination During
Human Embryonic Stem Cell Differentiation

49

[169] Dannenberg, J.H., et al., *mSin3A corepressor regulates diverse transcriptional networks governing normal and neoplastic growth and survival.* Genes Dev, 2005. 19(13): p. 1581-95.

[170] David, G., et al., *Specific requirement of the chromatin modifier mSin3B in cell cycle exit and cellular differentiation.* Proc Natl Acad Sci U S A, 2008. 105(11): p. 4168-72.

[171] Vaquero, A., *The conserved role of sirtuins in chromatin regulation.* Int J Dev Biol, 2009. 53(2-3): p. 303-22.

[172] Kuzmichev, A., et al., *Composition and histone substrates of polycomb repressive group complexes change during cellular differentiation.* Proc Natl Acad Sci U S A, 2005. 102(6): p. 1859-64.

[173] Fulco, M., et al., *Sir2 regulates skeletal muscle differentiation as a potential sensor of the redox state.* Mol Cell, 2003. 12(1): p. 51-62.

[174] Picard, F., et al., *Sirt1 promotes fat mobilization in white adipocytes by repressing PPAR-gamma.* Nature, 2004. 429(6993): p. 771-6.

[175] Prozorovski, T., et al., *Sirt1 contributes critically to the redox-dependent fate of neural progenitors.* Nat Cell Biol, 2008. 10(4): p. 385-94.

[176] McBurney, M.W., et al., *The mammalian SIR2alpha protein has a role in embryogenesis and gametogenesis.* Mol Cell Biol, 2003. 23(1): p. 38-54.

[177] Dambacher, S., M. Hahn, and G. Schotta, *Epigenetic regulation of development by histone lysine methylation.* Heredity, 2010. 105(1): p. 24-37.

[178] Barski, A., et al., *High-resolution profiling of histone methylations in the human genome.* Cell, 2007. 129(4): p. 823-37.

[179] Cui, K., et al., *Chromatin signatures in multipotent human hematopoietic stem cells indicate the fate of bivalent genes during differentiation.* Cell Stem Cell, 2009. 4(1): p. 80-93.

[180] Pauler, F.M., et al., *H3K27me3 forms BLOCs over silent genes and intergenic regions and specifies a histone banding pattern on a mouse autosomal chromosome.* Genome Res, 2009. 19(2): p. 221-33.

[181] Yagi, H., et al., *Growth disturbance in fetal liver hematopoiesis of Mll-mutant mice.* Blood, 1998. 92(1): p. 108-17.

[182] Yu, B.D., et al., *Altered Hox expression and segmental identity in Mll-mutant mice.* Nature, 1995. 378(6556): p. 505-8.

[183] Ernst, P., et al., *Definitive hematopoiesis requires the mixed-lineage leukemia gene.* Dev Cell, 2004. 6(3): p. 437-43.

[184] Glaser, S., et al., *Multiple epigenetic maintenance factors implicated by the loss of Mll2 in mouse development.* Development, 2006. 133(8): p. 1423-32.

[185] Glaser, S., et al., *The histone 3 lysine 4 methyltransferase, Mll2, is only required briefly in development and spermatogenesis.* Epigenetics Chromatin, 2009. 2(1): p. 5.

[186] Lee, J., et al., *Targeted inactivation of MLL3 histone H3-Lys-4 methyltransferase activity in the mouse reveals vital roles for MLL3 in adipogenesis.* Proc Natl Acad Sci U S A, 2008. 105(49): p. 19229-34.

[187] Heuser, M., et al., *Loss of MLL5 results in pleiotropic hematopoietic defects, reduced neutrophil immune function, and extreme sensitivity to DNA demethylation.* Blood, 2009. 113(7): p. 1432-43.

[188] O'Carroll, D., et al., *The polycomb-group gene Ezh2 is required for early mouse development.* Mol Cell Biol, 2001. 21(13): p. 4330-6.

[189] Ezhkova, E., et al., *Ezh2 orchestrates gene expression for the stepwise differentiation of tissue-specific stem cells.* Cell, 2009. 136(6): p. 1122-35.

[190] Margueron, R., et al., *Ezh1 and Ezh2 maintain repressive chromatin through different mechanisms.* Mol Cell, 2008. 32(4): p. 503-18.

[191] Su, I.H., et al., *Ezh2 controls B cell development through histone H3 methylation and Igh rearrangement.* Nat Immunol, 2003. 4(2): p. 124-31.

[192] Peters, A.H., et al., *Loss of the Suv39h histone methyltransferases impairs mammalian heterochromatin and genome stability.* Cell, 2001. 107(3): p. 323-37.

[193] Dodge, J.E., et al., *Histone H3-K9 methyltransferase ESET is essential for early development.* Mol Cell Biol, 2004. 24(6): p. 2478-86.

[194] Takada, I., et al., *A histone lysine methyltransferase activated by non-canonical Wnt signalling suppresses PPAR-gamma transactivation.* Nat Cell Biol, 2007. 9(11): p. 1273-85.

[195] Tachibana, M., et al., *Histone methyltransferases G9a and GLP form heteromeric complexes and are both crucial for methylation of euchromatin at H3-K9.* Genes Dev, 2005. 19(7): p. 815-26.

[196] Tachibana, M., et al., *G9a histone methyltransferase plays a dominant role in euchromatic histone H3 lysine 9 methylation and is essential for early embryogenesis.* Genes Dev, 2002. 16(14): p. 1779-91.

[197] Feldman, N., et al., *G9a-mediated irreversible epigenetic inactivation of Oct-3/4 during early embryogenesis.* Nat Cell Biol, 2006. 8(2): p. 188-94.

[198] Epsztejn-Litman, S., et al., *De novo DNA methylation promoted by G9a prevents reprogramming of embryonically silenced genes.* Nat Struct Mol Biol, 2008. 15(11): p. 1176-83.

[199] Wagschal, A., et al., *G9a histone methyltransferase contributes to imprinting in the mouse placenta.* Mol Cell Biol, 2008. 28(3): p. 1104-13.

[200] Pedersen, M.T. and K. Helin, *Histone demethylases in development and disease.* Trends Cell Biol, 2010. 20(11): p. 662-71.

[201] Shi, Y., *Histone lysine demethylases: emerging roles in development, physiology and disease.* Nat Rev Genet, 2007. 8(11): p. 829-33.

[202] Wang, J., et al., *The lysine demethylase LSD1 (KDM1) is required for maintenance of global DNA methylation.* Nat Genet, 2009. 41(1): p. 125-9.

[203] Ciccone, D.N., et al., *KDM1B is a histone H3K4 demethylase required to establish maternal genomic imprints.* Nature, 2009. 461(7262): p. 415-8.

[204] Fan, Z., et al., *BCOR regulates mesenchymal stem cell function by epigenetic mechanisms.* Nat Cell Biol, 2009. 11(8): p. 1002-9.

[205] Liu, Z., et al., *Jmjd1a demethylase-regulated histone modification is essential for cAMP-response element modulator-regulated gene expression and spermatogenesis.* J Biol Chem, 2010. 285(4): p. 2758-70.

[206] Okada, Y., et al., *Histone demethylase JHDM2A is critical for Tnp1 and Prm1 transcription and spermatogenesis.* Nature, 2007. 450(7166): p. 119-23.

[207] Loh, Y.H., et al., *Jmjd1a and Jmjd2c histone H3 Lys 9 demethylases regulate self-renewal in embryonic stem cells.* Genes Dev, 2007. 21(20): p. 2545-57.

[208] Lopez-Bigas, N., et al., *Genome-wide analysis of the H3K4 histone demethylase RBP2 reveals a transcriptional program controlling differentiation.* Mol Cell, 2008. 31(4): p. 520-30.

Role of Signaling Pathways and Epigenetic Factors in Lineage Determination During
Human Embryonic Stem Cell Differentiation

51

[209] Agger, K., et al., *UTX and JMJD3 are histone H3K27 demethylases involved in HOX gene regulation and development.* Nature, 2007. 449(7163): p. 731-4.

[210] Lan, F., et al., *A histone H3 lysine 27 demethylase regulates animal posterior development.* Nature, 2007. 449(7163): p. 689-94.

[211] Burgold, T., et al., *The histone H3 lysine 27-specific demethylase Jmjd3 is required for neural commitment.* PLoS One, 2008. 3(8): p. e3034.

[212] Jepsen, K., et al., *SMRT-mediated repression of an H3K27 demethylase in progression from neural stem cell to neuron.* Nature, 2007. 450(7168): p. 415-9.

[213] Sen, G.L., et al., *Control of differentiation in a self-renewing mammalian tissue by the histone demethylase JMJD3.* Genes Dev, 2008. 22(14): p. 1865-70.

[214] Huang, C., et al., *Dual-specificity histone demethylase KIAA1718 (KDM7A) regulates neural differentiation through FGF4.* Cell Res, 2010. 20(2): p. 154-65.

[215] Lan, J., et al., *DNA methyltransferases and methyl-binding proteins of mammals.* Acta Biochim Biophys Sin (Shanghai), 2010. 42(4): p. 243-52.

[216] Latham, T., N. Gilbert, and B. Ramsahoye, *DNA methylation in mouse embryonic stem cells and development.* Cell Tissue Res, 2008. 331(1): p. 31-55.

[217] Lei, H., et al., *De novo DNA cytosine methyltransferase activities in mouse embryonic stem cells.* Development, 1996. 122(10): p. 3195-205.

[218] Okano, M. and E. Li, *Genetic analyses of DNA methyltransferase genes in mouse model system.* J Nutr, 2002. 132(8 Suppl): p. 2462S-2465S.

[219] Okano, M., et al., *DNA methyltransferases Dnmt3a and Dnmt3b are essential for de novo methylation and mammalian development.* Cell, 1999. 99(3): p. 247-57.

[220] Watanabe, D., et al., *Stage- and cell-specific expression of Dnmt3a and Dnmt3b during embryogenesis.* Mech Dev, 2002. 118(1-2): p. 187-90.

[221] Watanabe, D., et al., *Expression of Dnmt3b in mouse hematopoietic progenitor cells and spermatogonia at specific stages.* Gene Expr Patterns, 2004. 5(1): p. 43-9.

[222] Watanabe, D., K. Uchiyama, and K. Hanaoka, *Transition of mouse de novo methyltransferases expression from Dnmt3b to Dnmt3a during neural progenitor cell development.* Neuroscience, 2006. 142(3): p. 727-37.

[223] Arima, T., et al., *Loss of the maternal imprint in Dnmt3Lmat-/- mice leads to a differentiation defect in the extraembryonic tissue.* Dev Biol, 2006. 297(2): p. 361-73.

[224] Webster, K.E., et al., *Meiotic and epigenetic defects in Dnmt3L-knockout mouse spermatogenesis.* Proc Natl Acad Sci U S A, 2005. 102(11): p. 4068-73.

[225] Hata, K., et al., *Dnmt3L cooperates with the Dnmt3 family of de novo DNA methyltransferases to establish maternal imprints in mice.* Development, 2002. 129(8): p. 1983-93.

[226] Kaneda, M., et al., *Essential role for de novo DNA methyltransferase Dnmt3a in paternal and maternal imprinting.* Nature, 2004. 429(6994): p. 900-3.

[227] Tsumura, A., et al., *Maintenance of self-renewal ability of mouse embryonic stem cells in the absence of DNA methyltransferases Dnmt1, Dnmt3a and Dnmt3b.* Genes Cells, 2006. 11(7): p. 805-14.

[228] Jackson, M., et al., *Severe global DNA hypomethylation blocks differentiation and induces histone hyperacetylation in embryonic stem cells.* Mol Cell Biol, 2004. 24(20): p. 8862-71.

[229] Saladi, S.V. and I.L. de la Serna, *ATP dependent chromatin remodeling enzymes in embryonic stem cells.* Stem Cell Rev, 2010. 6(1): p. 62-73.

[230] de la Serna, I.L., Y. Ohkawa, and A.N. Imbalzano, *Chromatin remodelling in mammalian differentiation: lessons from ATP-dependent remodellers*. Nat Rev Genet, 2006. 7(6): p. 461-73.

[231] Moshkin, Y.M., et al., *Functional differentiation of SWI/SNF remodelers in transcription and cell cycle control*. Mol Cell Biol, 2007. 27(2): p. 651-61.

[232] Bultman, S., et al., *A Brg1 null mutation in the mouse reveals functional differences among mammalian SWI/SNF complexes*. Mol Cell, 2000. 6(6): p. 1287-95.

[233] Guidi, C.J., et al., *Disruption of Ini1 leads to peri-implantation lethality and tumorigenesis in mice*. Mol Cell Biol, 2001. 21(10): p. 3598-603.

[234] Lickert, H., et al., *Baf60c is essential for function of BAF chromatin remodelling complexes in heart development*. Nature, 2004. 432(7013): p. 107-12.

[235] Wang, Z., et al., *Polybromo protein BAF180 functions in mammalian cardiac chamber maturation*. Genes Dev, 2004. 18(24): p. 3106-16.

[236] Kim, J.K., et al., *Srg3, a mouse homolog of yeast SWI3, is essential for early embryogenesis and involved in brain development*. Mol Cell Biol, 2001. 21(22): p. 7787-95.

[237] Ho, L., et al., *An embryonic stem cell chromatin remodeling complex, esBAF, is essential for embryonic stem cell self-renewal and pluripotency*. Proc Natl Acad Sci U S A, 2009. 106(13): p. 5181-6.

[238] Yan, Z., et al., *BAF250B-associated SWI/SNF chromatin-remodeling complex is required to maintain undifferentiated mouse embryonic stem cells*. Stem Cells, 2008. 26(5): p. 1155-65.

[239] Gao, X., et al., *ES cell pluripotency and germ-layer formation require the SWI/SNF chromatin remodeling component BAF250a*. Proc Natl Acad Sci U S A, 2008. 105(18): p. 6656-61.

[240] Schaniel, C., et al., *Smarcc1/Baf155 couples self-renewal gene repression with changes in chromatin structure in mouse embryonic stem cells*. Stem Cells, 2009. 27(12): p. 2979-91.

[241] Stopka, T. and A.I. Skoultchi, *The ISWI ATPase Snf2h is required for early mouse development*. Proc Natl Acad Sci U S A, 2003. 100(24): p. 14097-102.

[242] Banting, G.S., et al., *CECR2, a protein involved in neurulation, forms a novel chromatin remodeling complex with SNF2L*. Hum Mol Genet, 2005. 14(4): p. 513-24.

[243] Barak, O., et al., *Isolation of human NURF: a regulator of Engrailed gene expression*. EMBO J, 2003. 22(22): p. 6089-100.

[244] Landry, J., et al., *Essential role of chromatin remodeling protein Bptf in early mouse embryos and embryonic stem cells*. PLoS Genet, 2008. 4(10): p. e1000241.

[245] Gaspar-Maia, A., et al., *Chd1 regulates open chromatin and pluripotency of embryonic stem cells*. Nature, 2009. 460(7257): p. 863-8.

[246] Bosman, E.A., et al., *Multiple mutations in mouse Chd7 provide models for CHARGE syndrome*. Hum Mol Genet, 2005. 14(22): p. 3463-76.

[247] Pouponnot, C., L. Jayaraman, and J. Massague, *Physical and functional interaction of SMADs and p300/CBP*. J Biol Chem, 1998. 273(36): p. 22865-8.

[248] Itoh, S., et al., *The transcriptional co-activator P/CAF potentiates TGF-beta/Smad signaling*. Nucleic Acids Res, 2000. 28(21): p. 4291-8.

[249] Kahata, K., et al., *Regulation of transforming growth factor-beta and bone morphogenetic protein signalling by transcriptional coactivator GCN5*. Genes Cells, 2004. 9(2): p. 143-51.

[250] Frontelo, P., et al., *Suv39h histone methyltransferases interact with Smads and cooperate in BMP-induced repression*. Oncogene, 2004. 23(30): p. 5242-51.

Role of Signaling Pathways and Epigenetic Factors in Lineage Determination During
Human Embryonic Stem Cell Differentiation

53

[251] Gronroos, E., et al., *Control of Smad7 stability by competition between acetylation and ubiquitination.* Mol Cell, 2002. 10(3): p. 483-93.

[252] Bai, S. and X. Cao, *A nuclear antagonistic mechanism of inhibitory Smads in transforming growth factor-beta signaling.* J Biol Chem, 2002. 277(6): p. 4176-82.

[253] Lin, X., et al., *Smad6 recruits transcription corepressor CtBP to repress bone morphogenetic protein-induced transcription.* Mol Cell Biol, 2003. 23(24): p. 9081-93.

[254] Wu, K., et al., *DACH1 inhibits transforming growth factor-beta signaling through binding Smad4.* J Biol Chem, 2003. 278(51): p. 51673-84.

[255] Kida, Y., et al., *Chick Dach1 interacts with the Smad complex and Sin3a to control AER formation and limb development along the proximodistal axis.* Development, 2004. 131(17): p. 4179-87.

[256] Luo, K., et al., *The Ski oncoprotein interacts with the Smad proteins to repress TGFbeta signaling.* Genes Dev, 1999. 13(17): p. 2196-206.

[257] Akiyoshi, S., et al., *c-Ski acts as a transcriptional co-repressor in transforming growth factor-beta signaling through interaction with smads.* J Biol Chem, 1999. 274(49): p. 35269-77.

[258] Melhuish, T.A., C.M. Gallo, and D. Wotton, *TGIF2 interacts with histone deacetylase 1 and represses transcription.* J Biol Chem, 2001. 276(34): p. 32109-14.

[259] Hecht, A., et al., *The p300/CBP acetyltransferases function as transcriptional coactivators of beta-catenin in vertebrates.* EMBO J, 2000. 19(8): p. 1839-50.

[260] Takemaru, K.I. and R.T. Moon, *The transcriptional coactivator CBP interacts with beta-catenin to activate gene expression.* J Cell Biol, 2000. 149(2): p. 249-54.

[261] Sierra, J., et al., *The APC tumor suppressor counteracts beta-catenin activation and H3K4 methylation at Wnt target genes.* Genes Dev, 2006. 20(5): p. 586-600.

[262] Janknecht, R. and A. Nordheim, *MAP kinase-dependent transcriptional coactivation by Elk-1 and its cofactor CBP.* Biochem Biophys Res Commun, 1996. 228(3): p. 831-7.

[263] Kretzschmar, M., J. Doody, and J. Massague, *Opposing BMP and EGF signalling pathways converge on the TGF-beta family mediator Smad1.* Nature, 1997. 389(6651): p. 618-22.

[264] Kretzschmar, M., et al., *A mechanism of repression of TGFbeta/ Smad signaling by oncogenic Ras.* Genes Dev, 1999. 13(7): p. 804-16.

[265] Roelen, B.A., et al., *Phosphorylation of threonine 276 in Smad4 is involved in transforming growth factor-beta-induced nuclear accumulation.* Am J Physiol Cell Physiol, 2003. 285(4): p. C823-30.

[266] Sif, S., et al., *Mitotic inactivation of a human SWI/SNF chromatin remodeling complex.* Genes Dev, 1998. 12(18): p. 2842-51.

[267] Foster, K.S., et al., *Members of the hSWI/SNF chromatin remodeling complex associate with and are phosphorylated by protein kinase B/Akt.* Oncogene, 2006. 25(33): p. 4605-12.

[268] Gao, H., et al., *Akt/PKB interacts with the histone H3 methyltransferase SETDB1 and coordinates to silence gene expression.* Mol Cell Biochem, 2007. 305(1-2): p. 35-44.

[269] Cha, T.L., et al., *Akt-mediated phosphorylation of EZH2 suppresses methylation of lysine 27 in histone H3.* Science, 2005. 310(5746): p. 306-10.

[270] Huang, W.C. and C.C. Chen, *Akt phosphorylation of p300 at Ser-1834 is essential for its histone acetyltransferase and transcriptional activity.* Mol Cell Biol, 2005. 25(15): p. 6592-602.

[271] Pardo, M., et al., *An expanded Oct4 interaction network: implications for stem cell biology, development, and disease.* Cell Stem Cell, 2010. 6(4): p. 382-95.

[272] Dow, L.E. and P.O. Humbert, *Polarity regulators and the control of epithelial architecture, cell migration, and tumorigenesis.* Int Rev Cytol, 2007. 262: p. 253-302.

[273] Alarcon, V.B., *Cell polarity regulator PARD6B is essential for trophectoderm formation in the preimplantation mouse embryo.* Biol Reprod, 2010. 83(3): p. 347-58.

[274] Plusa, B., et al., *Downregulation of Par3 and aPKC function directs cells towards the ICM in the preimplantation mouse embryo.* J Cell Sci, 2005. 118(Pt 3): p. 505-15.

[275] Suzuki, A., et al., *Nanog binds to Smad1 and blocks bone morphogenetic protein-induced differentiation of embryonic stem cells.* Proc Natl Acad Sci U S A, 2006. 103(27): p. 10294-9.

3

Retinoid Signaling is a Context-Dependent Regulator of Embryonic Stem Cells

Zoltan Simandi and Laszlo Nagy
University of Debrecen
Hungary

1. Introduction

Although the beneficial effect of certain foods, such as liver, egg or carrot is known from ancient remedies, one of the common active substances, called Vitamin A, was not identified until 1913, when it has been independently discovered by Elmer McCollum at the University of Wisconsin–Madison, and Lafayette Mendel and Thomas Burr Osborne at Yale University. Since then numerous studies have come to light documenting the effect of vitamin A on the health of the individual from birth to adult age. Hale has demonstrated among the first that deprivation of vitamin A during pregnancy induces congenital ocular malformation (Hale, 1933). Wilson and Warkany later described several other congenital malformations that occurred in fetuses from vitamin A-deficient (VAD) rats affecting the genito-urinary tract, heart and great vessels, ocular and respiratory system (Wilson and Warkany 1947; Wilson and Warkany 1950; Warkany 1954).

In 1968 Saunders and Gasseling have shown that grafting a posterior margin zone (called zone of polarizing activity, ZPA) of a chick embryo limb bud to the anterior side is able to induce an extra set of limb structures (Saunders 1968). It suggested that the ZPA region contains a diffusible morphogen. Surprisingly, retinoic acid (RA), a derivative of vitamin A, has been found to have the same effect on the anterior side of the bud (Tickle, Alberts et al. 1982). There was a doubt that retinoic acid is responsible *in vivo* for the phenomenon, but in 1987 Thaller and Eichele demonstrated the graded distribution of endogenous retinoic acid from posterior to anterior in the limb bud (Thaller and Eichele 1987). This was the time when retinoic acid became known as the first morphogen. Part of the truth that later RA was found to act indirectly, via induction of sonic hedgehog (Shh), and actually Shh is the true morphogen signal peptide produced by the ZPA (Riddle, Johnson et al. 1993).

Our understanding on how vitamin A and its derivatives (called retinoids) are able to have such morpho-regulatory effect on the body has dramatically increased in parallel with the evolution of molecular biology methodologies. Development of cloning strategy, establishment of cDNA library made possible the identification of a receptor for the active derivative of vitamin A by the Evans and Chambon laboratories (Giguere, Ong et al. 1987; Petkovich, Brand et al. 1987). This opened the way to clarify the role of retinoids in embryonic development. Several aspects of the retinoid signaling have been described in the last two deacades using genetically modified mice. Excellent reviews are available summarizing these *in vivo* results (Duester 2008; Dolle 2009; Mark, Ghyselinck et al. 2009).

At the same time, *in vivo* system did not make it possible to understand the molecular mechanism in details. Thus, different cell lines were used, including embryonic carcinoma (EC) and embryonic stem (ES) cells. ES cells have the ability to resemble normal embryonic development much closer than any other cell lines and allow one to study the molecular mechanisms in the context of differentiation.

In this chapter we will focus on recent studies using embryonic stem cells as a model system to deconvolute the retinoid signaling in depth. The first section 'Retinoid signaling pathway' will introduce briefly the present accepted molecular mechanism of retinoid action. We will then go through the retinoid field in the context of ES cell pluripotency and in context of early differentiation. Unconventionally, we will discuss a set of genes that were identified in high-throughput methods as potentially retinoic acid regulated genes in ES cells, including many that were previously not implicated in RA regulation. The chapter intends to serve as a starting point to the better orientation in retinoid field and embryonic stem cells.

2. Retinoid signaling pathway

There are two sources of dietary vitamin A. Retinoids are immediately available to the body from intracellular stores. In contrast, precursors (such as carotenoids, mainly found in plants) first must be converted to active forms. The predominant retinoid present in the mammalian fasting circulation is the retinol. Retinol is bound to a 21 kDa retinol-binding protein (RBP4) since it is not soluble in aqueous environments (Noy 1992). Two active derivatives, all-*trans* retinoic acid (atRA) and 13-*cis*-retinoic acid can be also found in the fasting plasma (Horst, Reinhardt et al. 1995), however at much lower concentration (for instance, atRA is 7.3-9 nmol/l in rats) (Cullum and Zile 1985). Retinol is transported into the cytoplasm of the target cell through RBP receptor Stra6 (Kawaguchi, Yu et al. 2007). Cellular retinol binding proteins (CRBPI and II) are able to bind this cytosolic retinol in many cell types, functioning as storage of retinol. For biological effects retinol must be converted into its active forms, and that process involves two steps. Alcohol dehydrogenases (ADHs) and retinol dehydrogenases (RDHs) are catalyzing the first step, the oxidation of retinol to retinaldehyde (retinal). The second step is the oxidation of retinaldehyde to retinoic acid (RA) that is catalyzed by retinaldehyde dehydrogenases (Aldh1a1, Aldh1a2 and Aldh1a3). Retinoic acid is not produced by all cell of the body. Cells without active RA synthesis may have access to it, since it can be also taken up from the environment. RA can chemically exist as several different isomers including atRA, 9-cis-RA, 11-cis-RA, 13-cis-RA, etc, showing some tissue specific distribution. In the cytoplasm RA binds to intracellular retinoic acid binding protein 2 (Crabp2) and delivers to the nucleus where it serves as a ligand for the retinoic acid receptor – retinoid X receptor heterodimer (RAR:RXR) (reviews in (Blomhoff and Blomhoff 2006; Duester 2008; D'Ambrosio, Clugston et al. 2011).

RA acts via the activation of RAR:RXR heterodimer. RAR (RARα, RARβ and RARγ) and RXR (RXRα, RXRβ and RXRγ) are two families of nuclear receptors that bind DNA and directly regulate transcription (review in (Chambon 2005)). RARs and RXRs exhibit the conserved structure of nuclear receptors, including DNA-binding domain (DBD) and C-terminal ligand binding domain (LBD) (review in (Bain, Heneghan et al. 2007)). RARs bind atRA, and the RXR partner bind 9-*cis*-RA. However, 9-*cis*-RA is normally undetectable except when retinol is present in excess (Mic, Molotkov et al. 2003). When RA binds to the RAR partner of RAR:RXR heterodimers it binds to a regulatory DNA element, called RA response element (RARE) (Umesono, Giguere et al. 1988; Glass 1994). The excess of RA is further oxidized and degraded by Cyp26 enzymes (Cyp26a1, b1 and c1) (Figure 1). During embryonic development RA acts as a morpho-regulator, forming an anterior-posterior (A–P) concentration gradient (Casci 2008) and cross-talks with other key embryonic signals, especially fibroblast growth factors (FGFs) and sonic hedgehog (Shh) (Niederreither and Dolle 2008). Production by Aldh1a1-a3 and elimination together determine the local concentration of RA. Cells can read their position in the RA gradient (considering the gradient of other morphogenes) and differentiate accordingly to these signals. Knockout of both Aldh1a2 and Cyp26a1, the two key enzymes responsible to determine the local RA concentration, lead to early morphogenetic defects and embryonic lethality, indicating the importance of the precise regulation of RA concentration along the body (Niederreither, Subbarayan et al. 1999). Interestingly, Cyp26a1 expression itself is inducible by RA (Ray, Bain et al. 1997), and has two identified RARE (Loudig, Maclean et al. 2005), suggesting a negative feedback mechanism to control the RA concentration. After all, Cyp26a1 is not expressed posteriorly, where RA is the highest, raising the possibility that Cyp26a1 is controlled by another signals as well. Fibroblast growth factor (FGF) is one of the candidates that can be responsible for RA independent regulation. Accordingly, the elimination of FGF signaling was found to shift the expression of Cyp26a1 posteriorly (Casci 2008).

Present model proposes that unliganded RAR heterodimerizes with RXR and binds to DNA. In the absence of ligand the heterodimer is often complexed with corepressor proteins (such as SMRT, NCoR, etc.) (Nagy, Kao et al. 1997) and inhibits gene expression. Indeed, RA receptors are present not only where RA signaling is active, but also in anterior regions in which RA is fully absent. This is, as we will show later, true for undifferentiated embryonic stem cells, as well. Unliganded RAR:RXR thought to have a repressor function. Such active repression of RAR signaling has important regulatory role, for instance it is required for the proper head formation (Koide, Downes et al. 2001). Ligand binding stimulates a cascade of events resulting the release of corepressor complexes, recruitment of transcriptional coactivators (NCoA, CBP/p300, etc.) and thus initiation of transcription (Figure 1) (Glass and Rosenfeld 2000; Rochette-Egly 2005). Alternatively, ligand dependent repression of target genes is also known (Horlein, Naar et al. 1995).

Strikingly, while in embryonic carcinoma (EC) or HL60 cells RA induces cell cycle arrests and differentiation (Flynn, Miller et al. 1983; Mummery, van Rooijen et al. 1987) in hepatocytes RA promotes cell proliferation (Ledda-Columbano, Pibiri et al. 2004). Cell-type specific expression of coregulators may resolve this contradiction and provide an additional context-dependent level of RA-signaling control. Little is known about the expression of RA coregulators in ES cells and early differentiation. Gudas recently showed an example for the complexity of mechanism that control RA-mediated transcription in fibroblasts versus stem cells. It was found that while RARβ2 is induced in both cell types by RA; Hoxa1 and Cyp26a1 are induced only in F9 stem cells, but not in fibroblasts. Coactivators and RNA Pol II recruitment are following this pattern. Strikingly, recruitment of Suz12 (a polycomb protein), H3K27me3 (repressive epigenetic modification), H3K9 and K14 acetylation (activation) and methylated CpG islands are just partly able to explain this phenomenon (Kashyap and Gudas 2010). Thus, simple gene expressional studies are not enough to clarify the context-dependent role of coregulators in cell fate commitment. Combination of single cell analysis and genome-wide screen will be required to unexplore this level of regulation. Potential applications and an outlook will be discussed briefly at the end of this chapter, in the "Future directions".

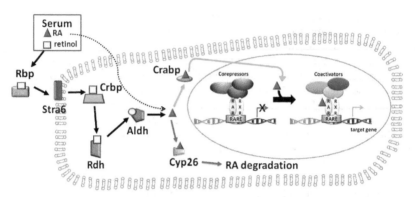

Fig. 1. Overview of retinoid signaling. Retinol is taken up from the serum by the cells via retinol binding protein (Rbp) receptor Stra6. Intracellular retinol is reversibly oxidized to retinal by retinol dehydrogenases (Rdh) and further oxidized to biologically active RA by retinal dehydrogenases (Aldh). Alternatively, cells can take up RA from the environment. Depending on the cell necessities the unwanted RA is eliminated by Cyp26 enzymes or transported into the nucleus and activate the transcription via RAR:RXR. According to the present model, unliganded RAR:RXR bind corepressor complexes while activating ligands replace them to coactivators and promote transcriptional activation.

3. Retinol in ES pluripotency

In standard mammalian cell cultures blood derived fetal bovine serum (FBS) or fetal calf serum (FCS) are widely used in 1-20% to supplement the basal media providing essential factors for the cells. Media for embryonic stem cell culturing contains notable, typically 15% FBS and other factors, provided by the feeder cells. Due to the requirement of these components, ES-cell self-renewal was thought to be dependent on multifactorial stimulations. However, serum-free condition and feeder-independent cultures have been developed in recent years with success. These cultures require addition of Bmp4 and LIF (Williams, Hilton et al. 1988; Qi, Li et al. 2004). LIF can act via activation of Jak-Stat3 signaling pathway, however a complex interplay of different signaling pathways and transcription factors, such as Nanog, Oct3/4, Fgf4, Sox2, etc. are all together responsible for the pluripotency. Recently, it was shown that inhibition of FGF receptor tyrosine kinases and the inhibition of ERK cascade in combination with LIF addition are able to maintain cellular growth capacity and self-renewal of ES cells, providing a ground state to ES cells (Ying, Wray et al. 2008). These studies excluded the requirement of other extrinsic signals, such as FBS content. However, developing embryo is in direct contact with the serum, thus further studies of FBS will help us to better understand its role in embryogenesis.

Certification of defined sera usually does not include the information of its retinol content. According to our data, an ES-qualified serum contains notable retinol (Simandi, Balint et al. 2010). It is questionable whether this high retinol content of serum is playing any role in maintenance of normal phenotype of undifferentiated ES cells. Jaspal S. Khillan and his research group have focused on whether retinol affects any key signaling pathways in ES pluripotency. Interestingly, they found that it can suppress the differentiation of ESCs by up-regulating the expression of Nanog (Chen, Yang et al. 2007). The activation of Nanog by retinol appears to be independent of previously described LIF/Stat3, Oct3/4-Sox2, bone morphogenic proteins (BMPs), and Wnt/beta-catenin pathways. Importantly, forced constitutive expression of Nanog was shown to sufficiently prevent ES cell differentiation and render self-renewal constitutive even in the presence of active FGF/Erk signaling (references in (Silva and Smith 2008)).

The ability of retinol to influence gene expression and cell fate commitment is thought to make possible by enzymes controlling the conversion steps of the biologically active forms. In other words, only that cell is able to respond to the retinol which is expressing the necessary enzymes and receptors, listed above in section 'Retinoid signaling pathway'. Using global gene expression analyses we found, that only RDHs, Crabp1, RARs (Rarγ, Rarβ) and RXRs (Rxrα, Rxrβ) are expressed unambiguously detectable levels in ES cells. RBPs, ALDHs and Cyp26s are present at very low mRNA levels in undifferentiated embryonic stem cells (Simandi, Balint et al. 2010). These results suggest that endogenous production of RA from the retinol content of serum is unlikely to take place in undifferentiated ES cells. Indeed, it has been demonstrated by HPLC analysis that retinol is not metabolized to RA in ES cells in the presence of LIF (Lane, Chen et al. 1999). Thus, presence of retinol in the serum is not in contrast with the importance of RA in differentiation, since endogenous RA synthesis is not taking place to induce retinoid signaling and differentiation. The fact, that RBP neutralizing antibody fail to prevent retinol-mediated up-regulation of Nanog, suggests a new and independent retinol mediated pathway. Indeed, retinol can activate PI3kinase directly via insulin-like growth factor-1 (IGF-1) receptor/IRS-1 (Chen and Khillan 2010). The exact mechanism by which retinol interacts with IGF-1 receptor is not clear at this stage. As the authors hypothesize, retinol may be required to preserve the integrity of stem cells in early-stage embryos before the lineage restricted differentiation is determined. Verifying this striking mechanism, IGF-1/IGFBP-1 has been already shown to facilitate the establishment of a stem-cell line (Lin, Yen et al. 2003). Further studies confirming the positive effect of retinol on stem cell culture may raise the adaptation of purified retinol in routine stem cell culturing and it may further revise the composition of serum-free media.

However active ligand of RAR is not produced in undifferentiated ES cells, important to note, that as the circulating serum, the FBS may also contain active derivatives of retinol, such as atRA or 13-cis RA in low but detectable concentration. AtRA, although fully ionized in free solution at pH 7.4, is uncharged when within a lipid environment (Noy 1992). Uncharged atRA is able to traverse the membrane and enter the cell (Figure 1) (Chen and Gudas 1996). It was discussed above that even ES cells express RARs and RXRs and Crabp, minimally required to respond for a stimuli. In our study we could detect atRA content of the cell culture serum and we could detect atRA by LC-MS in the cells, suggesting that atRA is taken up by the cells. Furthermore, we found that it has impact on basal gene expression level which could be inhibited by BMS493, an inverse RAR agonist (Simandi, Balint et al. 2010). In conclusion these data suggest that the artificial combination of retinol and RAR antagonist may enhance the quality of ES cultures.

4. Retinoid receptors in undifferentiated ES cells

Even in undifferentiated ES cells Rarγ, Rarβ, Rxrα and Rxrβ are expressed, however their function is not clear at this moment. According to the "unliganded receptor-repression" model their DNA binding influences the expression of adjacent genes. The binding site of the RAR:RXR heterodimer on the DNA is the so called RA response element (RARE). RARE is consisting two consensus half-sites separated by a variable length of DNA. The sequence of this consensus half-site is most typically 5'-**AGGTCA**-3' (Balmer and Blomhoff 2005). According to the relative direction of the half-sites, direct repeat, inverted repeat and everted repeat can be distinguished (Honkakoski and Negishi 2000). Type II nuclear receptors, such as RARs and RXRs typically bind to a direct repeat (DR), separated by 1, 2 or 5 nucleotides (called DR1, DR2, DR5, respectively). The RAREs tipically located in target genes, however large number of DR2-type elements are present within Alu repeats (Vansant and Reynolds 1995) (Figure 2 show some of the well known RA target genes and their RAREs).

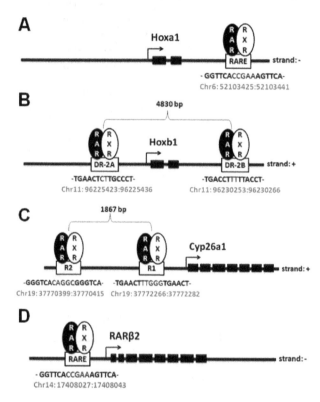

Fig. 2. RARE elements of well-known RA target genes. RAR binding occurs most typically on DR5 (Hoxa1, Cyp26a1, RARβ2) and DR2 (Hoxb1) elements.

Chromatin immunoprecipitation (ChIP) is a powerful and widely applied technique for detecting the association of individual proteins with specific genomic regions. ChIP can be combined with microarray technology to identify the location of specific proteins on a genome-wide basis (called ChIP-chip) (Aparicio, Geisberg et al. 2004). A recent study has performed ChIP-chip on mouse embryonic fibroblasts and ES cells overexpressing tagged Rarγ (Delacroix, Moutier et al. 2010). Rarγ is the dominantly expressed subtype of RAR in ES cells, thus it confirms the biological relevance of this analysis. 354 target loci bound by the RAR were identified in MEFs and 462 loci in undifferentiated ES cells. These sites obviously do not cover the full repertoire, but as this was the first large-scale study, it served many striking results. First, it was found that only a minority of the 354 MEF loci were present in ES cells, suggesting cell-specific occupancy of RAR binding. This can be an important mechanism contributing to the distinct of retinoid signaling seen in different cell types. Not unexpectedly, in ES cells RAR was found to occupy genes with a wide variety of functions: pluripotency (Oct3/4, Lin28, or Utf1), differentiation (Lefty1, Lefty2), important signaling pathways (Nodal, Notch4, sonic hedgehog pathway components, several FGF), a more systematic discussion of regulated genes will be provided in the next section. In MEF cells RAR occupancy (ChIP-chip data) and RA regulation (microarray) has been analyzed together, showing that only small subset of RAR bound genes were regulated by RA. In undifferentiated ES cells such dataset is still not available. It cannot be completely excluded that formaldehyde cross-linking or overexpression of Rarγ gives its artificial detection by ChIP. However, many of those RAR bound, but not regulated genes were found to be regulated by RA in other cell types, suggesting the good source of data and a highly cell type and context dependent regulation. Moreover, part of the genes, bound by unliganded RAR, showed H3K4me3 (associated with active chromatin) and expression. Data is lacking to show whether there is a partial repression in case of these genes or unliganded RAR binding do not influence their expression at all. Latter would suggest that unliganded RAR silences only small subsets of bounded target genes. This is at least partly in contrast with the previously mentioned "unliganded RAR – corepressors recruitment" model (shown on Figure 1) and confute one at this moment to unambiguously predict which gene and which cell type will respond to the stimuli. In the same study the sequence of RAR-bound loci has been compared. Interestingly, majority of the loci did not contain consensus DR1, -2 or -5 elements, rather compromised one or several anomalously spaced consensus half sites. Strikingly, there was no correlation between the presence/absence of recognizable DR elements and RA regulation. Bioinformatic analyses are considering the sequence diversity of RAR binding sites and the varying distance between the direct repeats only in a limited level. Genome-wide RAR binding studies in different cell types combined with advanced bioinformatic analysis of target loci may help to build a better prediction model and further investigate the biological aspects of different binding sites and the potential role of epigenetic state of these regions. One of such pioneer study (Mahony, Mazzoni et al. 2011) will be discussed in the next section.

5. Retinoic acid induced downregulation of stem cell pluripotency and differentiation induction

The moment that we revoke LIF from the media of undifferentiated ES cells results in the spontaneous differentiation of cells. This can be further induced by allowing them to form aggregates, called embryoid bodies (EB). We have looked for the early changes during the four day embryoid body formation using genome-wide expressional analysis and found ~1000 genes to be regulated. Important genes involved in retinoid signaling, such as Stra6, Aldh1a2, Rarβ, etc. are not among them, only the expression of the RA induced-RA eliminator Cyp26a1 is elevated, suggesting that RA signaling is not activated yet in this stage and the incidental RA level is actively cleared away. This is in correlation with the findings that presence of RA decreases the viability of blastocyst (Huang, Shen et al. 2003) and explain the importance of uterine Cyp26a1 activity in the maintenance of pregnancy, especially during the process of blastocyst implantation (Han, Xia et al. 2010). Potentially, an

RA-independent, FGF signaling controlled Cyp26a1 expression may be responsible for this for RA clearance in day 4 EBs. This explains why Cyp26a1 could upregulate in the presence of RAR inverse agonist BMS493. In contrast, following the post-implantation RA is sorely needed. Absence of RA in this stage cause serious malformations, including axial rotation, shortens along the anteroposterior axis, disturbed limb bud development, finally resulting early embryo death (Niederreither, Subbarayan et al. 1999).

Currently, the effector molecules and cascade signaling of the early retinoid signaling in the vertebrate embryo are barely known. Mechanistic studies showed that RA is not just initiating the differentiation, but also actively decrease the pluripotency via binding to RARE in Oct3/4 promoter (Pikarsky, Sharir et al. 1994) and regulation of LIF-signaling (Tighe and Gudas 2004). Indeed, Oct3/4 is not changing significantly between day 0 and day 4 in our data, but it is actively down-regulated following RA-treatment. In the same time, neural marker DCX becomes upregulated (Simandi, Balint et al. 2010). This suggests clearly the importance of retinoic acid-free (but not retinol-free) environment to the undifferentiated embryonic stem cells. The importance of RA in pluripotency can be studied from a different viewpoint, namely, whether retinoid signaling is able to influence the cell reprogramming. Yamanaka and contributors have shown that introduction of four factors (Oct3/4, C-Myc, Klf4 and Sox-2) into mouse embryonic fibroblast (MEF) cells induce the reprogramming of the differentiated cells and driving back them to embryonic stem cell-like cells, called induced pluripotent stem cells (iPSC) (Takahashi and Yamanaka 2006). A recent study has investigated how different nuclear receptors influence the iPS generation from MEFs. This screen included 19 nuclear receptors, among them Rarα, Rarγ and Rxrα. Surprisingly, none of the overexpressed retinoid receptors influenced significantly the obtained iPS colony numbers (Heng, Feng et al. 2010). Importantly, this study did not use ligands or antagonists to activate (or repress) the overexpressed receptors.

More is known about the ES differentiation promoting effect of RA. Over the years, many RA-regulated differentiation pathways have been discovered first in embryonic carcinoma (EC) and then adopted to ES cells as well. The most studied mouse EC cell lines include F9 cells, which can be induced by RA to differentiate into primitive, parietal, and visceral endodermal cells; and P19 cells, which can differentiate to endodermal and neuronal cells upon RA treatment. ES cells can be induced to differentiate into a number of different cell types; many of which require RA treatment (Soprano, Teets et al. 2007).

To understand in depth how retinoic acid is able to drive a given differentiation pathway, one should identify a set of regulated genes by high-throughput methods. Here, a very important issue is the applicable concentration of retinoic acid. Typically, a regulated gene shows dose dependent effect. From this dose dependent curve one can determine the half maximal effective concentration (EC_{50}) of the given gene. This value may vary in case of other target genes. Thus, it can happen that with the application of lower retinoic acid concentration one will induce only the most responsiveness genes (lower EC_{50}). A solution for this problem can be a high RA concentration that will give the maximal response (saturation). However, this posing is just partly correct. First, in the embryonic development RA grade has very important effect in the anterior-posterior patterning and deep impact on cell fate commitment. This can be true for stem cell differentiation as well. Strikingly, there is no systematic study available using different concentration of RA comparing sets of regulated genes genome-wide. Theoretically, a low concentration of RA results in the expression of "gene A", a higher concentration will also express "gene B", which may negatively affect the expression of "gene A" by a negative feedback mechanism.

Limited number of studies demonstrated the dose-dependent effect of RA on a given pathway. For instance, it was shown that higher concentrations of RA induce a dorsal phenotype, while lower concentrations of RA induced a more ventral phenotype during RA induced neural differentiation (Okada, Shimazaki et al. 2004). Not only the concentration, but also the timing of RA signal might be very important. According to the established protocols, different cell types (such as adipocyte, pancreatic cell, neural cells, primordial germ cells, etc.) requires RA signal in various time-points during their differentiation (Bost, Caron et al. 2002; Bibel, Richter et al. 2007; Eguizabal, Shovlin et al. 2009).

The exact molecular events that lead from a pluripotent stem cell to a fully differentiated cell following RA treatment are yet to be determined. Considering the above discussed time- and dose-dependent effect, gene expressional studies can determine the early signaling pathways induced by retinoic acid. We have performed such a study on 4 day-old embryoid bodies treated with 5 μM ATRA for 12 hours and identified 70 annotated genes that were regulated at least 2-fold. At first glance it seems a low number of genes, but another independent study could detect similarly only 96 significantly differently expressed genes (Mahony, Mazzoni et al. 2011). Gene expressional studies cannot clearly classify sets of genes that are directly regulated by RAR. A new method, namely ChIP-Seq, combines chromatin immunoprecipitation (ChIP) with parallel DNA sequencing to identify global binding sites for any protein of interest (Johnson, Mortazavi et al. 2007). A recently published paper investigated the ligand-dependent dynamics of RAR binding during early differentiation using ChIP-Seq. In the absence of RA, ChIP-Seq enrichment could be detected at 1822 sites in embryoid bodies. After 8 hours of exposure to RA this number did not really changed (enrichment at 1924 sites). The most frequent motifs were DR2 and DR5. Confirming the previously discussed ChIP-chip dataset, only 507 sites bound constitutively RAR. This is further query the accepted model of constitutively binding RARs. More strikingly, in the same study they could detect a ligand-dependent shift in RAR's preference from DR0 and DR1 (absence of ligand) to DR5 (presence of ligand).

6. Retinoic acid driven signaling pathways in embryonic stem cells

Vitamin A-deficient and genetic animal models revealed the importance of retinoic acid signaling in embryonic development and organogenesis. In early development, RA participates in the organization of the trunk by providing an instructive signal for posterior neuroectoderm, foregut endoderm and a permissive signal for trunk mesoderm differentiation. At later stages, RA contributes to the development of the eye and other organs (reviewed in (Duester 2008). Presumably, *in vitro* experiments in stem cell cultures are able to reveal the *in vivo* molecular targets of retinoid action during the development. Indeed, we will show hereinafter that genes identified in cell culture experiments match *in vivo* findings. However, one should assume that these *in vitro* cultures are not able to perfectly mimic the spatio-temporal events.

Binding of RA to its receptor induces differentiation mainly via one of the following mechanisms: 1) Initiate changes in interaction of RAR:RXR and co-regulators (SMRT, NCoR, NCoA, CBP/p300, etc.), resulting transcription of primary target genes; 2) Induces expression of transcription factors (Hox, Cdx, etc) and other signaling molecules, resulting transcription of secondary target genes. Regulation of non-coding RNAs may serve as additional level of retinoid action (Rossi, D'Urso et al. 2010); 3) Alters interactions with proteins involved in epigenetic regulation (Kashyap, Gudas et al. 2011). Furthermore, there are proteins that bind at or near RAREs resulting a more complex mechanism of retinoid action (for review, see (Gudas and Wagner 2011).

In the followings we will discuss the potential role of genes identified in ChIP-chip study of ES cells (Delacroix, Moutier et al. 2010), in day 2 EBs by ChIP-Seq study (Mahony, Mazzoni et al. 2011) or in our microarray study (Simandi, Balint et al. 2010), focusing especially on those which were found in more than one of these studies. In fact, the overlap between the results is remarkable. The results of these experiments provide a list about genes that are primary (ChIP-chip, ChIP-Seq) or secondary response to RA (microarray) considering the technical limitation of such experiments. Based on the published biological functions, we divided arbitrarily some of the genes into functional subgroups. An asterisk (*) mark genes where previously identified or predicted RARE could be identified. Following the gene name, an arrow marks the atRA effect for the expression of the given gene (↑, ↓), up and down, respectively.

6.1 Regulators of RA metabolism

The following genes are well known players in the retinoid metabolism (see Figure 1 and 3). At the same time many of them are involved in the proper eye function, and very likely important in its development. For more details about retinoid signaling in embryonic eye development look for recent reviews in (Duester 2009), (Cvekl and Wang 2009).

Cyp26a1* (cytochrome P450, family 26, subfamily a, polypeptide 1) (↑)

Cyp26 enzymes have been shown to restrict the availability of RA to the transcriptional machinery (review in (Pennimpede, Cameron et al. 2010). HPLC and LC-MS-MS identified 4-OH-RA, 4-oxo-RA and 18-OH-RA and other oxidized products formed as metabolites by Cyp26a1 (Chithalen, Luu et al. 2002). Cyp26a1 expression is directly regulated by RA, and presumably independently regulated by FGF (Casci 2008). Microarray analyses revealed that RA-treated Cyp26a1 $^{-/-}$ ES cells exhibited lower mRNA levels than wild-type ES cells for genes involved in differentiation, particularly in neural and smooth muscle differentiation (Langton and Gudas 2008). One intriguing possible role of Cyp26a1 is to regulate the formation of waves or pulses of RA during the dynamic development of some structures, most notably the hindbrain (Sirbu, Gresh et al. 2005).

Dhrs3 (dehydrogenase/reductase (SDR family) member 3), also known as retinal short-chain dehydrogenase/reductase (retSDR1) (↑)

It has been first described in cone photoreceptors suggesting its possible responsibility for reduction of all-trans-retinal in photoreceptor outer segments that serve as the first step in the regeneration of bleached visual pigments (Haeseleer, Huang et al. 1998). Furthermore, it was found to be expressed also in placenta, lung, liver, kidney, pancreas, and retina; many of these tissues known to actively metabolize retinol. Thus, it suggests that Dhrs3 acts as a generic all-trans-retinol dehydrogenase in many tissues, ensuring that deleterious levels of all-trans-retinal do not accumulate. It was later demonstrated that Dhrs3 is induced by RA in a wide array of cell lines derived from different human tissues and a recent study has shown that Dhrs3 respond oppositely to RA antagonists. Using morpholino knockdown and mRNA over-expression, this study demonstrated that Dhrs3 is required to limit RA levels in the embryo, primarily in the central nervous system (CNS) (Feng, Hernandez et al. 2010). These together suggest that Dhrs3 is an RA-induced feedback inhibitor of RA biosynthesis, and it acts very similarly than Cyp26a1. Whether the RA function is direct or indirect in

Dhrs3 regulation remained to be undetermined. Both ChIP-chip and ChIP-Seq analysis could identify Dhrs3; however typical binding site was not identifiable.

Rarb* (retinoic acid receptor, beta) (↑)

The various RAR subtypes (α, β, γ) are widely but differentially expressed during murine embryonic development, and most tissues express one or more of the subtypes and isoforms during development in different combinations (Dolle 2009). The expression of Rarβ gene is spatially and temporally restricted in certain structures in the developing embryo (segmented brain (r7), hypothalamus, ventricular neuroepithelium, pigmented epithelium, proximal bronchi, myocardium, etc.), suggesting that Rarβ could play specific roles during morphogenesis. In contrast, mice lacking all isoforms of Rarβ develop normally and there is no obvious alteration in the spatial pattern of expression of Hox genes (Luo, Pasceri et al. 1995). These experiments demonstrate that Rarβ is not absolutely required for embryonic development, maybe due to the redundancy in their role among the RAR isoforms.

Rbp1* (retinol binding protein 1, cellular), also known as CRBP1 (↑)

As it was discussed previously, retinol and retinaldehyde in the cytoplasm are associated with cellular retinol-binding proteins (CRBPs). CRBP1 is the most widespread, but it displays some tissue specificity (Dolle, Ruberte et al. 1990). Functional analysis of CRBP1 suggested its role in retinol storage and release where high levels of RA are required for specific morphogenetic processes (Ghyselinck, Bavik et al. 1999). However, CRBP1-deficient mice did not show any morphological defects, did not result altering organogenesis and CRBP1 ablation did not change RA-dependent gene expression, indicating that absence of CRBP1 is not life-threatening, at least under conditions of maternal vitamin A dietary sufficiency (Ghyselinck, Bavik et al. 1999).

Stra6 (stimulated by retinoic acid gene 6) (↑)

Existence of a cell-surface receptor for RBP has been predicted since the mid-1970s. In 2007, Kawaguchi and coworkers could identify Stra6 that acts as a high affinity cell surface receptor for RBP (Kawaguchi, Yu et al. 2007), however Stra6 is not expressed in all retinoid metabolizing tissues. Interestingly, cell culture experiments have shown that Stra6-expressing cells, preloaded with retinol, are able to release more retinol into the culture medium than cells without expresson of Stra6 (Isken, Golczak et al. 2008), suggesting that Stra6 acts as a bidirectional transporter of retinol. Potentially, Stra6 depending on intracellular retinol/retinoic acid concentration, coordinate retinol uptake /removal, thus avoiding cells to take up toxic amount of retinol. Stra6 mutation was found to lead severe congenital abnormalities in humans, including congenital heart defects, mental retardation and lung hypoplasia (Pasutto, Sticht et al. 2007).

6.2 Regulators of body axis patterning

Retinoic acid has been described as a first morphogen (Slack 1987). Indeed, it is responsible for the regulation of several genes implicated in body axis determination. However, the embryonic axis formation is a very complex process, regulated by additional factors, such as Wnt, Shh, Bmp and FGF signaling (Meyers and Martin 1999; Diez del Corral and Storey 2004). Final outcome of the differentiation is the resultant of these signaling pathways. Most of the following genes are well known RA signaling targets, the reason for listing them here is to demonstrate the role of RA in body axis determination.

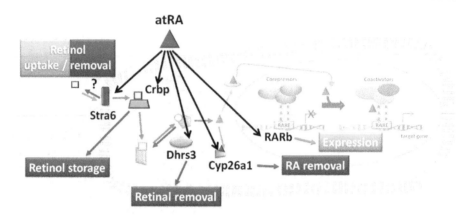

Fig. 3. Effect of all-trans retinoic acid treatment on the retinoid pathway in EBs. Addition of atRA induce its removal via multiple pathway (in red). Stra6 may responsible to eliminate the intracellular retinol, Crbp1 may hold back the retinol from further steps, Dhrs3 participates in retinal removal, while Cyp26a1 can degrade the produced RA. These mechanisms may have a role to protect the blastocyst from the toxic effect of retinoids.

Cdx1* (caudal type homeobox 1) (↑)

The Cdx genes (Cdx1, 2 and 4) are relatives of Hox genes (see below) and believed to derive from a common ProtoHox ancestral cluster (Chourrout, Delsuc et al. 2006). Cdx regulate anterior-posterior (AP) vertebral patterning, at least in part, through direct regulation of Hox gene expression via Cdx-binding sites, which are often found in clusters throughout the Hox cluster (Gaunt, Drage et al. 2008). Prior work has shown that Cdx1 is target of Wnt, RA and FGF signaling, suggesting that Cdx1 is responsible to convey the activity of these signaling molecules to Hox genes. Indeed, RARE and Lef/Tcf-response elements (LRE) has been identified in the proximal promoter of Cdx1. Interestingly, mutation of LRE greatly reduce the induction of Cdx1 by RA, demonstrating a requirement for Wnt signaling in the regulation of this gene by retinoids (Beland, Pilon et al. 2004). Retinoic acid plays a key role in early stages of Cdx1 expression at embryonic day 7.5. Surprisingly, Cdx1 -/- mice are viable and fertile, however showing anterior homeotic transformations of vertebrae (Subramanian, Meyer et al. 1995). These abnormalities are concomitant with posterior shifts of Hox gene expression domains in the somitic mesoderm.

In ES cell derived EBs Cdx1 expression is increasing, peaking between day 2 and day 3 which is the reported window of hemangioblast and blood fate specification (day 3 to day 4 of EB differentiation). Ectopic expression of Cdx1 in differentiating EBs up-regulated Hoxa and Hoxb posterior cluster genes (Hoxa6, Hoxb8, Hoxb9) (McKinney-Freeman, Lengerke et al. 2008).

Hox (homeobox) **genes** (* in the text) (↑)

Hox genes are organized in gene clusters (Hoxa, Hoxb, Hoxc, and Hoxd) and show a strict coordinated expression, reglated by among others Cdx genes. Retinoic acid is not only through the regulation of Cdx, but also directly a well-established regulator of Hox genes along the anterior-posterior axis in higher animals. Genes in the 3' ends of Hox clusters are induced by RA, while 5' Hox genes are not induced by RA (Langston and Gudas 1992;

Langston, Thompson et al. 1997). Indeed, microarray and ChIP-Seq studies identified several members of the Hox family (Hoxa1*, a2*, a3*, a4, a5*, a10 and Hoxb1*, b2*, b3*, b4*, b5*, b6*, Hoxc4 etc.). Hoxc and Hoxd clusters are not induced upon RA treatment in ES cells and day 2 or day 4 old EBs. Several RARE has been identified in the Hox cluster by ChIP-Seq, many of them have been described in previous publications (Popperl and Featherstone 1993; Dupe, Davenne et al. 1997; Packer, Crotty et al. 1998; Huang, Chen et al. 2002).

Lefty1 (left right determination factor 1) (↑)

A distinctive and essential feature of the vertebrate body is a pronounced left-right asymmetry (review in (Mercola and Levin 2001). Left-right asymmetric signaling molecules in mammals include three transforming growth factor beta (TGFbeta)-related factors, Nodal, Lefty1 and Lefty2 that are responsible for the mirror-image anatomy. They are all expressed on the left half of developing mouse embryos. Nodal acts as a left-side determinant by transducing signals through Smad and FAST and by inducing Pitx2 expression on the left side. Lefty proteins are antagonists that inhibit Nodal signaling (Hamada, Meno et al. 2001). Nodal and Lefty are expressed in the pancreas during embryogenesis and islet regeneration. *In vitro* studies demonstrated that Nodal inhibits, whereas Lefty enhances, the proliferation of a pancreatic cell line (Zhang, Sterling et al. 2008).

Meis1 and **Meis2*** (myeloid ecotropic viral integration site) (↑)

Homeodomain proteins of the Meis subfamily are expressed dynamically in several organs during embryogenesis and exert potent regulatory activity through their interaction with Hox proteins and other transcription factors. Meis1-deficient embryos have partially duplicated retinas and smaller lenses than normal. They also fail to produce megakaryocytes, display extensive hemorrhaging, and die by embryonic day 14.5 (Hisa, Spence et al. 2004). In addition, Meis1-deficient embryos lack well-formed capillaries, although larger blood vessels are normal. Definitive myeloerythroid lineages are present in the mutant embryos, but the total numbers of colony-forming cells are dramatically reduced (Azcoitia, Aracil et al. 2005).

Pbx2* (pre B-cell leukemia transcription factor 2) ((-), see in the text)

It has been found that Pbx2 -/- embryos are born at the expected Mendelian frequencies and exhibit no detectable abnormalities in development and organogenesis (Selleri, DiMartino et al. 2004), however they show limb abnormalities (Capellini, Di Giacomo et al. 2006). Supporting its role in this phenomenon, its elevated expression in limb buds after RA treatment has been demonstrated. Retinoic acid response element in the promoter of Pbx2 has been identified in both ChIP-chip and ChIP-Seq study, even without ligand activation. However it seems to be not regulated by atRA in ES cells or EBs according to the microarray data, suggesting a more context dependent regulation of this gene by RA. As Pbx proteins have been shown to dimerize with Hox proteins and act as a cofactor, we included here (Moens and Selleri 2006). Pbx2 is believed to be involved in the control of proximodistal axis formation in mouse (Capellini, Zewdu et al. 2008).

Tshz1 (teashirt zinc finger family member 1) (↑)

Tshz1 is detected from E9.5 in the somites, and also present in the spinal cord, limb buds and branchial arches. Tshz1 -/- mice exhibit Hox-like vertebral malformations and homeotic transformations in the cervical and thoracic regions, suggesting that Tshz1 and Hox genes are involved in common pathways to control skeletal morphogenesis (Core, Caubit et al.

2007). Previous studies suggested Tshz1 as an RA regulated gene, however direct evidence was not shown yet.

6.3 Testis development, spermatogenesis, female fertility

Generation of putative primordial germ cells (PGCs) has been reported during the differentiation of mouse and human ESCs in *in vitro* systems using RA (reviewed in (Zhou, Meng et al. 2010)). *In vivo* PGCs come from the proximal epiblast and migrate subsequently into the mesoderm, the endoderm and the posterior of the yolk sac (Bendel-Stenzel, Anderson et al. 1998). The mechanisms responsible for the pluripotent epiblast cells to become PGCs involve bone morphogenetic protein 2 (Bmp2), Bmp4, Bmp8b, Prdm1 and Prdm14 (Ying and Zhao 2001; Edson, Nagaraja et al. 2009). Migration of PGCs requires interferon-induced transmembrane proteins 1 and 3, Kit ligand and Cxcl12 (Molyneaux, Zinszner et al. 2003). Germ cells continue to proliferate by mitosis upon arriving in the genital ridge. Spermatogonial lineage does not enter meiosis before puberty, and the proliferation is inhibited by androgens. In contrast, germ cells in the female gonad continue to proliferate by mitosis and enter meiosis. These are raising the evidence of testicular meiosis-preventing and ovarian meiosis-inducing factors. Initiation of meiosis in the fetal ovary has been suggested to require retinoic acid (Bowles, Knight et al. 2006). Germ cells fail to enter meiosis and remain undifferentiated in embryonic vitamin A-deficient ovaries, suggesting that retinol regulates the initiation of meiosis I (Li and Clagett-Dame 2009). Another study revealed, that RA-degrading enzyme Cyp26b1 in fetal testis is responsible to delay meiosis until postnatal development (Koubova, Menke et al. 2006). However, RA acts too widely in mammalian development to account, by itself, for the cell-type and temporal specificity of meiotic initiation. The following RA regulated genes have been found related to germ cell development; many of them only partly characterized yet.

Agpat3* (1-acylglycerol-3-phosphate O-acyltransferase 3) also known LPAAT3 (↑)

Agpat3 was shown to have both lysophosphatidic acid acyltransferase (LPAAT) and lysophosphatidylinositol acyltransferase (LPIAT) activities. It is mainly expressed in the liver, kidney, and testis. Present studies suggest its role in PI (phosphatidylinositol) production of the testis. Interestingly, expression of Agpat3 in the testis is enhanced significantly in an age-dependent manner (Yuki, Shindou et al. 2009).

Nrip1 (Nuclear receptor interacting protein 1) also known as RIP140 (↑)

A nuclear protein that specifically interacts with the hormone-dependent activation domain AF2 of nuclear receptors. Mice null for Nrip1 gene are viable, but females are infertile because of complete failure of mature follicles to release oocytes at ovulation stage. Heterozygous females are only partially affected (White, Leonardsson et al. 2000).

Rec8* (REC8 homolog (yeast)) (↑)

Gene expression of Rec8 is strictly confined to spermatocytes and spermatids in male mouse and oocytes in female mouse. Restricted expression pattern of Rec8 mRNA implies its essential role in meiosis in both sexes of mammals (Lee, Yokota et al. 2002). It was found that Rec8 is a key component of the meiotic cohesin complex. During meiosis, cohesin is required for the establishment and maintenance of sister-chromatid cohesion, for the formation of the synaptonemal complex, and for recombination between homologous chromosomes. Importantly, Rec8 -/- mice are born in sub-Mendelian frequencies and both sexes have germ cell failure causing sterility (Xu, Beasley et al. 2005).

Stra8* (stimulated by retinoic acid 8) (↑)

Encodes a protein that is crucial for mammalian germ cells to enter into pre-meiotic stages. Microarray analysis of whole murine embryonic ovary and postnatal testis time course data revealed a single peak of Stra8 expression in each organ at the onset of meiosis; at E14.5 in the ovary and 10 days postpartum in the testis (Hogarth, Mitchell et al. 2011). Stra8 is specifically expressed in mammalian germ cells before their transition from mitosis to meiosis and its expression is observed only in the postnatal testis. Stra8 associates with DNA and possesses transcriptional activity (Tedesco, La Sala et al. 2009). Stra8 mRNA and protein were induced in cells treated by all-trans and 9-cis retinoic acids in P19 embryonal carcinoma cells (Oulad-Abdelghani, Bouillet et al. 1996), however using Aldh1a2 -/- mice (lacking RA synthesis) it was found that Stra8 expression is detectable even in the absence of RA (Kumar, Chatzi et al. 2011).

The following genes are also regulated by atRA and could be detected with ChIP-chip or ChIP-Seq. They are related to fertility, testis or germ cells, but due to the limited available data, they are not discussed here in details: **Wdr40b** (↑), **Nr0b1** (↑), **Cxcl12** (↑), **Kit** (↑), **Tcp11** (↑).

6.4 Neuroectodermal cell fate commitment

Other chapters of the book prominently construe with the neural differentiation of stem cells. Present protocols are widely using RA to induce the neural differentiation of stem cells; however the exact mechanisms remained largely unknown yet. The fact that endogenous RA is starting to synthetize in mouse embryo after forebrain and midbrain neuroectoderm induction is raising the possibility that RA is actually not required for neural induction (Duester 2008). However, RA induced Hoxa1 activity is clearly essential for the neuronal differentiation (Martinez-Ceballos and Gudas 2008).

The following genes were found to be related to the neural differentiation or functioning. They may have role in the neural specification only. Some of them are putatively involved in the eye development as well.

Ankrd43* (ankyrin repeat domain 43) (↑)

Very limited information is available for this gene. It is among those seven genes which were found to be differentially expressed in progenitors in the lateral and medial ganglionic eminences (LGE and MGE). LGE progenitors produce striatal projection neurons and olfactory bulb interneurons, whereas MGE as well as caudal ganglionic eminence (CGE) progenitors produce cortical and hippocampal interneurons. Thus, its RA regulation suggests the role of RA in neural specialization (Tucker, Segall et al. 2008).

Glra2 (glycine receptor chloride channel, alpha 2 subunit) (↑)

This gene mediates inhibitory neurotransmission in the spinal cord, brainstem and retina. During development, Glra2 is expressed in the retina, in the spinal cord, and throughout the brain. Mice with a targeted deletion of Glra2 show no gross morphological or molecular alterations in the nervous system. (Young-Pearse, Ivic et al. 2006).

Gpr124 (G protein-coupled receptor 124) (↑)

GPR124 is highly expressed in central nervous system (CNS) endothelium. Its deletion resulted embryonic lethality through CNS-specific angiogenesis arrest in forebrain and neural tube. Conversely, GPR124 overexpression throughout all adult vascular beds produced CNS-specific hyperproliferative vascular malformations (Kuhnert, Mancuso et al. 2010).

6.5 Adipocyte differentiation

Adipogenesis is a complex process by a multifaceted transcriptional regulatory cascade. In recent years data have emerged indicating a role of retinoids in adipose tissue. Retinoids has been shown to inhibit preadipocyte to adipocyte differentiation by repressing Pparγ and Rxrα activities (Ziouzenkova, Orasanu et al. 2007), however we should note that the embryonic stem cell derived adipogenesis requires RA in the very beginning (Bost, Caron et al. 2002). The role of such early RA signal in adipocyte differentiation remained largely unknown.

Cidea (cell death-inducing DNA fragmentation factor, alpha subunit-like effector A) (↑)

Cidea-null mice are lean and resistant to diet-induced obesity and diabetes, indicating a role for Cidea in energy balance and adiposity (Zhou, Yon Toh et al. 2003). Thus, Cidea can be a potential RA regulated gene in ES cell that influence the adipocyte differentiation.

Nrip1 (discussed also in "Regulators of RA metabolism" section) (↑)

Knockout male and female mice are smaller than wild-type littermates. Nrip1-null cells show elevated energy expenditure and express high levels of the uncoupling protein 1 gene (Ucp1), carnitine palmitoyltransferase 1b, and the cell-death-inducing DFF45-like effector A (Cidea) (Christian, Kiskinis et al. 2005).

Rbp1* (retinol binding protein 1, cellular), also known as CRBP1 (discussed also in "Regulators of RA metabolism" section) (↑)

Interestingly, a recent study showed that CRBP1-deficient mice fed with high-fat diet (HFD) lead to increased adiposity. Similarly, suppression of CRBP-I expression *in vitro* enhanced adipocyte differentiation (Zizola, Frey et al. 2010).

Rarb* (discussed also in "Regulators of RA metabolism" section) (↑)

Rarβ activation has been shown that both sufficient and necessary to trigger commitment of mES cells to adipocytes (Monteiro, Wdziekonski et al. 2009).

7. Future directions

Microarray completed with ChIP-chip or ChIP-Seq is useful to determine sets of RA regulated genes and map the binding sites of RAR:RXR heterodimer. We have shown that RA treatment of ES cells or EBs induces expression of genes involved in retinoid metabolism, body-axis regulation, gonad development and neural differentiation. Other recently introduced methods, such as RNA-Seq (Wang, Gerstein et al. 2009) and Gro-Seq (Core, Waterfall et al. 2008), still have not been used in retinoid research, and may serve more detailed picture about the direct effect of RA (detailed description of genome-wide approaches in aspect of stem cell research is reviewed in (Zhang and Huang 2010). Future experiments should be complemented with studies investigating the co-occupancy of RAR, RXR, RNA Pol II and coregulators (SMRT, NCoR, NCoA, CBP/p300, etc.) genome-wide to get information about the direct gene regulation and its temporal dynamics. Development of data processing methods and integration of system biology will be also required for analyzing the complexity underlying the regulatory networks in stem cells and during cell fate commitment (Macarthur, Ma'ayan et al. 2009).

There are other technical challenges limiting our recent possibilities. Several cell-type specific differentiation protocol has been published, many of them resulting heterogeneous cell population. This is mainly due to our poor understanding on interactions of different signal cascades. Uncontrolled content of FBS, heterogeneity during EB formation, not adequate ligand treatment may also affect the quality of cell culture. For instance, embryonic stem cell derived embryoid bodies often show heterogeneity in their size that may have impact on cell fate commitment (Mansergh, Daly et al. 2009). Adherent monolayer cultures have been used to get more homogenous differentiation. It has been successfully used for neural differentiation (Pachernik, Esner et al. 2002), however many of the lineage differentiation is still require the EB formation, implying the importance of a three-dimensional structure. Replacement of EBs by scaffolds can provide such three-dimensional environment in which cells have access to nutrients and space to grow. Recent studies are using scaffolds to induce high organization of stem cells during differentiation. For instance, one of the most recent study reported the dynamic, autonomous formation of the optic cup structure from a three-dimensional culture of mouse embryonic stem cell aggregates (Eiraku, Takata et al. 2011).

During development, morphogens are secreted locally and presented to embryonic cells in a spatially and temporally controlled manner to direct appropriate differentiation and tissue formation. This seems to be true for RA production as well. *In vitro* addition of RA to the media of differentiating EBs does not accurately replicate this process. In addition, the diffusion of RA into EBs may be restricted by the formation of an exterior shell composed of collagenous matrix and tight E-cadherin mediated cell–cell adhesions at the EB surface. Biodegradable microspheres to deliver morphogens directly within EBs may enable production of more homogeneous populations of differentiated cells (Bratt-Leal, Carpenedo et al. 2010). A study examined ESC differentiation in response to microsphere-mediated delivery of RA (Li, Davidovich et al. 2011). The authors found that after 10 days of differentiation, the RA microsphere-containing EBs formed large cystic structures that comprised the majority of the EBs. Genome-wide analysis revealed more pronounced up-regulation in visceral endoderm, epiblast, and early primitive streak markers and down-regulation in mesoderm and definitive endoderm differentiation. Thus, in the existing stem cell differentiation protocols we need to revisit the usefulness of cytokine/ligand delivering microspheres.

Finally, important to note that RT-PCR, western blot or even microarray analysis are able to reveal only the average response of the cell population to a given signal (Figure 4). This is clearly giving only limited information. Single cell analyzing methods will bring us closer to understand the dynamics of cell fate commitment. This field is expected to accelerate soon and will change recently used methodologies.

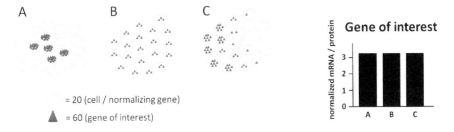

Fig. 4. Population measurements can obscure the heterogeneity of the cells within the embryoid body. For instance, western blot or RT-PCR are not able to determine whether only a few cell are expressing the gene of interest on high level (A), every cell on middle level (B) or there is a polarity (C).

8. Conclusions

Embryonic cells are widely used model system to understand the early steps of embryonic development. Over the last years, many RA-regulated pathways have been discovered in EC and ES cells using a diverse set of techniques. In this chapter we have summarized the results of recent studies using high-throughput approaches (microarray, ChIP-chip, ChIP-Seq) to understand the mechanistic of retinoid signaling in early embryonic development. However, many questions remained to be unanswered. We should face the new technical challenges to be able to work out these issues.

9. References

Aparicio, O., J. V. Geisberg, et al. (2004). "Chromatin immunoprecipitation for determining the association of proteins with specific genomic sequences in vivo." *Curr Protoc Cell Biol* Chapter 17: Unit 17 7.

Azcoitia, V., M. Aracil, et al. (2005). "The homeodomain protein Meis1 is essential for definitive hematopoiesis and vascular patterning in the mouse embryo." *Dev Biol* 280(2): 307-20.

Bain, D. L., A. F. Heneghan, et al. (2007). "Nuclear receptor structure: implications for function." *Annu Rev Physiol* 69: 201-20.

Balmer, J. E. and R. Blomhoff (2005). "A robust characterization of retinoic acid response elements based on a comparison of sites in three species." *J Steroid Biochem Mol Biol* 96(5): 347-54.

Beland, M., N. Pilon, et al. (2004). "Cdx1 autoregulation is governed by a novel Cdx1-LEF1 transcription complex." *Mol Cell Biol* 24(11): 5028-38.

Bendel-Stenzel, M., R. Anderson, et al. (1998). "The origin and migration of primordial germ cells in the mouse." *Semin Cell Dev Biol* 9(4): 393-400.

Bibel, M., J. Richter, et al. (2007). "Generation of a defined and uniform population of CNS progenitors and neurons from mouse embryonic stem cells." *Nat Protoc* 2(5): 1034-43.

Blomhoff, R. and H. K. Blomhoff (2006). "Overview of retinoid metabolism and function." *J Neurobiol* 66(7): 606-30.

Bost, F., L. Caron, et al. (2002). "Retinoic acid activation of the ERK pathway is required for embryonic stem cell commitment into the adipocyte lineage." *Biochem J* 361(Pt 3): 621-7.

Bowles, J., D. Knight, et al. (2006). "Retinoid signaling determines germ cell fate in mice." *Science* 312(5773): 596-600.

Bratt-Leal, A. M., R. L. Carpenedo, et al. (2010). "Incorporation of biomaterials in multicellular aggregates modulates pluripotent stem cell differentiation." *Biomaterials* 32(1): 48-56.

Capellini, T. D., G. Di Giacomo, et al. (2006). "Pbx1/Pbx2 requirement for distal limb patterning is mediated by the hierarchical control of Hox gene spatial distribution and Shh expression." *Development* 133(11): 2263-73.

Capellini, T. D., R. Zewdu, et al. (2008). "Pbx1/Pbx2 govern axial skeletal development by controlling Polycomb and Hox in mesoderm and Pax1/Pax9 in sclerotome." *Dev Biol* 321(2): 500-14.

Casci, T. (2008). "Developmental biology: Retinoic acid passes the morphogen test." *Nature Reviews Genetics* (9): 7-7.

Chambon, P. (2005). "The nuclear receptor superfamily: a personal retrospect on the first two decades." *Mol Endocrinol* 19(6): 1418-28.

Chen, A. C. and L. J. Gudas (1996). "An analysis of retinoic acid-induced gene expression and metabolism in AB1 embryonic stem cells." *J Biol Chem* 271(25): 14971-80.

Chen, L. and J. S. Khillan (2010). "A novel signaling by vitamin A/retinol promotes self renewal of mouse embryonic stem cells by activating PI3K/Akt signaling pathway via insulin-like growth factor-1 receptor." *Stem Cells* 28(1): 57-63.

Chen, L., M. Yang, et al. (2007). "Suppression of ES cell differentiation by retinol (vitamin A) via the overexpression of Nanog." *Differentiation* 75(8): 682-93.

Chithalen, J. V., L. Luu, et al. (2002). "HPLC-MS/MS analysis of the products generated from all-trans-retinoic acid using recombinant human CYP26A." *J Lipid Res* 43(7): 1133-42.

Chourrout, D., F. Delsuc, et al. (2006). "Minimal ProtoHox cluster inferred from bilaterian and cnidarian Hox complements." *Nature* 442(7103): 684-7.

Christian, M., E. Kiskinis, et al. (2005). "RIP140-targeted repression of gene expression in adipocytes." *Mol Cell Biol* 25(21): 9383-91.

Core, L. J., J. J. Waterfall, et al. (2008). "Nascent RNA sequencing reveals widespread pausing and divergent initiation at human promoters." *Science* 322(5909): 1845-8.

Core, N., X. Caubit, et al. (2007). "Tshz1 is required for axial skeleton, soft palate and middle ear development in mice." *Dev Biol* 308(2): 407-20.

Cullum, M. E. and M. H. Zile (1985). "Metabolism of all-trans-retinoic acid and all-trans-retinyl acetate. Demonstration of common physiological metabolites in rat small intestinal mucosa and circulation." *J Biol Chem* 260(19): 10590-6.

Cvekl, A. and W. L. Wang (2009). "Retinoic acid signaling in mammalian eye development." *Exp Eye Res* 89(3): 280-91.

D'Ambrosio, D. N., R. D. Clugston, et al. (2011). "Vitamin A Metabolism: An Update." 3(1): 63-103.

Delacroix, L., E. Moutier, et al. (2010). "Cell-specific interaction of retinoic acid receptors with target genes in mouse embryonic fibroblasts and embryonic stem cells." *Mol Cell Biol* 30(1): 231-44.

Diez del Corral, R. and K. G. Storey (2004). "Opposing FGF and retinoid pathways: a signalling switch that controls differentiation and patterning onset in the extending vertebrate body axis." *Bioessays* 26(8): 857-69.

Dolle, P. (2009). "Developmental expression of retinoic acid receptors (RARs)." *Nucl Recept Signal* 7: e006.

Dolle, P., E. Ruberte, et al. (1990). "Retinoic acid receptors and cellular retinoid binding proteins. I. A systematic study of their differential pattern of transcription during mouse organogenesis." *Development* 110(4): 1133-51.

Duester, G. (2008). "Retinoic acid synthesis and signaling during early organogenesis." *Cell* 134(6): 921-31.

Duester, G. (2009). "Keeping an eye on retinoic acid signaling during eye development." *Chem Biol Interact* 178(1-3): 178-81.

Dupe, V., M. Davenne, et al. (1997). "In vivo functional analysis of the Hoxa-1 3' retinoic acid response element (3'RARE)." *Development* 124(2): 399-410.

Edson, M. A., A. K. Nagaraja, et al. (2009). "The mammalian ovary from genesis to revelation." *Endocr Rev* 30(6): 624-712.

Eguizabal, C., T. C. Shovlin, et al. (2009). "Generation of primordial germ cells from pluripotent stem cells." *Differentiation* 78(2-3): 116-23.

Eiraku, M., N. Takata, et al. (2011). "Self-organizing optic-cup morphogenesis in three-dimensional culture." *Nature* 472(7341): 51-6.

Feng, L., R. E. Hernandez, et al. (2010). "Dhrs3a regulates retinoic acid biosynthesis through a feedback inhibition mechanism." *Dev Biol* 338(1): 1-14.

Flynn, P. J., W. J. Miller, et al. (1983). "Retinoic acid treatment of acute promyelocytic leukemia: in vitro and in vivo observations." *Blood* 62(6): 1211-7.

Gaunt, S. J., D. Drage, et al. (2008). "Increased Cdx protein dose effects upon axial patterning in transgenic lines of mice." *Development* 135(15): 2511-20.

Ghyselinck, N. B., C. Bavik, et al. (1999). "Cellular retinol-binding protein I is essential for vitamin A homeostasis." *EMBO J* 18(18): 4903-14.

Giguere, V., E. S. Ong, et al. (1987). "Identification of a receptor for the morphogen retinoic acid." *Nature* 330(6149): 624-9.

Glass, C. K. (1994). "Differential recognition of target genes by nuclear receptor monomers, dimers, and heterodimers." *Endocr Rev* 15(3): 391-407.

Glass, C. K. and M. G. Rosenfeld (2000). "The coregulator exchange in transcriptional functions of nuclear receptors." *Genes Dev* 14(2): 121-41.

Gudas, L. J. and J. A. Wagner (2011). "Retinoids regulate stem cell differentiation." *J Cell Physiol* 226(2): 322-30.

Haeseleer, F., J. Huang, et al. (1998). "Molecular characterization of a novel short-chain dehydrogenase/reductase that reduces all-trans-retinal." *J Biol Chem* 273(34): 21790-9.

Hamada, H., C. Meno, et al. (2001). "Role of asymmetric signals in left-right patterning in the mouse." *Am J Med Genet* 101(4): 324-7.

Han, B. C., H. F. Xia, et al. (2010). "Retinoic acid-metabolizing enzyme cytochrome P450 26a1 (cyp26a1) is essential for implantation: functional study of its role in early pregnancy." *J Cell Physiol* 223(2): 471-9.

Heng, J. C., B. Feng, et al. (2010). "The nuclear receptor Nr5a2 can replace Oct4 in the reprogramming of murine somatic cells to pluripotent cells." *Cell Stem Cell* 6(2): 167-74.

Hisa, T., S. E. Spence, et al. (2004). "Hematopoietic, angiogenic and eye defects in Meis1 mutant animals." *EMBO J* 23(2): 450-9.

Hogarth, C. A., D. Mitchell, et al. (2011). "Identification and expression of potential regulators of the mammalian mitotic-to-meiotic transition." *Biol Reprod* 84(1): 34-42.

Honkakoski, P. and M. Negishi (2000). "Regulation of cytochrome P450 (CYP) genes by nuclear receptors." *Biochem J* 347(Pt 2): 321-37.

Horlein, A. J., A. M. Naar, et al. (1995). "Ligand-independent repression by the thyroid hormone receptor mediated by a nuclear receptor co-repressor." *Nature* 377(6548): 397-404.

Horst, R. L., T. A. Reinhardt, et al. (1995). "Identification of 9-cis,13-cis-retinoic acid as a major circulating retinoid in plasma." *Biochemistry* 34(4): 1203-9.

Huang, D., S. W. Chen, et al. (2002). "Analysis of two distinct retinoic acid response elements in the homeobox gene Hoxb1 in transgenic mice." *Dev Dyn* 223(3): 353-70.

Huang, F. J., C. C. Shen, et al. (2003). "Retinoic acid decreases the viability of mouse blastocysts in vitro." *Hum Reprod* 18(1): 130-6.

Isken, A., M. Golczak, et al. (2008). "RBP4 disrupts vitamin A uptake homeostasis in a STRA6-deficient animal model for Matthew-Wood syndrome." *Cell Metab* 7(3): 258-68.

Johnson, D. S., A. Mortazavi, et al. (2007). "Genome-wide mapping of in vivo protein-DNA interactions." *Science* 316(5830): 1497-502.

Kashyap, V. and L. J. Gudas (2010). "Epigenetic regulatory mechanisms distinguish retinoic acid-mediated transcriptional responses in stem cells and fibroblasts." *J Biol Chem* 285(19): 14534-48.

Kashyap, V., L. J. Gudas, et al. (2011). "Epigenomic reorganization of the clustered Hox genes in embryonic stem cells induced by retinoic acid." *J Biol Chem* 286(5): 3250-60.

Kawaguchi, R., J. Yu, et al. (2007). "A membrane receptor for retinol binding protein mediates cellular uptake of vitamin A." *Science* 315(5813): 820-5.

Koide, T., M. Downes, et al. (2001). "Active repression of RAR signaling is required for head formation." *Genes Dev* 15(16): 2111-21.

Koubova, J., D. B. Menke, et al. (2006). "Retinoic acid regulates sex-specific timing of meiotic initiation in mice." *Proc Natl Acad Sci U S A* 103(8): 2474-9.

Kuhnert, F., M. R. Mancuso, et al. (2010). "Essential regulation of CNS angiogenesis by the orphan G protein-coupled receptor GPR124." *Science* 330(6006): 985-9.

Kumar, S., C. Chatzi, et al. (2011). "Sex-specific timing of meiotic initiation is regulated by Cyp26b1 independent of retinoic acid signalling." *Nat Commun* 2: 151.

Lane, M. A., A. C. Chen, et al. (1999). "Removal of LIF (leukemia inhibitory factor) results in increased vitamin A (retinol) metabolism to 4-oxoretinol in embryonic stem cells." *Proc Natl Acad Sci U S A* 96(23): 13524-9.

Langston, A. W. and L. J. Gudas (1992). "Identification of a retinoic acid responsive enhancer 3' of the murine homeobox gene Hox-1.6." *Mech Dev* 38(3): 217-27.

Langston, A. W., J. R. Thompson, et al. (1997). "Retinoic acid-responsive enhancers located 3' of the Hox A and Hox B homeobox gene clusters. Functional analysis." *J Biol Chem* 272(4): 2167-75.

Langton, S. and L. J. Gudas (2008). "CYP26A1 knockout embryonic stem cells exhibit reduced differentiation and growth arrest in response to retinoic acid." *Dev Biol* 315(2): 331-54.

Ledda-Columbano, G. M., M. Pibiri, et al. (2004). "Induction of hepatocyte proliferation by retinoic acid." *Carcinogenesis* 25(11): 2061-6.

Lee, J., T. Yokota, et al. (2002). "Analyses of mRNA expression patterns of cohesin subunits Rad21 and Rec8 in mice: germ cell-specific expression of rec8 mRNA in both male and female mice." *Zoolog Sci* 19(5): 539-44.

Li, H. and M. Clagett-Dame (2009). "Vitamin A deficiency blocks the initiation of meiosis of germ cells in the developing rat ovary in vivo." *Biol Reprod* 81(5): 996-1001.

Li, L., A. E. Davidovich, et al. (2011). "Neural lineage differentiation of embryonic stem cells within alginate microbeads." *Biomaterials*.

Lin, T. C., J. M. Yen, et al. (2003). "IGF-1/IGFBP-1 increases blastocyst formation and total blastocyst cell number in mouse embryo culture and facilitates the establishment of a stem-cell line." *BMC Cell Biol* 4: 14.

Loudig, O., G. A. Maclean, et al. (2005). "Transcriptional co-operativity between distant retinoic acid response elements in regulation of Cyp26A1 inducibility." *Biochem J* 392(Pt 1): 241-8.

Luo, J., P. Pasceri, et al. (1995). "Mice lacking all isoforms of retinoic acid receptor beta develop normally and are susceptible to the teratogenic effects of retinoic acid." *Mech Dev* 53(1): 61-71.

Macarthur, B. D., A. Ma'ayan, et al. (2009). "Systems biology of stem cell fate and cellular reprogramming." *Nat Rev Mol Cell Biol* 10(10): 672-81.

Mahony, S., E. O. Mazzoni, et al. (2011). "Ligand-dependent dynamics of retinoic acid receptor binding during early neurogenesis." *Genome Biol* 12(1): R2.

Mansergh, F. C., C. S. Daly, et al. (2009). "Gene expression profiles during early differentiation of mouse embryonic stem cells." *BMC Dev Biol* 9: 5.

Mark, M., N. B. Ghyselinck, et al. (2009). "Function of retinoic acid receptors during embryonic development." *Nucl Recept Signal* 7: e002.

Martinez-Ceballos, E. and L. J. Gudas (2008). "Hoxa1 is required for the retinoic acid-induced differentiation of embryonic stem cells into neurons." *J Neurosci Res* 86(13): 2809-19.

McKinney-Freeman, S. L., C. Lengerke, et al. (2008). "Modulation of murine embryonic stem cell-derived CD41+c-kit+ hematopoietic progenitors by ectopic expression of Cdx genes." *Blood* 111(10): 4944-53.

Mercola, M. and M. Levin (2001). "Left-right asymmetry determination in vertebrates." *Annu Rev Cell Dev Biol* 17: 779-805.

Meyers, E. N. and G. R. Martin (1999). "Differences in left-right axis pathways in mouse and chick: functions of FGF8 and SHH." *Science* 285(5426): 403-6.

Mic, F. A., A. Molotkov, et al. (2003). "Retinoid activation of retinoic acid receptor but not retinoid X receptor is sufficient to rescue lethal defect in retinoic acid synthesis." *Proc Natl Acad Sci U S A* 100(12): 7135-40.

Moens, C. B. and L. Selleri (2006). "Hox cofactors in vertebrate development." *Dev Biol* 291(2): 193-206.

Molyneaux, K. A., H. Zinszner, et al. (2003). "The chemokine SDF1/CXCL12 and its receptor CXCR4 regulate mouse germ cell migration and survival." *Development* 130(18): 4279-86.

Monteiro, M. C., B. Wdziekonski, et al. (2009). "Commitment of mouse embryonic stem cells to the adipocyte lineage requires retinoic acid receptor beta and active GSK3." *Stem Cells Dev* 18(3): 457-63.

Mummery, C. L., M. A. van Rooijen, et al. (1987). "Cell cycle analysis during retinoic acid induced differentiation of a human embryonal carcinoma-derived cell line." *Cell Differ* 20(2-3): 153-60.

Nagy, L., H. Y. Kao, et al. (1997). "Nuclear receptor repression mediated by a complex containing SMRT, mSin3A, and histone deacetylase." *Cell* 89(3): 373-80.

Niederreither, K. and P. Dolle (2008). "Retinoic acid in development: towards an integrated view." *Nat Rev Genet* 9(7): 541-53.

Niederreither, K., V. Subbarayan, et al. (1999). "Embryonic retinoic acid synthesis is essential for early mouse post-implantation development." *Nat Genet* 21(4): 444-8.

Noy, N. (1992). "The ionization behavior of retinoic acid in aqueous environments and bound to serum albumin." *Biochim Biophys Acta* 1106(1): 151-8.

Okada, Y., T. Shimazaki, et al. (2004). "Retinoic-acid-concentration-dependent acquisition of neural cell identity during in vitro differentiation of mouse embryonic stem cells." *Dev Biol* 275(1): 124-42.

Oulad-Abdelghani, M., P. Bouillet, et al. (1996). "Characterization of a premeiotic germ cell-specific cytoplasmic protein encoded by Stra8, a novel retinoic acid-responsive gene." *J Cell Biol* 135(2): 469-77.

Pachernik, J., M. Esner, et al. (2002). "Neural differentiation of mouse embryonic stem cells grown in monolayer." *Reprod Nutr Dev* 42(4): 317-26.

Packer, A. I., D. A. Crotty, et al. (1998). "Expression of the murine Hoxa4 gene requires both autoregulation and a conserved retinoic acid response element." *Development* 125(11): 1991-8.

Pasutto, F., H. Sticht, et al. (2007). "Mutations in STRA6 cause a broad spectrum of malformations including anophthalmia, congenital heart defects, diaphragmatic hernia, alveolar capillary dysplasia, lung hypoplasia, and mental retardation." *Am J Hum Genet* 80(3): 550-60.

Pennimpede, T., D. A. Cameron, et al. (2010). "The role of CYP26 enzymes in defining appropriate retinoic acid exposure during embryogenesis." *Birth Defects Res A Clin Mol Teratol* 88(10): 883-94.

Petkovich, M., N. J. Brand, et al. (1987). "A human retinoic acid receptor which belongs to the family of nuclear receptors." *Nature* 330(6147): 444-50.

Pikarsky, E., H. Sharir, et al. (1994). "Retinoic acid represses Oct-3/4 gene expression through several retinoic acid-responsive elements located in the promoter-enhancer region." *Mol Cell Biol* 14(2): 1026-38.

Popperl, H. and M. S. Featherstone (1993). "Identification of a retinoic acid response element upstream of the murine Hox-4.2 gene." *Mol Cell Biol* 13(1): 257-65.

Qi, X., T. G. Li, et al. (2004). "BMP4 supports self-renewal of embryonic stem cells by inhibiting mitogen-activated protein kinase pathways." *Proc Natl Acad Sci U S A* 101(16): 6027-32.

Ray, W. J., G. Bain, et al. (1997). "CYP26, a novel mammalian cytochrome P450, is induced by retinoic acid and defines a new family." *J Biol Chem* 272(30): 18702-8.

Riddle, R. D., R. L. Johnson, et al. (1993). "Sonic hedgehog mediates the polarizing activity of the ZPA." *Cell* 75(7): 1401-16.

Rochette-Egly, C. (2005). "Dynamic combinatorial networks in nuclear receptor-mediated transcription." *J Biol Chem* 280(38): 32565-8.

Rossi, A., O. F. D'Urso, et al. (2010). "Non-coding RNAs change their expression profile after Retinoid induced differentiation of the promyelocytic cell line NB4." *BMC Res Notes* 3: 24.

Saunders, J. W., JR and Gasseling, M. T. (1968). "Ectodermal-mesodermal interactions in the origin of limb symmetry." *Epithelial-Mesenchymal Interactions in Development*: pp. 78-79.

Selleri, L., J. DiMartino, et al. (2004). "The TALE homeodomain protein Pbx2 is not essential for development and long-term survival." *Mol Cell Biol* 24(12): 5324-31.

Silva, J. and A. Smith (2008). "Capturing pluripotency." *Cell* 132(4): 532-6.

Simandi, Z., B. L. Balint, et al. (2010). "Activation of retinoic acid receptor signaling coordinates lineage commitment of spontaneously differentiating mouse embryonic stem cells in embryoid bodies." *FEBS Lett* 584(14): 3123-30.

Sirbu, I. O., L. Gresh, et al. (2005). "Shifting boundaries of retinoic acid activity control hindbrain segmental gene expression." *Development* 132(11): 2611-22.

Slack, J. M. (1987). "Embryology: we have a morphogen!" *Nature* 327(6123): 553-4.

Soprano, D. R., B. W. Teets, et al. (2007). "Role of retinoic acid in the differentiation of embryonal carcinoma and embryonic stem cells." *Vitam Horm* 75: 69-95.

Subramanian, V., B. I. Meyer, et al. (1995). "Disruption of the murine homeobox gene Cdx1 affects axial skeletal identities by altering the mesodermal expression domains of Hox genes." *Cell* 83(4): 641-53.

Takahashi, K. and S. Yamanaka (2006). "Induction of pluripotent stem cells from mouse embryonic and adult fibroblast cultures by defined factors." *Cell* 126(4): 663-76.

Tedesco, M., G. La Sala, et al. (2009). "STRA8 shuttles between nucleus and cytoplasm and displays transcriptional activity." *J Biol Chem* 284(51): 35781-93.

Thaller, C. and G. Eichele (1987). "Identification and spatial distribution of retinoids in the developing chick limb bud." *Nature* 327(6123): 625-8.

Tickle, C., B. Alberts, et al. (1982). "Local application of retinoic acid to the limb bond mimics the action of the polarizing region." *Nature* 296(5857): 564-6.

Tighe, A. P. and L. J. Gudas (2004). "Retinoic acid inhibits leukemia inhibitory factor signaling pathways in mouse embryonic stem cells." *J Cell Physiol* 198(2): 223-9.

Tucker, E. S., S. Segall, et al. (2008). "Molecular specification and patterning of progenitor cells in the lateral and medial ganglionic eminences." *J Neurosci* 28(38): 9504-18.

Umesono, K., V. Giguere, et al. (1988). "Retinoic acid and thyroid hormone induce gene expression through a common responsive element." *Nature* 336(6196): 262-5.

Vansant, G. and W. F. Reynolds (1995). "The consensus sequence of a major Alu subfamily contains a functional retinoic acid response element." *Proc Natl Acad Sci U S A* 92(18): 8229-33.

Wang, Z., M. Gerstein, et al. (2009). "RNA-Seq: a revolutionary tool for transcriptomics." *Nat Rev Genet* 10(1): 57-63.

Warkany, J. (1954). "Disturbance of embryonic development by maternal vitamin deficiencies." *J Cell Physiol Suppl* 43(Suppl. 1): 207-36.

White, R., G. Leonardsson, et al. (2000). "The nuclear receptor co-repressor nrip1 (RIP140) is essential for female fertility." *Nat Med* 6(12): 1368-74.

Williams, R. L., D. J. Hilton, et al. (1988). "Myeloid leukaemia inhibitory factor maintains the developmental potential of embryonic stem cells." *Nature* 336(6200): 684-7.

Wilson, J. G. and J. Warkany (1947). "Anomalies of the genito-urinary tract induced by maternal vitamin A deficiency in fetal rats." *Anat Rec* 97(3): 376.

Wilson, J. G. and J. Warkany (1950). "Congenital anomalies of heart and great vessels in offspring of vitamin A-deficient rats." *Am J Dis Child* 79(5): 963.

Xu, H., M. D. Beasley, et al. (2005). "Absence of mouse REC8 cohesin promotes synapsis of sister chromatids in meiosis." *Dev Cell* 8(6): 949-61.

Ying, Q. L., J. Wray, et al. (2008). "The ground state of embryonic stem cell self-renewal." *Nature* 453(7194): 519-23.

Ying, Y. and G. Q. Zhao (2001). "Cooperation of endoderm-derived BMP2 and extraembryonic ectoderm-derived BMP4 in primordial germ cell generation in the mouse." *Dev Biol* 232(2): 484-92.

Young-Pearse, T. L., L. Ivic, et al. (2006). "Characterization of mice with targeted deletion of glycine receptor alpha 2." *Mol Cell Biol* 26(15): 5728-34.

Yuki, K., H. Shindou, et al. (2009). "Characterization of mouse lysophosphatidic acid acyltransferase 3: an enzyme with dual functions in the testis." *J Lipid Res* 50(5): 860-9.

Zhang, X. and J. Huang (2010). "Integrative genome-wide approaches in embryonic stem cell research." *Integr Biol (Camb)* 2(10): 510-6.

Zhang, Y. Q., L. Sterling, et al. (2008). "Nodal and lefty signaling regulates the growth of pancreatic cells." *Dev Dyn* 237(5): 1255-67.

Zhou, G. B., Q. G. Meng, et al. (2010). "In vitro derivation of germ cells from embryonic stem cells in mammals." *Mol Reprod Dev* 77(7): 586-94.

Zhou, Z., S. Yon Toh, et al. (2003). "Cidea-deficient mice have lean phenotype and are resistant to obesity." *Nat Genet* 35(1): 49-56.

Ziouzenkova, O., G. Orasanu, et al. (2007). "Retinaldehyde represses adipogenesis and diet-induced obesity." *Nat Med* 13(6): 695-702.

Zizola, C. F., S. K. Frey, et al. (2010). "Cellular retinol-binding protein type I (CRBP-I) regulates adipogenesis." *Mol Cell Biol* 30(14): 3412-20.

Part 2

Neural and Retinal Differentiation

4

Pluripotent Stem Cells as an *In Vitro* Model of Neuronal Differentiation

Irina Kerkis[1], Mirian A. F. Hayashi[2], Nelson F. Lizier[1], Antonio C. Cassola[3], Lygia V. Pereira[4] and Alexandre Kerkis[5]

[1]*Laboratory of Genetics, Butantan Institute and Department of Morphology and Genetics, Federal University of Sao Paulo,*
[2]*Departament of Pharmacology, Federal University of Sao Paulo,*
[3]*Department of Physiology and Biophysics, University of Sao Paulo,*
[4]*Institute of Biosciences, University of Sao Paulo,*
[5]*Celltrovet (Genética Aplicada), Ltda.*
Brazil

1. Introduction

Embryonic stem (ES) cells are derived directly from inner cell mass (ICM) of mouse or human preimplantation embryos (Evans & Kaufman 1981, Martin 1981, Thomson et al., 1998). They are pluripotent, once they are able to differentiate *in vitro* and *in vivo* into derivatives of the three embryonic germ cell lines: mesoderm, endoderm and ectoderm (Fig. 1). The establishment of protocols for direct *in vitro* differentiation of pluripotent stem cell (PSC) into desirable cell type is extremely important for their use in therapies, for the studies of human diseases, and also for biochemical, toxicological and pharmacological studies (Pederson 1999, Sukoyan et al., 2002, Wobus & Löser 2011). Therefore, focusing on the PSCs use in these studies, many efforts have been devoted to the establishment of stem cells models with a particular emphasis to their *in vitro* differentiation into mature and functional neurons.

The nervous system is the most complex system in the organism and its formation usually involves four stages: specification of the neural cells identity (neural or glia), neural migration and axon formation, synapse formation (with target neurons, muscle or gland cells) and synaptic connection refinement (elimination of axons branches and cells death) (Müller 2006). It is well-known that many genes are involved in the process of neuronal stem cells fate specification (Aiba et al., 2006). This process depends on the specific environment during organogenesis, after birth and during adult life. The temporal and spatial factors are essential for neuronal differentiation, due to the multilayer nature of cortex (Müller 2006). Although numerous publications have reported PSCs differentiation toward neurons, many important questions are not answered yet, especially in respect to the equivalency of the *in vitro* PSCs model and *in vivo* central nervous system (CNS) development. Accomplishments in these directions would represent a crucial starting point for the stem cell therapies and drug discovery. A number of important protocols have been set up for the differentiation of PSCs into neurons, which mainly lead to the coexistence in the culture of differentiated neurons and non-neural cells, together with neural precursors and undifferentiated PSCs (Okabe et al., 1996, Li et al., 1998, Mujtaba et al., 1999, Baharvand et al., 2007). Most of these protocols are short-lasting, which therefore does not allow a careful analysis of the neurons maturation, aging, and death processes.

In this chapter, we describe principal methods of PSCs differentiation into neurons *in vitro*. Next, we present a method developed by our group, which established a long-term culture of committed neuronal precursors and functional neurons from mouse embryonic stem (mES) cells. In addition, using this long-term protocol we demonstrated the temporal and spatial localization of microtubule-associated proteins, such as, Lis1 (Lissencephaly-1) and Ndel1 (nuclear distribution element-like) in neuronal precursors and differentiated neurons. These both proteins have been shown to be essential for neuronal differentiation during the CNS development. Regardless of the relevance of these proteins for neuronal differentiation, their expression during PSCs differentiation was marginally explored.

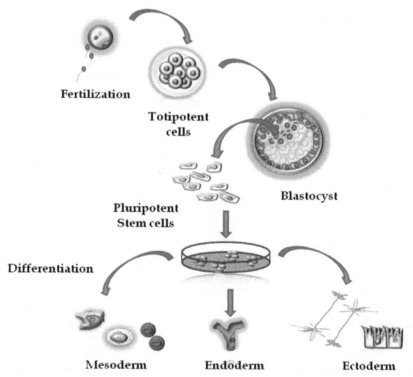

Fig. 1. ES cell isolation and differentiation.

2. Pluripotent stem cells as a model of *in vitro* differentiation

ES cells are powerful biological model, which can provide important information for our knowledge regarding the cell commitment and differentiation during development process (O'Shea 1999, Wobus & Boheler 2005). Multiple methods have been developed in order to induce *in vitro* PSCs differentiation and to obtain the desirable cell phenotype (Baharvand et al., 2004, Keller 2005). It has been found that ES cells are able to differentiate spontaneously within cell aggregates, when feeder layers and required factors to maintain pluripotency are removed. These aggregates, denominated embryoid bodies (EBs), resemble early post implantation embryos, although chaotically organized inside. It is assumed that EBs formation initiates spontaneous differentiation of ES cells to the three embryonic germ layers (Evans & Kaufman 1981). Innumerous studies have addressed the issue of cell specific differentiation of ES cells. In Figure 2 we summarize the main cell phenotypes, which can be induced to differentiate from ES cells *in vitro* under specific culture conditions. Those accomplishments are the result of a dynamic interaction between knowledge of embryonic development and empirical testing, targeted at reproducing *in vitro* cell specification conditions found in the developing embryo.

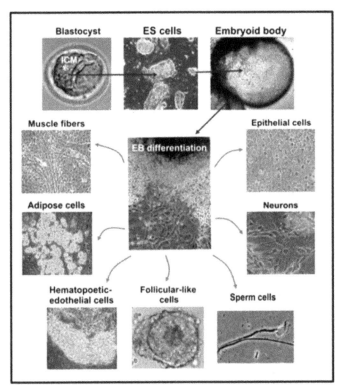

Fig. 2. ES cell differentiation *in vitro*. ES cells are isolated from the ICM of the blastocyst. These cells can be induced to form EBs, which are structures that contain representatives of the three embryonic germ layers. Under the appropriate culture condition, the EBs can be induced to differentiate into several types of cells *in vitro*.

2.1 Mesoderm specification

Mesoderm is the germ layer responsible for the development of muscle, bone, cartilage, blood, and connective tissue. Blood and endothelial cells are the first cell types to form in the developing vertebrate embryo at around six days of gestation. This event leads to the formation of the yolk sac, an extraembryonic membrane composed of adjacent mesodermal and primitive (visceral) endodermal cell layers, which give rise to blood and endothelial cells (Baron 2001). *In vitro* differentiation of ES cells in EBs allows the generation of blood islands containing erythrocytes and macrophages (Doetschman et al., 1985), whereas differentiation in semisolid medium is efficient for the formation of neutrophilis, macrophages, and erythroid lineages (Wiles & Keller 1991). In an attempt to identify potential inducers of the hematopoietic lineage, researchers indicated Wnt3 (Proto-oncogene protein) as an important signaling molecule that plays a significant role in enhancing hematopoietic commitment during *in vitro* differentiation of ES cells (Lako et al., 2001). The hematopoietic cells derived from ES cells have been characterized by specific gene expression patterns and by cell surface antigens (Wiles & Keller 1991, Wang et al., 1992). However, the most important aspect was to characterize these cells in the functional capacity, by demonstrating long-term multilineage hematopoietic repopulating properties in an animal model (Palacios et al., 1995).

Cardiomyocytes readily differentiate from aggregates composed of mES cells in the presence of high concentration of serum (around 20%), and display properties comparable to those observed *in vivo*: they express similar cardiac gene expression patterns, present sarcomeric structures, and demonstrate contractility triggered by cardiac-specific ion currents, as well as the expression of membrane-bound ion channels. This type of differentiation can develop spontaneously or be induced by differentiation factors including dimethyl sulfoxide (DMSO) and retinoic acid (RA), or small molecules, such as Dynorphin B and cardiogenol derivatives (Fassler et al., 1996). Human ES cells also hold the ability to differentiate into cardiomyocytes, which show similar properties to those derived from mES cells (Kehat et al., 2001). Furthermore, it is well established that ES cells can efficiently differentiate into several other mesodermal cells types, including mesenchymal cell-derived adipogenic (Dani et al., 1997), chondrogenic (Kramer et al., 2000), osteoblast (Buttery et al., 2001), and myogenic cells (Rohwedel et al., 1994). In all of these experiments, the cell type derivation was induced by specific differentiation factors.

2.2 Endoderm specification

Endoderm is responsible for deriving the pancreas and liver. Regarding the therapeutic interest for the treatment of hepatic failure and diabetes mellitus, hepatic and pancreatic cells are of special interest. Thus, since these cells could be derived from ES cells new hope has emerged (Soria 2001). These *in vitro* derived cells showed hepatic-restricted transcripts and proteins, and were able to integrate and to function in a host liver following transplantation (Chinzei et al., 2002). Recently, researchers demonstrated that hepatocyte-like endodermal markers were also detected in ES cell derivatives (Yamada et al., 2002).

The potential use of ES cells for treatment of diabetes was enhanced by the perspective of deriving insulin-producing pancreatic endocrine cells. Researchers at NovoCell, Inc., a biotechnology company in the USA, have developed an *in vitro* differentiation process that mimics pancreatic organogenesis. By directing cells through stages resembling definitive endoderm, gut-tube endoderm, pancreatic endoderm and endocrine precursor, they were able to convert human ES cells to endocrine cells capable of synthesizing the pancreatic hormones insulin, glucagon, somatostatin, pancreatic polypeptide and ghrelin (D'Amour et al., 2006). Moreover, in pre-clinical trials, the same group showed that those ES-derived pancreatic cells efficiently generated glucose-responsive endocrine cells after implantation into mice, and those insulin producing cells, in turn protected animals from streptozotocin-induced hyperglycemia (Kroon et al., 2008).

2.3 Ectoderm specification

The embryonic ectoderm is an embryonic germ layer, which can produce various cell lineages during development. Of particular interest, the differentiation of ES cells into neuronal cells was published independently by three groups in 1995 (Bain et al., 1995, Fraichard et al., 1995, Strubing et al., 1995). Gene expression and electrophysiological studies of cell derivatives from PSCs indicated the presence of the all three major cell types of the brain: astrocytes, oligodendrocytes, and neurons (dopaminergic, GABAergic (gamma-aminobutyric-acid-releasing), serotonergic, glutamatergic and cholinergic neurons) (Lee et al., 2000, Rolletschek at al., 2001, Aubert et al., 2002) (Fig. 3). Thus, these studies opened first perspectives regarding ES cell models for the study of neurodegenerative disorders. Human ES cells are also able to generate the neural epithelium (Thomson et al., 1998, Reubinoff et al., 2000, Zhang et al., 2001). However, although neural progenitors derived from ES cells could be enriched and directed to differentiate into mature neurons, astrocytes, and oligodendrocytes (Carpenter et al., 2001), experimental data obtained until recently could not demonstrate the formation of a given neuron subtype (Lee et al., 2000, Rolletschek at al., 2001, Aubert et al., 2002). The possibility of generating neurons *in vitro* signals for a first step towards exploring the therapeutic potential of ES cells for Parkinson's disease (Svendsen, 2008).

PCSs

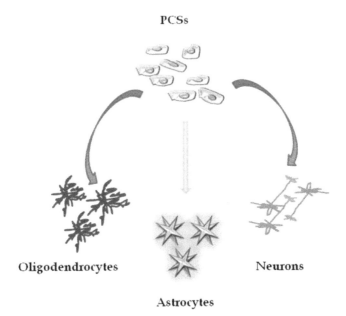

Oligodendrocytes   Neurons

Astrocytes

Fig. 3. All three major cell types of CNS derivative from PSCs: oligodendrocytes, astrocytes, and neurons.

2.3.1 Three dimensional (3-D) model of PSCs differentiation

Currently, common protocol comprises three steps: EBs (3-D model) formation, derivation of primitive neuroepithelial cells from EBs and generation of differentiated neural cell types. The most widely used method to induce neuronal differentiation is to enzymatically or mechanically lift the PSCs colonies and place them into low-adherence culture dishes or flasks without substrate, feeder cells, or mitogens, where they form EBs (Carpenter et al., 2001, Colombo et al., 2006, Baharvand et al., 2007). The culture media formulations for EBs vary significantly between different works (Ng et al., 2005, Yoon et al., 2006). Next, EBs are transferred to serum-free culture media and are plated onto laminin (poly-lysine)-coated dishes in order to generate an adherent culture and to differentiate into neuroepithelial cells. The EBs undergo spontaneous differentiation and the formation of clusters of small elongated cells surrounding a central zone, free of cells, so-called neural rosettes was showed (Pankratz et al., 2007, Pankratz & Zhang 2007). These rosettes resemble the morphology of the primitive neural tube and express early neural marker antigens such as Nestin (type VI intermediate filament (IF) protein) and Musashi-1 (RNA-binding proteins expressed in the CNS), but not markers of more mature neural cells. These rosettes were observed in majority of the studies of induction of neural differentiation of PSCs. PSCs neuroepithelial differentiation method are widely used to generate neural progenitors and mature neural cell types. The neuroepithelial cells obtained by this approach express the neuroepithelial transcription factors, such as PAX6 (Paired box gene 6), Sox1 (Sex determining region Y-box 1), and Sox2 (sex determining region Y-box 2), in about 90% of the total differentiated progenies (Li et al., 2007, Pankratz & Zhang 2007). Neuronal differentiation can also occur without EBs formation. In this case, specific growth factors or the co-culture of PSCs with cells of a particular origin that have been found to produce factors of neuronal cell specification are used to accelerate the differentiation towards one cell type or lineage of interest.

RA is an important regulator of the nervous system development, regeneration and maintenance (Zhang 2006, Maden 2007). Although, rosette formation occurrs during spontaneous *in vitro* differentiation of PSC-derived EBs, addition of RA enhances significantly the yielding of rosettes and mature neurons. Therefore, the predominant number of studies uses RA alone or in combination with other factors, e.g. bFGF (*basic fibroblast growth factor*). Additionally, neural differentiation can also be induced by the withdrawal of bFGF/EGF (*epithelial growth factor*) and exposure to BDNF (*brain-derived neurotrophic factor*), NGF (*neuronal growth factor*) or other factors into the culture medium.

The above described protocol and its modifications commonly produce mixed population of neuronal cells, which contain precursors, neurons and glial cells. This mixed population needs the application of further protocols for selection and enrichment, in order to obtain almost pure population of precursors or neurons, suitable for pharmacological screening or therapeutic applications.

2.3.2 Bi-dimensional (2-D) model of PSCs differentiation

Primary neural stem cells (NSC) can proliferate *in vitro*, forming multicellular floating spherical clusters, commonly referred as neurospheres, which are mainly composed by committed progenitor cells. When adhered on substrate, these neurospheres differentiate into functional neurons (Reynolds & Weiss, 1992; Chojnacki & Weiss, 2008). Our group aimed at developing a protocol for PSCs differentiation into neurons, which resemble the differentiation pattern of NSC-derived adherent neurosphere (AN). This protocol comprises five steps: EBs formation, culturing of floating EBs in the presence of RA, EBs adherence, formation of AN (2-D model), composed by commuted neuronal precursors and generation of neurons from AN. We further referred adherent EBs as ANs. It is worth mentioning that this protocol avoids the formation of rosettes.

The details of 2-D protocol are presented in Figure 4. An enzymatic digestion with trypsin of mES cells were used in order to obtain a feeder-free cell suspension. The mES cells were plated in culture flask, which allows rapid adherence of feeder cells. The EBs were obtained in low serum (5%) basal culture medium, following routine protocol of hanging drop method. Next, EBs were transferred into low-adherence culture dishes without substrate that allows adherence, and the neuronal differentiation was induced by the addition of RA (at final concentration of 0.1 μM). The EBs were maintained under non-adherent serum-free culture conditions (neurobasal (NB) medium supplemented with B27), for additional 4 days. Next, RA was removed and the EBs was transferred to poly-lysine treated plastic dishes in order to form ANs. The ANs were maintained in serum-free conditions for additional 7 days. At this moment of neuronal differentiation, outgrowth of neuron-like cells on the periphery of ANs was clearly observed (Fig. 5). These ANs were caught in small pieces and mechanically transferred into another Petri dish. After 3-4 days, these small ANs start to produce outgrowth of neurons. This process of ANs mechanical splitting and transfer can be repeated several times continuously producing ANs and neurons.

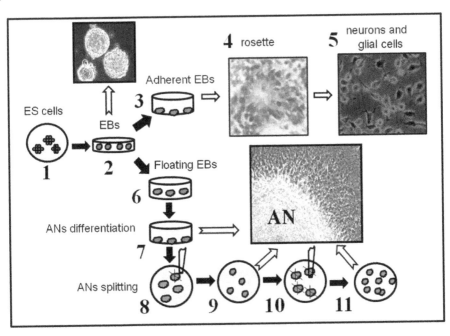

Fig. 4. Differentiation of ES cells towards neurons. 1-2: EBs formation; 3-6: 3-D model; 7-11:2-D model. (1) Pluripotent ES cells in basal culture medium. (2) EBs formation using suspension cell culture or hanging drop protocol. (3-5) Adherence of EBs, in serum-free medium with or without RA, production of neuroepithelial cells, (4) rosette formation, (5) neurons (white-brilliant) and glial cells (black) production. (6-11) culture of floating EBs in serum-free medium in the presence of RA, (7, 9, 10) RA removal, EBs adherence and ANs formation, production of neuronal precursor and mature neurons, (8, 10) ANs mechanical splitting and transfer using glass pipette. White arrows showed in (2) EBs (phase contrast), in (3) rosette (Hematoxylin & Eosin staining) in (5) neurons (phase contrast), in (7, 9, 11) AN with outgrowing neurons (phase contrast).

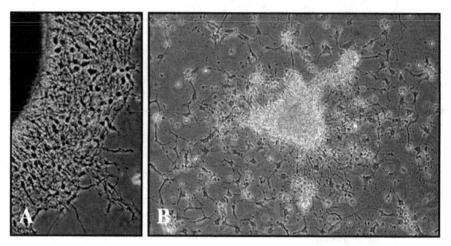

Fig. 5. Differentiation of PSC-derived adherent neurospheres. A) AN (black) producing a network of connected neurons. B) AN (white) after mechanical splitting and transfer. Migration of neurons also can be observed. Light microscopy (phase contrast).

These ANs present expression of the neural progenitor cell markers, such as Sox1 and Nestin just after plating. Following differentiation, the inner part of the AN, continuously expressed Sox 1 and Nestin proteins, while outgrowing neurons, which form an extensive neurite net around the AN expressed beta III-tubulin (neuron-specific marker) (Fig. 6).

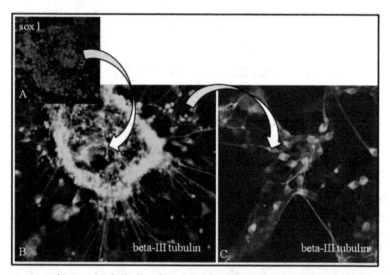

Fig. 6. Expression of neuroepithelial and neuronal markers in AN. A) Expression of Sox 1 protein (red), which express in the nucleus of progenitor cells localized in the inner part of AN. B) Expression of beta-III tubulin protein (green) at the periphery of AN and in outgrowing neurons. C) Higher magnification of extensive neurite net in (B) showing interconnected neurons.

The expression of other neuron-specific proteins, such as MAP2 (microtubule-associated protein 2), NF-M (neurofilament medium protein), Tau (a microtubule-associated protein), NeuN (neuronal nuclei marker), GABA and 5-HT (5-hydroxytryptamin), was observed in neurons derived from ANs each time after splitting and mechanical transfer, which was maintained during three months. Electrophysiological analysis, by using the patch-clamp technique, in long-lasting culture of AN-derived mature neurons, showed the presence of ionic channels and membrane electrical potentials typical of electrically excitable cells, which is a characteristic feature of functional CNS neurons.

This method of mechanical splitting and transfer of ANs is advantageous because it avoids the trauma associated to the trypsin treatments and mechanical dissociation and, so forth, may improve the survival of committed precursors able to differentiate into neurons. It is well-known that CNS precursors are localized in stem cell niche of organisms, which guarantees their continuous growth and renewing, and also the production of differentiated cells. In our model, ANs provide a constant microenvironment (*in vitro* niche) for the neuronal progenitor cells, which can be maintained for at least twelve weeks in culture, following repetitive mechanical splitting and transfer. Since expression of GFAP (Glial fibrillary acidic protein) gene has not been detected, it seems that AN direct the fate of non-committed precursors toward the neurons generation.

2.3.3 Importance of lineage selection for transplantation studies in regenerative medicine

A majority of available protocols for neural differentiation result in the generation of multiple cell types of committed neural precursor to a fully differentiated, post-mitotic neural cell. The selection and expansion of ES-derived neural precursors is a material for transplantation studies focusing on diseases as Parkinson's or Alzheimer's disease, or neural damage following stroke or injury. Such protocol is important due to the elimination of PSCs from the transplanted cell population, which can generate teratocarcinomas (Zhang et al., 1996, Deacon et al., 1998, Bjorklund et al., 2002). Commonly genetic engineering methods are used for lineage selection on differentiating ES cells to purify neural precursors. These techniques rely on the introduction of a reporter/selection cassette into a locus with restricted expression in the desired cell type by homologous recombination. Thus, to address lineage selection of neuronal precursor one copy of the pan-neural gene Sox1 has been replaced by the dual selection/reporter cassette egfpIRESpac in ES cell line, which confers cell-autonomous green fluorescence and puromycin resistance to cells that express Sox1. This gene is not expressed in ES cells. Its expression is limited to neuroectodermal cell, and undifferentiated ES cells are not fluorescent. Upon neural differentiation, Sox1 is activated and the cells produce green fluorescence enabling further purification of both neural and non-neural cells generated during differentiation. Fluorescence-activated cell sorting (FACS) is used for the isolation of both Sox1–GFP-positive and -negative cells allowing further analysis (Li et al., 1998, Pevny et al., 1998, Wood et al., 1999, Ying et al., 2003).

The comparison of AN and the above described techniques demonstrated that we succeeded to establish very simple and long-term protocol for generation of Sox1 positive cells. It is useful to note that 3 months of several mechanical splitting, Sox1-positive cells maintain the expression and continuously produce outgrowing beta III-tubulin-positive cells, while expression of GFAP gene has not been detected (Hayashi et al., 2010). Quantification of precursors and mature neurons demonstrated stable production of both Sox1 and beta III-tubulin proteins during the first 2 months. At the end of the third month, Sox1-nestin-positive cells were maintained at a similar level as before (~83%), whereas the number of immature neurons (~45%) decreased 1.5-fold, suggesting delay of the maturation process (~32%). Moreover, we showed that under the described conditions, dopaminergic, GABAergic, and serotonergic neurons can be produced. Therefore, generation of 2-D model is of great importance because allows expansion of neural progenitor without genetic modification from primary ES cell culture. Our AN protocol is especially advantageous for the future of regenerative medicine and treatment of neurodegenerative diseases, which will provide more tools for a safety clinical protocol with the advantage of lacking the intermediate effects from non-neural cells.

2.3.4 Importance of microtubule associated proteins for neuronal differentiation

Neuronal migration has been studied extensively in diverse mammalian species and the sequence of events that occurs during cortical development is shared by all mammals. (Gleeson & Walsh 2000, Walsh & Goffinet 2000). During neurogenesis, neural precursors are generated, which proliferate and differentiate into immature postmitotic neurons. These immature cells migrate from the ventricular zone (VZ) to preplate, a layer at the surface of the developing cerebral cortex, splitting the preplate and forming the cortical plate, which further develops into the cortex. Following immature neurons migration from the VZ, cortical lamination is established in an inside-out fashion. In the deep of the cortex, the earliest-born neurons end up, while later-born neurons localize at more superficial layers of the cortex residing near the pial surface. Synaptogenesis and apoptosis of neurons occur at the final stages of cortical development. Indeed, the migration of neurons requires the same steps, which is necessary for migration of any cell type. The signals of environment for attraction and repulsion; the nucleus dislocation from central position to the periphery, a process called nucleokinesis; and a mechanism for migration end up. Microtubule associated proteins (MAPs), for instance, Lis1 and Ndel1, have been shown to be essential for neuronal differentiation and cell migration during the CNS development and also in the adult nervous system.

2.3.4.1 Lis1 and Ndel1

Haploinsufficiency of Lis1 results in lissencephaly, a human neuronal migration disorder (Reiner et al., 1993, Saillour et al., 2009). Patients with type 1 Lissencephaly disorder, have a reduction in brain folding, and aberrant distribution and orientation of neurons in several brain regions. Lis1 binds with high affinity to a protein called Ndel1. Both proteins can complex with cytoplasmic dynein, the retrograde microtubule motor. Lis1 and Ndel1 are proposed to be important for the regulation of dynein-related events in mitosis and migration (Shu et al., 2004, Yamada et al., 2008, Youn et al., 2009, Hippenmeyer et al., 2010, Zyłkiewicz et al., 2011). Thus, PSCs can provide an important model to study migration defects related to MAPs.

Lis1 is a central component of a protein complex, evolutionarily conserved from fungus to human that regulates nuclear migration (Morris, 2000). Lis1 is able to regulate neuronal migration efficiency in a dose-dependent manner (Gambello et al., 2003). Reduced Lis1 activity results in severe defects in the radial migration of multiple types of neurons, including neocortical projection neurons (Tsai et al., 2005).

Ndel1 is important for normal cortical development and it is involved in microtubule organization, nuclear translocation, and neuronal positioning, in concert with various other proteins, including Lis1 (Shu et al., 2004, Youn et al., 2009). Mutations in the mammals Lis1 gene result in neuronal migration defects (Reiner et al., 1993, Youn et al., 2009, Saillour et al., 2009), while knockdown or ablation of cortical Ndel1 function also results in impaired migration of neocortical projection neurons (Sasaki et al., 2005, Youn et al., 2009). Lis1 and Ndel1 co-localize predominantly in the centrosome in early neuroblasts, and later, redistributes to axons during neuronal development (Shu et al., 2004, Guo et al., 2006, Bradshaw et al., 2008, Hayashi et al., 2010). Thus, Lis1 and Ndel1 are essential for normal cortical neuronal migration and neurite outgrowth.

Currently, Lis1 and Ndel1 were shown to have additional, important functions in the cytoplasmic dynein pathway. They participate in nuclear and centrosomal transport in migrating neurons (Shu et al., 2004, Tsai et al., 2005). Additionally, they influence a centrosome positioning in migrating non-neuronal cells (Dujardin et al., 2003, Stehman et al., 2007, Shen et al., 2008) as well as chromosome alignment, and mitotic spindle orientation (Faulkner et al., 2000, Siller et al., 2005, Liang et al., 2007, Stehman et al., 2007, Vergnolle & Taylor 2007). McKenney and co-authors (2010), using biochemical and biophysical approaches, investigated whether and how Lis1 and NudE (Ndel1) affect dynein motor activity. Results obtained in this work apparently explain the requirement for Lis1 and NudE in the transport of nuclei, centrosomes, chromosomes, and the microtubule cytoskeleton. Additionally, they provide new insight into the molecular basis for lissencephaly, and the mechanism of action of these proteins in a broad range of biological functions.

2.3.4.2 Expression of Lis1 and Ndel1 in ANs

Regardless of the relevance of these proteins for neuronal differentiation, their expression during PSCs differentiation is not well explored yet. Our group was the first to analyze intracellular localization of both proteins in mES cells, undifferentiated and during *in vitro* neural differentiation (Hayashi et al., 2010). The expression of both Lis1 and Ndel1 proteins was observed in undifferentiated cells, which presented co-localization within the perinuclear region (Fig. 7). At early stages of differentiation, just after formation of ANs, Lis1 expression was observed in the cytoplasm, while Ndel1 was in the perinuclear region of committed cells. Following differentiation, when ANs grow in size, the expression of both proteins was no more observed in the area of committed cells. Both Lis1 and Ndel1 proteins were visualized in outgrowing neuritis. Additionally, they co-localized with Tau, which is a marker of MAPs, involved in the microtubule assembly and stabilization. In the same way, Ndel1 and MAP2 were also co-localized. In non-rosette MAP2 positive neurons, Lis1 and Ndel1 proteins co-localized in neuronal cell body and growing axons (Fig. 7).

In attempt to mimic the development of cortical layers *in vitro* and to study the cell migration during the differentiation process, which can be assessed by the analysis of the expression pattern of these proteins, the ANs were allowed to grow for 15 days without splitting. Significant variation in spatial distribution of Lis1 and Ndel1 proteins were observed within 2-D ANs. The expression of Lis1 was observed in the inner part of ANs, in the cells presenting rosette morphology. Unexpectedly, Ndel1 was not expressed in rosette forming cells. Both proteins were co-localized in the cytoplasm of the cells showing neuroblast-like morphology, which were found close to the periphery of AN. Lis1 protein was expressing in the cells very closely localized to Ndel1 expressing cells, which, in turn, were close to the region of outgrowing neurons. Co-localization of Lis1 and Ndel1 expression was detected in cells from upper layer of ANs. Ndel1 was found to interact with centrosomes, suggesting that these cells are early neuroblasts (Fig. 8).

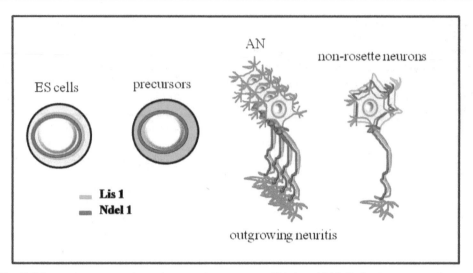

Fig. 7. Schematic presentation of expression pattern of Lis1 and Ndel1 during neuronal differentiation of PSCs. In undifferentiated ES cells, both Lis1 and Ndel1 show a perinuclear co-localization. In neuronal precursors, Lis1 presents a cytoplasmatic and Ndel1 a perinuclear localization. In neurons, at the periphery of ANs, both Lis1 and Ndel1 co-localize in the outgrowing neurites. In non-rosette neurons, these proteins co-localize in neuronal body and neurites.

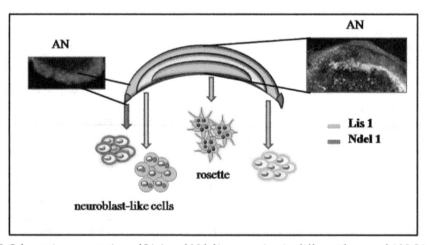

Fig. 8. Schematic presentation of Lis1 and Ndel1 expression in different layers of AN. Lis1 (green) expression was observed in the inner part of AN in the cells organized in rosettes. Intermediate layer (yellow) is composed by the neuroblast-like cells, which express both proteins, Lis1 (green) in the cytoplasm and Ndel1 in centriolos (red) and less in cytoplasm. Upper layer is composed mainly by Lis1 and at the periphery of AN by Ndel1 expressing cells. Proteins expression is also demonstrated by immunofluorescence within AN located on both sides of schematic presentation (Confocal microscopy + Fluorescence).

Interaction of Lis1 and Ndel1 with other cytosolic proteins had been well studied using cultured non-neuronal and/or neuronal cells and the expression of both Ndel1 and Lis1 genes in early neuroblasts derived from embryonic and adult tissues was observed (Sasaki et al., 2000, Shu et al., 2004). Our data demonstrated an expression of only Ndel1 without Lis1 expression in the centrosome region in neuroblast-like cells within differentiated AN. Variation of spatial distribution of Lis1 and Ndel proteins expression was also observed. The ES cells isolated from, for instance, Lis1 or Ndel1 knockout mice, followed by their differentiation into neuronal cells using the present protocol, will permit the elucidation of the real role of each protein during the neuronal differentiation process. Our data suggest that further analysis involving other important MAPs are necessary to allow a better comprehension of the migration mechanism(s) and of the specification fate of neuronal cells during differentiation.

3. Conclusions

PSCs have the capacity to differentiate *in vitro* into neuronal cells spontaneously through EBs formation or in monolayer culture. EBs 3-D model is shown to be more efficient model, which can be improved using serum-free culture conditions and inductors of differentiation (e.g. RA). Following this protocol, neuroepithelial cells could be obtained, which formed rosettes. Further selection and enrichment protocols are needed to isolate culture of committed neuronal precursor, neurons and/or glial cells. This 3-D model provides short-term culture of neuronal cells, which did not allow analysis of neurons migration and survival. It is of note that these AN can be maintained even in the absence of growth factors, without lacking the capacity to produce functional neurons.

Our study demonstrated that ANs is a long-term protocol, which can be used to analyze the process of neuronal differentiation in dynamics. Plating of intact ANs also provides a window of time to the precursor cells for establishing their fate in a 2-D environment. ANs model avoid a stage of rosettes formation directly producing committed progenitors and non-rosette neurons, mimicking process of differentiation of neurospheres form CNS. Mature neurons, obtained from ANs, display ionic channels and membrane electrical potential, which are typical of electrically excitable cells and are also a characteristic feature of functional CNS neurons.

Following mechanical splitting and transfer, these ANs grow continuously, confirming their auto-renewing properties similarly to progenitors of CNS. When maintained untouched during prolonged period (at least 15 days), progenitors inside growing ANs undergo further cell specification. As we demonstrated by the analyses of expression of Lis1 and Ndel1 proteins, both presented differential spatial distribution within the ANs. The discrepancy between patterns of expression of these proteins in neuroblasts isolated from embryonic or adult mouse neuronal tissues, and in those AN-derived cells was observed. AN-derived neuroblasts demonstrated only Ndel1 location in centrosome region, instead of showing the location of both proteins in this region. This indicates that miss expression of proteins, which are responsible for neuronal cells division and migration, can occur during *in vitro* differentiation.

Thus, our protocol provides an efficient experimental model for studying neuronal *in vitro* differentiation mimicking early development, as well as it represents a novel source of functional cells that can be used as tools for testing the effects of drugs on functional neuronal cells.

4. Acknowledgments

The authors thank Dr. Antonio C.M. Camargo and Dr. Juliano R. Guerreiro from Butantan Institute for their contribution in our research, as well as Alexsander Seixas de Souza for his technical assistance with confocal microscopy; and Dr. Toshie Kawano (in memoriam), Laboratory of Parasitology of Butantan Institute, for allowing the free access to the microscope whenever necessary. This work was financially supported by FAPESP.

5. References

Aiba, K.; Sharov, A.A.; Carter, M.G.; Foroni, C.; Vescovi, A.L.; Ko, M.S. (2006). Defining a developmental path to neural fate by global expression profiling of mouse embryonic stem cells and adult neural stem/progenitor cells. *Stem Cells 24(4)*, pp. 889-895.

Aubert, J.; Dunstan, H.; Chambers, I. & Smith, A. (2002). Functional gene screening in embryonic stem cells implicates Wnt antagonism in neural differentiation. *Nat. Biotechnol. 20*, pp.1240-1245.

Baharvand, H.; Ashtiani, S.K.; Valojerdi, M.R.; Shahverdi, A.; Taee, A.; Sabour, D. (2004). Establishment and in vitro differentiation of a new embryonic stem cell line from human blastocyst. *Differentiation 72*, pp. 224-229.

Baharvand, H.; Mehrjardi, N.Z.; Hatami, M.; Kiani, S.; Rao, M.; Haghighi, M.M. (2007). Neural differentiation from human embryonic stem cells in a defined adherent culture condition. *Int. J. Dev. Biol. 51(5)*, pp. 371–378.

Bain, G.; Kitchens, D.; Yao, M.; Huettner, J.E. & Gottlied, D.I. (1995). Embryonic stem cells express neuronal properties in vitro. *Dev. Biol. 168*, pp. 342-357.

Baron, M. (2001). Induction of embryonic hematopoietic and endothelial stem/progenitor cells by hedgehog-mediated signals. *Differentiation 68*, pp.175-185.

Bjorklund, L.M.; Sanchez-Pernaute, R.; Chung, S.; Andersson, T.; Chen, I.Y.; McNaught, K.S.; Brownell, A.L.; Jenkins, B.G.; Wahlestedt, C.; Kim, K.S.; and Isacson, O. (2002). Embryonic stem cells develop into functional dopaminergic neurons after transplantation in a Parkinson rat model. *Proc. Natl. Acad. Sci. USA. 99*, pp. 2344–2349.

Bradshaw, N.J.; Ogawa, F.; Antolin-Fontes, B.; Chubb, J.E.; Carlyle, B.C.; Christie, S.; Claessens, A.; Porteous, D.J.; Millar J.K. (2008). DISC1, PDE4B, and NDE1 at the centrosome and synapse. *Biochem. Biophys. Res. Commun. 377(4)*, pp. 1091-1096. Erratum in: *Biochem Biophys Res Commun. 3, 384(3)*, p. 400 (2009).

Buttery, L.D.; Bourne, S.; Xynos, J.D. et al. (2001). Differentiation of osteoblasts and in vitro bone formation from murine embryonic stem cells. *Tissue Eng. 7*, pp. 89-99.

Carpenter, M.K.; Inokuma, M.S.; Denham, J.; Mujtaba, T.; Chiu, C.P. & Rao, M.S. (2001). Enrichment of neurons and neural precursors from human embryonic stem cells. *Exp. Neurol. 172*, pp. 383-397.

Chinzei, R.; Tanaka, Y.; Shimizu-Saitou, K.; et al. (2002). Embryoid-body cells derived from a mouse embryonic stem cell line show differentiation into functional hepatocytes. *Hepatology 36*, pp. 22-29.

Chojnacki, A. & Weiss, S. (2008). Production of neurons, astrocytes and oligodendrocytes from mammalian CNS stem cells. *Nat. Protoc. 3*, pp. 935.

Colombo, E.; Giannelli, S.G.; Galli, R.; Tagliafico, E.; Foroni, C.; Tenedini, E.; et al. (2006). Embryonic stem-derived versus somatic neural stem cells: a comparative analysis of their developmental potential and molecular phenotype. *Stem Cells 24*, pp. 825-834.

D'Amour, K.A.; Bang, A.G.; Eliazer, S.; Kelly, O.G.; et al. (2006). Production of pancreatic hormone–expressing endocrine cells from human embryonic stem cells. *Nat. Biotechnology 24*, pp. 1392-1401.

Dani, C.; Smith, A.G.; Dessolin, S.; et al. (1997). Differentiation of embryonic stem cells into adipocytes in vitro. *J. Cell Sci.110*, pp. 1279-1285.

Deacon, T.; Dinsmore, J.; Costantini, L.C.; Ratliff, J. and Isacson, O. (1998). Blastula-stage stem cells can differentiate into dopaminergic and serotonergic neurons after transplantation. *Exp. Neurol. 149*, pp.28–41.

Doetschman, T.C.; Eistetter, H.; Katz, M.; Schmidt, W. & Kemler, R. (1985). The in vitro development of blastocyst-derived embryonic stem cell lines: formation of visceral yolk sac, blood islands and myocardium. *J. Embryol. Exp. Morphol. 87*, pp. 27-45.

Dujardin, D.L.; Barnhart, L.E.; Stehman, S.A.; Gomes, E.R.; Gundersen, G.G. and Vallee, R. B. (2003). A role for cytoplasmic dynein and LIS1 in directed cell movement. *J. Cell Biol. 163*, pp. 1205-1211.

Evans, M.J. & Kaufman, M.H. (1981). Establishment in culture of pluripotential cells from mouse embryos. *Nature 292*, pp. 154–156.

Fassler, R.; Rohwedel, J.; Maltsev, V.; et al (1996). Differentiation and integrity of cardiac muscle cells are impaired in the absence of beta 1 integrin. *J. Cell Sci. 109*, pp. 2989-2999.

Faulkner, N. E.; Dujardin, D. L.; Tai, C. Y.; Vaughan, K. T.; O'Connell, C. B.; Wang, Y. and Vallee, R. B. (2000). A role for the lissencephaly gene LIS1 in mitosis and cytoplasmic dynein function. *Nat. Cell Biol. 2*, pp. 784-791.

Fraichard, A.; Chassande, O.; Bilbaut, G.; Dehay, C.; Savatier, P. & Samarut, J. (1995). In vitro differentiation of embryonic stem cells into glial cells and functional neurons. *J. Cell Sci. 108*, pp. 3181-3188.

Gambello, M.J.; Darling, D.L.; Yingling, J.; Tanaka, T.; Gleeson, J.G.; Wynshaw-Boris, A. (2003). Multiple dose-dependent effects of Lis1 on cerebral cortical development. *J. Neurosci. 23(5)*, pp. 1719-1729.

Gleeson, J.G. & Walsh, C.A. (2000). Neuronal migration disorders: From genetic diseases to developmental mechanisms. *Trends Neurosci. 23(8)*, pp. 352-359.

Guo, J.; Yang, Z.; Song, W.; Chen, Q.; Wang, F.; Zhang, Q.; Zhu, X. (2006). Nudel contributes to microtubule anchoring at the mother centriole and is involved in both dynein-dependent and -independent centrosomal protein assembly. *Mol. Biol. Cell 17(2)*, pp. 680-689.

Hayashi, M.A.; Guerreiro, J.R.; Cassola, A.C.; Lizier, N.F.; Kerkis, A.; Camargo, A.C.; Kerkis, I. (2010). Long-term culture of mouse embryonic stem cell-derived adherent neurospheres and functional neurons. *Tissue Eng. Part C Methods 16(6)*, pp. 1493-1502.

Hippenmeyer, S.; Youn, Y.H.; Moon, H.M.; Miyamichi, K.; Zong, H.; Wynshaw-Boris, A.; Luo, L. (2010). Genetic mosaic dissection of Lis1 and Ndel1 in neuronal migration. *Neuron 68(4)*, pp. 695-709.

Kehat, I.; Kenyagin-Karsenti, D.; Snir, M.; et al. (2001). Human embryonic stem cells can differentiate into myocytes with structural and functional properties of cardiomyocytes. *J. Clin. Invest. 108*, pp. 407-414.

Keller, G. (2005). Embryonic stem cell differentiation: emergence of a new era in biology and medicine. *Genes and Devel. 19*, pp. 1129-1155.

Kramer, J.; Hegert, C.; Guan, K.; Wobus, A.M.; Muller, P.K. & Rohwedel, J. (2000). Embryonic stem cell-derived chondrogenic differentiation in vitro: activation by BMP-2 and BMP-4. *Mech. Dev. 92*, pp.193-205.

Kroon, E.; Martinson, L.A.; Kadoya, K.; Bang, A.G.; et al. (2008). Pancreatic endoderm derived from human embryonic stem cells generates glucose-responsive insulin-secreting cells in vivo. *Nat. Biotechnology 26*, pp. 443-452.

Lako, M.; Lindsay, S.; Lincoln, J.; Cairns, P.M.; Armstrong, L. & Hole, N. (2001). Characterization of Wnt gene expression during the differentiation of murine embryonic stem cells in vitro: role of Wnt3 in enhancing haematopoietic differentiation. *Mech. Dev. 103*, pp.49-59.

Lee, J.B.; Lumelsky, N.; Studer, L.; Auerbach, J.M. & McKay, R.D. (2000). Efficient generation of midbrain and hindbrain neurons from mouse embryonic stem cells. *Nat. Biotechnol. 18*, pp. 675-679.

Li, M.; Pevny, L.; Lovell-Badge, R.; Smith, A. (1998). Generation of purified neural precursors from embryonic stem cells by lineage selection. *Curr Biol 8*, pp. 971–974.

Li, X.J.; Yang, D.; Zhang, S.C. (2007). Motor Neuron and Dopamine Neuron Differentiation. In: Loring, JF., Wesselschmidt, RL., Schwartz, PH., editors. *Human Stem Cell Manual*. 1 ed. Elsevier. pp. 199-209.

Liang, Y.; Yu, W.; Li, Y.; Yu, L.; Zhang, Q.; Wang, F.; Yang, Z.; Du, J.; Huang, Q.; Yao, X. et al. (2007). Nudel modulates kinetochore association and function of cytoplasmic dynein in M phase. *Mol. Biol. Cell 18*, pp. 2656-2666.

Maden, M. (2007). Retinoic acid in the development, regeneration and maintenance of the nervous system. *Nat. Rev. Neurosci. 8(10)*, pp. 755–65.

Martin, G.R. (1981). Isolation of a pluripotent cell line from early mouse embryos cultured in medium conditioned by teratocarcinoma stem cells. *PNAS 78*, pp. 7634–7638.

McKenney, R.J.; Vershinin, M.; Kunwar, A.; Vallee, R.B.; Gross, S.P. (2010). LIS1 and NudE induce a persistent dynein force-producing state. *Cell. 141(2)*, pp. 304-14.

Morris, N.R. (2000). Nuclear migration. From fungi to the mammalian brain. *J. Cell Biol. 148*, pp. 1097–1101.

Mujtaba, J.; Piper, D.; Groves, A.; Kalyani, A.; Lucero, M.; Rao, M.S. (1999). Lineage restricted precursors can be isolated from both the mouse neural tube and cultured ES cells. *Dev. Biol. 214*, pp. 113-127.

Müller, T. (2006). Neural Development. *Encyclopedic Reference of Genomics and Proteomics in Molecular Medicine Part 14*, pp. 1258-1266.

Ng, E.; Davis, R.; Azzola, L.; et al. (2005). Forced aggregation of defined numbers of human embryonic stem cells into embryoid bodies fosters robust, reproducible hematopoietic differentiation. *Blood 106*, pp. 1601-1603.

O'Shea, K.S. (1999). Embryonic stem cell models of development. *Anat. Rec. 257*, pp. 32–41.

Okabe, S.; Nilsson, K.F.; Spiro, A.C.; Segal, M.; McKay, R.D.G. (1996). Development of neuronal precursor cells and functional postmitotic neurons from embryonic stem cells in vitro. *Mech. Dev. 59*, pp. 89–102.

Palacios, R.; Golunski, E.; Samaridis, J. (1995). In vitro generation of hematopoietic stem cells from an embryonic stem cell line. *Proc. Natl. Acad. Sci. USA 92(16)*, pp. 7530-7534.

Pankratz, M.T. & Zhang, S.C. (2007). Embryoid Bodies and Neuroepithelial Development. In: Loring, JF., Wesselschmidt, RL., Schwartz, PH., editors. *Human Stem Cell Manual*. 1 ed.. Elsevier. pp. 185-198.

Pankratz, M.T.; Li, X.J.; Lavaute, T.M.; Lyons, E.A.; Chen, X.; Zhang, S.C. (2007). Directed neural differentiation of human embryonic stem cells via an obligated primitive anterior stage. *Stem Cells 25(6)*, pp.1511–1520.

Pederson, R. (1999). Embryonic stem cells for medicine. *Scientific American 284*, pp. 69–73.

Pevny, L.H.; Sockanathan, S.; Placzek, M. and Lovell-Badge, R. (1998). A role for SOX1 in neural determination. *Development 125*, pp. 1967–1978.

Reiner, O.; Carrozzo, R.; Shen, Y.; Wehnert, M.; Faustinella, F.; Dobyns, W.B.; Caskey, C.T.; Ledbetter, D.H. (1993). Isolation of a Miller-Dieker lissencephaly gene containing G protein beta-subunit-like repeats. *Nature 364*, pp. 717–721.

Reubinoff, B.E.; Itsykson, P.; Turetsky, T. *et al.* (2000). Neural progenitors from human embryonic stem cells. *Nat. Biotechnol.19*, pp. 1134-1140.

Reynolds, B.A. & Weiss, S. (1992). Generation of neurons and astrocytes from isolated cells of the adult mammalian central nervous system. *Science 255*, pp. 1707.

Rohwedel, J.; Maltsev, V.; Bober, E.; Arnold, H.H.; Hescheler, J. & Wobus, A.M. (1994). Muscle cell differentiation of embryonic stem cells reflects myogenesis in vivo: developmentally regulated expression of myogenic determination genes and functional expression of ionic currents. *Dev. Biol. 164*, pp. 87-101.

Rolletschek, A.; Chang, H.; Guan, K.; Czyz, J.; Meyer, M. & Wobus, A.M. (2001). Differentiation of embryonic stem cell-derived dopaminergic neurons is enhanced by survival-promoting factors. *Mech. Dev. 105*, pp. 93-104.

Saillour, Y.; Carion, N.; Quelin, C.; Leger, P.L.; Boddaert, N.; Elie, C.; Toutain, A.; Mercier, S.; Barthez, M.A.; Milh, M.; Joriot, S.; des Portes, V.; Philip, N.; Broglin, D.; Roubertie, A.; Pitelet, G.; Moutard, M.L.; Pinard, J.M.; Cances, C.; Kaminska, A.; Chelly, J.; Beldjord, C.; Bahi-Buisson, N. (2009). LIS1-related isolated lissencephaly: spectrum of mutations and relationships with malformation severity. *Arch. Neurol. 66(8)*, pp. 1007-1015.

Sasaki, S.; Shionoya, A.; Ishida, M.; Gambello, M.J.; Yingling, J.; Wynshaw-Boris, A.; and Hirotsune, S. (2000). A LIS1/NUDEL/ cytoplasmic dynein heavy chain complex in the developing and adult nervous system. *Neuron 28*, pp. 681.

Sasaki, S.; Mori, D.; Toyo-oka, K.; Chen, A.; Garrett-Beal, L.; Muramatsu, M.; Miyagawa, S.; Hiraiwa, N.; Yoshiki, A.; Wynshaw-Boris, A.; Hirotsune, S. (2005). Complete loss of Ndel1 results in neuronal migration defects and early embryonic lethality. *Mol. Cell Biol. 25(17)*, pp. 7812-7827.

Shen, Y.; Li, N.; Wu, S.; Zhou, Y.; Shan, Y.; Zhang, Q.; Ding, C.; Yuan, Q.; Zhao, F.; Zeng, R. et al. (2008). Nudel binds Cdc42GAP to modulate Cdc42 activity at the leading edge of migrating cells. *Dev. Cell 14*, pp. 342-353.

Shu, T.; Ayala, R.; Nguyen, M.D.; Xie, Z.; Gleeson, J.G.; Tsai, L.H. (2004). Ndel1 operates in a common pathway with LIS1 and cytoplasmic dynein to regulate cortical neuronal positioning. *Neuron 44(2)*, pp. 263-277.

Siller, K.; Serr, M.; Steward, R.; Hays, T. and Doe, C. (2005). Live imaging of *Drosophila* brain neuroblasts reveals a role for Lis1/dynacitn in spindle assembly and mitotic checkpoint control. *Mol. Biol. Cell 16*, pp. 5127-5140.

Soria, B. (2001). In-vitro derivation of pancreatic beta-cells. *Differentiation 68*, pp. 205-219.

Stehman, S. A.; Chen, Y.; McKenney, R. J. and Vallee, R. B. (2007). NudE and NudEL are required for mitotic progression and are involved in dynein recruitment to kinetochores. *J. Cell Biol. 178*, pp. 583-594.

Strubing, C.; Ahnert-Hilger, G.; Shan, J.; Wiedenmann, B.; Hescheler, J. & Wobus, A.M. (1995). Differentiation of pluripotent embryonic stem cells into neuronal lineage in vitro gives rise to mature inhibitory and excitatory neurons. *Mech. Dev. 53*, pp.275-287.

Sukoyan, M.A.; Kerkis, A.Y.; Mello, M.R.B.; Kerkis, I.E.; Visintin, J.A. and Pereira, L.V. (2002). Establishment of new murine embryonic stem cell lines for the generation of mouse models of human genetic diseases. *Braz. J. Med. Biol. Res. 35(5*, pp. 535-542.

Svendsen, C. (2008). Stem cells and Parkinson's disease: toward a treatment, not a cure. *Cell Stem Cell 2*, pp. 412-413.

Thomson, J.A.; Itskovitz-Eldor, J.; Shapiro, S.S.; Waknitz, M.A.; Swiergiel, J.J.; Marshall, V.S. & Jones, J.M. (1998). Embryonic stem cell lines derived from human blastocysts. *Science 282*, pp. 1145 – 1147.

Tsai, J.W. ; Chen, Y. ; Kriegstein, A.R. ; Vallee, R.B. (2005). LIS1 RNA interference blocks neural stem cell division, morphogenesis, and motility at multiple stages. *J. Cell Biol. 170(6)*, pp. 935-945.

Vergnolle, M. & Taylor, S. (2007). Cenp-F links kinetochores to Ndel1/Nde1/Lis1/dynein microtubule motor complexes. *Curr. Biol. 17*, pp. 1173-1179.

Walsh, C.A. & Goffinet, A.M. (2000). Potential mechanisms of mutations that affect neuronal migration in man and mouse. *Curr. Opin. Genet. Dev. 10*, pp. 270–274.

Wang, R.; Clark, R. & Bautch, V.L. (1992). Embryonic stem cell-derived cystic embryoid bodies form vascular channels: an in vitro model of blood vessel development. *Development 114*, pp. 303-316.

Wiles, M.V. & Keller, G. (1991). Multiple hematopoietic lineages develop from embryonic stem (ES) cells in culture. *Development 111*, pp. 259-267.

Wobus, A. M. & Löser, P. (2011). Present state and future perspectives of using pluripotent stem cells in toxicology research. *Arch. Toxicol. 85(2)*, pp. 79–117.

Wobus, A.M. & Boheler, K.R. (2005). Embryonic stem cells: prospects for developmental biology and cell therapy. *Physiol. Rev. 85*, pp. 635-678.

Wood, H.B. & Episkopou, V. (1999). Comparative expression of the mouse Sox1, Sox2 and Sox3 genes from pre-gastrulation to early somite stages. *Mech. Dev. 86*, pp. 197–201.

Yamada, T.; Yoshikawa, M.; Kanda, S.; et al. (2002). In vitro differentiation of embryonic stem cells into hepatocyte-like cells identified by cellular uptake of indocyanine green. *Stem Cells 20*, pp. 146-154.

Yamada, M.; Toba, S.; Yoshida, Y.; Haratani, K.; Mori, D.; Yano, Y.; Mimori-Kiyosue, Y.; Nakamura, T.; Itoh, K.; Fushiki, S.; Setou, M.; Wynshaw-Boris, A.; Torisawa, T.; Toyoshima, Y.Y.; Hirotsune, S. (2008). LIS1 and NDEL1 coordinate the plus-end-directed transport of cytoplasmic dynein. *EMBO J. 27(19)*, pp. 2471-2483.

Ying, Q.L.; Stavridis, M.; Griffiths, D.; Li, M. and Smith, A. (2003). Conversion of embryonic stem cells into neuroectodermal precursors in adherent monoculture. *Nat. Biotechnol. 21(2)*, pp. 183-186.

Yoon, B.; Yoo, S.; Lee, J.; et al. (2006). Enhanced differentiation of human embryonic stem cells into cardiomyocytes by combing hanging drop culture and 5-azacytidine treatment. *Differentiation 74*, pp. 149-159.

Youn, Y.H.; Pramparo, T.; Hirotsune, S.; Wynshaw-Boris, A. (2009). Distinct dose-dependent cortical neuronal migration and neurite extension defects in Lis1 and Ndel1 mutant mice. *J. Neurosci. 29(49)*, pp. 15520-15530.

Zhang, K.Z.; Westberg, J.A.; Holtta, E. and Andersson, L.C. (1996). Bcl2 regulates neural diffentiation. *Proc. Natl. Acad. Sci. USA. 93*, pp. 4504–4508.

Zhang, S.C.; Wernig, M.; Duncan, I.D.; Brustle, O. and Thomson, J.A. (2001). In vitro differentiation of transplantable neural precursors from human embryonic stem cells. *Nat. Biotechnol. 19*, pp. 1129–1133.

Zhang, S.C. (2006). Neural subtype specification from embryonic stem cells. *Brain Pathol. 16(2)*, pp. 132–142.

Zyłkiewicz, E.; Kijańska, M.; Choi, W.C.; Derewenda, U.; Derewenda, Z.S.; Stukenberg, P.T. (2011). The N-terminal coiled-coil of Ndel1 is a regulated scaffold that recruits LIS1 to dynein. *J. Cell Biol. 192(3)*, pp. 433-445.

5

Oligodendrocyte Fate Determination in Human Embryonic Stem Cells

Siddharth Gupta[1], Angelo All[1,4] and Candace Kerr[2,3]
[1]Department of Biomedical Engineering
[2]Department of Obstetrics and Gynecology
[3]Institute for Cell Engineering
[4]Department of Neurology
Johns Hopkins University School of Medicine, Baltimore, MD
United States of America

1. Introduction

Oligodendrocytes (OL) are cells of the glial lineage which play a critical role in the central nervous system (CNS) by producing the multilamellar protein, myelin. Oligodendrocytes extend processes which wrap around the axons of several neurons. This myelin sheath increases neuronal conduction by decreasing ion leakage and capacitance of the axonal membrane and increasing saltatory conduction. Damage to oligodendrocytes results in loss of myelin and consequent functional impairment due to loss or decay of neuronal conduction. Demyelination in the CNS is the hallmark of conditions such as spinal cord injury (**SCI**), transverse myelitis and multiple sclerosis – resulting in functional impairment across the sensory, motor and cognitive domains. Current research on treatment of SCI focuses on the implantation of oligodendrocyte progenitor cells (OPC) into the injured region to achieve remyelination of the spared axons and potentially repair the sensory and motor pathways. However, this approach requires a large and relatively pure population of OPCs, which are differentiated from other multipotent cell lineages. Human embryonic stem cells have been used in several studies for this purpose and hence, it is important to understand the molecular mechanisms regulating the differentiation of pluripotent hESCs to oligodendrocytes. Elucidation of such mechanisms may lead to the development of more efficient differentiation protocols and the derivation of cells with improved myelination potential for implantation in injured spinal cords.

While the molecular basis for hESC differentiation into OL lineage cells is not completely understood, several recent studies have filled some of the gaps in our knowledge of the field. The journey from a pluripotent state to commitment to the OL fate is characterized by a complex interplay between genetic regulation and epigenetic modifiers such as histone modification, DNA methylation and microRNAs (miRNAs). Global miRNA expression profiling of OL differentiation from hESCs has revealed that a significant number of the differentially expressed miRNAs have targets hypothesized to be involved in myelination and OL development. Such studies are complemented by histone modification analyses in ESCs which show that specific histone acetyltransferases (HATs) and histone deacetylases (HDACs) are up- or down-regulated during different time points in OL differentiation to guide myelin production. This review focuses on the role of miRNAs in oligodendrocyte development from human embryonic stem cells and elucidates a new protocol developed to obtain oligodendrocytes from human embryonic stem cells with high yield and purity.

2. MicroRNA regulation of oligodendrocyte development

To date, many studies have attempted to unravel mechanisms of stem cell fate determination by studying gene expression by measuring messenger RNA (**mRNA**) expression. However, in the early-mid 90's a novel class of RNA molecules was discovered that regulated gene expression at the level of translation in C. *elegans*. These RNAs were shown to regulate the translation of a target mRNA, by directly base-pairing to its 3'-untranslated region (3' UTR) (Lee, Feinbaum & Ambros 1993, Wightman, Ha & Ruvkun 1993). Nevertheless, the broad significance of these small RNAs was not fully appreciated until only a few years ago when many similar molecules were further identified in C. *elegans*, Drosophila, and in some mammals (Lee, Ambros 2001, Lagos-Quintana et al. 2001), and these newly recognized regulatory RNAs were termed microRNAs (**miRNAs or miRs**). To date, sequencing libraries of cloned small RNAs and bioinformatic analyses of genomic sequences have led to the identification of ~500 verified mammalian miRNAs while studies exploiting the high degree of conservation of miRNAs across mammalian genomes have suggested that as many as 1000 human miRNAs are likely to exist (Berezikov et al. 2005, Bentwich et al. 2005). Despite these great advances in the identification of miRNAs, our understanding of their roles in cellular processes remains at a very early stage although there is evidence suggesting that miRNA dysfunction contributes significantly to oncogenesis and stem cell self-renewal.

MiRNAs are found in plants, viruses and animals and are generated via a multi-stage process. In mammals they are first transcribed as long precursor transcripts (~60-80 nucleotides) known as primary (pri)-miRNAs containing a hairpin loop (Lee et al. 2002). Pri-miRNAs are then processed into shorter hairpin shaped precursors (pre)-miRNAs in the nucleus and transported to the cytoplasm. There, the RNase-III enzyme Dicer performs a second cleavage to generate a double-stranded 21-23 nucleotide RNA molecule (Bernstein et al. 2001, Grishok et al. 2001, Hutvágner et al. 2001, Ketting et al. 2001, Knight, and Bass 2001). A large protein complex known as the RNA-induced silencing complex, or RISC, associates with this RNA duplex and unwinds it. Generally, only one strand is stably incorporated into RISC while the other is discarded and rapidly degraded (Meister et al. 2004). After the RISC is formed the miRNAs guide it to the target mRNA that is subsequently cleaved or translationally silenced. The degree of complementarity between a miRNA and its target dictates the mechanism of silencing (Meister et al. 2004, Hutvágner et al. 2004, Brennecke et al. 2003)

While degradation occurs predominantly in plants, in mammals the predominant mechanism appears to be through imperfect base-pairing between a miRNA and its target, resulting in translational silencing through a complex mechanism that appears to involve inhibition of both translation initiation and elongation (Pillai, Bhattacharyya & Filipowicz 2007).

MiRNAs are attractive candidates for regulating stem cell identity, which includes self-renewal and cell fate decisions, as their ability to simultaneously regulate many targets provides a means for coordinated control of gene action (Chen et al. 2007). Although direct functional roles in stem cell biology are just emerging, corroborating evidence from expression patterns, predicted targets, and from overexpression studies suggests miRNAs are key regulators (Cheng et al. 2005). For example, the loss of Dicer1 in mice has been demonstrated to cause embryonic lethality as well as loss of stem cell populations implicating a role for miRNAs in stem cell self-renewal (Bernstein et al. 2003, Murchison et al. 2005). Based on several reports from mouse and human studies, distinct sets of miRNAs are expressed specifically in pluripotent stem cells and not in adult tissues further implicating their role in stem cell self-renewal. In addition, Argonaute family proteins, which are key components of the RISC complex, have also been shown to be required in the maintenance of germline stem cells in different organisms (Carmell et al. 2002).

The role of miRNAs in oligodendrocyte fate determination has been a recent field of research and a few studies have reviewed the state of the current knowledge on the subject (He et al. 2011, Emery 2010, Dugas, Notterpek 2011).. This chapter aims to review the advances made in understanding oligodendrocyte fate determination by miRNAs and elucidate a novel protocol to derive OLs from embryonic stem cells in vitro to study their development.

2.1 MicroRNAs in glial fate determination

Zheng et al first reported that miRNAs were essential for the "developmental switch from neurogenesis to gliogenesis" (Zheng et al. 2010). The authors deleted Dicer, a protein necessary for functional miRNA synthesis, in the mouse ventral spinal neuroepithelium, where embryonic gliogenesis occurs. Neural patterning and motor neuron development occurred even in the absence of miRNA formation, showing that they are probably not involved in neuron maturation. However, oligodendrogenesis in the ventral spinal cord was blocked in the absence of Dicer, as confirmed by the complete absence of PDGFRα+ cells and a huge reduction in Sox10+ cells in the spinal cord parenchyma of Dicer mutants. On similar lines, astrogliogenesis was also found to be miRNA-dependent, as the study found that Dicer deletion led to the complete block of the development of a subset of astrocytes from the ventral neuroepithelium. This was confirmed by the lack of GFAP immunostaining of a small region flanking the floor plate when compared to the control. However, this study did not implicate any specific miRNA species as being involved in the regulation of gliogenesis in the developing spinal cord.

2.2 MicroRNAs in oligodendrocyte development

A 2009 study by Shin et al definitively established that miRNAs were involved in epigenetic regulation of oligodendrocyte function. This was performed by the OL-specific knockout of *Dicer* in postnatal mice. The Dicer protein is essential for synthesis of functional miRNAs and it was found that its elimination in postnatal OLs led to demyelination, oxidative damage, inflammatory astrocytosis and microgliosis in the brain. This phenotype resulted primarily from the disruption of miR-217 and consequent upregulation of its target ELOVL7 (elongation of very long chain fatty acids protein 7). Overexpression of ELOVL7 leads to lipid accumulation in the myelin rich regions of the brain and significant decrease in peroxisomal β-oxidation activity (Shin et al. 2009).

In the first study to analyze the global miRNA expression pattern in oligodendrocytes, Lau et al identified 98 miRNAs expressed by developing oligodendrocytes in the postnatal rat brain and found that 37 of these have an mRNA bias (Lau et al. 2008). In addition, the predicted protein targets of 13 miRNAs were dynamically regulated during OL development. In particular, the study identified miR-9 as a candidate miRNA with an important regulatory role during the transition from OPC (A2B5+/GalC−) to premyelinating OL (A2B5+/GalC+) and it was found that miR-9 downregulated the expression of the peripheral myelin protein (**PMP**) 22. PMP22 is expressed by Schwann cells and is a component of the compact myelin of the peripheral nervous system. Interestingly, miR-9 is not expressed by Schwann cells.

Another study identified miR-23 and its target, Lamin B1 (**LMNB1**) as a regulatory component of OL differentiation (Lin, Fu 2009). Genomic duplication of *LMNB1* has been implicated in autosomal dominant leukodystrophy (Padiath et al. 2006), a disease characterized by severe myelin loss in the CNS. Nuclear lamins such as LMNB1 interact with heterochromatin to regulate DNA synthesis and transcription and LMNB1 specifically regulates OL function; this was confirmed by the repression of transcription of OL-specific genes such as myelin basic protein (**MBP**), proteolipid protein (**PLP**) and myelin oligodendrocyte glycoprotein (**MOG**) by overexpression of LMNB1. The Lin et al study showed that miR-23 downregulates LMNB1 in normal OLs and that downregulation of LMNB1 by miR-23 was important for the development of OLs from glial cell cultures (Lin, Fu 2009). The effect of LMNB1 on differentiation was confirmed by the observation that increased *LMNB1* gene dosage caused an arrest in differentiation and led to the development of an MBP and PLP negative phenotype. This was hypothesized to be due to either faulty transcription of these genes or defective nuclear export.

A 2010 study by Zhao et al identified miR-219 and miR-338 as OL-specific miRNAs. This was confirmed by the complete absence of these two miRNAs in the spinal cord of Olig1 mutant mice. Fluorescent in situ hybridization revealed that miR-219 and miR-338 positive cells were found only in the white matter of the spinal cord, which is where OLs reside. Further, it was found that these two miRNAs promoted OPC maturation in vitro and in vivo. Transfection of OPC-enriched cultures with these miRNAs led to a significant increase in the number of MBP+ cells (a marker of mature OLs) and a slight decrease in the number of PDGFRα+ OPCs. MiR-219 and miR-338 were also found to be necessary for OL maturation. The study also identified Sox6 and Hes5 as potential protein targets of these miRNAs. These two transcription factors are inhibitors of OL maturation and have been shown to downregulate myelin gene expression and oligodendrocyte maturation (Kondo, Raff 2000, Liu et al. 2006). Sox6 and Hes5 are downregulated by miR-219 and miR-338. The authors suggest that commitment to the oligodendroglial lineage would require downregulation of transcription factors which induce differentiation to other neural cell fates and this was confirmed by the observation that miR-219 and miR-338 also downregulated other proneurogenic transcription factors such as NeuroD1, Isl1 and Otx2. In summary, these two miRs promote OL maturation by simultaneously inhibiting the inhibitors of OL differentiation and transcription factors which promote differentiation to non-OL neural cell fates.

Another recent study confirmed the importance of miR-219 and miR-338 in OL differentiation and maturation (Dugas et al. 2010). In addition, it also found miR-138 to be strongly upregulated during OL differentiation. Among the three, miR-219 was found to be the strongest inducer of OL differentiation and its transfection in a purified OPC population increased the number of differentiated OLs expressing both early (CNP, MBP) and late (MOG) OL markers. OLs induced by transfection with miR-138 only expressed early OL markers. As expected, OL-specific miRNAs were found to target genes that are repressed during OL differentiation. In addition, this study also found that miR-219 downregulates inhibitors of OL differentiation. The validated targets of miR-219 were found to include

PDGFRα, Sox6, FoxJ3 and ZFP238. PDGF has been known to be an OPC mitogen for multiple decades (Besnard et al. 1987). ZFP238 and FoxJ3 had previously not been functionally characterized in OPCs and this study confirmed that FoxJ3 and ZFP238 are inhibitors of OL differentiation by constitutively expressing these genes in OPCs and observing significantly reduced differentiation to the mature OL stage.

A study by Letzen et al was the first to perform a global miRNA analysis of cells isolated from 8 developmental stages from the pluripotent embryonic stem cell state to a mature, myelinating OL state (Letzen et al. 2010). Significantly, this study analyzed the expression of miRNAs in human cells as opposed to rodent models used in prior investigations. The study detected 183 miRNAs over the eight stages of oligodendrocyte maturation and also identified the highest differentially expressed miRNAs at each transition in the pluripotent-to-mature OL differentiation scheme. These differentially-expressed miRNAs were then matched to potential protein targets which revealed proteins such as chromosome 11 open reading frame 9 (**C11orf9**), claudin-11 (**Cldn11**), myelin transcription factor 1-like (**Mytl1**), myelin-associated oligodendrocyte basic protein (**Mobp**), myelin protein zero-like 2 (**Mpzl2**), and discoidin domain receptor tyrosine kinase 1 (**Ddr1**). The study focused on two miRNAs – miR-199a-5p and miR145, both of which show a decreasing expression level during the early to mid OP transition. C11orf9, which appears to be the human analog of the mouse myelin regulatory factor (MRF) was the target protein predicted for these 2 miRNAs. MRF has been shown to be necessary for myelination and OL maturation (Emery et al. 2009). It is thought that the decrease in miR199a-5p levels during OPC maturation may be parallel to the observed increase in MRF expression during the same time window, implying that miR-199a-5p may be one of the regulators of myelination and OPC maturation. MiR-214 was also observed to be strongly downregulated during the early-to-mid OPC transition and its predicted target is myelin-associated oligodendrocyte basic protein (MOBP), an important structural component of myelin.

2.3 Oligodendrocytes, miRNA and disease

Dysfunctional oligodendrocytes due to misregulation by miRNAs have recently been implicated in diseases of the central nervous system. For instance, mutations in several miRNAs have been discovered in the pathogenesis of multiple sclerosis (**MS**) (Junker, Hohlfeld & Meinl 2010). Specifically, miR-219 and miR-338 showed the maximum relative reduction in expression when the entire microRNAome of healthy, mature OLs was compared with chronic, inactivated MS tissue lesions (Junker et al. 2009). Other reports have also shown that miRNAs provide a mechanism for resistance against viral infection, and that miR-122 levels were significantly reduced in OLs infected with the Borna disease virus. This is significant as the Borna disease virus causes neurological disease in animals, and recent findings have implicated that it may also play a role in some human neurological and psychiatric conditions including bipolar disorder and depression (VandeWoude et al. 1990). In this case, overexpression of miR-122 inhibited viral protein synthesis and viral gene transcription and translation (Qian et al. 2010).

In one study to examine the possible role of miRNAs in the development of schizophrenia, the expression levels of 435 miRNAs in postmortem brain samples of schizophrenic patients were compared with those of psychiatric healthy controls (Moreau et al. 2011). In this study, 19% of the miRNAs analyzed showed misexpression in the schizophrenic samples, with these miRNAs mostly being downregulated compared to the healthy controls. On the other hand, a previous study identified differential expression of 28 miRNAs in the postmortem dorsolateral prefrontal cortex (Brodmanns Area) of schizophrenic individuals (Santarelli et al. 2011). 89% of these 28 miRNAs were upregulated and quantitative PCR was used to validate this finding for miR-328, miR-17-5p, miR-134, miR-652, miR-382, and miR-107. This elevation was linked to the observed upregulation of Dicer activity in these samples. The role of miRNAs in other neurological disorders has been reviewed (Xu, Karayiorgou & Gogos 2010).

3. Methods of oligodendrocyte differentiation

Unlike animal models, the study of oligodendrocyte development in humans has been generally limited in scope by the lack of models both in vivo and vitro that can be utilized to study this process. However, human embryonic stem cells provide an exciting model to help identify mechanisms that regulate the differentiation of oligodendrocytes. This includes elucidating the role of miRNAs in regulating the oligodendrocyte fate. This section describes a novel protocol for generating oligodendrocyte fated cells from human embryonic stem cells which have been developed in part from several published protocols (Nistor et al. 2005, Kerr et al. 2010).

3.1 Materials
3.1.1 Buffers and solutions
PBS: Phosphate buffered saline, without Ca^{+2} and Mg^{+2}, pH 7.0 (Invitrogen).
Trypsin/EDTA: HBSS containing 0.05% trypsin and 0.53 mM EDTA (Sigma).
Collagenase: 1mg/ ml collagenase IV (Invitrogen) in PBS, filtered.

3.1.2 Culture media
Basic culture medium for **MEF**: (Mouse embryonic fibroblast line PMEF-CF1 from Millipore): DMEM high glucose, supplemented with 10% Fetal Bovine Serum (Invitrogen), 2 mM glutamax (Invitrogen), 5 U/ml penicillin–streptomycin (Invitrogen), and 0.1 mM non-essential amino acids (**NEAA**).
Basic culture medium for undifferentiated human embryonic stem cells: DMEM/F12 (Invitrogen), supplemented with 20% Knockout Serum Replacement (Invitrogen), 2 mM glutamax (Invitrogen), 5 U/ml penicillin–streptomycin (Invitrogen), 0.1 mM non-essential amino acids and 3.5 µl β-mercaptoethanol supplemented with basic fibroblast growth factor (**FGF2**).
Basic culture medium for neural and oligodendrocyte progenitors: Neural Basal Media, supplemented with 10% Bovine Serum Albumin in PBS, filtered (Gibco), 0.5% N2 supplement (Invitrogen), 0.1 mM β-mercaptoethanol (Sigma) and 25 ug/ml gentamicin (Invitrogen).

3.1.3 Fixatives
4% Paraformaldehyde: 4g paraformaldehyde in 100 ml PBS. To dissolve the paraformaldehyde, the PBS was preheated at 90°C and sodium hydroxide (NaOH) added drop-wise slowly until the solution turns clear. The solution was cooled down before use.

3.2 Cell culture
Human ESCs were maintained on irradiated mouse embryonic fibroblasts (**MEFs**) in ESC growth media. Prior to differentiation, ESCs were separated from the feeder layer using a

solution of 1 mg/ml collagenase and plated on a 4% matrigel (BD Biosciences) substrate for 5 to 7 days and fed feeder-conditioned media daily. Cells were subsequently differentiated into embryoid bodies (**EBs**), neural progenitors (**NPC**), glial restricted precursors (**GPC**), and oligodendrocyte precursors (**OPC**) and finally mature oligodendrocytes (**OL**).

3.2.1 Preparation of MEF feeder layers

MEFs were maintained in basic MEF culture medium. The feeder cells were prepared the day before ESCs are expanded. The MEFs were plated at a density of 10×10^4 cells/cm² onto 0.1% w/v gelatin (Stem Cell Technologies) -coated culture dishes. Next morning, the feeder plates were γ-irradiated with a dose of 50 Gy (5000 rads) to induce cell cycle arrest. After irradiation, the culture medium was replaced. MEFs can also be mitotically-inactivated by treatment with mitomycin C (Sigma) at a concentration of 10 µg/ml for 4 hours at 37°C. The ESCs were plated on top of the MEF feeder layer using collagenase as described below. The medium was replaced daily with fresh medium supplemented with growth factors.

3.2.2 Human embryonic stem cells

The derivation and maintenance of human embryonic stem cells has been covered at length and details can be found in the following reviews (Park et al. 2003, Draper et al. 2004, Lu et al. 2006, Suemori et al. 2006, Ludwig et al. 2006, Hoffman, and Carpenter 2005). In brief, a culture plate with mitotically inactivated MEF feeder cells was prepared 24 h before use with ESCs with MEF basic culture media. The medium was removed from a culture dish of ESCs and the dish was washed with PBS. ESC can be expanded using either collagenase or trypsin. In both cases, however, over trypsinization of the colonies should be avoided because it will reduce cell viability. This could occur by incubating cells too long with enzyme and/or over triturating. For one 10 cm plate of ESCs, 1 ml of collagenase or trypsin solution was added and placed in incubator at 37°C for 5 to 10 min. The plate was removed from the incubator, the bottom of the plate scraped with a 5 ml pipette, making sure that all colonies had been lifted off, and then triturated slowly until only very small clumps were obtained. The colonies were not broken up into single cells as unlike their mouse counterparts, human ESCs do not survive well as single cells. The cell suspension was transferred into a 15 ml conical tube, 10 ml complete medium added and centrifuged for 5 to 10 min at 200 g at room temperature (**RT**). The pellet was resuspended in complete medium and placed onto mitotically-inactivated MEF feeder cell plate containing ESC complete medium with FGF2. The medium was replaced daily until ESC colonies reached optimal size for further passage. ESCs usually expanded by 5 fold after 5-7 days.

3.2.3 Embryoid body formation

Neural differentiation of ESCs was initiated via embryoid body (EB) suspensions. Embryonic stem cells were plated and dissociated onto 10 cm matrigel-coated tissue culture dishes as described above for passaging ESCs onto 10 cm plates with MEF. When ESCs were transferred onto matrigel they were grown in basic ESC culture media that had been conditioned on MEFs (live or irradiated) for 24 hours (12 ml of media per 10cm of confluent feeders), filtered and supplemented with 4 ng/ml FGF2. MEF-conditioned media was replaced on a daily basis until colonies were large and tight, almost near confluency in the wells.

To generate embryoid bodies, the medium was removed from a culture dish of ESCs and the dish washed with PBS. For one six well plate of ESCs, the cells were incubated in 0.5 ml of 1 mg/ml collagenase in PBS (avoid trypsinization as it can affect cell viability) and placed into the incubator at 37°C for 5 to 10 min. After removing the tube from the incubator, the cells were scraped with a cell scraper or lifter. The cell suspension was transferred to a centrifuge tube very gently, 10 ml of neural basal media supplemented with 200 ng/ml noggin, 20 ng/ml FGF2, and 20 ng/ml FGF4 (all growth factors from R&D Systems) was added and centrifuged for 5 min at 200 g, (RT). The supernatant was removed and the pellet gently resuspended into complete medium and placed onto a non-adherent or low adhesive 10 cm culture plate (Corning).

Neural EBs were fed daily by sedimentation. This was performed by tilting the dish at a 45 degree angle, waiting 5 minutes, and carefully aspirating with a 5ml pipette only half of the media so as to not discard the EBs floating in suspensions. EBs were grown for 10-25 days until they produced a transparent morphology. EBs were characterized by their loss of pluripotent markers, AP, OCT4, and NANOG and initiation of early markers of neuroectodermal fate including SSEA1, SOX1, PAX6 and Islet1 (**Figure 1**). The time may vary for different cell lines to reach this stage. Thus, the time at which is takes EBs to express these markers is dependent on the ESC line employed and so the cells should always be characterized at this point before proceeding forward. This can be performed by RT-PCR and by immunohistochemistry by freezing EBs in cryoprotectant mount media such as O.C.T. (Sakura Finetek TissueTek) and antibody staining (**Table 1**). The timeline provided here is based on our experiences using ESC lines H1 and H9 generated by Thomson et al (Thomson et al. 1998).

Human Oligodendrocyte Development Markers

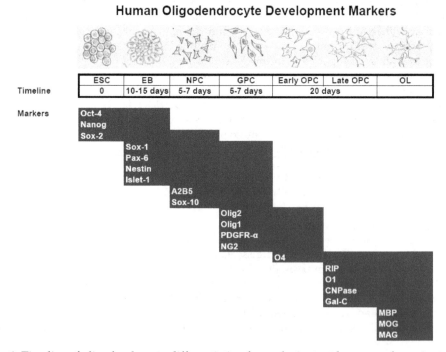

Fig. 1. Timeline of oligodendrocyte differentiation from pluripotent human embryonic stem cells, showing the expression of relevant cellular markers at each stage.

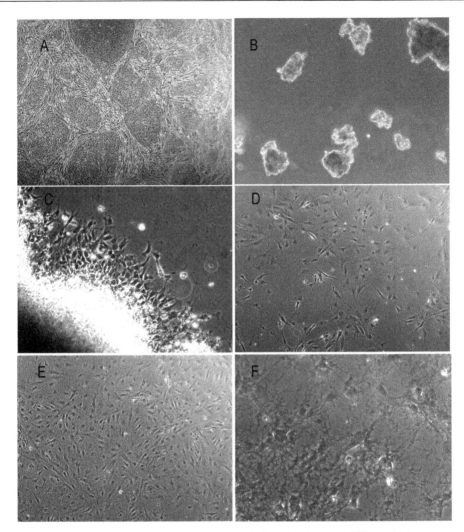

Fig. 2. **Phase contrast images of various stages of oligodendrocyte differentiation.**
A. Pluripotent human embryonic stem cells on MEFs, B. EBs one day after being generated
by the scraping method, C. NPCs sprouting from the periphery of a plated EB on matrigel
after 24 hrs, D. OPC 9 days after 2 expansions in OPC inducing medium, and OLs one week
after being exposed to OL inducing media.

3.2.4 Neural progenitor cells

10 cm tissue culture plates were coated with 3 ml of 4% matrigel in neural basal media for
one hour prior to plating EBs. Human ESC Qualified Matrigel Matrix was thawed overnight
at 4°C then diluted 1:24 (approximately 4% Matrigel) in cold neural basal medium.
Afterwards, the matrigel was removed and EBs plated in 10 ml of neural basal media
supplemented with 20 ng/ml FGF2 for 5 to 10 days. In this time, EBs spread over the plate

and became confluent. Most cells expressed neural fated markers including nestin and neural surface marker (A2B5) (**Figure 1**). NPCs at this stage were capable of deriving cells with both neuronal and glial fates. NPCs were fed daily.

3.2.5 Glial progenitor cells
NPCs were passaged in 1 to 3 splits for expansion using collagenase as described below (*Passaging Cells*) and replated on matrigel coated plates for differentiation into glial progenitor fate. Twenty-four hours after replating, media was changed to neural basal media supplemented with 20ng/ml EGF. Cells were fed daily for 10-14 days. GPCs began to express NG2, PDGFRα, and Olig1 (**Figure 1**). These cells can differentiate into either astrocytes or oligodendrocytes at this stage depending on the growth factors employed.

3.2.6 Oligodendrocyte progenitor cells
To promote differentiation into OPC, the media was supplemented with 20 ng/ml PDGF-AA. Cells were fed daily and begin to express OPC markers O1, O4, CNP, RIP, and GalC after one week (**Figure 1**). After 7–10 days the OPC morphology could be detected and was visible on the culture dish (**Figure 2**). By two weeks greater than 95% pure OPC could be obtained. Pure populations of OPCs can be obtained by FACs or MACs using O1 and O4 antibody selection using standard procedures. Once an OPC line is derived, cells can be expanded using 1 mg/ml collagenase in PBS onto gelatin-coated plates for several months before they reach senescence.

3.2.7 Oligodendrocytes
Terminal differentiation to mature oligodendrocytes was initiated by the addition of 50 ng/ml T3 (triiodothyronine, Sigma) and removal of PDGF-AA from the neural basal medium. Mature OLs demonstrate complex morphology after 3-5 days and express myelin-associated proteins such as MAG, MOG, MOBP, and MBP (**Figure 1**). These cells do not survive as long as the progenitor cells and begin to die off after the first week. In total, their survival under these culture conditions is between 1-3 weeks after maturity.

3.2.8 Passaging cells
3 ml of 0.1% matrigel is placed on a 10cm tissue culture plate. The medium is removed from a culture dish of OL-fated cells and the dish washed with PBS. For one six well plate, the cells were incubated in 0.5 ml of 1 mg/ml collagenase in PBS (avoid trypsinization as it can affect cell viability) and cells placed into the incubator at 37°C for 5 to 10 min. After removing the tube from the incubator, the cells were scraped with cell scraper or lifter. The suspension was mixed by gently pipetting up and down the cell clumps until a single-cell suspension was obtained. Importantly, to reduce cell mortality, the extent of cell disruption was controlled by pipetting only 5 to 10 times and with a 5ml pipette. The cell suspension was transferred to a centrifuge tube and centrifuge for 5 min at 200g at RT. The supernatant was removed and pellet resuspended in complete medium and placed onto the matrigel-coated plates. Medium was replaced daily until the cells were confluent before passaging onto a larger culture dish plate.

3.2.9 Freezing cells
From one confluent 6-well ESCs, NPCs, GPCs or OPCs were dissociated using collagenase as described above. These were rinsed in neural basal media for neural cells and ESC media

for ESCs at 200g for 5 min. The supernatant was aspirated and the pellet resuspended in freshly prepared 1X Freezing Media (for neural cells: 50% Neural Basal Media, 40% FCS, 10% DMSO; ESC freezing media: 50% Fetal Bovine Serum (Defined, Hyclone), 40% Neural Basal Media (Invitrogen) and 10% DMSO (Sigma), filtered). 1 ml of freezing media was added dropwise, mixing well after each addition. The suspension was transferred into sterile freezing vials, and placed into cryovessels. The cells were frozen overnight at -80°C, and then transferred to the liquid nitrogen freezer after 24 hours.

3.2.10 Thawing out cells

The vial of frozen cells was removed from the nitrogen freezer and transferred to a 37°C heat water bath to thaw by gentle shaking (thawing generally takes only 1-2 minutes). The suspension was transferred into 15 cc conical tube and 10 ml of culture media added and centrifuged at 200g for 5 min. The supernatant was removed, culture medium added, and plated directly onto a fresh matrigel coated plate for NPs, GPCs and OPCs or feeder plate for ESCs.

Name	Company	Product Code
Oct-4	BD Biosciences	611203
Nanog	EBioscience	14-5768-82
Sox-2	Abcam	ab15830-100
Sox-1	Abcam	ab22572
Pax-6	Abcam	ab5790
Nestin	Millipore	mab5326
Islet-1	DSHB	394D5
A2B5	Millipore	mab312r
Sox-10	Santa Cruz Bio.	sc17343
Olig1	Millipore	mab5540
PDGFR-a	Abcam	ab61219
NG2	Millipore	ab5320
O4	Millipore	mab345
O1	Millipore	mab344
RIP	Abcam	ab2035
CNPase	Millipore	mab326r
MBP	Abcam	ab7349-2

Table 1. Specific antibodies for oligodendrocyte characterization

3.3 Cell characterization

The identity of a cell in the differentiation pathway from pluripotent embryonic stem cells to mature oligodendrocytes is most commonly studied by its morphology, its gene expression and by analyzing the expression of protein markers by immunodetection.

Morphologically, undifferentiated ESCs generate colonies on top of feeders, NPC are more columnar or cuboidal in shape while GPCs and OPCs generate bipolar cells. Mature OLs demonstrate a complex network of dendritic processes (**Figure 2**).

Immunofluorescence (**IF**) staining of plated cells is more accurate morphology and the simplest method of analyzing protein expression to define the different stages of OL potential (**Table 1** lists sources of reliable antibodies for OL characterization). Here we present a standard protocol for IF staining for OL fated cells. **Figure 3** demonstrates staining at various stages of OL differentiation.

Cells were plated onto 24-well culture plates. Before cells became confluent, cells were washed twice in PBS and the excess PBS was removed. Cells were fixed in 4% PFA in PBS for 10 minutes at RT. The fixative solution was removed and wells washed twice with PBS for 5 min each. Cells were permeabilized and blocked with PBS solution containing 0.2% (w/v) Triton X-100 and bovine serum albumin (BSA; Sigma) at a concentration 1% (w/v) in PBS and incubated for 5 minutes at RT (for cells surface markers this step was skipped). Primary antibody (1:50 dilution) was added after dilution in antibody dilution buffer (PBS with 0.1% (w/v) BSA) and incubated for 1 hr at RT. Sample was washed three times with PBS for 5 minutes each. Appropriate secondary antibody was added (Alexa488 or Alexa546 conjugated antibodies, 1:200; Molecular Probes) in antibody dilution buffer and incubated in a humidified dark chamber for 1 hr at RT. Washed three times with PBS for 5 min each. Nuclei were stained with DAPI solution (Sigma) for 10 min at RT in a humidified chamber in the dark. DAPI solution was aspirated and 0.5 ml PBS was added to each well. Samples were examined under a fluorescence microscope with appropriate filters within 24 hrs as signal diminishes very rapidly. After 2 to 3 days most of the fluorescence signal is bleached. Sealant tape and aluminum foil was applied around the plates and stored in the dark at 4°C (short term storage only).

4. Results

4.1 Morphological analysis of differentiated cells

As shown in **Figure 2**, oligodendrocytes were successfully differentiated from human embryonic stem cells by our protocol described above. Embryoid bodies (Fig. 2b) were generated from pluripotent embryonic stem cells colonies (Fig. 2a). Plating these embryoid bodies on matrigel led to their adhesion and appearance of neural progenitor cells (Fig. 2c), which were then differentiated to glial progenitors (Fig. 2d) and subsequently oligodendrocyte progenitor cells (Fig 2e). Removal of all growth factors from the media led to the appearance of mature oligodendrocytes (Fig. 2e).

4.2 Immunocytochemistry of differentiated cells

EBs were characterized by their loss of pluripotent markers, AP, OCT4, and NANOG and initiation of early markers of neuroectodermal fate including SSEA1, SOX1, PAX6 and Islet1 (**Figure 1**). Upon contact with matrigel, EBs spread over the plate and became confluent. Most cells expressed neural fated markers including nestin and neural surface marker (A2B5)(**Figure 1**). After 5-7 days in NP media and addition of EGF, GPCs appeared and began to express NG2, PDGFRα, and Olig1 (**Figure 1**). Subsequent addition of PDGF-AA after 7 days led to the appearance of OPC markers O1, O4, CNP, RIP, and GalC (**Figure 1**). Finally, mature oligodendrocytes express myelin-associated proteins such as MAG, MOG, MOBP, and MBP (**Figure 1**).

Immunofluorescent images for a few of these markers are shown in **Figure 3.**

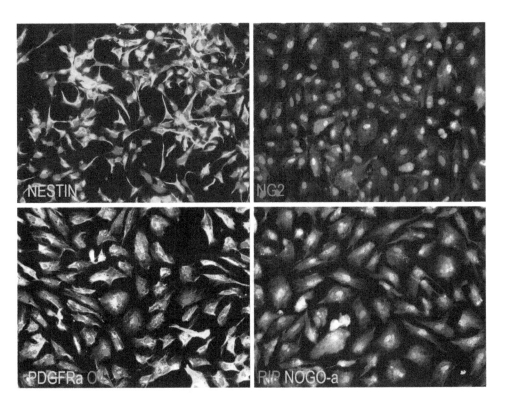

Fig. 3. Indirect immunofluorescence microscopy to examine differentiation of human ESCs into the oligodendrocyte lineage. The nuclei are stained blue by DAPI. Nestin (green) is shown for neural progenitors while NG2 (red), PDGFRa (green) O4 (red), RIP (red) and NOGO-a (green) are expressed by 5-day old oligodendrocyte progenitor cells.

5. Conclusion

In conclusion, a novel protocol adapted from previously published ones for oligodendrocyte development from pluripotent human embryonic stem cells has been developed. The cells express the established neural, glial and oligodendroglial markers as they advance along the differentiation timeline and we have confirmed this using indirect immunofluorescent microscopy.

Also, we have reviewed the current state of knowledge about microRNA regulation of oligodendrocyte differentiation from pluripotent cells and myelination of CNS neurons by those cells. It is hoped that the protocol for obtaining OLs in high purity will aid in the unraveling of more mechanisms of miRNA regulation of myelination so that this knowledge can eventually be used for the development of a more efficient approach to the stem cell based therapy of spinal cord injuries and other demyelinating disorders.

6. References

Bentwich, I., Avniel, A., Karov, Y., Aharonov, R., Gilad, S., Barad, O., Barzilai, A., Einat, P., Einav, U. & Meiri, E. 2005, "Identification of hundreds of conserved and nonconserved human microRNAs", *Nature genetics,* vol. 37, no. 7, pp. 766-770.

Berezikov, E., Guryev, V., van de Belt, J., Wienholds, E., Plasterk, R.H.A. & Cuppen, E. 2005, "Phylogenetic shadowing and computational identification of human microRNA genes", *Cell,* vol. 120, no. 1, pp. 21-24.

Bernstein, E., Caudy, A.A., Hammond, S.M. & Hannon, G.J. 2001, "Role for a bidentate ribonuclease in the initiation step of RNA interference", *Nature,* vol. 409, no. 6818, pp. 363-365.

Bernstein, E., Kim, S.Y., Carmell, M.A., Murchison, E.P., Alcorn, H., Li, M.Z., Mills, A.A., Elledge, S.J., Anderson, K.V. & Hannon, G.J. 2003, "Dicer is essential for mouse development", *Nature genetics,* vol. 35, no. 3, pp. 215-217.

Besnard, F., Perraud, F., Sensenbrenner, M. & Labourdette, G. 1987, "Platelet-derived growth factor is a mitogen for glial but not for neuronal rat brain cells in vitro", *Neuroscience letters,* vol. 73, no. 3, pp. 287-292.

Brennecke, J., Hipfner, D.R., Stark, A., Russell, R.B. & Cohen, S.M. 2003, "bantam encodes a developmentally regulated microRNA that controls cell proliferation and regulates the proapoptotic gene hid in Drosophila", *Cell,* vol. 113, no. 1, pp. 25-36.

Carmell, M.A., Xuan, Z., Zhang, M.Q. & Hannon, G.J. 2002, "The Argonaute family: tentacles that reach into RNAi, developmental control, stem cell maintenance, and tumorigenesis", *Genes & development,* vol. 16, no. 21, pp. 2733.

Chen, C., Ridzon, D., Lee, C.T., Blake, J., Sun, Y. & Strauss, W.M. 2007, "Defining embryonic stem cell identity using differentiation-related microRNAs and their potential targets", *Mammalian Genome,* vol. 18, no. 5, pp. 316-327.

Cheng, A.M., Byrom, M.W., Shelton, J. & Ford, L.P. 2005, "Antisense inhibition of human miRNAs and indications for an involvement of miRNA in cell growth and apoptosis", *Nucleic acids research,* vol. 33, no. 4, pp. 1290.

Draper, J.S., Moore, H.D., Ruban, L.N., Gokhale, P.J. & Andrews, P.W. 2004, "Culture and characterization of human embryonic stem cells", *Stem Cells and Development,* vol. 13, no. 4, pp. 325-336.

Dugas, J.C., Cuellar, T.L., Scholze, A., Ason, B., Ibrahim, A., Emery, B., Zamanian, J.L., Foo, L.C., McManus, M.T. & Barres, B.A. 2010, "Dicer1 and miR-219 are required for normal oligodendrocyte differentiation and myelination", *Neuron,* vol. 65, no. 5, pp. 597-611.

Dugas, J.C. & Notterpek, L. 2011, "MicroRNAs in Oligodendrocyte and Schwann Cell Differentiation", *Developmental neuroscience, .*

Emery, B. 2010, "Regulation of oligodendrocyte differentiation and myelination", *Science,* vol. 330, no. 6005, pp. 779.

Emery, B., Agalliu, D., Cahoy, J.D., Watkins, T.A., Dugas, J.C., Mulinyawe, S.B., Ibrahim, A., Ligon, K.L., Rowitch, D.H. & Barres, B.A. 2009, "Myelin gene regulatory factor is a critical transcriptional regulator required for CNS myelination", *Cell,* vol. 138, no. 1, pp. 172-185.

Grishok, A., Pasquinelli, A.E., Conte, D., Li, N., Parrish, S., Ha, I., Baillie, D.L., Fire, A., Ruvkun, G. & Mello, C.C. 2001, "Genes and mechanisms related to RNA interference regulate expression of the small temporal RNAs that control C. elegans developmental timing", *Cell,* vol. 106, no. 1, pp. 23-34.

He, X., Yu, Y., Awatramani, R. & Lu, Q.R. 2011, "Unwrapping Myelination by MicroRNAs", *The Neuroscientist,.*

Hoffman, L.M. & Carpenter, M.K. 2005, "Characterization and culture of human embryonic stem cells", *Nature biotechnology,* vol. 23, no. 6, pp. 699-708.

Hutvágner, G., McLachlan, J., Pasquinelli, A.E., Bálint, É., Tuschl, T. & Zamore, P.D. 2001, "A cellular function for the RNA-interference enzyme Dicer in the maturation of the let-7 small temporal RNA", *Science,* vol. 293, no. 5531, pp. 834.

Hutvágner, G., Simard, M.J., Mello, C.C. & Zamore, P.D. 2004, "Sequence-specific inhibition of small RNA function", *PLoS Biology,* vol. 2, no. 4, pp. e98.

Junker, A., Hohlfeld, R. & Meinl, E. 2010, "The emerging role of microRNAs in multiple sclerosis", *Nature Reviews Neurology,* vol. 7, no. 1, pp. 56-59.

Junker, A., Krumbholz, M., Eisele, S., Mohan, H., Augstein, F., Bittner, R., Lassmann, H., Wekerle, H., Hohlfeld, R. & Meinl, E. 2009, "MicroRNA profiling of multiple sclerosis lesions identifies modulators of the regulatory protein CD47", *Brain,* vol. 132, no. 12, pp. 3342.

Kerr, C.L., Letzen, B.S., Hill, C.M., Agrawal, G., Thakor, N.V., Sterneckert, J.L., Gearhart, J.D. & All, A.H. 2010, "Efficient differentiation of human embryonic stem cells into oligodendrocyte progenitors for application in a rat contusion model of spinal cord injury", *International Journal of Neuroscience,* vol. 120, no. 4, pp. 305-313.

Ketting, R.F., Fischer, S.E.J., Bernstein, E., Sijen, T., Hannon, G.J. & Plasterk, R.H.A. 2001, "Dicer functions in RNA interference and in synthesis of small RNA involved in developmental timing in C. elegans", *Genes & development,* vol. 15, no. 20, pp. 2654.

Knight, S.W. & Bass, B.L. 2001, "A role for the RNase III enzyme DCR-1 in RNA interference and germ line development in Caenorhabditis elegans", *Science,* vol. 293, no. 5538, pp. 2269.

Kondo, T. & Raff, M. 2000, "Basic helix-loop-helix proteins and the timing of oligodendrocyte differentiation", *Development,* vol. 127, no. 14, pp. 2989.

Lagos-Quintana, M., Rauhut, R., Lendeckel, W. & Tuschl, T. 2001, "Identification of novel genes coding for small expressed RNAs", *Science,* vol. 294, no. 5543, pp. 853.

Lau, P., Verrier, J.D., Nielsen, J.A., Johnson, K.R., Notterpek, L. & Hudson, L.D. 2008, "Identification of dynamically regulated microRNA and mRNA networks in developing oligodendrocytes", *Journal of Neuroscience,* vol. 28, no. 45, pp. 11720.

Lee, R.C. & Ambros, V. 2001, "An extensive class of small RNAs in Caenorhabditis elegans", *Science,* vol. 294, no. 5543, pp. 862.

Lee, R.C., Feinbaum, R.L. & Ambros, V. 1993, "The C. elegans heterochronic gene lin-4 encodes small RNAs with antisense complementarity to lin-14", *Cell,* vol. 75, no. 5, pp. 843-854.

Lee, Y., Jeon, K., Lee, J.T., Kim, S. & Kim, V.N. 2002, "MicroRNA maturation: stepwise processing and subcellular localization", *The EMBO journal,* vol. 21, no. 17, pp. 4663-4670.

Letzen, B.S., Liu, C., Thakor, N.V., Gearhart, J.D., All, A.H., Kerr, C.L. & Linden, R. 2010, "MicroRNA expression profiling of oligodendrocyte differentiation from human embryonic stem cells", *PLoS One,* vol. 5, no. 5, pp. e10480.

Lin, S.T. & Fu, Y.H. 2009, "miR-23 regulation of lamin B1 is crucial for oligodendrocyte development and myelination", *Disease Models & Mechanisms,* vol. 2, no. 3-4, pp. 178.

Liu, A., Li, J., Marin-Husstege, M., Kageyama, R., Fan, Y., Gelinas, C. & Casaccia-Bonnefil, P. 2006, "A molecular insight of Hes5-dependent inhibition of myelin gene expression: old partners and new players", *The EMBO journal,* vol. 25, no. 20, pp. 4833-4842.

Lu, J., Hou, R., Booth, C.J., Yang, S.H. & Snyder, M. 2006, "Defined culture conditions of human embryonic stem cells", National Acad Sciences, .

Ludwig, T.E., Bergendahl, V., Levenstein, M.E., Yu, J., Probasco, M.D. & Thomson, J.A. 2006, "Feeder-independent culture of human embryonic stem cells", *Nature methods*, vol. 3, no. 8, pp. 637-646.

Meister, G., Landthaler, M., Dorsett, Y. & Tuschl, T. 2004, "Sequence-specific inhibition of microRNA-and siRNA-induced RNA silencing", *Rna*, vol. 10, no. 3, pp. 544.

Moreau, M.P., Bruse, S.E., David-Rus, R., Buyske, S. & Brzustowicz, L.M. 2011, "Altered microRNA expression profiles in postmortem brain samples from individuals with schizophrenia and bipolar disorder", *Biological psychiatry*, vol. 69, no. 2, pp. 188-193.

Murchison, E.P., Partridge, J.F., Tam, O.H., Cheloufi, S. & Hannon, G.J. 2005, "Characterization of Dicer-deficient murine embryonic stem cells", *Proceedings of the National Academy of Sciences of the United States of America*, vol. 102, no. 34, pp. 12135.

Nistor, G.I., Totoiu, M.O., Haque, N., Carpenter, M.K. & Keirstead, H.S. 2005, "Human embryonic stem cells differentiate into oligodendrocytes in high purity and myelinate after spinal cord transplantation", *Glia*, vol. 49, no. 3, pp. 385-396.

Padiath, Q.S., Saigoh, K., Schiffmann, R., Asahara, H., Yamada, T., Koeppen, A., Hogan, K., Ptácek, L.J. & Fu, Y.H. 2006, "Lamin B1 duplications cause autosomal dominant leukodystrophy", *Nature genetics*, vol. 38, no. 10, pp. 1114-1123.

Park, J.H., Kim, S.J., Oh, E.J., Moon, S.Y., Roh, S.I., Kim, C.G. & Yoon, H.S. 2003, "Establishment and maintenance of human embryonic stem cells on STO, a permanently growing cell line", *Biology of reproduction*, vol. 69, no. 6, pp. 2007.

Pillai, R.S., Bhattacharyya, S.N. & Filipowicz, W. 2007, "Repression of protein synthesis by miRNAs: how many mechanisms?", *Trends in cell biology*, vol. 17, no. 3, pp. 118-126.

Qian, J., Zhai, A., Kao, W., Li, Y., Song, W., Fu, Y., Chen, X., Zhang, Q., Wu, J. & Li, H. 2010, "Modulation of miR-122 on persistently Borna disease virus infected human oligodendroglial cells", *Antiviral Research*, vol. 87, no. 2, pp. 249-256.

Santarelli, D.M., Beveridge, N.J., Tooney, P.A. & Cairns, M.J. 2011, "Upregulation of Dicer and MicroRNA Expression in the Dorsolateral Prefrontal Cortex Brodmann Area 46 in Schizophrenia", *Biological psychiatry*, vol. 69, no. 2, pp. 180-187.

Shin, D., Shin, J.Y., McManus, M.T., Ptcek, L.J. & Fu, Y.H. 2009, "Dicer ablation in oligodendrocytes provokes neuronal impairment in mice", *Annals of Neurology*, vol. 66, no. 6, pp. 843-857.

Suemori, H., Yasuchika, K., Hasegawa, K., Fujioka, T., Tsuneyoshi, N. & Nakatsuji, N. 2006, "Efficient establishment of human embryonic stem cell lines and long-term maintenance with stable karyotype by enzymatic bulk passage", *Biochemical and biophysical research communications*, vol. 345, no. 3, pp. 926-932.

Thomson, J.A., Itskovitz-Eldor, J., Shapiro, S.S., Waknitz, M.A., Swiergiel, J.J., Marshall, V.S. & Jones, J.M. 1998, "Embryonic stem cell lines derived from human blastocysts", *Science*, vol. 282, no. 5391, pp. 1145.

VandeWoude, S., Richt, J.A., Zink, M.C., Rott, R., Narayan, O. & Clements, J.E. 1990, "A Borna virus cDNA encoding a protein recognized by antibodies in humans with behavioral diseases", *Science*, vol. 250, no. 4985, pp. 1278.

Wightman, B., Ha, I. & Ruvkun, G. 1993, "Posttranscriptional regulation of the heterochronic gene lin-14 by lin-4 mediates temporal pattern formation in C. elegans", *Cell*, vol. 75, no. 5, pp. 855-862.

Xu, B., Karayiorgou, M. & Gogos, J.A. 2010, "MicroRNAs in psychiatric and neurodevelopmental disorders", *Brain research*, vol. 1338, pp. 78-88.

Zheng, K., Li, H., Zhu, Y., Zhu, Q. & Qiu, M. 2010, "MicroRNAs Are Essential for the Developmental Switch from Neurogenesis to Gliogenesis in the Developing Spinal Cord", *Journal of Neuroscience*, vol. 30, no. 24, pp. 8245.

6

Characterization of Embryonic Stem (ES) Neuronal Differentiation Combining Atomic Force, Confocal and DIC Microscopy Imaging

Maria Elisabetta Ruaro, Jelena Ban and Vincent Torre
International School for Advanced Studies
(SISSA-ISAS), via Bonomea 265, Trieste
Italy

1. Introduction

The nervous system development is of tremendous fundamental importance, but it is immensely challenging because of the complexity of both its architecture and function (Staii et al., 2011). Understanding the formation of this ordered complexity is one of the greatest challenges of modern science. Mechanisms by which progenitor cells differentiate and acquire their cell identity are just beginning to be fully understood (Gilbert, 2000; Lai & Johnson, 2008).

A potent tool for studying differentiation and development *in vitro* has been offered to researchers by the isolation of mouse embryonic stem (ES) cells derived from the inner cell mass of blastocyst-stage embryos more than 20 years ago (Evans & Kaufman, 1981; Martin, 1981). Two unique characteristics distinguish them from all other organ-specific stem cells identified to date. First, they can be maintained and expanded as pure populations of undifferentiated cells for extended periods of time retaining normal karyotypes. Second, they are pluripotent, capable to generate every cell type in the body. The pluripotent nature of mouse ES cells was formally demonstrated by their ability to contribute to all tissues of adult mice, including the germline, following their injection into host blastocysts (Bradley et al., 1984). In addition to their developmental potential *in vivo*, ES cells display a remarkable capacity to form all differentiated cell types in culture (Keller, 2005).

In vitro differentiation of embryonic stem (ES) cells recapitulates early events in the development of the mammalian nervous system: ES cells can both generate and respond *in vitro* to signals that normally regulate embryonic development (Fraichard et al., 1995; Keller, 2005). This knowledge has been transported *in vitro* designing several different protocols that have evolved to promote neuroectoderm differentiation (Cai & Grabel, 2007; Keller, 2005). Each of the three major neural cell types of the central nervous system—neurons, astrocytes, and oligodendrocytes—can be generated, and relatively pure populations of each can be isolated when cultured under appropriate conditions (Okabe et al., 1996; Barberi et al., 2003). In addition to the generation of these different neural populations, conditions have been established for the development of different subtypes of neurons. Thus neurons of different parts of the neural tube were successfully generated including spinal motoneurons, midbrain dopaminergic neurons, spinal cord interneurons, Purkinje and granule cells of cerebellum, hypothalamus and finally cortical pyramidal cells (Gaspard & Vanderhaeghen, 2010).

These neurons do not only have the correct morphology and express specific markers but they are also functional: electrophysiological data from ES-derived neurons with different protocols validate their functional differentiation *in vitro* and there are evidence of the formation of synapse between ES-derived neurons or between an ES-derived neuron and a mature neuron in organotypic slices as well as integration of ES-derived neurons *in vivo*. Moreover, networks formed by ES-derived neurons display functional properties remarkably similar to those of hippocampal neurons (Ban et al., 2007 and references herein). The isolation of human ES cells in 1998 (Thomson et al., 1998) dramatically elevated the interest in the therapeutic promises of ES cells differentiation, in particular for brain repair. Therefore ES have emerged as a powerful tool in neurobiology, helping address longstanding questions in an entirely novel way (Gaspard & Vanderhaeghen, 2011).

If the cell is to become a neuron, the next decision is what type of neuron it will be. After fate is determined, still another decision gives the neuron a specific target (Gilbert, 2000). Neurons find their targets by protruding axons driven by the motile apparatus of growth cones. The surface of growth cones contains receptors for extracellular guidance cues that integrate this information into directional movement towards the target cell (Grzywa et al., 2006). Filamentous (F)-actin is the primary cytoskeletal element that maintains the growth cone shape and is essential for proper axon guidance, whereas microtubules are essential for giving the axon structure and serve an important function in axon elongation (Dent & Gertler, 2003). Thus growth cones act as sensors, signal transducers and motility devices and understanding their fate is a key question.

While the role of guidance molecules (Dickson, 2002) for growth cone movements, underlying signalling of both the F-actin and microtubules is well established (Dent & Gertler, 2003; Schaefer et al., 2002), relatively little is known about the three-dimensional structure of growth cones, which is difficult to determine *in vivo* in the mouse embryo and impossible in the human embryo (Keller, 2005).

Cellular three-dimensional structures can be analyzed with different imaging techniques. Despite the enormous advancements brought about by electron and scanning probe microscopy, about 80% of all microscopy investigations in the life sciences are still carried out with conventional lenses and visible light. Taking advantage of the optical transparency of cells, light microscopy uniquely provides noninvasive imaging of the interior of cells (Hell, 2007).

Discovered and first patented in 1957 by Marvin Minsky, confocal microscope, a predecessor to today's widely used **confocal laser scanning microscopy (CLSM)** has allowed a major advance in biological imaging of cell structure and physiology in thick specimens, in three dimensions and in time. CLSM offers high-quality three-dimensional fluorescent images over conventional wide-field optical microscopy, due to its ability to control the depth of a focal plane to eliminate out-of-focus light or glares in specimens and its capability to collect serial (i.e., z-stack) optical images for thick specimens without the need for physical sectioning of the tissue. In this way, thin, optical sections with greater resolution and contrast and with greater sensitivity than conventional, wide-field microscopes are produced (Dailey et al., 1999; Park et al., 2010; Pawley, 2006).

Characterization of Embryonic Stem (ES) Neuronal Differentiation Combining Atomic Force, Confocal and
DIC Microscopy Imaging

117

Confocal laser scanning microscopy (CLSM) utilizes the optical pathway of a regular optical microscope and in combination with immunofluorescence histochemistry has been widely used to simultaneously map the distribution and localization of different cellular components (extracellular and intracellular macro-molecules, including proteins, nucleic acids and lipids, as well as intracellular ions such as calcium) helping to understand intracellular mechanisms (Dailey et al., 1999; Rajwa et al., 2004). Moreover, it is possible to monitor the process and dynamics of living cells with high temporal resolution (Hell, 2007; Park et al., 2010).

The 200 nm resolution limit of the CLSM is restricted by the diffraction limits of the microscope objective and does not permit accurate evaluation of the sample height. The z-resolution of CLSM for any given wavelength is always at least 2 times less than the corresponding xy-resolution thus restricting a detailed structural image that can be achieved when exploring biological samples (Doak et al., 2008; Rajwa et al., 2004).

Great advances in optical microscopy such as near field scanning optical microscopy (NSOM), stimulated emission depletion microscopy (STED), photoactivated localization microscopy (PALM), and stochastic optical reconstruction microscopy (STORM) have been achieved to overcome the optical diffraction limit (Hell, 2007 and 2009; Schermelleh et al., 2010), but there are still constraints for realizing time-resolved dynamics or three dimensional imaging (Park et al., 2010). These techniques provide an excellent spatial resolution in the xy plane also in live specimens but relying on the presence of fluorophores cannot provide information on the overall morphology of cells.

State-of-the-art transmission and scanning electron microscopy techniques are technically demanding, relatively costly, and time-consuming. Moreover, the possibility to specifically label and visualize multiple cellular structures or components in one specimen is still limited. Furthermore, chemical fixation, contrasting procedures and/or physical sectioning can cause artifacts and exclude the option to observe living cells (Schermelleh et al., 2010).

With the discovery of **Atomic force microscopy (AFM)**, amazing progress has been made in the imaging of biomolecules with sub-nanometer resolution (Binnig et al., 1986; Engel et al. 1997; Fotiadis et al., 2002; Kasas et al, 1993; Lal & John, 1994; Müller et al., 1999), comparable to scanning electron microscopy. To date, AFM has been used increasingly and is progressively becoming a usual benchtop technique. The volume of scientific publications citing AFM increases continuously and papers with a biological emphasis reached more than 21% of total publications (as in 2006) (Parot et al., 2007).

AFM is a scanning probe device, which generates an image by systematically scanning a sharp tip mounted on the end of a flexible cantilever over the samples' surface. The tip interacts with the surface causing the cantilever to bend. A laser beam acting as an optical lever is deflected from the end of the cantilever to a position sensitive photo-diode that measures the cantilever deflection. In this way a topographic map of the surface is generated (Doak et al., 2008).

AFM can be used in ambient air or under liquid and provides an unprecedented way to image the morphological structure of the surfaces of cells and other biological samples, i.e. it images the surfaces where most of the regulatory biochemical and other signals are directed (Lal & John, 1994). By functionalizing the cantilever tip with appropriate molecules, (Reddy et al., 2004; Li et al., 2006), it is possible to localize specific molecules on the surface of the cell and to obtain a high resolution map of their localization. Furthermore, AFM, by measuring forces within and between biological molecules, can provide additional biophysical information on molecular characteristics by acting as a sensor that quantifies the interaction forces between the tip and sample as they are brought into and out of contact (Butt et al., 2005, as cited in Doak et al., 2008).

In the case of neurons, the majority of AFM imaging has focused on the cell body, axon, and synaptic vesicles, whereas less attention has been paid to the growth cone and its underlying cytoskeletal structures (Grzywa et al., 2006; Laishram et al., 2009; McNally et al., 2005; Parpura et al., 1993; Xiong et al., 2009; Yunxu et al., 2006). In particular the morphological characterization at nanometer scale of ES-derived growth cones with AFM is largely unexplored.

As a stand-alone technique, AFM can provide unique biophysical and ultra-structural information on a sample, but a limitation is the difficulty in correlating structural or mechanical features with functionality (Kellermayer et al., 2006; Doak et al., 2008). Therefore it is necessary to combine AFM imaging with other techniques to obtain functional information. In particular, with fluorescent confocal microscopy specific subcellular components can be stained allowing functional studies.

AFM microscopy is a scanning method and therefore cannot be used to investigate the motion of large biological samples at a high temporal resolution, which are better viewed with conventional video imaging with CCD cameras (Cojoc et al., 2007; Niell and Smith, 2004; Schaefer et al., 2002) or time-lapse confocal microscope (Dailey et al., 1999; Fishell et al., 1995). It is possible to follow moving biological structures with AFM only when small details such as filopodia are imaged (McNally et al., 2005), or the temporal resolution is substantially decreased (Yunxu et al., 2006).

Here we describe how combining three different imaging techniques (time-lapse DIC imaging, AFM on both fixed and living neurons and fluorescence confocal microscopy) used separately, at different times, on different instruments - but on the same samples it was possible to provide a morphological characterization of ES-derived growth cones related to their movement (Ban et al., 2011) and hypothesize a possible functional role of the fragmented structures observed only in a fraction of growth cones.

2. Combined AFM, confocal and DIC imaging for characterization of ES-derived neuronal growth cones

2.1 Morphological characterization of ES-derived growth cones

AFM imaging on more that one hundred fixed cells (n=119) revealed different morphologies of ES-derived growth cones, as shown in Figure 1.

ES-derived neuronal precursors were obtained using the protocol described previously (Ban et al., 2007). Cells were plated on coverslips and induced to differentiate for 24 hours. During this period of culture, ES-derived neurons extended neurites with growth cones moving forward, retracting and exploring the environment with their filopodia. The structure of the differentiating growth cones was analyzed by AFM in contact mode in liquid. Cells were plated at a density of 3×10^4 cells/cm^2 in order to obtain isolated growth cones to avoid overlapping structures. This low density, however, is sufficient for the neuronal survival in culture.

At this stage of differentiation, very different structures were observed with the diameter of growth cones that varied from 1.5 to 28 μm and height that varied from 65 to 593 nm. They could be classified in three different morphological groups: in the first one (Figure 1D-I) they appeared swollen and smooth, with several filopodia spreading from the central domain. The

height differed substantially from one growth cone to another but in this group (68% of
growth cones analyzed) it always exceeded 200nm. In the second group (21% of cases) growth
cones were flat with few or no filopodia (Figure 1A-C) and their height was consistently below
200nm. In the third group (11% of cases) growth cones showed a ruffled and fragmented
structure with several holes (Figure 1J-L). The height of these growth cones was also below
200nm, and their thickness almost vanished in some regions. All these structural details were
not recognizable with optical microscope due to their small dimensions.

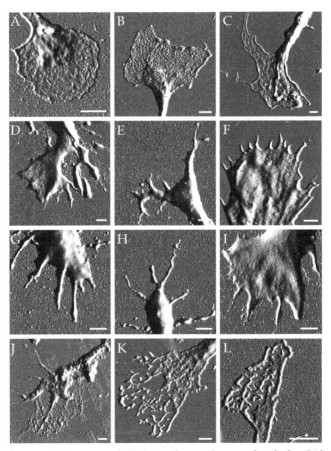

Fig. 1. High resolution AFM images of ES-derived growth cones fixed after 24 h of
differentiation. Growth cones could have flat and rough (A-C), swollen and smooth (D-I) or
fragmented (J-L) structures. Scale bar, 2μm.

Although during image acquisition the AFM tip interacts with the cell surface and could
modify or damage the cell membrane, we demonstrated that the fragmented structures were
not an artifact of AFM scanning by acquiring a series of images of a compact growth cone at
increasing tapping forces of 200, 1000 and 3000 pN respectively. In 4 independent
experiments performed, the height profile of the growth cones at varying forces showed a
decrease in height caused by a compression of the cell structures, probably due to the

residual cell elasticity, after the fixation procedure. However, when the imaging force was restored to the initial value of 200pN, the cell morphology was exactly the same as in the first scan and no damage was introduced (Ban et al., 2011).

Holes and fragments of growth cones were not fixation artefacts. In fact, using three different fixation methods both fragmented and compact growth cones were present on the same coverslip and sometimes on neighbouring cells. Fragmented structures were also observed in growth cones of living neurons analyzed by AFM: in 6 out of 23 imaged cells the growth cones retracted leaving behind fragments with variable dimensions. In 3 cases holes in the growth cones were observed and in one case the holes were already present at the first scan. The physiological dynamics was poorly affected by AFM scans and the cantilever tip did not damage the growth cones since in majority of cases (14 out of 23 imaged cells) their compact structure was preserved during the scanning period even though cycles of protrusion and retraction were observed. Moreover, fragmentation observed under living conditions (13% of cases) had comparable proportion in respect to what observed with fixed cells (11% of cases). Altogether, these observations suggested that the fragments observed on the fixed cells were originated before fixation and that fragmentation is a physiological phenomenon (Ban et al., 2011).

We hypothesized that the different morphologies observed in the growth cones might correlate with different types of movement. For doing so we took advantage of the 3 techniques described to study the motion of living growth cones and trying to correlate it with structure and expression of specific subcellular components.

2.2 Preparation of coverslips

To be able to collect images with all these techniques (each of them with different performaces, resolution and collection modes) but from the same cell it was necessary to have a position marker on the sample.

In our case we prepared a home-made coverslips on which ES-derived neuronal precursors were plated and induced to differentiate. But commercial coverslips with numerical grid could serve the same purpose.

Coverslips with printed markers were prepared by optical lithography and metal evaporation on 24mm diameter glass coverslips. A polymeric photoresist was deposited on one side of the coverslips by spin coating. The indexed pattern was produced by UV exposure through a patterned optical mask. A 20nm titanium layer was finally deposited and stripped by lift-off techniques (Figure 2A).

In the free space between printed markers the movement of neurons and their growth cones could be clearly monitored (Figure 2B). Time-lapse DIC and AFM imaging can be performed on living cells while immunofluorescence assays (Figure 2C) and high resolution AFM (Figure 2D) can be done at very different time intervals after fixation (from few hours up to many months if samples are kept at +4°C in paraformaldehyde).

2.3 Correlation between movement and structure/function

Theoretically movement and structure could be analyzed imaging living cells with AFM. When performing AFM on living cells images could be obtained in tapping mode at 0.6 scan line per second and with a maximum of 256 scan lines. In this way the acquisition of AFM images required several minutes and, due to the movement of growth cones and to the fluidity of the membrane, a high resolution AFM image could not be achieved. Giving higher temporal resolution, time-lapse differential interference contrast (DIC) imaging was

Characterization of Embryonic Stem (ES) Neuronal Differentiation Combining Atomic Force, Confocal and
DIC Microscopy Imaging

121

used. Images with resolution between 512x512 and 1024x1024 pixels were acquired every 10 seconds, for a total of 80 frames (total duration 13 minutes and 20 seconds) and the motion of more than 100 growth cones was collected.

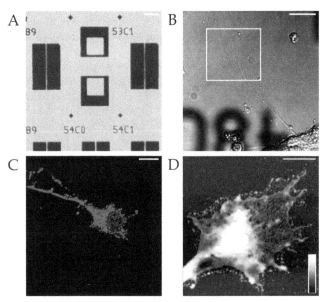

Fig. 2. (A) An example of a coverslip with printed markers and numbers. Scale bar, 100 μm. (B) ES-derived growth cone (inset) imaged with DIC using a confocal microscope. Scale bar, 25 μm. (C) Confocal image (1024x1024 pixels) of a growth cone stained for with an antibody against neural cell adhesion molecule (NCAM). Scale bar, 10 μm. (D) AFM image (1024x1024 pixels) of the same growth cone. Scale bar, 5 μm. Color bar from 0 to 350nm (From Kondra et al., 2009, Journal of Neuroscience Methods, ELSEVIER).

From the time-lapse analysis 4 different types of movements were observed: exploring (43/104), growing (16/104), retracting (17/104) and stasis (28/104). 29 of these cells were imaged with AFM. Cells were fixed immediately after video imaging, AFM with a resolution between 512x512 and 1024x1024 pixels was performed followed by staining with appropriate antibodies.

Filopodia of exploring growth cones (9 out of 29 cells) moved with a velocity up to 80 nm s^{-1} with an average value of 25±7 nm s^{-1} exploring very efficiently the surrounding free space independently in all directions. Some filopodia were continuously extending and retracting, changing rapidly in their length, while some others were freely exploring maintaining their shape. AFM imaging revealed a smooth and compact surface. The growth cones had average height of 852 ± 235 nm and their filopodia had a height varying between 67 and 219 nm (n=40; average height 98.8 ± 48.3nm).

Neurites of growing growth cones (5 out of 29 cells) could grow by 1-5 μm in 2-10 minutes and in two cases a neurite grew up to 14 μm in less than 2 minutes. As for exploring growth cones, in all cases AFM showed a compact and smooth surface. Filopodia height reached almost 2 μm and their average length was 3.5 μm (n=20).

Retracting growth cones (7 out of 29 cells) moved with a velocity ranging from 80 to 135 nm/sec, retracting their filopodia and the whole neurites from the original position. After fixation, AFM scanning revealed the presence of fragments near the tip of fast retracting growth cones. The confirm that these fragments were actual parts of the growth cone left behind by the neuron came from AFM imaging of living neurons. In all 6 retracting growth cones observed, fragments with an average diameter of 85 ± 27 nm and an average height of 75 ± 28 nm were detected.

Growth cones were classified as static (8 out of 29 cells) when the external contour of the growth cone remained in the same position and the length of their neurite did not change during DIC observation. These growth cones had an apparently intact shape when viewed with time-lapsed DIC images (Figure 2B), but their 3D shape was highly fragmented when viewed with AFM (Figure 2D). Static growth cones were thinner and rarely reached 200nm height.

When the same growth cone was analyzed with immunofluorescence - with actin and tubulin to follow cytoskeletal component underlying growth cone movement or neural cell adhesion molecule (NCAM) to visualize cell membrane contours - the two images were difficult to compare due to the different resolution (Figure 2C and D). Moreover, AFM and CLSM images contain different information: every pixel at location (x,y) in the AFM images provides a direct measurement in nm of the sample height while fluorescence images acquired with a confocal laser scanning microscope characterize the emitted fluorescence at the same location.

In order to integrate the information derived from AFM and immunofluorescence analyses it is important to properly align or superimpose these different images. This problem has been extensively studied in Computer Vision, where it is referred as "Registration" of different images (Kondra et al., 2009).

2.4 Image registration

Image registration is the process of overlaying two or more images of the same scene taken at different times, different viewpoints, and/or by different imaging modalities. Differences between images are introduced because of different imaging conditions, such as different viewing points or light conditions or because of the use of two different microscopes, as in the case under consideration. Registration transforms one image – usually the sensed image – so that it becomes aligned to the reference image. Image registration is a crucial step in image analysis and can be solved using methods used in computer vision (Trucco & Verri, 1998), in which the final information is obtained by integrating various data sources like in image fusion (Zitova & Flusser, 2003). Images taken from different modalities may undergo a linear deformation in scale, translation, rotation and sometimes shearing i.e. affine deformation.

The word registration is used with two different meanings (Hill et al., 2001). The first meaning is to determine a transformation of one image so that features in the sensed image can be put in a one-to-one correspondence to features in the reference image. The symbol T is used to represent this type of transformation. The second meaning of registration enables also the comparison of the intensity at corresponding positions. The symbol T_i is used to describe this second meaning of registration, which incorporates the concepts of re-sampling and interpolation.

T is a spatial mapping. The more complete mapping T_i maps both position and associated intensity value from image A to image B. Therefore T_i maps an image to an image, whereas T maps between coordinates of image A into coordinates of image B. To overlay two images that have been registered, or to subtract one from another, is necessary to know T_i, not just

T. T_i is only defined in the region of overlap of the image fields of view, and has to take into account of image sampling and spatial resolution.

Before doing the registration, it is necessary to select the correct type of transformation required for the images under consideration. The most widely used transformations are Linear, Affine and Projective. The linear transformation is used when shapes in the sensed image are unchanged, but are distorted by some combination of translation, rotation, and scaling. Straight lines remain straight, and parallel lines are still parallel. This is the case of the same biological sample viewed by two microscopes using different objectives and imaging systems, such as an AFM (Figure 2D) and a CLSM (Figure 2C). Registration using affine transformation is necessary when shapes in the sensed image are distorted also by shearing or a linear deformation. In this case, straight lines remain straight, and parallel lines remain parallel, but rectangles become parallelograms. Projective transformation is used when the scene appears tilted. Straight lines remain straight, but parallel lines converge toward vanishing points that might or might not fall within the image.

If we consider two images of the same biological sample, the first one acquired using AFM and the second using a CLSM, the two imaging systems differ because of different scale factors, by a rigid translation of their origin and a possible rotation of their axis. It is assumed that the two imaging systems do not introduce any deformation. Registration of the two images consists in the determination of the transformation parameter by aligning properly the two images.

The unknown parameters in the transformation matrix can be estimated either by matching a selected number of points or landmarks in the two images or by matching entire contours in the two images. The first method is used when it is possible to identify in the two images enough points corresponding to the same physical structure, such as the tip of a dendrite, or a small vesicle. The second method is used in presence of rounded biological structures, with no obvious marks and it is more convenient to put in correspondence two contours than isolated points.

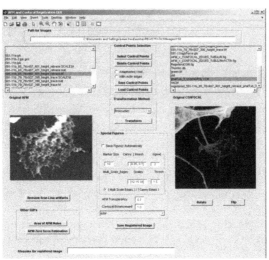

Fig. 3. Snapshot of the graphical user interface (From Kondra et al., 2009, Journal of Neuroscience Methods, ELSEVIER).

To apply these methods to the images derived from different microscopes we have implemented our Registration program using Matlab7.1 (The MathWorks Inc. http://www.mathworks.com) a standard tool common in the computer vision and biomedical community for statistical analysis and production of figures and images of analyzed data and results.

For a more detailed mathematical description of the different transformations and description of the program see Kondra et al., 2009, Appendix 1, 2 and 3).

Corresponding points or contours in AFM image and confocal image were marked by hand using a friendly graphical user interface developed for this particular purpose (Figure 3).

Registration by points selection method is illustrated in Figure 4. The operator identifies N (minimum 3) points in the AFM image (Figure 4A) that are put in correspondence with N points in the confocal image (Figure 4B). Corresponding points in Figure 4A and B are indicated by the same number. By using these correspondences the parameters determining the transformation T are obtained by solving a system of linear equation and the confocal image can be registered. In this way same physical points in the original AFM and in the new registered confocal image, shown in Figure 4C, have the same location.

To make more user friendly the selection of points, confocal image can be rotated in a sequence of 90 degrees and/or flipped to make a approximate alignment with AFM image (compare Figure 2C with Figure 4B). Control Point Selection Tool in Matlab was used to mark the control point pairs in the image to be registered, the input image (Figure 4B), and the image to which you are comparing it, the base image (Figure 4A) corresponding points were initially specified by pointing and clicking in the input and base images so that each point specified in the input image had a match in the base image.

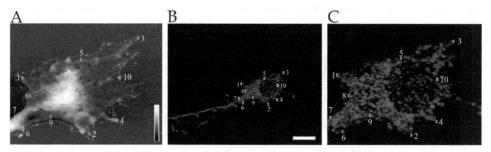

Fig. 4. Example of registering images using points selection method. (A) AFM image of ES-derived growth cone. Color bar from 0 to 350nm. (B) Confocal image of the same ES-derived growth cone. Scale bar, 10 μm. (C) Registered confocal image (From Kondra et al., 2009, Journal of Neuroscience Methods, ELSEVIER).

The advantage of this tool is that, after the first three pairs are selected, it is sufficient to select a point in the input image and the Control Point Selection Tool estimates its match point in the base image or *vice versa* automatically, based on the geometric relationship of the previously selected control points. Another advantage of this tool is that if the image is not registered properly, it is possible to change the position of control points to get the exact superimposition.

The alternative method is registration by aligning contours with Procrustes Analysis. Procrustes was a robber in Greek mythology. He would offer travellers hospitality in his road-side house, and the opportunity to stay the night in his bed that would perfectly fit each visitor. As the visitors discovered to their cost, however, it was the guest who was altered to fit the bed, rather than the bed that was altered to fit the guest (Hill et al., 2001). Let us consider that the AFM image is like the bed and is the guest. So using the Procrustes' method means that confocal image is altered by scaling and/or rotating it to approximately fit AFM image.

The number of landmarks available depends on the structure of the image, and there may be differences in opinion between scientists as to which landmarks are consistent and locatable. Marking of the corresponding points thus becomes difficult when there are few corners in the structure, and thus exact location of the points is impossible and can differ from observer to observer. This problem can be solved by marking many points along the contour of the structure in both images. The contours are then interpolated so that both of them contain the same number of equally spaced points (for mathematical description of transformation see Kondra et al., 2009).

An example of this method is illustrated in Figure 5. A contour was marked by continuously clicking on points following the borderline of the structure of interest in AFM image (Figure 5A) and in the confocal image as well (Figure 5B). As a consequence of Procrustes analysis, confocal image was properly transformed and put in correspondence with AFM image (Figure 5C).

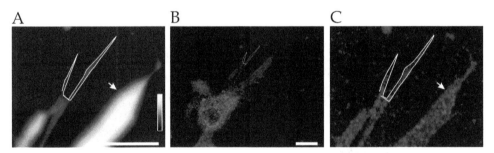

Fig. 5. Example of registering images using Procrustes Analysis. (A) AFM image of ES-derived growth cone. Scale bar, 10µm. Color bar from 0 to 2200 nm. (B) Confocal image of the same ES-derived growth cone stained for neural cell adhesion molecule (NCAM). Scale bar, 10µm. (C) Registered confocal image of membrane protein NCAM (From Kondra et al., 2009, Journal of Neuroscience Methods, ELSEVIER).

2.5 Identification of nanometric structures and subcellular component in static fragmented growth cones

With registration of confocal and AFM images it was possible to further analyze the composition of fragments characteristic of static and retracting growth cones. Their structure seemed compact when viewed with time-lapsed DIC images (Figure 6A), instead AFM (Figure 6B) revealed highly fragmented 3D shape. Profiles of AFM images of static growth cones showed isolated fragments with height that varied from 50 to 150 nm (Figure 6E). Registered confocal images demonstrated that they contain actin filaments but not tubulin and they are positive for neural cell adhesion molecule (NCAM) indicating that fragments left behind by growth cones are formed by chunks of actin filaments enveloped by the cell membrane (Figure 6C and D).

Height of fragments and of filopodia had a similar distribution varying from less than 30 nm up to 300 nm (Ban et al., 2011). Immobile growth cones not only were surrounded by detached fragments, but they also had holes. Growth cone regions surrounding these holes had a height varying from 20 to 90 nm and holes had an area varying between 0.03 to 0.650 μm^2. Fragments had a height varying from 40 to 400 nm with an area varying between 0.4 to 6μm^2.

During the time-lapse DIC imaging none of the neurons with static growth cones showed signs of membrane blebbing or cell shrinking typical of apoptotic cell indicating that the observed fragmentation was not associated with apoptosis. Moreover, nuclear staining by Hoechst revealed that none of the eight cells that were also analyzed by AFM and immunofluorescence after fixation had an apoptotic nucleus. We can therefore conclude that growth cone fragmentation is not part of the apoptotic process.

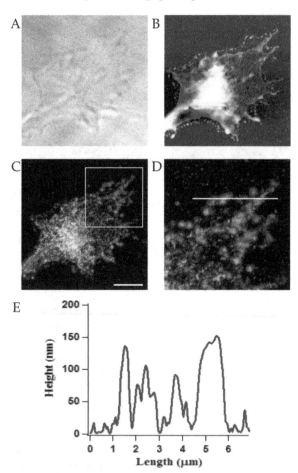

Fig. 6. Static growth cones. (A) DIC, (B) AFM topography and (C) registered confocal image of the same growth cone stained for F-actin (green), NCAM (red) and β-tubulin III (blue). Scale bar, 5 μm. (D) Confocal image of the inset shown in C. (E) Height profile along the white line shown in D.

Characterization of Embryonic Stem (ES) Neuronal Differentiation Combining Atomic Force, Confocal and
DIC Microscopy Imaging

127

3. Discussion

Three different imaging techniques used separately, at different times, on different instruments - but on the same samples and the possibility to compare AFM and confocal images due to the development of the registration method (Kondra et al., 2009) allowed us to obtain a morphological characterization of ES-derived growth cones.

Integrated AFM and CLSM instrument has been developed and it offers the advantage of parallel analysis of the same sample with nanometer-scale spatial resolution, frame/second temporal resolution, and chemical identification through fluorescence detection can be done simultaneously for live cells (Doak et al., 2008; Park et al., 2010).

In addition to optical microscopy, AFM can be combined with other instruments and techniques, such as microfluidic liquid cell (Schoenwald et al., 2010), patch-clamp (Pamir et al., 2008) or ultramicrotome (Efimov et al., 2007) providing a novel insights to further understanding of cellular structure-function relationships getting down to the scale of single molecule.

Although there are several studies where AFM is combined with confocal microscope (Doak et al, 2008; Moreno Flores & Toca-Herrera., 2009; Kassies et al., 2005; Owen et al., 2006; Park et al., 2010), our method is useful in cases where combined fluorescence (confocal) and atomic force microscope is not available. In addition, performing different assays separately permitted optimization of sample preparation for each experiment. For example, AFM on fixed cells was performed in contact mode, in liquid (phosphate buffer saline (PBS)) while for immunofluorescence assays, coverslips were mounted with commercial mounting medium, in order to reduce photobleaching during the repetitive number of confocal scans required to zoom in the region corresponding to the growth cone. Our AFM microscope was provided with fluorescence setup and we collected some fluorescent images while performing AFM. However, in PBS the samples bleached rapidly and the resulting images had poor definition.

The combination of AFM and fluorescence confocal microscopy on fixed cells, and of time-lapse DIC and AFM imaging on living cells allowed us to correlate morphology of ES-derived growth cones to their movement prior fixation providing therefore both structural and functional insights.

Growth cones actively exploring the environment before fixation had a smooth external surface. In contrast, growth cones which were immobile before fixation revealed a fragmented shape, composed of several nanoscale structures either partly attached or completely isolated from the rest of the growth cone. In addition, by using AFM on live specimen, fragmentation was observed in some of the retracting growth cones. Therefore the morphology of ES-derived growth cones depends on their overall motility.

Growth cones with micrometric size holes of retinal ganglion cell axons were previously observed *in vivo* (Godement et al., 1994; Mason & Erskin, 2000). They appear in the spread growth cones and are predicted to form from the fusion or contact of lamellar extensions of the growth cone as they enfold radial glial processes. However, although morphologically similar, these two findings reflect a different biological phenomenon: first because our observations were the result of a technical approach measuring at nanometric level and second, because we never found fragmented structures in growing growth cones.

The fragmentation can be related to growth cones pruning that occurs during the early development of the central nervous system, where an excessive outgrowth of projections need to be refined to achieve precise connectivity (Faulkner et al., 2007). The selective elimination of neuronal cell processes, or neurites, is an essential step during normal development and occurs through retraction, degeneration, or a combination of both (Franze et al., 2009).

This phenomenon resembles the growth cone collapse induced by several factors like mercury (Leong et al., 2001), X-ray (Al-Jahdari et al., 2008) or semaphorin in the absence of growth factors (Tamagnone & Comoglio, 2004). The fragmentation of the growth cone we observed is a local phenomenon, similar to what observed for Lysophosphatidic acid (LPA) induction of collapse *in vitro* which, in contrast with other collapsing treatments, is reversible and not toxic (Saito, 1997). However, to our knowledge, this is the first time that this collapse-like phenomenon was observed to occur spontaneously.

Previous investigations have shown the formation of migration tracks resulting from the release of cellular material onto glass surfaces and artificial matrices for a number of cell types (Fuhr et al., 1998; Kirfel et al., 2004; Richter et al., 2000; Zimmermann et al., 2001). Macroaggregates left behind migrating keratinocytes contain high amounts of β1 integrin and parts of the fibronectin and laminin receptors. They lack, however, of any cytosolic proteins including actin and of the adhesion complex constituents talin and vinculin. In our experimental conditions, fragments left behind by growth cones are composed of cell membrane but also of cytoplasmic proteins such as F-actin, as it was reported for other migrating cells (Fuhr et al., 1998). Fragments could correspond to filopodia originally present on the growth cone in that position also because the height distribution of filopodia and fragments was similar, suggesting that they may be composed of similar building/dismantling blocks. The existence of building blocks could agree with a previous study (Parpura et al., 1993) where it was found that the height of an hippocampal growth cones corresponds to a multiple of the heights of individual filopodia possibly due to overlying actin bundles arising from different filopodia.

The release of a fragment might be energetically advantageous for faster retraction and/or change in growing direction compared to recycling of distal elements. However it cannot be excluded that fragments might act as guidance signals for neighboring neurons.

Vertebrate semaphorins are either secreted or associated with the cell surface. *In vitro* and *in vivo* experiments have implicated semaphorins in the guidance of elongating axons and dendrites, as well as in axon branching, pruning and degeneration (Tamagnone & Comoglio, 2004). The primary role of Sema 3A in the nervous system is to repel growth cones from inappropriate areas and to help steer both axons and migrating cells along the correct trajectory (Brown & Bridgman, 2009). When added in bath, they cause rapid collapse of growth cones, followed by axon retraction (Kolpak et al., 2009).

The fragmentation of growth cones that have not established contact or by pruned contact here observed could therefore serve as a migrating track for other neurons, by exposing semaphorins or other membrane proteins that act as receptors and/or ligands for axon guidance.

4. Conclusion

The combination of AFM and fluorescence confocal microscopy on fixed cells, and of time-lapse DIC and AFM imaging on living cells allowed us to obtain a morphological characterization of ES-derived growth cones related to their movement providing both structural and functional insights.

Characterization of Embryonic Stem (ES) Neuronal Differentiation Combining Atomic Force, Confocal and DIC Microscopy Imaging

129

In particular the registration method allowed to superimpose images taken from different modalities. Registration, however, is not restricted to confocal and AFM images but is a versatile tool for combined studies. The main advantage is that there is no need for sophisticated and combined microscopes but with conventional instruments and AFM, structural information at nanometer scale is combined with functional studies.

5. Acknowledgment

This work was supported by the EU projects: NEURO Contract n. 012788 (FP6-STREP, NEST) and NanoScale Contract n.214566 (FP7-NMP-2007-SMALL-1). In addition we need to acknowledge the financial support of a FIRB grant D.M.31/03/05 from the Italian Government, of Contr. RICN no.011936 BINASP from the European Community, of funds from the Istituto Italiano di Tecnologia (Research Unit IIT) and of the GRAND Grant from CIPE/FVG by the Friuli Venezia Giulia region.

6. References

Al-Jahdari, W.S.; Suzuki, Y.; Yoshida, Y.; Noda, S.E.; Shirai, K.; Saito, S; Goto, F. & Nakano, T. (2008). Growth cone collapse and neurite retractions: an approach to examine X-irradiation affects on neuron cells, *Journal of Radiation Research (Tokyo)*, Vol.49, No.5, (September 2008), pp. 481-489

Ban, J.; Bonifazi, P.; Pinato, G.; Broccard, F.D.; Studer, L.; Torre V. & Ruaro, M.E. (2007). Embryonic stem cell-derived neurons form functional networks in vitro. *Stem Cells*, Vol.25, No.3, (March 2007), pp. 738-749

Ban, J.; Migliorini, E.; Di Foggia, V.; Lazzarino, M.; Ruaro, M.E. & Torre, V. (2011). Fragmentation as a Mechanism for Growth Cone Pruning and Degeneration. *Stem Cells and Development*, Vol.20, No.6, (June 2011), pp.1031-1041

Barberi, T.; Klivenyi, P.; Calingasan, N.Y.; Lee, H.; Kawamata, H.; Loonam, K.; Perrier, A.L.; Bruses, J.; Rubio, M.E.; Topf, N.; Tabar, V.; Harrison, N.L.; Beal, M.F.; Moore, M.A. & Studer, L. (2003). Neural subtype specification of fertilization and nuclear transfer embryonic stem cells and application in parkinsonian mice. *Nature Biotechnology*, Vol. 21, No. 10, (October 2003), pp.1200-1207

Binnig, G.; Quate, C.F. & Gerber, C. (1986). Atomic force microscope. *Physical Review Letters*, Vol.56, No.9, (March 1986), pp. 930-933

Bradley, A.; Evans, M.; Kaufman, M.H. & Robertson, E. (1984). Formation of germ-line chimaeras from embryo-derived teratocarcinoma cell lines. *Nature*, Vol.309, No.5965, (May 1984), pp. 255-256

Brown, J.A. & Bridgman, P.C. (2009). Disruption of the cytoskeleton during Semaphorin 3A induced growth cone collapse correlates with differences in actin organization and associated binding proteins. *Developmental Neurobiology*, Vol.69, No.10 (September 2009), pp.633-646

Cai, C. & Grabel, L. (2007). Directing the differentiation of embryonic stem cells to neural stem cells. *Developmental Dynamics*, Vol.236, No.12, (December 2007), pp. 3255-3266

Cojoc, D.; Difato, F.; Ferrari, E.; Shahapure, R.B.; Laishram, J.; Righi, M.; Di Fabrizio, E.M. & Torre, V. (2007). Properties of the force exerted by filopodia and lamellipodia and the involvement of cytoskeletal components. *PLoS ONE*, Vol.24, No.10, (October 2007), e1072

Dailey, M.; Marrs, G.; Satz, J. & Waite, M. (1999). Concepts in imaging and microscopy. Exploring biological structure and function with confocal microscopy. *Biological Bullettin*, Vol.197, No.2, (October 1999), pp. 115-122

Dent, E.W. & Gertler, F.B. (2003). Cytoskeletal dynamics and transport in growth cone motility and axon guidance. *Neuron*, Vol. 40, No.2 (October 2003), pp. 209-227

Dickson, B.J. (2002). Molecular mechanisms of axon guidance. *Science*, Vol.298, No.5600, (December 2002), pp. 1959-1964. Erratum in: *Science*, Vol.299, No.5606, (January 2003), pp. 515

Doak, S.H.; Rogers, D.; Jones, B.; Francis, L.; Conlan, R.S. & Wright, C. (2008). High-resolution imaging using a novel atomic force microscope and confocal laser scanning microscope hybrid instrument: essential sample preparation aspects. *Histochemistry and Cell Biology*, Vol.130, No.5, (November 2008), pp. 909-916

Efimov, A.E.; Tonevitsky, A.G.; Dittrich, M. & Matsko, N.B. (2007). Atomic force microscope (AFM) combined with the ultramicrotome: a novel device for the serial section tomography and AFM/TEM complementary structural analysis of biological and polymer samples. Journal of Microscopy, Vol.226, Pt3, (June 2007), pp. 207-217

Engel, A.; Schoenenberger, C.-A. & Muller, D.J. (1997). High resolution imaging of native biological sample surfaces using scanning probe microscopy. *Current Opinion in Structural Biology*, Vol.7, No.2, (April 1997), pp. 279-284

Evans, M.J. & Kaufman, M.H. (1981). Establishment in culture of pluripotential cells from mouse embryos. *Nature*, Vol.292, No.5819, (Jul 1981), pp. 154-156

Faulkner, R.L.; Low, L.K. & Cheng, H.J. (2007). Axon pruning in the developing vertebrate hippocampus. *Developmental Neuroscience*, Vol.29, No.1-2 (December 2006), pp. 6-13

Fishell, G.; Blazeski, R.; Godement, P.; Rivas, R.; Wang, L.C. & Mason, C.A. (1995). Optical microscopy. 3. Tracking fluorescently labeled neurons in developing brain. *FASEB Journal*, Vol.9, No.5, (March 1995), pp. 324-34

Fotiadis, D.; Scheuring, S.; Müller, S.A.; Engel, A. & Müller, D.J. (2002). Imaging and manipulation of biological structures with the AFM. *Micron*, Vol.33, No.4, (January 2002), pp. 385-397

Fraichard, A.; Chassande, O.; Bilbaut, G.; Dehay, C.; Savatier, P. & Samarut, J. (1995). In vitro differentiation of embryonic stem cells into glial cells and functional neurons. *Journal of Cell Science*, Vol.108, No.10, (October 1995), pp. 3181-3188

Franze, K.; Gerdelmann, J.; Weick, M.; Betz, T.; Pawlizak, S.; Lakadamyali, M.; Bayer, J.; Rillich, K.; Gögler, M.; Lu, Y.B.; Reichenbach, A.; Janmey, P. & Käs, J. (2009). Neurite branch retraction is caused by a threshold-dependent mechanical impact. *Biophysical Journal*, Vol.97, No.7, (October 2009), pp. 1883-1890

Fuhr, G.; Richter, E.; Zimmermann, H.; Hitzler, H.; Niehus, H. & Hagedorn, R. (1998). Cell traces--footprints of individual cells during locomotion and adhesion. *Biological Chemistry*, Vol.379, No.8-9 (August-September 1998), pp. 1161-1173

Gaspard, N. & Vanderhaeghen, P. (2010). Mechanisms of neural specification from embryonic stem cells. *Current Opinion in Neurobiology*, Vol.20, No.1, (February 2010), pp. 37-43

Characterization of Embryonic Stem (ES) Neuronal Differentiation Combining Atomic Force, Confocal and DIC Microscopy Imaging

131

Gaspard, N. & Vanderhaeghen, P. (2011). From stem cells to neural networks: recent advances and perspectives for neurodevelopmental disorders. *Developmental Medicine & Child Neurology*, Vol.53, No.1, (January 2011), pp. 13-17

Gilbert, S.F. (2000). Neural crest cells and axonal specificity, In: *Developmental Biology*. Sunderland, MA, Sinauer, pp. 407-441. ISBN-10: 0-87893-243-7

Godement, P.; Wang, L.C. & Mason, C.A. (1994). Retinal axon divergence in the optic chiasm: dynamics of growth cone behaviour at the midline. *Journal of Neuroscience*, Vol.14, No.11 Pt2 (November 1994), pp. 7024-7039. Erratum in: *Journal of Neuroscience*, Vol.15, No.3 Pt1, (March 1995), followi

Grzywa, E.L.; Lee, A.C.; Lee, G.U. & Suter, D.M. (2006). High-resolution analysis of neuronal growth cone morphology by comparative atomic force and optical microscopy. *Journal of Neurobiology*, Vol.66, No.14, (December 2006), pp.1529-1543

Hell, S.W. (2007). Far-field optical nanoscopy. *Science*, Vol.316, No. 5828, (May 2007), pp. 1153-1158

Hell, S.W. (2009). Microscopy and its focal switch. *Nature Methods*, Vol.6, No.1, (January 2009), pp. 24-32

Hill, D.L.; Batchelor, P.G.; Holden, M. & Hawkes, D.J. (2001) Medical image registration. *Physics in Medicine and Biology*, Vol46, No.3, (March 2001), pp. R1-45

Kasas, S.; Gotzos, V. & Celio, M.R. (1993). Observation of living cells using the atomic force microscope. *Biophysical Journal*, Vol.64, No.2, (February 1993), pp. 539-544

Kassies, R.; van der Werf, K.O.; Lenferink, A.; Hunter, C.N.; Olsen, J.D.; Subramaniam, V. & Otto, C. (2005). Combined AFM and confocal fluorescence microscope for applications in bio-nanotechnology. *Journal of Microscopy*, Vol.217, No. 1 (January 2005), pp. 109-116

Keller, G. (2005). Embryonic stem cell differentiation: emergence of a new era in biology and medicine. *Genes &Development*, Vol.19, No.10, (May 2005), pp. 1129-1155

Kellermayer, M.S.; Karsai, A.; Kengyel, A.; Nagy, A.; Bianco, P.; Huber, T.; Kulcsár, A.; Niedetzky, C.; Proksch, R. & Grama, L. (2006). Spatially and temporally synchronized atomic force and total internal reflection fluorescence microscopy for imaging and manipulating cells and biomolecules. *Biophysical Journal*, Vol.91, No.7, (October 2006), pp.2665-2677

Kirfel, G.; Rigort, A; Borm, B. & Herzog, V. (2004). Cell migration: mechanisms of rear detachment and the formation of migration tracks. *European Journal of Cell Biology*, Vol.83, No.11-12, (December 2004), pp.717-724

Kolpak, A.L.; Jiang, J.; Guo, D.; Standley, C.; Bellve, K.; Fogarty, K. & Bao, Z.Z. (2009). Negative guidance factor-induced macropinocytosis in the growth cone plays a critical role in repulsive axon turning. *Journal of Neuroscience*, Vol.29, No.34 (August 2009), pp.10488-10498

Kondra, S.; Laishram, J.; Ban, J.; Migliorini, E.; Di Foggia, V.; Lazzarino, M.; Torre, V. & Ruaro, M.E. (2009). Integration of confocal and atomic force microscopy images. *Journal of Neuroscience Methods*, Vol.177, No.1, (February 2009), pp. 94-107

Lai, H.C. & Johnson, J.E. (2008). Neurogenesis or neuronal specification: phosphorylation strikes again! *Neuron*, Vol.58, No.1, (April 2008), pp.3-5

Laishram., J.; Kondra, S.; Avossa, D.; Migliorini, E.; Lazzarino, M. & Torre, V. (2009). A morphological analysis of growth cones of DRG neurons combining atomic force and confocal microscopy. *Journal of Structural Biology*, Vol.168, No.3, (December 2009), pp. 366-377

Lal, R. & John, S.A. (1994). Biological applications of atomic force microscopy. *American Journal of Physiology*, Vol.266, No.1, (January 1994), pp. C1-21

Leong, C.C.; Syed, N.I. & Lorscheider, F.L. (2001). Retrograde degeneration of neurite membrane structural integrity of nerve growth cones following in vitro exposure to mercury. *Neuroreport*, Vol.12, No.4, (March 2001), pp. 733-737

Li, G.; Xi, N. & Wang, D.H. (2006). Probing membrane proteins using atomic force microscopy. *Journal of Cellular Biochemistry*, Vol.97, No.6, (April 2006), pp. 1191-1197

Martin, G.R. (1981). Isolation of a pluripotent cell line from early mouse embryos cultured in medium conditioned by teratocarcinoma stem cells. *Proceedings of the National Academy of Sciences of the United States of America*, Vol.78, No.12, (December 1981), pp. 7634-7638

Mason, C. & Erskine, L. (2000). Growth cone form, behavior, and interactions in vivo: retinal axon pathfinding as a model. *Journal of Neurobiology*, Vol.44, No.2 (August 2000), pp. 260-270. Erratum in: *Journal of Neurobiology*, Vol.45, No.2, (November 2000), p. 134

McNally, H.A.; Rajwa, B.; Sturgis, J. & Robinson, J.P. (2005). Comparative three-dimensional imaging of living neurons with confocal and atomic force microscopy. *Journal of Neuroscience Methods*, Vol.142, No.2, (March 2005), pp. 177-184

Moreno Flores, S. & Toca-Herrera, J.L. (2009). The new future of scanning probe microscopy: Combining atomic force microscopy with other surface-sensitive techniques, optical microscopy and fluorescence techniques. *Nanoscale*, Vol.1, No.1, (October 2009), pp. 40-49

Müller, D.J.; Fotiadis, D.; Scheuring, S.; Müller, S.A. & Engel, A. (1999). Electrostatically balanced subnanometer imaging of biological specimens by atomic force microscope. *Biophysical Journal*, Vol.76, No.2, (February 1999), pp. 1101-1111

Niell, C.M. & Smith, S.J. (2004). Live optical imaging of nervous system development. *Annual Review of Physiology*, Vol.66, (March 2004), pp. 771-798

Okabe, S.; Forsberg-Nilsson, K.; Spiro, A.C.; Segal, M. & McKay, R.D. (1996). Development of neuronal precursor cells and functional postmitotic neurons from embryonic stem cells in vitro. *Mechanisms of Development*, Vol.59, No.1, (September 1996), pp. 89-102

Owen, R.J.; Heyes, C.D.; Knebel, D.; Röcker, C. & Nienhaus, G.U. (2006). An integrated instrumental setup for the combination of atomic force microscopy with optical spectroscopy. *Biopolymers*, Vol.82, No.4, (July 2006), pp. 410-414

Pamir, E.; George, M.; Fertig, N. & Benoit, M. (2008). Planar patch-clamp force microscopy on living cells. *Ultramicroscopy*, Vol.108, No.6, (May 2008), pp. 552-557

Park, J.W.; Park, A.Y.; Lee, S.; Yu, N.K.; Lee, S.H. & Kaang, B.K. (2010). Detection of TrkB receptors distributed in cultured hippocampal neurons through bioconjugation between highly luminescent (quantum dot-neutravidin) and (biotinylated anti-TrkB antibody) on neurons by combined atomic force microscope and confocal laser scanning microscope. *Bioconjugate Chemistry*, Vol.21, No.4, (Aprile 2010), pp. 597-603

Characterization of Embryonic Stem (ES) Neuronal Differentiation Combining Atomic Force, Confocal and DIC Microscopy Imaging

133

Parot, P.; Dufrêne, Y.F.; Hinterdorfer, P.; Le Grimellec, C.; Navajas, D.; Pellequer, J.L. & Scheuring, S. (2007). Past, present and future of atomic force microscopy in life sciences and medicine. *Journal of Molecular Recognition*, Vol.20, No.6, (November 2007), pp. 418-431

Parpura, V.; Haydon, P.G. & Henderson, E. (1993). Three-dimensional imaging of living neurons and glia with the atomic force microscope. *Journal of Cell Science*, Vol.104, Pt2, (February 1993), pp. 427-32

Pawley, J.B. (2006). Handbook of biological confocal microscopy, Third Edition, Springer, available from: http://www.springerlink.com/content/978-0-387-25921-5#section=746525&page=1&locus=0

Rajwa, B.; McNally, H.A.; Varadharajan, P.; Sturgis, J. & Robinson, J.P. (2004). AFM/CLSM data visualization and comparison using an open-source toolkit. *Microscopy Research and Technique*, Vol.64, No.2, (June 2004), pp. 176-184

Reddy, C.V.; Malinowska, K.; Menhart, N. & Wang, R. (2004). Identification of TrkA on living PC12 cells by atomic force microscopy. *Biochimica et Biophysica Acta*, Vol.1667, No.1, (November 2004), pp. 15-25

Richter, E.; Hitzler, H.; Zimmermann, H.; Hagedorn, R. & Fuhr, G. (2000). Trace formation during locomotion of L929 mouse fibroblasts continuously recorded by interference reflection microscopy (IRM). *Cell Motility and the Cytoskeleton*, Vol.47, No.1, (September 2000), pp.38-47

Saito S. (1997). Effects of lysophosphatidic acid on primary cultured chick neurons. *Neuroscience Letters*, Vol.229, No.2, (June 1997), pp. 73-76

Schaefer, A.W.; Kabir, N. & Forscher, P. (2002). Filopodia and actin arcs guide the assembly and transport of two populations of microtubules with unique dynamic parameters in neuronal growth cones. *Journal of Cell Biology*, Vol.158, No.1, (July 2002), pp. 139-152

Schermelleh, L.; Heintzmann, R. & Leonhardt, H. (2010). A guide to super-resolution fluorescence microscopy. *Journal of Cell Biology*, Vol.190, No.2, (July 2010), pp. 165-175

Schoenwald, K.; Peng, Z.C.; Noga, D.; Qiu, S.R. & Sulchek, T. (2010). Integration of atomic force microscopy and a microfluidic liquid cell for aqueous imaging and force spectroscopy. *Review of Scientific Instruments*, Vol.81, No.5, (May 2010):053704

Staii, C.; Viesselmann, C.; Ballweg, J.; Williams, J.C.; Dent, E.W.; Coppersmith, S.N. & Eriksson, M.A. (2011). Distance dependence of neuronal growth on nanopatterned gold surfaces. Langmuir, Vol.27, No.1, (January 2011), pp. 233-239

Tamagnone, L. & Comoglio, P.M. (2004). To move or not to move? Semaphorin signalling in cell migration. *EMBO Reports*, Vol.5, No.4, (April 2004), pp. 356-361

Thomson, J.A.; Itskovitz-Eldor, J.; Shapiro, S.S.; Waknitz, M.A.; Swiergiel, J.J.; Marshall, V.S. & Jones, J.M. (1998). Embryonic stem cell lines derived from human blastocysts. *Science*, Vol.282, No.5391, (November 1998), pp. 1145-1147. Erratum in: *Science*, Vol.282, No.5395, (December 1998), p. 1827

Trucco, E. & Verri, A. (1998). Introductory Techniques for 3-D Computer Vision. 1998; Prentice Hall, New Jersey, USA.

Xiong, Y.; Lee, A.C.; Suter, D.M. & Lee, G.U. (2009). Topography and nanomechanics of live neuronal growth cones analyzed by atomic force microscopy. *Biophysical Journal*, Vol.96, No.12, (June 2009), pp. 5060-5072

Yunxu, S.; Danying, L.; Yanfang, R.; Dong, H. & Wanyun, M. (2006). Three-dimensional structural changes in living hippocampal neurons imaged using magnetic AC mode atomic force microscopy. *Journal of Electron Microscopy (Tokyo)*, Vol.55, No.3, (June 2006), pp. 165-172

Zimmermann, H.; Richter, E.; Reichle, C.; Westphal, I.; Geggier, P.; Rehn, U.; Rogaschewski, S.; Bleiss, W. & Fuhr, G. (2001). Mammalian cell traces: morphology, molecular composition, artificial guidance and biotechnological relevance as a new type of "bionanotube". *Applied Physics*, Vol.73, No.1 , (May 2001), pp. 11-26

Zitova, B. & Flusser, J. (2003). Image registration methods: a survey. *Image and Vision Computing*, Vol.21, No.11, (October 2003), pp. 977-100

7

Stem-Cell Therapy for Retinal Diseases

Rubens Camargo Siqueira
São Paulo University - Ribeirão Preto
Rubens Siqueira Research Center
Retina Cell
Brazil

1. Introduction

1.1

Stem cell (SC) therapy is not a new concept. In the aftermath of the bombings of Hiroshima and Nagasaki in 1945, researchers discovered that bone marrow transplanted into irradiated mice produced hematopoiesis (Lorenz, 1951). Hematopoietic stem cells (HSCs) were first identified in 1961 and their ability to migrate and differentiate into multiple cell types was documented (Till, 1961).

Distinct SC types have been established from embryos and identified in the fetal tissues and umbilical cord blood (UCB) as well as in specific niches in many adult mammalian tissues and organs such as bone marrow (BM), brain, skin, eyes, heart, kidneys, lungs, gastrointestinal tract, pancreas, liver, breast, ovaries, prostate and testis (Siqueira, 2010). All SCs are undifferentiated cells that exhibit unlimited self renewal and can generate multiple cell lineages or more restricted progenitor populations which can contribute to tissue homeostasis by replenishing the cells or to tissue regeneration after injury (Lanza, 2004; Mimeault, 2006).

Several investigations (Mimeault, 2006; Ortiz-Gonzalez, 2004; Trounson, 2006) have been carried out with isolated embryonic, fetal and adult SCs in a well-defined culture microenvironment to define the sequential steps and intracellular pathways that are involved in their differentiation into the specific cell lineages. More particularly, different methods have been developed for the *in vitro* culture of SCs, including the use of cell feeder layers, cell-free conditions, extracellular matrix molecules such as collagen, gelatin and laminin and diverse growth factors and cytokines (Mimeault, 2004; Siqueira, 2010).

1.2 Overview of the retinal anatomy

The retina is approximately 0.5 mm thick and lines the back of the eye. The **optic nerve** contains ganglion cell axons running to the brain and incoming blood vessels that open into the retina to vascularize the retinal layers and neurons. A radial section of a portion of the retina reveals that the **ganglion cells** (the output neurons of the retina) lie innermost in the retina closest to the lens and front of the eye, and the photosensors (the **rods** and **cones**) lie outermost in the retina against the retinal-pigment epithelium (RPE) and choroid. Light must, therefore, travel through the thickness of the retina before striking and activating the rods and cones. Subsequently, the absorption of photons by the visual pigment of the photoreceptors is translated first into a biochemical message and then into an electrical message that stimulates all of the succeeding neurons of the retina. The retinal message concerning the photic input and some preliminary organization of the visual image into several forms of sensation are transmitted to the brain from the spiking discharge pattern of the ganglion cells (Kolb, 2005).

RPE cells support photoreceptor survival and are involved in, for example, ion and nutrient transport, formation of the blood-retina barrier and light absorption.

They are also responsible for phagocytosis of the photoreceptor outer segments, which is important for the renewal of photoreceptor membranes. Interestingly, it has been demonstrated in a chicken model that, RPE in the postnatal stage of life is similar to that found in the embryonic retina with regard to specific gene expression.

Furthermore, the generation and *ex vivo* expansion of RPE from human embryonic stem cells (hESCs) has been extensively studied and characterized. Moreover, hESC-derived RPE cells have been demonstrated to be functional in *ex vivo* conditions. More recently, the *in vitro* differentiation of RPE and photoreceptors from human induced pluripotent stem (iPS) cell cultures provid another potential tool for transplantation purposes and additionally enables avoidance of host immune reactions (Machalinska, 2009).

1.3 Retinal diseases

Age-related macular degeneration (AMD), glaucoma and diabetic retinopathy are the three most common causes of visual impairment and legal blindness in developed countries (Bunce, 2006). One common denominator of these conditions is progressive loss of the neural cells of the eye [photoreceptors, interneurons and retinal ganglion cells (RGC)] and essential supporting cells such as the RPE. Retinal dystrophies [retinitis pigmentosa (RP), Stargardt's disease, Best disease, Leber congenital amaurosis, etc.] all evolve with early loss of photoreceptors and subsequent loss of RGC. Recent years have seen enormous progress in the treatment options that stop the progression of AMD from a neovascular state to fibrosis, that slow down the progression of glaucoma by reducing intraocular pressure, and that prevent progression of diabetic retinopathy by optimizing glycemic control and treat retinal neovascularization early (Chakravarthy, 2010; Maier, 2005; O'Doherty, 2008; Mohamed, 2007). However, irreversible visual loss still occurs in a significant proportion of cases. Research is aimed at developing novel treatments using neuroprotective and regenerative strategies.

SCs can potentially be used for both neuroprotection and cell replacement. Intravitreal delivery of neurotrophic factors slows down photoreceptor degeneration in rodent models of RP, RGC loss in glaucoma models and optic nerve and optic tract trauma, but the effect may be temporary. Slow-release preparations and gene therapy approaches used to induce retinal cells to secrete neurotrophic factors are two ways to induce longer-term effects. A third option is to use SC as long-term delivery agents, possibly encapsulated in a device, because many SC either secrete neurotrophins naturally or can be genetically engineered to do so (Otani, 2004; Dahlmann-Noor, 2010).

Progress has also been made in the field of photoreceptor, RPE and RGC replacement by SC and progenitor cells, although long-term restoration of visual function has been confirmed. The recent discoveries that human fibroblasts can be "reprogrammed" to behave like embryonic SC and that adult eyes harbor retinal progenitor cells, also increase the potential availability of SC for transplantation, including autologous transplantation and stimulate intrinsic "self-regeneration, " which could potentially overcome a lot of the problems associated with non-autologous transplantation in humans (Dahlmann-Noor, 2010).

2. Potential sources of stem cells for cell therapy in retinal diseases

2.1 Bone marrow-derived stem cells

Bone marrow-derived SCs have been proposed as a potential source of cells for regenerative medicine (Machalinska, 2009; Enzmann, 2009). This is based on the assumption that HSCs isolated from BM are plastic and are able to "transdifferentiate" into tissue-committed SCs for other organs (e. g., heart, liver or brain). Unfortunately, the concept of SC plasticity was not confirmed in recent studies and previously encouraging data demonstrating this phenomenon *in vitro* could be explained by a phenomenon of cell fusion or, as believed by our group, by the presence, of heterogeneous populations of SCs in BM (Müller-Sieburg, 2002; Spangrude 1988). The identification of very small, embryonic-like SCs in BM supports the notion that this tissue contains a population of primitive SCs, which, if transplanted together with HSCs, would be able to regenerate damaged tissues in certain experimental settings. Cells from BM are easily and safely aspirated. After administering local anesthesia, about 10 mL of the BM is aspirated from the iliac crest using a sterile BM aspiration needle; subsequently mononuclear bone marrow SCs are separated using the Ficoll density separation method (Siqueira, 2010) (Figure 1).

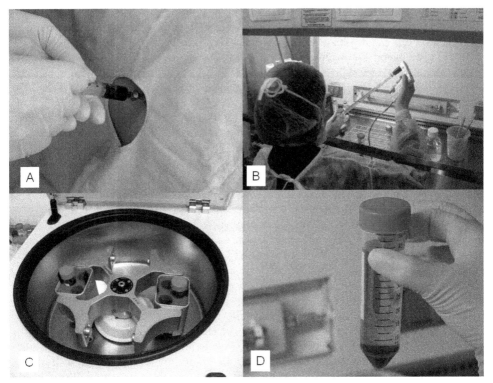

Fig. 1. Sequence of photos showing the collection of bone marrow (A) and the initial separation of the mononuclear cells using Ficoll-Hypaque gradient centrifugation (B) (C) (D) (Siqueira RC 2010)

SC-based therapy has been tested in animal models for several diseases including neurodegenerative disorders, such as Parkinson disease, spinal cord injury, and multiple sclerosis. The replacement of lost neurons that are not physiologically replaced is pivotal for therapeutic success. In the eye, degeneration of neural cells in the retina is a hallmark of such widespread ocular diseases as AMD and RP. In these cases the loss of photoreceptors that occurs as a primary event as in RP or secondary to loss of RPE, as in AMD, leads to blindness (Machalinska 2009; Siqueira 2010).

BM is an ideal tissue for studying SCs because of its accessibility and because proliferative dose-responses of bone marrow-derived SCs can be readily investigated. Furthermore, there are a number of well-defined mouse models and cell surface markers that allow effective studies of hematopoiesis in healthy and injured mice. Because of these characteristics and the experience of BM transplantation in the treatment of hematological cancers, bone marrow-derived SCs have also become an important tool in regenerative medicine. The BM harbors at least two distinct SC populations: HSCs and multipotent marrow stromal cells (MSC).

2.1.1 Hematopoietic stem cells

HSCs are multipotent SCs that give rise to all the blood cell types including myeloid (monocytes and macrophages, neutrophils, basophils, eosinophils, erythrocytes, megakaryocytes/platelets, dendritic cells), and lymphoid lineages (T-cells, B-cells, NK-cells).

HSCs are found in the BM of adults, which includes in femurs, hips, ribs, the sternum and other bones. Cells can be obtained directly from the hip using a needle and syringe (Figure 1), or from the blood following pretreatment with cytokines, such as G-CSF (granulocyte colony stimulating factors), that induce cells to be released from the BM compartment. Other sources for clinical and scientific use include UCB and placenta (Ratajczak, 2004; Müller-Sieburg 2002).

In reference to phenotype, HSCs are identified by their small size, lack of lineage markers, low staining (side population) by vital dyes such as rhodamine 123 (rhodamine-dull, also called rholo) or Hoechst 33342 and presence of various surface antigenic markers, many of which belong to the cluster of differentiation series: CD34, CD38, CD90, CD133, CD105, CD45 and also c-kit and SC factor receptor (Müller-Sieburg, 2002; Nielsen, 2009; Kuçi, 2009; Challen 2009 ; Voltarelli 2000; Voltarelli 2003). Otani (2004) demonstrated that whenever a fraction of mouse or human adult bone marrow–derived SCs [lineage-negative hematopoietic stem cells (Lin-HSCs)] containing endothelial precursors stabilizes and rescues retinal blood vessels that would ordinarily completely degenerate, a dramatic neurotrophic rescue effect is also observed. Retinal nuclear layers are preserved in two mouse models of retinal degeneration, rd1 and rd10, and detectable, albeit severely abnormal, electroretinogram recordings are observed in rescued mice at times when they are never observed in control-treated or untreated eyes. The normal mouse retina consists predominantly of rods, but the rescued cells after treatment with Lin-HSCs are nearly all cones. Microarray analysis of rescued retinas demonstrates significant upregulation of many antiapoptotic genes, including small heat shock proteins and transcription factors.

Some reports have demonstrated the clinical feasibility of the intravitreal administration of autologous bone marrow-derived mononuclear cells (ABMC) in patients with advanced degenerative retinopathies (Jonas, 2008 and 2010). More recently, our group conducted a prospective phase I trial to investigate the safety of intravitreal ABMC in patients with retinitis pigmentosa or cone-rod dystrophy, with promising results (Siqueira, 2011).

2.1.2 Multipotent Mesenchymal Stromal Cells (Mesenchymal Stem Cells)

Mesenchymal stem cells (MSCs) are progenitors of all connective tissue cells. In adults of multiple vertebrate species, MSCs have been isolated from BM and other tissues, expanded in culture and differentiated into several tissue-forming cells such as bone, cartilage, fat, muscle, tendon, liver, kidney, heart, and even brain cells.

According to the International Society for Cellular Therapy (Horwitz, 2005), there are three minimum requirements for a population of cells to be classified as MSCs. The first is that MSCs are isolated from a population of mononuclear cells on the basis of their selective adherence to the surface of the plastic of culture dishes, differing in this respect to bone marrow hematopoietic cells, a disadvantage of this method of identification is the possible contamination by hematopoietic cells and cellular heterogeneity with respect to the potential for differentiation. The second criteria is that CD105, CD73 and CD90 are present and that CD34, CD45, CD14 or CD11b, CD79, or CD19 and HLA-DR are not expressed in more than 95% of the cells in culture. Finally, the cells can be differentiated into bone, fat and cartilage (Phinney, 2007).

A number of studies have shown that bone-marrow-derived MSCs can differentiate into cells expressing photoreceptor proteins when injected into the subretinal space (Gong, 2008; Castanheira, 2008). Interestingly, it has been suggested that rat MSCs can be made to express photopigment (rhodopsin) *in vitro* simply by adding epidermal growth factor to the culture media (Zhang, 2008). Additionally, though other retina-relevant cell types have been engineered, a number of studies have shown that BM or adipose tissue MSCs are converted to RPE (Gong, 2008; Arnhold, 2006; Vossmerbaeumer 2009). As with work on other neuronal phenotypes, however, there has now been a reassessment of the ability of MSCs to differentiate into functionally useful retinal cells. Some studies have shown that transplanted bone marrow MSCs do not differentiate into neural retinal cells (YU, 2006). In an *in vitro* rat retina-explant model, untreated MSCs seemed to transdifferentiate into microglia109 in a way reminiscent of earlier work on MSC transplants in other neurological tissue (Azizi 1998). Some limited improvement was seen with pre-treatment with BDNF, NGF, and bFGF in terms of morphological differentiation into retinal neurons and expression of NF200, GFAP, PKC-alpha, and recoverin, but these cells did not express Rhodopsin (Erices, 2000).

In an ischemic retina rodent model, MSCs injected into the vitreous cavity have been shown to mature (with expression of neuron-specific enolase and neurofilament) and secrete CNTF, bFGF, and BDNF for at least 4 weeks (Li, 2009). Animal studies have also demonstrated that subretinal transplantation of MSCs delays retinal degeneration and preserves retinal function through a trophic response (Inoue, 2007). UCB-derived MSCs have also been shown to be neuroprotective of rat ganglion cells (Zwart, 2009). Very recently, the intravenous administration of bone marrow-derived MSCs was shown to prevent photoreceptor loss and preserve visual function in the RCS rat model of RP.

A role for genetically-modified MSCs may emerge in the treatment of subretinal neovascularization. It has been shown that bone-marrow-derived MSCs accumulate around subretinal membranes induced by retinal laser burns.

Intravenous injection of mouse bone-marrow MSCs genetically engineered to secrete pigment epithelium derived factor resulted in smaller neovascular complexes (Hou, 2010).

2.2 Induced pluripotent stem cells

Current methods of producing SCs from adult somatic cells offer an alternative cell source for transplantation. Induced pluripotent stem (iPS) cells are morphologically identical to embryonic SCs, display similar gene expression profiles and epigenetic status and have the potential to form any cell in the body (Takahashi, 2006 and 2007; Yu, 2007). These cells have been employed to generate cells for the treatment of various diseases including diabetes, cardiovascular disease, sickle cell anemia, Parkinson's disease and hemophilia (Zhang, 2009; Hanna, 2007; Xu, 2009; Wernig, 2008). Meyer et al. 2009 recently showed that iPS cells can differentiate into retinal cell types whilst a paper by Buchholz et al. 2009 showed that human iPS cells can be differentiated into retinal pigment epithelial cells which display functionality in vitro.

Carr (2009) demonstrated that iPS cells can be differentiated into functional iPS-RPE and that transplantation of these cells can facilitate the short-term maintenance of photoreceptors through phagocytosis of photoreceptor outer segments. Long-term visual function is maintained in this model of retinal disease even though the xenografted cells are eventually lost, suggesting a secondary protective host cellular response.

While this particular line of iPS-RPE cells cannot be used as a direct therapy due to viral insertions of pluripotency genes, recent advances in iPS cell reprogramming technology, including the use of small molecules (Huangfu, 2008; Shi, 2008; Li, 2009), piggyBac transposition (Woltjen, 2009; Kaji, 2009), non-integrating episomal vectors (Yu, 2009) and manipulation of endogenous transcription factors (Balasubramanian, 2009) should eliminate the risks associated with the integration of SC genes into the genome. Furthermore, the finding that blood cells can be used to derive iPS cells (Loh, 2009) may remove the need for the invasive biopsies required to collect somatic cells and accelerate the ethical production of SC-derived tissue for therapeutic use.

2.3 Human Embryonic Stem Cells

The human embryonic stem cell (hESC) is defined as a cell that can both renew itself by repeated division and differentiate into any one of the 200 or more adult cell types in the human body. An hESC cell arises from the eight-cell stage morula. Outside of normal development, hESCs have been differentiated in vitro into neural cell types and even pigmented epithelium, although controlling their differentiation has proven challenging. Several hESC lines exist and are supported by public research funds. The use of hESCs has significant limitations, including ethical issues, and a risk of teratoma formation, but the chief problem is that we are still struggling to understand the developmental cues that differentiate hESCs into the specific adult cell types required to repair damaged tissues (MacLaren, 2007).

Nistor et al. (2010) showed for the first time that three-dimensional early retinal progenitor tissue constructs can be derived from hESCs. Three-dimensional tissue constructs were developed by culturing hESC-derived neural retinal progenitors in a matrix on top of hESC-derived RPE cells in a cell culture insert. An osmolarity gradient maintained the nutrition of the three-dimensional cell constructs. Cross-sections through hESC-derived tissue constructs were characterized by immunohistochemistry for various transcription factors and cell markers. Tissue constructs derived from hESC expressed transcription factors characteristic of retinal development, such as pax6, Otx2, Chx10, retinal RAX; Brn3b (necessary for differentiation of retinal ganglion cells) and crx and nrl (role in photoreceptor development). Many cells expressed neuronal markers including nestin, beta-tubulin and microtubule-associated protein.

Assessments of safety and efficacy are crucial before hESC therapies can move into the clinic. Two important early potential hESC applications are the use of retinal pigment epithelium (RPE) for the treatment of age-related macular degeneration and Stargardt's disease, an untreatable form of macular dystrophy that leads to early-onset blindness. Long-term safety and function of RPE from hESCs in preclinical models of macular degeneration was demonstrated by Lu et al. (2009).

They showed long-term functional rescue using hESC-derived RPE in both RCS rats and Elov14 mice, which are animal models of retinal degeneration and Stargardt's disease, respectively. Good manufacturing practice-compliant hESC-RPE survived subretinal transplantation in RCS rats for prolonged periods (> 220 days). The cells sustained visual function and photoreceptor integrity in a dose-dependent fashion without teratoma formation or untoward pathological reactions.

Near-normal functional measurements were recorded at > 60 days survival in RCS rats. To further address safety concerns, a Good laboratory practice-compliant study was carried out in the NIH III immune-deficient mouse model. Long-term data (spanning the life of the animals) showed no gross or microscopic evidence of teratoma/tumor formation after subretinal hESC-RPE transplantation.

These results suggest that hESCs could serve as a potentially safe and inexhaustible source of RPE for the efficacious treatment of a range of retinal degenerative diseases.

In 2010, the US Food and Drug Administration (FDA) granted Orphan drug designation for RPE cells of Advanced Cell Technology, Inc. (ACT) to initiate its Phase 1/2 clinical trials

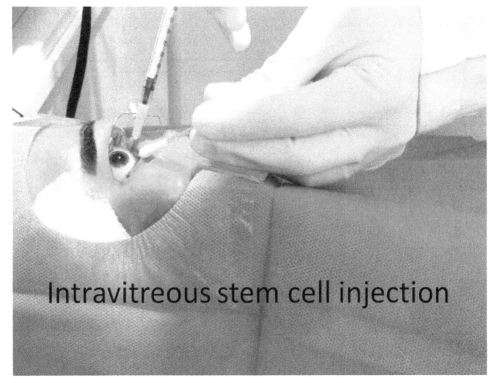

Fig. 1. Intravitreal injection of autologous bone marrow–derived stem cells in a patient with retinitis pigmentosa (Siqueira RC, 2010)

using retinal pigment epithelial (RPE) cells derived from hESCs to treat patients with Stargardt's Macular Dystrophy (SMD). Moreover, in 2011 the company received a positive opinion from the Committee for Orphan Medicinal Products (COMP) of the European Medicines Agency (EMA) towards designation of this product as an orphan medicinal product for the treatment of Stargardt's disease.

	Type of study	Type of injury or illness	Route used	Type and source of cells
Atsushi Otani et al.	Experimental study in animals	Mice with retinal degenerative disease	Intravitreous transplantation	Adult bone marrow–derived lineage-negative hematopoietic stem cells
Wang S et al.	Experimental study in animals	Retinitis pigmentosa	Tail vein	Pluripotent bone marrow-derived mesenchymal stem cells
Li Na & Li Xiao-rong & Yuan Jia-qin	Experimental study in animals	Rat injured by ischemia/reperfusion	Intravitreous transplantation	Bone marrow mesenchymal stem cells
Uteza Y, Rouillot JS, Kobetz A, et al.	Experimental study in animals	Photoreceptor cell degeneration in Royal College of Surgeon rats	Intravitreous transplantation	Encapsulated fibroblasts
Zhang Y, Wang W	Experimental study in animals	Light-damaged retinal structure	Subretinal space	Bone marrow mesenchymal stem cells
Tomita M	Experimental study in animals	Retinas mechanically injured using a hooked needle	Intravitreous transplantation	Bone marrow-derived stem cells
Meyer JS et al.	Experimental study in animals	Retinal degeneration	Intravitreous transplantation	Embryonic stem cells
Siqueira RC et al.	Experimental study in animals	Chorioretinal injuries caused by laser red diode 670N-M	Intravitreous transplantation	Bone marrow-derived stem cells
Wang HC et al.	Experimental study in animals	Mice with laser-induced retinal injury	Intravitreous transplantation	bone marrow-derived stem cells
Johnson TV et al.	Experimental study in animals	Glaucoma	Intravitreous transplantation	Bone marrow-derived mesenchymal stem cell
Castanheira P et al.	Experimental study in animals	Rat retinas submitted to laser damage	Intravitreous transplantation	Bone marrow-derived mesenchymal stem cell
Jonas JB et al.	Case report	Patient with atrophy of the retina and optic nerve	Intravitreous transplantation	bone marrow-derived mononuclear cell transplantation

	Type of study	Type of injury or illness	Route used	Type and source of cells
Jonas JB et al.	Case report	Three patients with diabetic retinopathy, age related macular degeneration and optic nerve atrophy (glaucoma)	Intravitreous transplantation	bone marrow-derived mononuclear cell transplantation
Siqueira RC et al. gov clinical trial. NCT01068561	Clinical Trial Phase I	Five patients with retinitis pigmentosa	Intravitreous transplantation	bone marrow-derived mononuclear cell transplantation
Siqueira RC et al. Ethics committee of Brazil. Register: 16018	Clinical trial Phase II	50 patients with retinitis pigmentosa	Intravitreous transplantation	bone marrow-derived mononuclear cell transplantation
Siqueira RC et al. Ethics committee of Brazil. Register 15978	Clinical trial Phase I/II	Ten patients with macular degeneration	Intravitreous transplantation	bone marrow-derived mononuclear cell transplantation
Advanced Cell Technology http://www. advancedcell. com/	Clinical trial Phase I/II	12 patients with Stargardt's Macular Dystrophy	Subretinal transplantation	retinal pigment epithelial (RPE) cells derived from human embryonic stem cells (hESCs)

Table 1. Clinical and experimental studies using cell therapy for retinal diseases

3. Conclusion

Stem cells maintain the balance between somatic cell populations in various tissues and are responsible for organ regeneration. The remarkable progress of regenerative medicine in the last few years indicates promise for the use of stem cells in the treatment of ophthalmic disorders. Based on the above mentioned mechanisms, experimental and human studies with intravitreal bone marrow-derived stem cells have begun (Table 1). The history starts to be written in this very promising therapeutic field.

4. Acknowledgment

Júlio Cesar Voltarelli, André Marcio Vieira Messias, Rodrigo Jorge from São Paulo University - USP, Ribeirão Preto, SP, Brazil.

5. References

[1] Lorenz E, Congdon C, Uphoff ED, R. Modification of acute irradiation injury in mice and guinea-pigs by bone marrow injections. Radiology. 1951; 58:863-77.
[2] Till JE, McCulloch EA. A direct measurement of the radiation sensitivity of normal mouse bone marrow cells. Radiat Res. 1961; 14:213-22.
[3] Lanza R, Rosenthal N. The stem cell challenge. Sci Am. 2004; 290:93-9.

[4] Mimeault M, Batra SK. Concise review: recent advances on the significance of stem cells in tissue regeneration and cancer therapies. Stem Cells. 2006; 24 (11):2319-45.

[5] Ortiz-Gonzalez XR, Keene CD, Verfaillie C, Low WC. Neural induction of adult bone marrow and umbilical cord stem cells. Curr Neurovasc Res. 2004; 1 (3):207-13.

[6] Trounson A. The production and directed differentiation of human embryonic stem cells. Endocr Rev. 2006; 27 (2):208-19. Review.

[7] Schuldiner M, Yanuka O, Itskovitz-Eldor J, Melton DA, Benvenisty N. Effects of eight growth factors on the differentiation of cells derived from human embryonic stem cells. Proc Natl Acad Sci U S A. 2002; 97 (21):11307-12.

[8] Siqueira RC, Voltarelli JC, Messias AM, Jorge R. Possible mechanisms of retinal function recovery with the use of cell therapy with bone marrow-derived stem cells. Arq Bras Oftalmol. 2010 Oct; 73 (5):474-9.

[9] Siqueira RC, Messias A, Voltarelli JC, Scott I, Jorge R. Autologous bone marrow-derived stem cells transplantation for retinitis pigmentosa. Cytotherapy. 2010; 12 Suppl 1:58.

[10] ClinicalTrials. gov. [Internet]. Autologous Bone Marrow-Derived Stem Cells Transplantation for Retinitis Pigmentosa. NCT01068561. [cited 2010 July 30]. Available at: http://clinicaltrial.gov/

[11] Siqueira RC. Autologous transplantation of retinal pigment epithelium in age related macular degeneration]. Arq Bras Oftalmol. 2009; 72 (1):123-30

[12] Siqueira RC, Abad L, Benson G, Sami M. Behaviour of stem cells in eyes of rabbits with chorioretinal injuries caused by laser red diode 670N-M. In: Annual Meeting of the Association for Research in Vision and Ophthalmology (ARVO), 2008, Fort Lauderdale. Invest Ophthalmol Vis Sci. 2008; 49:536.

[13] Siqueira RC. Cell therapy in ophthalmology diseases. Rev. Bras. Hematol. Hemoter. 2009, vol. 31, suppl. 1, pp. 120-127.

[14] Kolb H. Simple Anatomy of the Retina. The Organization of the Retina and Visual System [Internet]. Salt Lake City (UT): University of Utah Health Sciences Center; 1995-. 2005 May 1.

[15] Machalinska A, Baumert B, Kuprjanowicz L, Wiszniewska B, Karczewicz D, Machalinski B. Potential application of adult stem cells in retinal repair--challenge for regenerative medicine. Curr Eye Res. 2009 Sep; 34 (9):748-60. Review.

[16] Dahlmann-Noor A, Vijay S, Jayaram H, Limb A, Khaw PT. Current approaches and future prospects for stem cell rescue and regeneration of the retina and optic nerve. Can J Ophthalmol. 2010 Aug; 45 (4):333-41.

[17] Bunce C, Wormald R. Leading causes of certification for blindness and partial sight in England & Wales. BMC Public Health 2006; 6:58.

[18] Chakravarthy U, Evans J, Rosenfeld PJ. Age related macular degeneration. BMJ 2010; 340:c981.

[19] Maier PC, Funk J, Schwarzer G, Antes G, Falck-Ytter YT. Treatment of ocular hypertension and open angle glaucoma: meta-analysis of randomised controlled trials. BMJ 2005; 331:134.

[20] O'Doherty M, Dooley I, Hickey-Dwyer M. Interventions for diabetic macular oedema: a systematic review of the literature. Br J Ophthalmol 2008; 92:1581-90.

[21] Mohamed Q, Gillies MC, Wong TY. Management of diabetic retinopathy: a systematic review. JAMA 2007; 298:902-16.

[22] Enzmann V, Yolcu E, Kaplan HJ, Ildstad ST. Stem cells as tools in regenerative therapy for retinal degeneration. Arch Ophthalmol. 2009; 127 (4):563-71.

[23] Crisostomo PR, Markel TA, Wang Y, Meldrum DR. Surgically relevant aspects of stem cell paracrine effects. Surgery. 2008; 143 (5):577-81.

[24] Vandervelde S, van Luyn MJ, Tio RA, Harmsen MC. Signaling factors in stem cell-mediated repair of infarcted myocardium. J Mol Cell Cardiol. 2005; 39 (2):363-76.

[25] Oh JY, Kim MK, Shin MS, Lee HJ, Ko JH, Wee WR, Lee JH. The anti-inflammatory and anti-angiogenic role of mesenchymal stem cells in corneal wound healing following chemical injury. Stem Cells. 2008; 26 (4):1047-55.

[26] Gomei Y, Nakamura Y, Yoshihara H, Hosokawa K, Iwasaki H, Suda T, Arai F. Functional differences between two Tie2 ligands, angiopoietin-1 and -2, in the regulation of adult bone marrow hematopoietic stem cells. Exp Hematol. 2010; 38 (2):82-9.

[27] Li N, Li XR, Yuan JQ. Effects of bone-marrow mesenchymal stem cells transplanted into vitreous cavity of rat injured by ischemia/reperfusion. Graefes Arch Clin Exp Ophthalmol. 2009; 247 (4):503-14.

[28] Markel TA, Wang Y, Herrmann JL, Crisostomo PR, Wang M, Novotny NM, et al. VEGF is critical for stem cell-mediated cardioprotection and a crucial paracrine factor for defining the age threshold in adult and neonatal stem cell function. Am J Physiol Heart Circ Physiol. 2008; 295 (6):H2308-14.

[29] Markel TA, Crisostomo PR, Wang M, Herring CM, Meldrum DR. Activation of individual tumor necrosis factor receptors differentially affects stem cell growth factor and cytokine production. Am J Physiol Gastrointest Liver Physiol. 2007; 293 (4): G657-62

[30] Harris JR, Brown GA, Jorgensen M, Kaushal S, Ellis EA, Grant MB, Scott EW. Bone marrow-derived cells home to and regenerate retinal pigment epithelium after injury. Invest Ophthalmol Vis Sci. 2006; 47 (5):2108-13.

[31] Zhang P, Li J, Liu Y, Chen X, Kang Q, Zhao J, Li W. Human neural stem cell transplantation attenuates apoptosis and improves neurological functions after cerebral ischemia in rats. Acta Anaesthesiol Scand. 2009; 53 (9):1184-91.

[32] Cheng AS, Yau TM. Paracrine effects of cell transplantation: strategies to augment the efficacy of cell therapies. Semin Thorac Cardiovasc Surg. 2008; 20 (2):94-101.

[33] Harris JR, Fisher R, Jorgensen M, Kaushal S, Scott EW. CD133 progenitor cells from the bone marrow contribute to retinal pigment epithelium repair. Stem Cells. 2009; 27 (2):457-66.

[34] Tomita M, Adachi Y, Yamada H, Takahashi K, Kiuchi K, Oyaizu H, et al. Bone marrow-derived stem cells can differentiate into retinal cells in injured rat retina. Stem Cells. 2002; 20 (4):279-83.

[35] Otani A, Dorrell MI, Kinder K, Moreno SK, Nusinowitz S, Banin E, et al. Rescue of retinal degeneration by intravitreally injected adult bone marrow-derived lineagenegative hematopoietic stem cells. J Clin Invest. 2004; 114 (6):765-74. Comment in:J Clin Invest. 2004; 114 (6):755-7.

[36] Otani A, Kinder K, Ewalt K, Otero FJ, Schimmel P, Friedlander M. Bone marrow-derived stem cells target retinal astrocytes and can promote or inhibit retinal angiogenesis. Nat Med. 2002; 8 (9):1004-10. Comment in: Nat Med. 2002; 8 (9): 932-4.

[37] Meyer JS, Katz ML, Maruniak JA, Kirk MD. Embryonic stem cell-derived neural progenitors incorporate into degenerating retina and enhance survival of host photoreceptors. Stem Cells. 2006; 24 (2):274-83.

[38] Binder S, Stanzel BV, Krebs I, Glittenberg C. Transplantation of the RPE in AMD. Prog Retin Eye Res. 2007 Sep; 26 (5):516-54. Epub 2007 Mar 6. Review.

[39] Lu B, Malcuit C, Wang S, Girman S, Francis P, Lemieux L, Lanza R, Lund R. Long-term safety and function of RPE from human embryonic stem cells in preclinical models of macular degeneration. Stem Cells. 2009 Sep; 27 (9):2126-35.

[40] Takahashi K, Yamanaka S. Induction of pluripotent stem cells from mouse embryonic and adult fibroblast cultures by defined factors. *Cell.* 2006; 126:663-676.

[41] Takahashi K, Tanabe K, Ohnuki M, Narita M, Ichisaka T, et al. Induction of pluripotent stem cells from adult human fibroblasts by defined factors. *Cell.* 2007; 131:861-872.

[42] Yu J, Vodyanik MA, Smuga-Otto K, Antosiewicz-Bourget J, Frane JL, et al. Induced pluripotent stem cell lines derived from human somatic cells. *Science.* 2007; 318:1917-1920.

[43] Zhang D, Jiang W, Liu M, Sui X, Yin X, et al. Highly efficient differentiation of human ES cells and iPS cells into mature pancreatic insulin-producing cells. *Cell Res.* 2009; 52:615-621.

[44] Zhang J, Wilson GF, Soerens AG, Koonce CH, Yu J, et al. Functional cardiomyocytes derived from human induced pluripotent stem cells. *Circ Res.* 2009; 104:e30-41.

[45] Hanna J, Wernig M, Markoulaki S, Sun CW, Meissner A, et al. Treatment of sickle cell anemia mouse model with iPS cells generated from autologous skin. *Science.* 2007; 318:1920-1923.

[46] Xu D, Alipio Z, Fink LM, Adcock DM, Yang J, et al. Phenotypic correction of murine hemophilia A using an iPS cell-based therapy. *Proc Natl Acad Sci U S A.* 2009; 106:80

[47] Wernig M, Zhao JP, Pruszak J, Hedlund E, Fu D, et al. Neurons derived from reprogrammed fibroblasts functionally integrate into the fetal brain and improve symptoms of rats with Parkinson's disease. *Proc Natl Acad Sci U S A.* 2008; 105:5856-5861.

[48] Meyer JS, Shearer RL, Capowski EE, Wright LS, Wallace KA, et al. Modeling early retinal development with human embryonic and induced pluripotent stem cells. *Proc Natl Acad Sci U S A.* 2009; 106:

[49] Buchholz DE, Hikita ST, Rowland TJ, Friedrich AM, Hinman CR, et al. Derivation of Functional Retinal Pigmented Epithelium from Induced Pluripotent Stem Cells. *Stem Cells.* 2009; 27:2427-2434.

[50] Carr AJ, Vugler AA, Hikita ST, Lawrence JM, Gias C, Chen LL, Buchholz DE, Ahmado A, Semo M, Smart MJ, Hasan S, da Cruz L, Johnson LV, Clegg DO, Coffey PJ. Protective effects of human iPS-derived retinal pigment epithelium cell transplantation in the retinal dystrophic rat. PLoS One. 2009 Dec 3; 4 (12):e8152.

[51] Huangfu D, Osafune K, Maehr R, Guo W, Eijkelenboom A, et al. Induction of pluripotent stem cells from primary human fibroblasts with only Oct4 and Sox2. *Nat Biotechnol.* 2008; 26:1269-1275.

[52] Shi Y, Desponts C, Do JT, Hahm HS, Scholer HR, et al. Induction of pluripotent stem cells from mouse embryonic fibroblasts by Oct4 and Klf4 with small-molecule compounds. *Cell Stem Cell.* 2008; 3:568-574.]

[53] Li W, Zhou H, Abujarour R, Zhu S, Joo JY, et al. Generation of Human Induced Pluripotent Stem Cells in the Absence of Exogenous Sox2. *Stem Cells* 2009.

[54] Woltjen K, Michael IP, Mohseni P, Desai R, Mileikovsky M, et al. piggyBac transposition reprograms fibroblasts to induced pluripotent stem cells. *Nature.* 2009; 458:766–770.

[55] Kaji K, Norrby K, Paca A, Mileikovsky M, Mohseni P, et al. Virus-free induction of pluripotency and subsequent excision of reprogramming factors. *Nature.* 2009; 458:771–775.

[56] Yu J, Hu K, Smuga-Otto K, Tian S, Stewart R, et al. Human Induced Pluripotent Stem Cells Free of Vector and Transgene Sequences. *Science.* 2009; 324:797–801.

[57] Müller-Sieburg CE, Cho RH, Thoman M, Adkins B, Sieburg HB. Deterministic regulation of hematopoietic stem cell self-renewal and differentiation. Blood. 2002; 100 (4):1302-9.

[58] Balasubramanian S, Babai N, Chaudhuri A, Qiu F, Bhattacharya S, et al. Non Cell-Autonomous Reprogramming of Adult Ocular Progenitors: Generation of Pluripotent Stem Cells Without Exogenous Transcription Factors. *Stem Cells* 2009.

[59] Loh YH, Agarwal S, Park IH, Urbach A, Huo H, et al. Generation of induced pluripotent stem cells from human blood. *Blood.* 2009; 113:5476–5479.

[60] Spangrude GJ, Heimfeld S, Weissman IL. Purification and characterization of mouse hematopoietic stem cells. Science. 1988; 241 (4861):58-62. Erratum in: Science. 1989;244 (4908):1030.

[61] Ratajczak MZ, Kucia M, Reca R, Majka M, Janowska-Wieczorek A, Ratajczak J. Stem cell plasticity revisited: CXCR4-positive cells expressing mRNA for early muscle, liver and neural cells 'hide out' in the bone marrow. Leukemia. 2004; 18 (1):29-40.

[62] Müller-Sieburg CE, Cho RH, Thoman M, Adkins B, Sieburg HB. Deterministic regulation of hematopoietic stem cell self-renewal and differentiation. Blood. 2002; 100 (4):1302-9.

[63] Nielsen JS, McNagny KM. CD34 is a key regulator of hematopoietic stem cell trafficking to bone marrow and mast cell progenitor trafficking in the periphery. Microcirculation. 2009; 16 (6):487-96.

[64] Kuçi S, Kuçi Z, Latifi-Pupovci H, Niethammer D, Handgretinger R, Schumm M, et al. Adult stem cells as an alternative source of multipotential (pluripotential) cells inregenerative medicine. Curr Stem Cell Res Ther. 2009; 4 (2):107-17.

[65] Challen GA, Boles N, Lin KK, Goodell MA. Mouse hematopoietic stem cell identificationand analysis. Cytometry A. 2009; 75 (1):14-24. Review.

[66] Voltarelli JC, Ouyang J. Hematopoietic stem cell transplantation for autoimmune diseases in developing countries: current status and future prospectives. Bone Marrow Transplant. 2003; 32 Suppl 1:S69-71.

[67] Voltarelli JC. Applications of flow cytometry to hematopoietic stem cell transplantation. Mem Inst Oswaldo Cruz. 2000; 95 (3):403-14.

[68] Horwitz EM, Le Blanc K, Dominici M, Mueller I, Slaper-Cortenbach I, Marini FC, Deans RJ, Krause DS, Keating A; International Society for Cellular Therapy. Clarification of the nomenclature for MSC: The International Society for Cellular Therapy position statement. Cytotherapy. 2005; 7 (5):393-5.

[69] Phinney DG, Prockop DJ. Concise review: mesenchymal stem/multipotent stromal cells: the state of transdifferentiation and modes of tissue repair-current views. Stem Cells. 2007; 25 (11):2896-902.

[70] Gong L, Wu Q, Song B, et al. Differentiation of rat mesenchymal stem cells transplanted into the subretinal space of sodium iodate-injected rats. *Clin Experiment Ophthalmol.* 2008; 36:666–671.

[71] Castanheira P, Torquetti L, Nehemy MB, et al. Retinal incorporation and differentiation of mesenchymal stem cells intravitreally injected in the injured retina of rats. *Arq Bras Oftalmol.* 2008; 71:644–650.

[72] Zhang ZQ, Dong FT. In vitro differentiation of rat mesenchymal stem cells into photoreceptors. *Zhonghua Yan Ke Za Zhi.* 2008; 44:540–544.

[73] Vossmerbaeumer U, Ohnesorge S, Kuehl S, et al. Retinal pigment epithelial phenotype induced in human adipose tissue-derived mesenchymal stromal cells. *Cytotherapy.* 2009; 11:177–188.

[74] Arnhold S, Heiduschka P, Klein H, et al. Adenovirally transduced bone marrow stromal cells differentiate into pigment epithelial cells and induce rescue effects in RCS rats. *Invest Ophthalmol Vis Sci.* 2006; 47:4121–4129.

[75] Yu S, Tanabe T, Dezawa M, et al. Effects of bone marrow stromal cell injection in an experimental glaucoma model. *Biochem Biophys Res Commun.* 2006; 344:1071–1079.

[76] Azizi SA, Stokes D, Augelli BJ, et al. Engraftment and migration of human bone marrow stromal cells implanted in the brains of albino rats—Similarities to astrocyte grafts. *Proc Natl Acad Sci U S A.* 1998; 95:3908–3913.

[77] Erices A, Conget P, Minguell JJ. Mesenchymal progenitor cells in human umbilical cord blood. *Br J Haematol.* 2000; 109:235–242.

[78] Li N, Li XR, Yuan JQ. Effects of bone-marrow mesenchymal stem cells transplanted into vitreous cavity of rat injured by ischemia/reperfusion. *Graefes Arch Clin Exp Ophthalmol.* 2009; 247:503–514.

[79] Inoue Y, Iriyama A, Ueno S, et al. Subretinal transplantation of bone marrow mesenchymal stem cells delays retinal degeneration in the RCS rat model of retinal degeneration. *Exp Eye Res.* 2007; 85:234–241.

[80] Zwart I, Hill AJ, Al-Allaf F, et al. Umbilical cord blood mesenchymal stromal cells are neuroprotective and promote regeneration in a rat optic tract model. *Exp Neurol.* 2009; 216:439–448.

[81] Hou HY, Liang HL, Wang YS, et al. A Therapeutic strategy for choroidal neovascularization based on recruitment of mesenchymal stem cells to the sites of lesions. *Mol Ther.* 2010 Jul 20. [Epub ahead of print]

[82] Jonas JB, Witzens-Harig M, Arseniev L, Ho AD. Intravitreal autologous bone marrow-derived mononuclear cell transplantation: a feasibility report. Acta Ophthalmol. 2008; 86 (2):225-6.

[83] Jonas JB, Witzens-Harig M, Arseniev L, Ho AD. Intravitreal autologous bone marrow-derived mononuclear cell transplantation. Acta Ophthalmol. 2010; 88 (4):e131-2.

[84] Siqueira RC, Messias A, Voltarelli JC, Scott IU, Jorge R. Intravitreal injection of autologous bone marrow-derived mononuclear cells for hereditary retinal dystrophy: a phase I trial. Retina. 2011 feb 2. [epub ahead of print]

[85] Nistor G, Seiler MJ, Yan F, Ferguson D, Keirstead HS. Three-dimensional early retinal progenitor 3D tissue constructs derived from human embryonic stem cells. J Neurosci Methods. 2010 Jun 30; 190 (1):63-70. Epub 2010 May 4.

[86] MacLaren R E, Pearson R A. Stem cell therapy and the retina. *Eye* (2007) 21, 1352–1359

Part 3

Cardiac and Other Myogenic Differentiation

8

Transcriptional Networks of Embryonic Stem Cell-Derived Cardiomyogenesis

Diego Franco, Estefania Lozano-Velasco and Amelia Aránega
Cardiovascular Development Group,
Department of Experimental Biology,
University of Jaén, Jaén
Spain

1. Introduction

Embryonic stem cells are pluripotent cells that, if cultured under specific conditions, give rise to clusters of beating cardiomyocytes. Beating cardiomyocytes, also dubbed beating areas, display gene expression profiles and functional properties similar to adult cardiomyocytes. In line with this, a wide heterogeneity has been observed in embryonic stem cell-derived cardiomyocytes, resembling thus the distinct characteristics of atrial, ventricular and conductive cardiomyocytes.

It has been recently demonstrated that two distinct cardiogenic precursor cells contribute to the developing heart. The first heart field contributes to the cardiac linear straight tube while a second population of cells adds cells to both arterial and venous pole of the cardiac tube, delimiting thus the second heart field. As cardiogenesis advances the first heart field mainly gives rise to the left ventricle, whereas the second heart field contributes to the right ventricle, outflow tract and the atrial chambers. A third population of cells, with distinct gene expression fingerprint has been demonstrated to form the inflow tract, suggesting the possible existence of a third heart field.

Over the last years we have gained insights about the transcriptional mechanisms that govern the distinct heart fields, however, our understanding about if such endogenous program is recapitulated in embryonic stem cell-derived cardiomyogenesis remains elusive. Within this review we elaborate about the current state-of-the-art of the transcriptional networks that operate during embryonic stem cell-derived cardiomyogenesis, with special emphasis on the development of heart field transcriptional networks.

2. Cardiogenic potential of embryonic stem cells

Embryonic stem cells are pluripotent stem cells derived from the inner cell mass of the developing blastocyst. *In vitro* culture of embryonic stem cells, if nurtured under specific conditions, can give rise to distinct cell types of endodermal, mesodermal and ectodermal lineages, including thus beating cardiomyocytes (Miller-Hance et al. 1993). Such capabilities have raised the possibility of using embryonic stem cells as a source to heal the damaged heart (Chinchilla & Franco, 2006; Franco et al., 2007). However, several constrains has obstructed this purpose. Leaving apart ethical concerns, mainly applicable to human embryonic stem cells, technical and scientific obstacles also have contributed to slow down this quest. We shall update in this book chapter the state-of-the-art progress made to conquer the challenging aim of converting embryonic stem cells into beating cardiomyocytes as suitable therapeutical tools.

It is incredible to observe that a subset of cells hunted from the inner mass cells of the developing blastocyst, set in appropriate cell culture conditions, are able to progressively proceed *in vitro*, differentiating into neurons, fibroblasts, cardiomyocytes as well as in several other cells types (Lanza et al., 2004). The real question is then; does this occur mimicking the early step of embryogenesis? Several studies have demonstrated that upon the initial phases of *in vitro* embryonic stem cells culture, the aggregating cells that form the embryonic bodies in the hanging drops acquire a rather well organized three-dimensional structure, by which externally located cells express ectodermal markers, while internally located cells express mesodermal and endodermal makers (Doetschman et al., 1985, Wobus & Boheler, 1999; Boheler et al., 2002). Thus, these findings support the notion that cell specification and determination of embryonic stem cells into a discrete cell type would mainly follow the endogenous signal pathways. Therefore, in order to understand how stem cells can lead to cardiomyocytes, efforts should be made to learn the natural routing of a mesodermal cell that will contribute to the heart. In essence we need to learn how cardiac development is achieved.

3. Transcriptional control of cardiac muscle development

Over the last two decades, our understanding of the cellular and molecular mechanisms that govern cardiac development has greatly advanced. Initial steps of mesoderm commitment from the lateral plate mesoderm to the forming heart are mainly directed by interplay between Bmp, Fgf and Wnt signaling (Barron et al., 2000; Lopez-Sanchez et al., 2002; Marques et al., 2008). As soon as the cardiogenic mesoderm is committed, several transcription factors, such as Nkx2.5, Gata4, Srf, Hand2 and Mef2c are activated, which play crucial roles during cardiogenesis as revealed by loss-of-function experiments in mice (Lyons et al., 1995; Srivastava et al., 1995; Kuo et al., 1997; Lin et al., 1997). Cardiogenesis proceeds by the formation of two concentrical tissue layers, an external myocardial and internal endocardial layer. To date it remains elusive how each cardiogenic lineage is distinctly established and whether they share a common progenitor (Linask & Lash, 1993; Eisenberg & Bader, 1995) or, on the contrary, they are distinctly derived from separate precursors (Cohen-Gould & Mikawa, 1996; Wei & Mikawa, 2000). As the myocardium is configured, it has been recently demonstrated that two distinct cell populations contribute to the developing heart; the first heart field (FHF) will contribute to the linear heart tube and subsequently will give rise mainly to the left ventricle (Kelly & Buckingham, 2002), whereas a second population of cells is subsequently recruited, namely the second heart field (SHF), contributing to the rest of the developing heart (Kelly et al., 2001; Cai et al., 2001; Waldo et al., 2001; Kelly & Buckingham, 2002). FHF derivatives express Nkx2.5 but are negative from islet-1, while SHF cells express both Nkx2.5 and islet-1. In addition, SHF derivates can be subdivided in two distinct regions, according to their entry site to the developing heart; a) anterior SHF leads to the formation of the right ventricle and outflow tract, and its contribution is governed by signaling emanating from Fgf8- and Fgf10-expressing cells (Watanabe et al. 2010), as well as contribution from Tbx1 signaling at the arterial/pharyngeal pole of the heart (Huynh et al., 2007; Liao et al., 2008), b) posterior SHF will contribute to the atrioventricular canal as well as right and left atria, and its contribution is directed by Fgf10 signaling at the venous pole of the heart (Kelly et al., 2001). In addition, complex regulatory networks are operative in the embryonic heart providing differentiation cues to the developing myocardium, as illustrated by the complex expression pattern of T-box genes, including therein Tbx2, Tbx3, Tbx5, Tbx18 and Tbx20 (Singh & Kispert, 2010; Greulich et al., 2011), Hand1 and Hand2 providing systemic *vs* pulmonary cues (Srivastava et al., 1995; Thomas et al., 1995) as well as left/right positional cues as illustrated by Pitx2 (Franco & Campione, 2003; Chinchilla et al., 2011). Thus, shared and distinct transcriptional pathways are governing first and second heart field deployment, leading in both cases to activation of a core cardiac transcriptional regulatory network as illustrated in **Figure 1**.

In addition, a third population of cells, with distinct gene expression hallmark as compared to first and second heart field cardiac precursors, has been demonstrated to form the inflow tract of the heart, suggesting the possible existence of a third heart field (Mommersteeg et al., 2010). Nkx2.5 /islet-1 negative cells, but positive for Tbx18, contribute to the formation of the caval veins (Mommersteeg et al., 2010). However, recent Cre-based lineage tracing experiments have challenged this notion, since all myocardial component of the venous pole, including the atrial appendages and the caval and pulmonary veins, have been reported to be derived from islet-1 and Nkx2-5 positive cells (Ma et al., 2008).

Concomitant with the deployment of the first and second heart field precursor cells, differentiation into distinct cardiomyocyte cell types is occurring, providing thus distinct working chamber and conduction system myocardium. Tbx2 and Tbx3 have been reported to play a fundamental role controlling gene expression pattern within the atrioventricular node (Bakker et al., 2008; Aanhaanen et al., 2009, 2011). Shox2, Tbx3 and Tbx18 have been demonstrated to play a crucial role on the sinoatrial node formation (Hoogaars et al., 2007; Wiese et al., 2009; Espinoza-Lewis et al. 2009). Furthermore, cardiomyocyte subtypes progressively emerge during cardiogenesis, such as distinct atrial and ventricular chamber myocardium, although the transcriptional regulation of such cell identities remains rather elusive. In chicken, Irx4 plays a crucial role in this step (Bao et al., 1999; Bruneau et al. 2000), however such function is not conserved in mice (Bruneau et al., 2001), which might be partially taken by Coup-tfII (Pereira et al., 1999; Wu et al., 2011). Similar events also are applicable for the cardiac conduction system, in which nodal and bundle branch fascicles are developed, each of them with distinct functional capabilities, yet their transcriptional regulation remains rather unexplored (Franco & Icardo, 2001; Miquerol et al. 2011).

In the adult heart, some of the developmental differences are progressively smoothened, in such a way that we can consider the adult heart being composed of two types of working myocardium (atrial and ventricular) and three distinct types of conductive cells (SAN and AVN node, His and bundle branches, and Purkinje fibers). Curiously, novel transmural differences emerge in the adult ventricular myocardium (Yan & Antzelevitch et al., 1996, 1999; de Castro et al., 2005), which are crucial for correct function of the heart (Constantini et al. 2005).

In its important to highlight that during cardiogenesis, the heart is progressively acquiring novel functional capabilities, which are reflected on the progressive onset of expression of contractile, conductive and cytoskeleton proteins. At the contractile level, sarcomeric genes such as myosins, actins and troponins, and cytoskeleton proteins as tropomyosin and actinins are differently expressed already at early stages of development (Lyons et al., 1990; Franco et al., 1998) providing functional heterogeneity to the developing myocardium, as

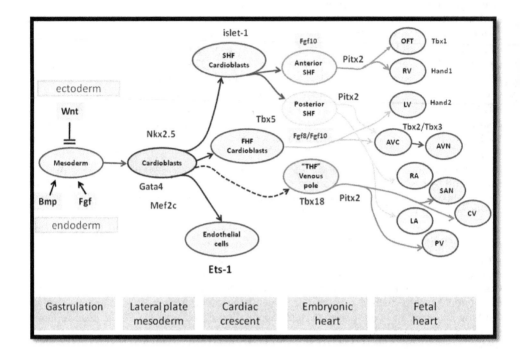

Fig. 1. **Schematic representation of embryonic cardiac development.** At gastrulation, nascent precardiac mesoderm listens to signal emanating from the surrounding ectodermal and endodermal tissues, committing the cells into the cardiogenic lineage, i.e. cardioblasts. Cardioblasts are characterized by the expression of core cardiac transcription factors, including Nkx2.5, Gata4 and Mef2c. Soon thereafter, cardiomyocyte and endothelial cell lineages emerged and within the cardiomyocyte lineage, two distinct populations of cells can be recognized, first heart field (FHF) and second heart field (SHF) cells. A third population of cells is originating soon thereafter, which lacks Nkx2.5 or islet-1 expression, yet, lineage tracing evidences using Cre/LoxP system suggested they have had a common ancestry (Cai et al., 2003; Zhou et al., 2008). FHF contributes mainly to the left ventricle and the atrioventricular canal (AVC). AVC will eventually be remodeled as septation proceeds, contributing therein to the formation of the atrioventricular node, which is characterized by Tbx2 and Tbx3 expression. Interestingly, SHF have two distinct components, an anterior SHF contributing to the outflow tract and right ventricle, listing to signal emanating from the pharyngeal arches domain, such as Fgf8 and Fgf10, and a posterior SHF leading to the right and left atrial chambers, listing to signals such as Fgf10. The "third" heart field contributes to the sinous venosus, forming therefore the caval veins and the sinoatrial node, and to the pulmonary myocardium which constitutes the atrial septa and the pulmonary veins (Franco et al., 2000). Importantly, almost all previously mentioned cardiac lineages listen to left/right signaling clues provided by the homeobox transcription factor Pitx2 (Campione et al., 1999; Franco & Campione, 2003).

detailed in **Table 1**. Similarly, ion channels and gap junctional proteins are progressively expressed in distinct regions of the developing heart (Gros & Jongsma, 1996; Franco et al. 2001; de Castro et al., 2005)(**Table 1**), providing the bases for the onset of a persitaltoid contraction in first instance and subsequently of synchronous contraction at late embryonic stage, displaying thus an apex-to-base pattern of activation. In essence, if we take thus as a reference our knowledge about cardiac development, it sounds reasonable that such information could be applicable to embryonic stem cells in order to obtain beating cardiomyocytes.

	OFT	RV	LV	AVC*	RA	SAN	LA	CV	PV
Transcription factors									
Mef2a									
Mef2b									
Mef2c									
Mef2d									
Hand1									
Hand2									
Tbx1									
Tbx2									
Tbx3									
Tbx5									
Tbx18									
Tbx20									
islet-1									
Pitx2									
Srf									
Nkx2.5									
Gata4									
Gata5									
Gata6									
Sarcommeric proteins									
α-cardiac actin									
skeletal actin									
sm-actin									
mlc1a									
mlc1v									
mlc2a									
mlc2v									
α-Mhc									
β-Mhc									
c troponin I									
sk troponin I									
c troponin T									
sk troponin T									
a-tropomyosin									
Ion channels									
Scn5a									
Scn1b									
Kcnq1									

	OFT	RV	LV	AVC*	RA	SAN	LA	CV	PV
Kcnh2									
Kcne1									
Kcne2									
Kcne3									
Kcne4									
Kcne5									
Kcnj2									
Kncj4									
Kcnj12									
Kv4.2									
Kv4.3									
KChiP2									
Hcn1									
Hcn2									
Hcn4									
Gap junctions									
Cx40									
Cx43									
Cx45									
Cx30.2									
Others									
Nppa									

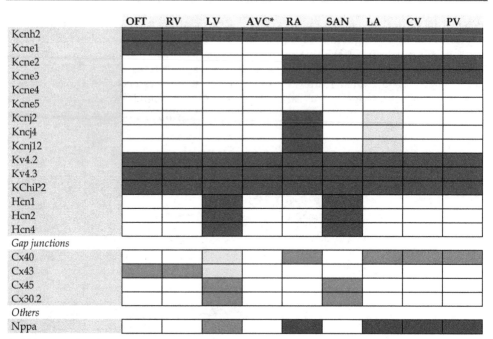

Table 1. Graphical respresentation of the expression profiles of cardiac-enriched transcription factors, sarcomeric proteins, ion channels and gap junctional proteins during embryonic heart development, in distinct regions of the embryonic/fetal heart. OFT, outflow tract; RV, right ventricle, LV, left ventricle, AVC, atrioventricular canal, RA, right atrium, LA, left atrium, SAN, sinoatrial node, CV, caval veins, PV, pulmonary veins. *AVC will lead in the adult heart to the atrioventricular node.

4. Understanding transcriptional control of *in vitro* cardiogenesis

The formation of beating cardiomyocytes from undifferentiated embryonic stem cell has been an important focus of scientific research, as it can be witnessed by the number of publication in this front. Several of the signaling pathways involved in *in vivo* cardiogenesis are also recapitulated *in vitro*, as depicted in **Figure 2**. Importantly, initial reports provided evidences that embryonic stem cell-derived cardiomyocytes display morphological, molecular and functional characteristics similar to adult cardiomyocytes, displaying therefore expression of sarcomeric and gap junctional proteins (Sachinidis et al., 2003; van Kempen et al., 2003; Fijnvandraaf et al., 2003ab). Additional experiments, demonstrated that most ion channels that are natively configure the cardiac action potential are also expressed during embryonic stem cell-derived cardiomyocytes (van Kempen et al., 2003). Furthermore, elegant spatio-temporal studies also nicely illustrate the progressive onset of the core transcriptional cardiac and ion channel expression during embryonic stem cell-derived cardiomyogenesis (Fijnvandraaf et al., 2003ab, van Kempen et al., 2003). However, several caveats were soon arising. Firstly, the fact that embryonic stem cell cultures, although capable of providing a source of cardiomyocytes, yield on average to a low percentage (<20%). Secondly, beating areas display distinct contraction rates, suggesting that large heterogeneity was observed from beating area to beating area, which might have gone unappreciated since most studies were done using RT-PCR methods. Thirdly, it was unclear if all cells within a beating area were equally differentiated. Sorting out these key questions is compulsory before any therapeutical strategy could be envisioned since a large number of cardiomyocytes is required, which will need to be morphologically homogeneous in order to avoid the chance of generating arrhythmias, and sufficiently and adequately differentiated in order to limit the oncogenic propagation of undifferentiated or poorly differentiated embryonic stem cells.

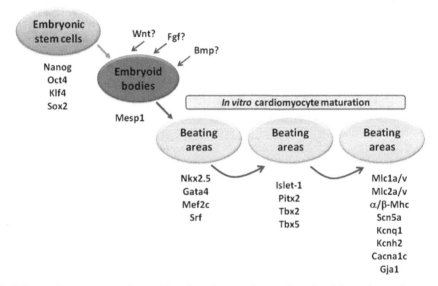

Fig. 2. **Schematic representation of the signaling pathways involved in embryonic stem cell–derived cardiogenesis.** Pluripotency makers such as Nanog, Oct4, Klf4 and Sox2 are expressed in undifferentiated embryonic stem cells. As soon as differentiation is initiated, these makers are down-regulated and mesoderm specification genes such as Mesp1 are expressed. Soon thereafter, as the beating areas are conformed, core cardiac transcriptional regulatory genes are up-regulated, and progressively the nascent cardiomyocytes acquire sacormeric and ion channel proteins, as depicted in **Table 2**.

First approaches to increase the efficiency of converting embryonic stem cells into cardiomycytes has been obtained by mimicking the inductive signals that naturally convert precardiogenic mesodermal cells into nascent cardioblasts (Hidai et al., 2003; Holtzinger et al., 2010). Bin et al. (2006) demonstrates that Bmp2 treatment of mouse embryonic stem cells increased the efficiency of obtaining beating areas, providing evidences that core transcriptional factor Nkx2.5 and structural proteins such as troponin-T and alpha-MHC were increased. Further evidences on the pivotal role of Bmp signaling in embryonic stem cell-derived cardiomyogenesis were reported by Rajasingh et al. (2007). More recently, Kim et al. (2008) provides similar evidences using human embryonic stem cells. However, other authors have reported that Bmp2 overexpression can also lead to induction of other mesodermal lineages such as smooth muscle cells (Blin et al., 2010) or condroblasts,

	OFT	RV	LV	AVC*	RA	SAN	LA	CV	PV
Transcription factors									
Mef2a									
Mef2b									
Mef2c									
Mef2d									
Hand1									
Hand2									
Tbx1									
Tbx2									
Tbx3									
Tbx5									
Tbx18									
Tbx20									
islet-1									
Pitx2	*	*	*	*					
Srf									
Nkx2.5									
Gata4									
Gata5									
Gata6									
Sarcommeric proteins									
α-cardiac actin									
skeletal actin									
sm-actin									
mlc1a									
mlc1v									
mlc2a									
mlc2v									
α-Mhc									
β-Mhc									
c troponin I									
slow troponin I									
fast troponin I									
c troponin T									
a-tropomyosin									
Ion channels									
Scn5a									
Scn1b									
Kcnq1									
Kcnh2									
Kcne1									
Kcne2									
Kcne3									
Kcnj2									
Kncj4									
Kcnj12									
Kv4.2									
Kv4.3									
KChiP2									

	OFT	RV	LV	AVC*	RA	SAN	LA	CV	PV
Hcn1									
Hcn2			■			■			
Hcn4									
Gap junctions								
Cx40									
Cx43									
Cx45									
Cx30.2									
Others								
Nppa									

Table 2. Graphical respresentation of the expression profiles of cardiac-enriched transcription factors, sarcomeric proteins, ion channels and gap junctional proteins during embryonic stem cell differentiation. ESC, embryonic stm cells, EB, embryoid bodies, BA2, beating areas at 2 days of culture, BA7, beating areas at 7 days of culture, EB14, beating areas at 14 days of cultures.

osteoblasts and adipoblasts, if cultures with supplementary co-factors (zur Nieden et al., 2005). Thus, these data suggest that combinatorial treatments might even further enhance embryonic stem cell-derived cardiomyogenesis. In this context, Evseenko et al. (2010) has elegantly evaluated the initial stages of mesoderm commitment during human embryonic stem cell differentiation, demonstrating the presence of endogenous cardiogenic morphogens such as activin A, Bmp4, Vegf and Fgf2. Laflamme et al. (2007) demonstrate that Bmp4 treatment increased *in vitro* cardiomyogenesis using human embryonic stem cells and Paige et al. (2010) has elegantly shown a balanced interplay between activin A/Bmp4 and Wnt/β-catenin is needed to efficiently induce mesodermal lineage formation and subsequent cardiomyocyte development in human embryonic stem cells. Similar findings are also observed using mouse embryonic stem cells (Taha et al., 2006, 2007; Taha & Valojerdi, 2008; Takei et al., 2009; Verma & Lenka, 2010). In addition to the role of Bmp signaling, several studies have reported the pivotal role of Fgf signaling controlling mouse embryonic stem cell-derived cardiomyogenesis (Dell'Era et al., 2003; Ronca et al. 2009). Importantly, Fgf signaling, in conjunction with Bmp signaling enhances cardiomyocyte formation of other stem cell sources, such as bone marrow stem cells (Degeorge et al., 2008) or P19 carcinoma cell line (Hidai et al., 2003), reinforcing the notion that Fgf signaling is necessary (embryonic stem cells) and sufficient (other sources) to induce cardiomyocyte development. Curiously, novel signaling pathways, such as Sdf-1/Cxcr4 (Chiriac et al., 2010) and Vegf (Chen et al., 2006) also play a determinant role in cardiogenesis, although their links to Bmp, Fgf and Wnt signaling remains unexplored.

Understanding of the embryonic stem cell-derived cardiomyogenesis has also been largely unraveled by manipulation of several cardiac enriched transcription factors. Gata4 and Gata6 deficient mice suggested a pivotal role of this transcription factor in early cardiogenesis (Kuo et al., 1997; Xin et al., 2006). Gata4 deficient embryonic stem cells have been reported to disrupt visceral endoderm formation and thus hematopoiesis (Soudais et al., 1995; Bielinska et al., 1996, 1997; Morrisey et al., 2000; Pierre et al., 2009). Similar findings are also observed in Gata6 deficient embryonic stem cells (Pierre et al., 2009). Importantly, cardiomyogenesis is not affected in Gata4 deficient embryonic stem cells (Narita et al., 1997) but over-expression of Gata4 in embryonic stem cells enhances cardiogenesis (Grepin et al.,

1997) and visceral endoderm (Holtzinger et al. 2009) suggesting that Gata4 is not necessary but is sufficient to induce cardiomyocyte differentiation. Nkx2.5 deficient mice display cardiac embryonic lethality (Lyons et al., 1995), supporting a pivotal role for Nkx2.5 in cardiomyogenesis. In this context, over-expression of Nkx2.5 in embryonic stem cells increases the expression of cardiogenic markers at the expenses of hematopoietic markers such as Gata-1 (Caprioli et al., 2011). Similarly, enhanced expression of Mef2c in embryonic stem cells increases cardiomyogenic differentiation (Puceat et al., 2003), in line with its determinant role during heart development as demonstrated by genetic deletion in mice (Lin et al., 1997). Comparable over-expression approaches in embryonic stem cells have been described for the homeobox transcription factor Pitx2, a left-right signaling pathway determinant (Campione et al., 1999, 2002). Enhanced expression of Pitx2 leads to increased expression of cardiac markers (Lozano-Velasco et al., 2011) supporting a role of this transcription factor in cardiogenesis. In addition, overexpression of Tbx5, a pivotal transcription factor associated with Holt-Oram syndrome (Li et al., 1997), in P19 embryonic carcinoma cells (Fijnvandraat et al., 2003abc) display similar findings. Overall, these studies illustrate the pivotal role of distinct transcription factors with reported enhanced expression during cardiogenesis, as well as it also provides the entry to previously unknown transcription factors as key elements for cardiomyogenic lineage differentiation, as it is the case for the transcription factors hhLIM (Zheng et al., 2006) and Rb (Papadimou et al., 2005) or the GTPase Rac1 (Puceat et al., 2003).

Importantly, although these reports provided evidence of enhancing cardiomyocte formation by the usage of discrete growth factors and/or transcription factors, and subsequently identifying cardiac specific molecular markers such as Nkx2.5, Gata4 and sarcomeric proteins (i.e troponin T and alpha-actinin), it remains elusive if cardiomyocyte heterogeneity in terms of lineage origin (FHF, SHF), gene expression (atrial/ventricular/nodal) or function (working/conductive) is observed. We have recently reported that mouse embryonic stem cell-derived cardiomyocytes display a dynamic temporal expression of FHF and SHF makers which are reminiscent of the *in vivo* cell lineage deployment (Lozano-Velasco et al. 2011). In addition, large heterogeneity in gene expression, displaying distinct atrial-, ventricular- and nodal-like patterns (Fijnvandraat et al. 2002, 2003abc) and functional heterogeneity (van Kempen et al., 2003) displaying distinct cardiac action potential configurations, have been extensively reported. In this context, is it important to highlight that overexpression of Pitx2 mainly directs the expression of SHF cardiomyocytes, since both islet-1 and Mef2c were up-regulated, whereas FHF marker Nkx2.5 was unaltered (Lozano-Velasco et al., 2011). Furthermore overexpression of Pitx2 enhances Tbx5 expression and thus Nppa (Anf) and Gja5 (Cx40)(Lozano-Velasco et al., 2011), in line with previous Tbx5 over-expression findings (Fijnvandraaf et al., 2003). Thus, it is plausible that enhance cardiomyocyte commitment by distinct inductive signals might generate cellular heterogeneity in a similar fashion as in the developing heart. If so, these observations might hindrance their therapeutical usage since, for example, engrafting nodal-like cells in the ventricular chambers might lead to ectopic electrical foci and thus to arrhythmias. In this context, searching for transcriptional factor cocktail which might homogenize the cardiomyocyte outcome is a plausible strategy, as recently reported to convert induced pluripotent fibroblasts into cardiomyocytes (Ieda et al. 2010) or hepatocytes (Huang et al., 2011).

Differentiation of embryonic stem cells into beating cardiomyocytes can therefore be naively observed by simply developing embryoid bodies or enhanced by supplementing these embryonic stem cells and/or embryoid bodies with a subset of growth factors and/or transcription factors. **Table 2** summarizes the current state of the art knowledge about the dynamic expression of distinct transcription factors, sarcommeric proteins, ion channels and gap junctions during embryonic stem cell-derived cardiomyogenesis. However, the question arising is: are all beating areas differentiated into cardiomyocytes or are there remaining non-differentiated embryonic stem cells or contaminating cells that might differentiate into other embryonic lineages? This is a crucial question if we aim to use them *in vivo*. We have recently reported that fine-dissection of beating areas have minor contamination of endodermal- or ectodermal cells (Lozano-Velasco et al., 2011) at distinct developmental stages. Thus, it seems that a rather homogeneously differentiated cluster of cells is normally achieved. It remains to be elucidated if undifferentiated embryonic stem cells remain in those areas. *In vivo* approaches suggest that indeed this might be the case, yet titering the number of engrafted cells results in absence of teratomas at the long run (Behfar et al., 2005, 2007; Yamada et al. 2009).

5. Conclusions and perspectives

Over the last decade we have started to understand the molecular mechanisms that govern cardiac formation and we are translating these findings to the manipulation of embryonic stem cells opening promising avenues to enhance cardiomyocyte differentiation. We have learnt how to increase the number of cardiomyocyte produced, and we have learnt that embryonic development is faithfully recapitulated *in vitro*, including the onset of first and second heart field transcriptional programs. Manipulation of these transcriptional machinaries will be therefore the upcoming challenges for the next years to come in order to facilitate the generation of fully differentiated, structurally similar and functionally homogeneous cardiomyocytes. Searching for transcription factor cocktails or opening new strategies such as those emerging from the microRNA world (Ivey et al. 2008; Chinchilla et al., 2011) constitutes the next goals, as recently illustrated for miR-499 (Wilson et al., 2010). Thus, in summary, an important part of the route has been walked, and the way ahead seems promising with the reward of achieving therapeutically usable embryonic stem cell-derived cardiomyocytes.

6. Acknowledgments

We thank Jorge N. Dominguez for critical reading the manuscript. This work is supported by VI EU grant Heart Failure and Cardiac Repair (LSHM-2005-CT-018630) to DF, grants from the Ministry of Science and Innovation of the Spanish Government to DF (MICINN 2009-11566) and AA (MICINNN 2008-01217) and grants from the Junta de Andalucia Regional Council to DF (CTS-1614, CVI-06556) and AA (CTS-03878, CTS-446).

7. References

Aanhaanen WT, Boukens BJ, Sizarov A, Wakker V, de Gier-de Vries C, van Ginneken AC, Moorman AF, Coronel R, Christoffels VM. Defective Tbx2-dependent patterning of the atrioventricular canal myocardium causes accessory pathway formation in mice. J Clin Invest. 2011; 121(2):534-44.

Aanhaanen WT, Brons JF, Domínguez JN, Rana MS, Norden J, Airik R, Wakker V, de Gier-de Vries C, Brown NA, Kispert A, Moorman AF, Christoffels VM. The Tbx2+

primary myocardium of the atrioventricular canal forms the atrioventricular node and the base of the left ventricle. Circ Res. 2009; 104(11):1267-74.

Bakker ML, Boukens BJ, Mommersteeg MT, Brons JF, Wakker V, Moorman AF, Christoffels VM. Transcription factor Tbx3 is required for the specification of the atrioventricular conduction system. Circ Res. 2008; 102(11):1340-9.

Bao ZZ, Bruneau BG, Seidman JG, Seidman CE, Cepko CL. Regulation of chamber-specific gene expression in the developing heart by Irx4. Science. 1999; 283(5405):1161-4.

Barron M, Gao M, Lough J. Requirement for BMP and FGF signaling during cardiogenic induction in non-precardiac mesoderm is specific, transient, and cooperative. Dev Dyn. 2000; 218:383-393.

Behfar A, Hodgson DM, Zingman LV, Perez-Terzic C, Yamada S, Kane GC, Alekseev AE, Pucéat M, Terzic A. Administration of allogenic stem cells dosed to secure cardiogenesis and sustained infarct repair. Ann N Y Acad Sci. 2005; 1049:189-98.

Behfar A, Perez-Terzic C, Faustino RS, Arrell DK, Hodgson DM, Yamada S, Puceat M, Niederländer N, Alekseev AE, Zingman LV, Terzic A. Cardiopoietic programming of embryonic stem cells for tumor-free heart repair. J Exp Med. 2007; 204(2):405-20. Epub 2007 Feb 5.

Bielinska M, Narita N, Heikinheimo M, Porter SB, Wilson DB. Erythropoiesis and vasculogenesis in embryoid bodies lacking visceral yolk sac endoderm. Blood. 1996; 88(10):3720-30.

Bielinska M, Wilson DB. Induction of yolk sac endoderm in GATA-4-deficient embryoid bodies by retinoic acid. Mech Dev. 1997; 65(1-2):43-54.

Bin Z, Sheng LG, Gang ZC, Hong J, Jun C, Bo Y, Hui S. Efficient cardiomyocyte differentiation of embryonic stem cells by bone morphogenetic protein-2 combined with visceral endoderm-like cells. Cell Biol Int. 2006; 30(10):769-76.

Blin G, Nury D, Stefanovic S, Neri T, Guillevic O, Brinon B, Bellamy V, Rücker-Martin C, Barbry P, Bel A, Bruneval P, Cowan C, Pouly J, Mitalipov S, Gouadon E, Binder P, Hagège A, Desnos M, Renaud JF, Menasché P, Pucéat M. A purified population of multipotent cardiovascular progenitors derived from primate pluripotent stem cells engrafts in postmyocardial infarcted nonhuman primates. J Clin Invest. 2010; 120(4):1125-39.

Boheler KR, Czyz J, Tweedie D, Yang HT, Anisimov SV, Wobus AM. Differentiation of pluripotent embryonic stem cells into cardiomyocytes. Circ Res. 2002; 91(3):189-201.

Bruneau BG, Bao ZZ, Fatkin D, Xavier-Neto J, Georgakopoulos D, Maguire CT, Berul CI, Kass DA, Kuroski-de Bold ML, de Bold AJ, Conner DA, Rosenthal N, Cepko CL, Seidman CE, Seidman JG. Cardiomyopathy in Irx4-deficient mice is preceded by abnormal ventricular gene expression. Mol Cell Biol. 2001; 21(5):1730-6.

Bruneau BG, Bao ZZ, Tanaka M, Schott JJ, Izumo S, Cepko CL, Seidman JG, Seidman CE. Cardiac expression of the ventricle-specific homeobox gene Irx4 is modulated by Nkx2-5 and dHand. Dev Biol. 2000; 217(2):266-77.

Cai CL, Liang X, Shi Y, Chu PH, Pfaff SL, Chen J, Evans S. Isl1 identifies a cardiac progenitor population that proliferates prior to differentiation and contributes a majority of cells to the heart. Dev Cell. 2003; 5(6):877-89

Campione M, Acosta L, Martínez S, Icardo JM, Aránega A, Franco D. Pitx2 and cardiac development: a molecular link between left/right signaling and congenital heart disease. Cold Spring Harb Symp Quant Biol. 2002; 67:89-95.

Campione M, Steinbeisser H, Schweickert A, Deissler K, van Bebber F, Lowe LA, Nowotschin S, Viebahn C, Haffter P, Kuehn MR, Blum M. The homeobox gene Pitx2: mediator of asymmetric left-right signaling in vertebrate heart and gut looping. Development. 1999; 126(6):1225-34.

Caprioli A, Koyano-Nakagawa N, Iacovino M, Shi X, Ferdous A, Harvey RP, Olson EN, Kyba M, Garry DJ. Nkx2-5 represses gata1 gene expression and modulates the cellular fate of cardiac progenitors during embryogenesis. Circulation. 2011; 123(15):1633-41.

Chen Y, Amende I, Hampton TG, Yang Y, Ke Q, Min JY, Xiao YF, Morgan JP. Vascular endothelial growth factor promotes cardiomyocyte differentiation of embryonic stem cells. Am J Physiol Heart Circ Physiol. 2006; 291(4):H1653-8.

Chinchilla A, Daimi H, Lozano-Velasco E, Dominguez JN, Caballero R, Delpón E, Tamargo J, Cinca J, Hove-Madsen L, Aranega AE, Franco D. PITX2 Insufficiency Leads to Atrial Electrical and Structural Remodeling Linked to Arrhythmogenesis. Circ Cardiovasc Genet. 2011 Apr 21. [Epub ahead of print]

Chinchilla A, Franco D. Regulatory mechanisms of cardiac development and repair. Cardiovasc Hematol Disord Drug Targets. 2006; 6(2):101-12.

Chinchilla A, Lozano E, Daimi H, Esteban FJ, Crist C, Aranega AE, Franco D. MicroRNA profiling during mouse ventricular maturation: a role for miR-27 modulating Mef2c expression. Cardiovasc Res. 2011; 89(1):98-108.

Chiriac A, Terzic A, Park S, Ikeda Y, Faustino R, Nelson TJ. SDF-1-enhanced cardiogenesis requires CXCR4 induction in pluripotent stem cells. J Cardiovasc Transl Res. 2010; 3(6):674-82.

Cohen-Gould L, Mikawa T. The fate diversity of mesodermal cells within the heart field during chicken early embryogenesis. Dev Biol. 1996; 177(1):265-73.

Costantini DL, Arruda EP, Agarwal P, Kim KH, Zhu Y, Zhu W, Lebel M, Cheng CW, Park CY, Pierce SA, Guerchicoff A, Pollevick GD, Chan TY, Kabir MG, Cheng SH, Husain M, Antzelevitch C, Srivastava D, Gross GJ, Hui CC, Backx PH, Bruneau BG. The homeodomain transcription factor Irx5 establishes the mouse cardiac ventricular repolarization gradient. Cell. 2005; 123(2):347-58.

de Castro MP, Acosta L, Domínguez JN, Aránega A, Franco D. Molecular diversity of the developing and adult myocardium: implications for tissue targeting. Curr Drug Targets Cardiovasc Haematol Disord. 2003; 3(3):227-39.

Degeorge BR Jr, Rosenberg M, Eckstein V, Gao E, Herzog N, Katus HA, Koch WJ, Frey N, Most P. BMP-2 and FGF-2 synergistically facilitate adoption of a cardiac phenotype in somatic bone marrow c-kit+/Sca-1+ stem cells. Clin Transl Sci. 2008; 1(2):116-25.

Dell'Era P, Ronca R, Coco L, Nicoli S, Metra M, Presta M. Fibroblast growth factor receptor-1 is essential for in vitro cardiomyocyte development. Circ Res. 2003; 93(5):414-20.

Doetschman TC, Eistetter H, Katz M, Schmidt W, Kemler R. The in vitro development of blastocyst-derived embryonic stem cell lines: formation of visceral yolk sac, blood islands and myocardium. J Embryol Exp Morphol. 1985; 87:27-45.

Eisenberg, C. A., and Bader, D. QCE-6: A clonal cell line with cardiac myogenic and endothelial cell potentials. Dev. Biol. 1995; 167:469– 481.

Espinoza-Lewis RA, Yu L, He F, Liu H, Tang R, Shi J, Sun X, Martin JF, Wang D, Yang J, Chen Y. Shox2 is essential for the differentiation of cardiac pacemaker cells by repressing Nkx2-5. Dev Biol. 2009; 327(2):376-85.

Evseenko D, Zhu Y, Schenke-Layland K, Kuo J, Latour B, Ge S, Scholes J, Dravid G, Li X, MacLellan WR, Crooks GM. Mapping the first stages of mesoderm commitment during differentiation of human embryonic stem cells. Proc Natl Acad Sci U S A. 2010; 107(31):13742-7.

Fijnvandraat AC, De Boer PA, Deprez RH, Moorman AF. Non-radioactive in situ detection of mRNA in ES cell-derived cardiomyocytes and in the developing heart. Microsc Res Tech. 2002; 58(5):387-94.

Fijnvandraat AC, Lekanne Deprez RH, Christoffels VM, Ruijter JM, Moorman AF. TBX5 overexpression stimulates differentiation of chamber myocardium in P19C16 embryonic carcinoma cells. J Muscle Res Cell Motil. 2003; 24(2-3):211-8.

Fijnvandraat AC, Lekanne Deprez RH, Moorman AF. Development of heart muscle-cell diversity: a help or a hindrance for phenotyping embryonic stem cell-derived cardiomyocytes. Cardiovasc Res. 2003; 58(2):303-12.

Fijnvandraat AC, van Ginneken AC, de Boer PA, Ruijter JM, Christoffels VM, Moorman AF, Lekanne Deprez RH. Cardiomyocytes derived from embryonic stem cells resemble cardiomyocytes of the embryonic heart tube. Cardiovasc Res. 2003; 58(2):399-409.

Fijnvandraat AC, van Ginneken AC, Schumacher CA, Boheler KR, Lekanne Deprez RH, Christoffels VM, Moorman AF. Cardiomyocytes purified from differentiated embryonic stem cells exhibit characteristics of early chamber myocardium. J Mol Cell Cardiol. 2003; 35(12):1461-72.

Franco D, Campione M, Kelly R, Zammit PS, Buckingham M, Lamers WH, Moorman AF. Multiple transcriptional domains, with distinct left and right components, in the atrial chambers of the developing heart. Circ Res. 2000; 87(11):984-91.

Franco D, Campione M. The role of Pitx2 during cardiac development. Linking left-right signaling and congenital heart diseases. Trends Cardiovasc Med. 2003; 13(4):157-63.

Franco D, Demolombe S, Kupershmidt S, Dumaine R, Dominguez JN, Roden D, Antzelevitch C, Escande D, Moorman AF. Divergent expression of delayed rectifier K(+) channel subunits during mouse heart development. Cardiovasc Res. 2001; 52(1):65-75.

Franco D, Icardo JM. Molecular characterization of the ventricular conduction system in the developing mouse heart: topographical correlation in normal and congenitally malformed hearts. Cardiovasc Res. 2001; 49(2):417-29.

Franco D, Lamers WH, Moorman AF. Patterns of expression in the developing myocardium: towards a morphologically integrated transcriptional model. Cardiovasc Res. 1998; 38(1):25-53.

Franco D, Moreno N, Ruiz-Lozano P. Non-resident stem cell populations in regenerative cardiac medicine. Cell Mol Life Sci. 2007; 64(6):683-91.

Grépin C, Nemer G, Nemer M. Enhanced cardiogenesis in embryonic stem cells overexpressing the GATA-4 transcription factor. Development. 1997; 124(12):2387-95.

Greulich F, Rudat C, Kispert A. Mechanisms of T-box gene function in the developing heart. Cardiovasc Res. 2011 Apr 14. [Epub ahead of print]

Gros DB, Jongsma HJ. Connexins in mammalian heart function. Bioessays. 1996; 18(9):719-30.

Hidai C, Masako O, Ikeda H, Nagashima H, Matsuoka R, Quertermous T, Kasanuki H, Kokubun S, Kawana M. FGF-1 enhanced cardiogenesis in differentiating embryonal carcinoma cell cultures, which was opposite to the effect of FGF-2. J Mol Cell Cardiol. 2003; 35(4):421-5.

Holtzinger A, Rosenfeld GE, Evans T. Gata4 directs development of cardiac-inducing endoderm from ES cells. Dev Biol. 2010; 337(1):63-73.

Hoogaars WM, Engel A, Brons JF, Verkerk AO, de Lange FJ, Wong LY, Bakker ML, Clout DE, Wakker V, Barnett P, Ravesloot JH, Moorman AF, Verheijck EE,Christoffels VM. Tbx3 controls the sinoatrial node gene program and imposes pacemaker function on the atria. Genes Dev. 2007; 21(9):1098-112.

Huang P, He Z, Ji S, Sun H, Xiang D, Liu C, Hu Y, Wang X, Hui L. Induction of functional hepatocyte-like cells from mouse fibroblasts by defined factors.Nature. 2011 May 11. [Epub ahead of print]

Huynh T, Chen L, Terrell P, Baldini A. A fate map of Tbx1 expressing cells reveals heterogeneity in the second cardiac field. Genesis. 2007; 45(7):470-5.

Ieda M, Fu JD, Delgado-Olguin P, Vedantham V, Hayashi Y, Bruneau BG, Srivastava D. Direct reprogramming of fibroblasts into functional cardiomyocytes by defined factors. Cell. 2010; 142(3):375-86.

Ivey KN, Muth A, Arnold J, King FW, Yeh RF, Fish JE, Hsiao EC, Schwartz RJ, Conklin BR, Bernstein HS, Srivastava D. MicroRNA regulation of cell lineages in mouse and human embryonic stem cells. Cell Stem Cell. 2008; 2(3):219-29.

Kelly RG, Brown NA, Buckingham ME. The arterial pole of the mouse heart forms from Fgf10-expressing cells in pharyngeal mesoderm. Dev Cell. 2001; 1(3):435-40.

Kelly RG, Buckingham ME. The anterior heart-forming field: voyage to the arterial pole of the heart. Trends Genet. 2002; 18(4):210-6.

Kim YY, Ku SY, Jang J, Oh SK, Kim HS, Kim SH, Choi YM, Moon SY. Use of long-term cultured embryoid bodies may enhance cardiomyocyte differentiation by BMP2. Yonsei Med J. 2008; 49(5):819-27.

Kuo CT, Morrisey EE, Anandappa R, Sigrist K, Lu MM, Parmacek MS, Soudais C, Leiden JM. GATA4 transcription factor is required for ventral morphogenesis and heart tube formation. Genes Dev. 1997; 11(8):1048-60.

Laflamme MA, Chen KY, Naumova AV, Muskheli V, Fugate JA, Dupras SK, Reinecke H, Xu C, Hassanipour M, Police S, O'Sullivan C, Collins L, Chen Y, Minami E, Gill EA, Ueno S, Yuan C, Gold J, Murry CE. Cardiomyocytes derived from human embryonic stem cells in pro-survival factors enhance function of infarcted rat hearts. Nat Biotechnol. 2007; 25(9):1015-24.

Lanza R, Gearhart J, hogan B, Melton D, Pedersen R, Thomson J, West M. Handbook of Stem Cells. 2004. Elsevier Academic Press, Burlington, MA, USA.

Li QY, Newbury-Ecob RA, Terrett JA, Wilson DI, Curtis AR, Yi CH, Gebuhr T, Bullen PJ, Robson SC, Strachan T, Bonnet D, Lyonnet S, Young ID, Raeburn JA, Buckler AJ, Law DJ, Brook JD. Holt-Oram syndrome is caused by mutations in TBX5, a member of the Brachyury (T) gene family. Nat Genet. 1997; 15(1):21-9.

Liao J, Aggarwal VS, Nowotschin S, Bondarev A, Lipner S, Morrow BE. Identification of downstream genetic pathways of Tbx1 in the second heart field. Dev Biol. 2008 15; 316(2):524-37.

Lin Q, Schwarz J, Bucana C, Olson EN. Control of mouse cardiac morphogenesis and myogenesis by transcription factor MEF2C. Science. 1997; 276:1404-1407.

Linask KK, Lash JW. Early heart development: Dynamics of endocardial cell sorting suggests a common origin with cardiomyocytes. Dev Dyn. 1993;195: 62-69.

Lopez-Sanchez C, Climent V, Schoenwolf GC, Alvarez IS, Garcia-Martinez V. Induction of cardiogenesis by Hensen's node and fibroblast growth factors. Cell Tissue Res. 2002; 309:237-249.

Lozano-Velasco E, Chinchilla A, Martínez-Fernández S, Hernández-Torres F, Navarro F, Lyons GE, Franco D, Aránega AE. Pitx2c Modulates Cardiac-Specific Transcription Factors Networks in Differentiating Cardiomyocytes from Murine Embryonic Stem Cells. Cells Tissues Organs. 2011 Mar 9. [Epub ahead of print]

Lyons GE, Schiaffino S, Sassoon D, Barton P, Buckingham M. Developmental regulation of myosin gene expression in mouse cardiac muscle. J Cell Biol. 1990; 111(6 Pt 1):2427-36.

Lyons I, Parsons LM, Hartley L, Li R, Andrews JE, Robb L, et al. Myogenic and morphogenetic defects in the heart tubes of murine embryos lacking the homeo box gene Nkx2-5. Genes Dev. 1995;9:1654-1666.

Ma Q, Zhou B, Pu WT. Reassessment of Isl1 and Nkx2-5 cardiac fate maps using a Gata4-based reporter of Cre activity. Dev Biol. 2008; 323(1):98-104.

Marques SR, Lee Y, Poss KD, Yelon D. Reiterative roles for FGF signaling in the establishment of size and proportion of the zebrafish heart. Dev Biol. 2008; 321:397-406.

Martínez-Estrada OM, Lettice LA, Essafi A, Guadix JA, Slight J, Velecela V, et al. Wt1 is required for cardiovascular progenitor cell formation through transcriptional control of Snail and E-cadherin. Nat Genet. 2010; 42:89-93.

Miller-Hance WC, LaCorbiere M, Fuller SJ, Evans SM, Lyons G, Schmidt C, Robbins J, Chien KR. In vitro chamber specification during embryonic stem cell cardiogenesis. Expression of the ventricular myosin light chain-2 gene is independent of heart tube formation. J Biol Chem. 1993;268(33):25244-52.

Miquerol L, Moreno-Rascon N, Beyer S, Dupays L, Meilhac SM, Buckingham ME, Franco D, Kelly RG. Biphasic development of the mammalian ventricular conduction system. Circ Res. 2010; 107(1):153-61.

Mommersteeg MT, Domínguez JN, Wiese C, Norden J, de Gier-de Vries C, Burch JB, Kispert A, Brown NA, Moorman AF, Christoffels VM. The sinus venosus progenitors separate and diversify from the first and second heart fields early in development. Cardiovasc Res. 2010; 87(1):92-101.

Morrisey EE, Musco S, Chen MY, Lu MM, Leiden JM, Parmacek MS. The gene encoding the mitogen-responsive phosphoprotein Dab2 is differentially regulated by GATA-6 and GATA-4 in the visceral endoderm. J Biol Chem. 2000; 275(26):19949-54.

Narita N, Bielinska M, Wilson DB. Cardiomyocyte differentiation by GATA-4-deficient embryonic stem cells. Development. 1997; 124(19):3755-64.

Paige SL, Osugi T, Afanasiev OK, Pabon L, Reinecke H, Murry CE. Endogenous Wnt/beta-catenin signaling is required for cardiac differentiation in human embryonic stem cells. PLoS One. 2010; 5(6):e11134.

Papadimou E, Ménard C, Grey C, Pucéat M. Interplay between the retinoblastoma protein and LEK1 specifies stem cells toward the cardiac lineage. EMBO J. 2005; 24(9):1750-61.

Pereira FA, Qiu Y, Zhou G, Tsai MJ, Tsai SY. The orphan nuclear receptor COUP-TFII is required for angiogenesis and heart development. Genes Dev. 1999; 13(8):1037-49.

Pérez-Pomares JM, Phelps A, Sedmerova M, Carmona R, González-Iriarte M, Muñoz-Chápuli R, et al. Experimental studies on the spatiotemporal expression of WT1 and

RALDH2 in the embryonic avian heart: a model for the regulation of myocardial and valvuloseptal development by epicardially derived cells (EPDCs). Dev Biol. 2002; 247:307-326.

Pierre M, Yoshimoto M, Huang L, Richardson M, Yoder MC. VEGF and IHH rescue definitive hematopoiesis in Gata-4 and Gata-6-deficient murine embryoid bodies. Exp Hematol. 2009; 37(9):1038-53.

Pucéat M, Travo P, Quinn MT, Fort P. A dual role of the GTPase Rac in cardiac differentiation of stem cells. Mol Biol Cell. 2003; 14(7):2781-92.

Rajasingh J, Bord E, Hamada H, Lambers E, Qin G, Losordo DW, Kishore R. STAT3-dependent mouse embryonic stem cell differentiation into cardiomyocytes: analysis of molecular signaling and therapeutic efficacy of cardiomyocyte precommitted mES transplantation in a mouse model of myocardial infarction. Circ Res. 2007; 101(9):910-8.

Ronca R, Gualandi L, Crescini E, Calza S, Presta M, Dell'Era P. Fibroblast growth factor receptor-1 phosphorylation requirement for cardiomyocyte differentiation in murine embryonic stem cells. J Cell Mol Med. 2009; 13(8A):1489-98.

Singh R, Kispert A. Tbx20, Smads, and the atrioventricular canal. Trends Cardiovasc Med. 2010; 20(4):109-14.

Soudais C, Bielinska M, Heikinheimo M, MacArthur CA, Narita N, Saffitz JE, Simon MC, Leiden JM, Wilson DB. Targeted mutagenesis of the transcription factor GATA-4 gene in mouse embryonic stem cells disrupts visceral endoderm differentiation in vitro. Development. 1995; 121(11):3877-88.

Srivastava D, Cserjesi P, Olson EN. A subclass of bHLH proteins required for cardiac morphogenesis. Science. 1995; 270:1995-1999.

Taha MF, Valojerdi MR, Mowla SJ. Effect of bone morphogenetic protein-4 (BMP-4) on cardiomyocyte differentiation from mouse embryonic stem cell. Int J Cardiol. 2007 9; 120(1):92-101.

Taha MF, Valojerdi MR, Mowla SJ. Effect of bone morphogenetic protein-4 (BMP-4) on adipocyte differentiation from mouse embryonic stem cells. Anat Histol Embryol. 2006; 35(4):271-8.

Taha MF, Valojerdi MR. Effect of bone morphogenetic protein-4 on cardiac differentiation from mouse embryonic stem cells in serum-free and low-serum media. Int J Cardiol. 2008;127(1):78-87.

Takei S, Ichikawa H, Johkura K, Mogi A, No H, Yoshie S, Tomotsune D, Sasaki K. Bone morphogenetic protein-4 promotes induction of cardiomyocytes from human embryonic stem cells in serum-based embryoid body development. Am J Physiol Heart Circ Physiol. 2009; 296(6):H1793-803.

Thomas T, Yamagishi H, Overbeek PA, Olson EN, Srivastava D. The bHLH factors, dHAND and eHAND, specify pulmonary and systemic cardiac ventricles independent of left-right sidedness. Dev Biol. 1998 Apr 15; 196(2):228-36.

van Kempen M, van Ginneken A, de Grijs I, Mutsaers N, Opthof T, Jongsma H, van der Heyden M. Expression of the electrophysiological system during murine embryonic stem cell cardiac differentiation. Cell Physiol Biochem. 2003; 13(5):263-70.

Verma MK, Lenka N. Temporal and contextual orchestration of cardiac fate by WNT-BMP synergy and threshold. J Cell Mol Med. 2010; 14(8):2094-108.

Waldo KL, Kumiski DH, Wallis KT, Stadt HA, Hutson MR, Platt DH, Kirby ML. Conotruncal myocardium arises from a secondary heart field. Development. 2001; 128(16):3179-88.

Watanabe Y, Miyagawa-Tomita S, Vincent SD, Kelly RG, Moon AM, Buckingham ME. Role of mesodermal FGF8 and FGF10 overlaps in the development of the arterial pole of the heart and pharyngeal arch arteries. Circ Res. 2010; 106(3):495-503.

Wei Y, Mikawa T. Fate diversity of primitive streak cells during heart field formation in ovo. Dev Dyn. 2000; 219(4):505-13.

Wiese C, Grieskamp T, Airik R, Mommersteeg MT, Gardiwal A, de Gier-de Vries C, Schuster-Gossler K, Moorman AF, Kispert A, Christoffels VM. Formation of the sinus node head and differentiation of sinus node myocardium are independently regulated by Tbx18 and Tbx3. Circ Res. 2009; 104(3):388-97.

Wilson KD, Hu S, Venkatasubrahmanyam S, Fu JD, Sun N, Abilez OJ, Baugh JJ, Jia F, Ghosh Z, Li RA, Butte AJ, Wu JC. Dynamic microRNA expression programs during cardiac differentiation of human embryonic stem cells: role for miR-499. Circ Cardiovasc Genet. 2010; 3(5):426-35.

Wobus AM, Boheler KR. Embryonic Stem Cells as Developmental Model in vitro. Preface. Cells Tissues Organs. 1999; 165(3-4):129-30.

Wu Sp, Ather S, Wehrens XL, Tsai MJ, Tsai SY. Regulation of atrial chamber identity bu COUP-TFII. Weinstein Cardiovascular Conference 2011 Cincinnati, Abstract book S3.2

Xin M, Davis CA, Molkentin JD, Lien CL, Duncan SA, Richardson JA, Olson EN. A threshold of GATA4 and GATA6 expression is required for cardiovascular development. Proc Natl Acad Sci U S A. 2006; 103(30):11189-94.

Yamada S, Nelson TJ, Crespo-Diaz RJ, Perez-Terzic C, Liu XK, Miki T, Seino S, Behfar A, Terzic A. Embryonic stem cell therapy of heart failure in genetic cardiomyopathy. Stem Cells. 2008; 26(10):2644-53.

Yan GX, Antzelevitch C. Cellular basis for the Brugada syndrome and other mechanisms of arrhythmogenesis associated with ST-segment elevation. Circulation. 1999; 100(15):1660-6.

Yan GX, Antzelevitch C. Cellular basis for the electrocardiographic J wave. Circulation. 1996; 93(2):372-9.

Zheng B, Wen JK, Han M. hhLIM is involved in cardiomyogenesis of embryonic stem cells. Biochemistry (Mosc). 2006;71 Suppl 1:S71-6, 6.

Zhou B, von Gise A, Ma Q, Rivera-Feliciano J, Pu WT. Nkx2-5- and Isl1-expressing cardiac progenitors contribute to proepicardium. Biochem Biophys Res Commun. 2008; 375(3):450-3.

zur Nieden NI, Kempka G, Rancourt DE, Ahr HJ. Induction of chondro-, osteo- and adipogenesis in embryonic stem cells by bone morphogenetic protein-2: effect of cofactors on differentiating lineages. BMC Dev Biol. 2005;5:1.

9

Human Pluripotent Stem Cell-Derived Cardiomyocytes: Maturity and Electrophysiology

Ville Kujala, Mari Pekkanen-Mattila and Katriina Aalto-Setälä
University of Tampere, Institute of Biomedical Technology, Tampere,
Finland

1. Introduction

Human pluripotent stem cells comprise embryonic and induced pluripotent stem cells. Both of these are able to give rise to all cell types of an individual, including heart muscle cells or cardiomyocytes. First stable human embryonic stem cell (hESC) lines were derived in 1998 by James A. Thomson and his co-workers (Thomson et al., 1998). First cardiomyocytes derived from hESCs were made in 2001 by Kehat and co-workers (Kehat et al., 2001) and after that many research groups have derived and studied human pluripotent stem cell derived cardiac cells and their properties. In 2007 the first human induced pluripotent stem cells (hiPSCs) were produced by Shinya Yamanaka's (Takahashi et al., 2007) and James A. Thomson's (Yu et al., 2007) groups from dermal fibroblasts, and hiPSCs have subsequently also been shown to be able to give rise to cardiomyocytes (Zhang et al., 2009, Zwi et al., 2009). Pluripotent stem cell derived cardiac cells have a great potential for cardiotoxicity testing, for preclinical testing of new chemical entities for the pharmaceutical industry and hopefully in the future for cell therapy in myocardial infarction and heart failure. However, before these goals are achieved thorough characterization of the cardiomyocytes is needed to ensure their feasibility for these applications.

2. Differentiation of cardiomyocytes from pluripotent stem cells

Cardiomyocytes can be differentiated from pluripotent stem cells by multiple methods and the differentiation event is quite rapid, 10-20 days. However, all the differentiation methods have common problems, which include uncontrolled differentiation, low differentiation rate and heterogeneous differentiated cell population. In addition, the cardiomyocyte differentiation efficiency has been shown to vary markedly between different hESC lines (Pekkanen-Mattila et al., 2009). The differentiation methods are described in more detailed manner below and summarized in Figure 1.

2.1 Spontaneous differentiation in embryoid bodies
Cardiomyocyte differentiation from hESCs and hiPSCs in EBs has been described in many reports (Figure 1 A) (Itskovitz-Eldor et al., 2000, Kehat et al., 2001, Burridge et al., 2007, Zhang et al., 2009). In addition to cardiomyocyte generation, EB differentiation is widely

used also in production of other cell types such as neuronal cells, hematopoietic cells, adipocytes and chondrocytes (Pera & Trounson, 2004). For the whole existence of hESCs, EB differentiation has been widely used differentiation method for its relatively simple and inexpensive nature regardless the low differentiation rate. For example, if aiming at cardiac differentiation, under 10% of the EBs formed contain beating areas (Kehat et al., 2001).

2.2 Differentiation with mouse visceral endoderm –like cells

A little more directed way to differentiate cardiomyocytes from hESCs is in co-culture with mouse endodermal-like (END-2) cells (Figure 1B) (Mummery et al., 2003, Passier et al., 2005). The differentiation inducing factors are secreted from END-2 cells and therefore END-2 conditioned medium can also be used in cardiomyocyte differentiation (Graichen et al., 2008). With END-2 methods, cardiogenic differentiation potential can be enhanced with serum-free medium supplemented with ascorbic acid (Passier et al., 2005) or adding cyclosporine A to the culture medium (Fujiwara et al., 2011).

END-2 cells support the differentiation towards endodermal and mesodermal derivatives (Mummery et al., 2003, Passier et al., 2005, Beqqali et al., 2006). This is in accordance with embryonal development studies, which have shown that anterior visceral endoderm is essential in normal heart development (Lough & Sugi, 2000). The specific mechanism or the specific factors inducing cardiac differentiation by END-2 cells are, however, not clearly known. It has been suggested that removal of insulin by END-2 cells could have a role in this differentiation method. Insulin inhibits cardiac differentiation by suppressing endoderm and mesoderm formation and favouring ectoderm differentiation (Freund et al., 2008) therefore the elimination of insulin from the medium by END-2 cells could favour the cardiac differentiation. Additionally, another more promising mechanism inducing cardiac differentiation by END-2 cells has been suggested to be prostaglandin I2 (PGI2) (Xu et al., 2008).

2.3 Cardiac differentiation with defined growth factors

The combination of activin A and BMP-4 with matrigel has been used in differentiation protocols for cardiomyocytes (Figure 1C) (Laflamme et al., 2007). These factors enhance mesoendoderm formation, an early precursor cell lineage which gives rise to mesoderm and endoderm (Laflamme et al., 2007). Mesoderm is the origin of cardiac cells , but cardiac differentiation inducing signals are in large extent arising from endoderm (Lough & Sugi, 2000).

A stepwise differentiation protocol has also been developed by Gordon Keller's group (Yang et al., 2008, Kattman et al., 2011). This protocol involves induction of primitive streak-like population, in addition to formation of cardiac mesoderm and expansion of cardiac lineages. The protocol is based on EB differentiation and is comprised of three stages. Growth factors BMP-4, FGF, activin A, vascular endothelial growth factor (VEGF) and dickkoptf homolog 1 (DKK1) were used in varying combinations. Mesoendoderm formation has also been induced by Wnt3A, an activator of the canonical Wnt/β-catenin signalling pathway (Tran et al., 2009).

3. Characteristics of differentiated cardiomyocytes

Cardiac differentiation can be followed by multiple markers at gene and protein expression levels. During early stages of differentiation mesoderm formation is detectable by the elevated mRNA level of Brachyury T. Brachyury T expression peak is detected at day 3 in

END-2 co-cultures (Beqqali et al., 2006, Pekkanen-Mattila et al., 2009) and a day later in EBs (Bettiol et al., 2007, Pekkanen-Mattila et al., 2010). The cardiac differentiation cascade can be

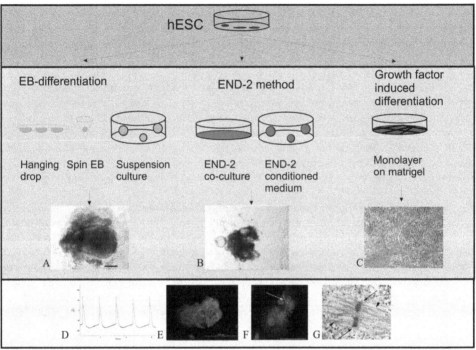

Fig. 1. Differentiation methods for hESC derived cardiomyocytes (middle column) and characteristics of the differentiated cells (undermost column). *EB-differentiation* can be performed in three ways, EBs can be formed either in hanging drops: enzymatically dissociated stem cells are pipetted in suspension into small drops on petri dish which is then inverted. EBs form in these drops and they can be plated down afterwards. EBs can be formed also in 96-well-plate wells, where single cell suspension is added and EB formation is forced by sentrifuging. Traditional was to EB formation is however the suspension method, where EBs form spontaneously in suspension from enzymatically dissociated hESCs. The picture A represents a 12-day old EB is attached to the bottom of cell culture dish. *Differentiation with END-2-cells* can be performed in two ways; hESC are plated onto END-2 cell layer and differentiated as co-culture or hESC are differentiated as EBs in END-2 conditioned medium. The picture B is taken from END-2 co-culture after one week of differentiation. Third way presented here is to culture hESCs on matrigel and initiate differentiation towrads cardiac lineage with *growth factors*, such as Activin-A and BMP-4. Differentiation is performed in a monolayer of cells (C).
The first sign for differentiated cardiomyocytes is the formation of beating areas. hESC-CM have the ability to contract spontaneously and in addition to fire spontaneously action potentials (D). Differentiated cells are stained positively with troponin T (E) and connexin 45 can be seen in the border areas of two troponin T positive cells (F). Electronmicroscopy (G) reveals sarcomere structures with Z-bands (marked with arrows) in the differentiated hESC-CMs.

followed further by the expression of the cardiac regulatory transcription factors such as Islet-1 (ISL-1), Mesp 1, GATA-4, NKX2.5 and Tbx6 (Graichen et al., 2008, Yang et al., 2008). The first clear indication for emergence of cardiomyocytes is the formation of spontaneously beating aggregates or areas in the cell culture dish (Kehat et al., 2001, Mummery et al., 2003). The number of beating areas has been used in quantifying differentiation efficiency even though the beating areas contain varying numbers of cardiomyocytes (Passier et al., 2005, Pekkanen-Mattila et al., 2009, Pekkanen-Mattila et al., 2010). The amount of cardiomyocytes has also been quantitated using flow cytometry (Kattman et al., 2011). Electron microscopy studies reveal that the differentiated cardiomyocytes contain myofibrils which are first organized randomly throughout the cytoplasm. However, organized sarcomeric structures occur at later stages of differentiation with A, I, and Z bands (Figure 1G). In the vicinity of the sarcomeres, mitochondria are also present. In addition, cells have intercalated disks with gap junctions and desmosomes (Kehat et al., 2001, Snir et al., 2003, Pekkanen-Mattila et al., 2009). Cardiac structural proteins such as troponin I, T or C (Figure 1 E), myosins and α-actinin are also present in differentiated beating cells (Kehat et al., 2001, Mummery et al., 2003).

The beating function of heart muscle is the result of chain reactions between many ionic currents through cell membranes and sarcomeric proteins in the cytoplasm. Cardiomyocytes express ion channels and gap junction proteins on the cell membrane and these proteins are needed for transmission of electrical stimuli from cell to another (Figure 1 F) (He et al., 2003, Sartiani et al., 2007). Furthermore, there are intracellular channels such as ryanodine receptor 2 (RyR2) which are responsible for the calcium-induced calcium release (CICR) from the sarcoplasmic reticulum (Fabiato, 1983, Dolnikov et al., 2006, Satin et al., 2008). All these channels function in a cascade which results in synchronous contraction of the heart mediated by sarcoplasmic proteins.

4. Cardiomyocytes during embryonic development and stem cell differentiation

The development of the heart is composed of series of complicated differentiation events and morphogenetic changes (Buckingham et al., 2005). Additionally, electrical activities of cardiac cell change during development. For example, the average beating rate of human neonatal cardiomyocytes is ~140 beats per minute and in adult cardiomyocytes ~80 beats per minute (Huang et al., 2007). The data of human cardiac embryology is, however, very restricted and, thus, most information is based on animal models. Microelectrode recordings from chick embryo revealed that the first contracting cardiomyocytes have pacemaker like action potentials. According to these measurements, the membrane diastolic potential in the first pacemaker like cells is in the range of -35 mV, action potential amplitude is relatively small and Ca^{2+} dependent action potential upstroke is slow (Sperelakis & Shigenobu, 1972).

Similar postnatal development changes are seen in rabbit models. The beating rate decreases, action potential duration increases and the maximal diastolic potential (MDP) reaches more negative values during development (Toda, 1980). Allah and co-workers investigated in rabbits mRNA levels of several ion channels and Ca^{2+} handling proteins such as hyperpolarization activated cyclic nucleotide-gated potassium channel 4 (HCN4), $Na_{V1.5}$, $Ca_{V1.3}$, NCX 1, $K_{V1.5}$, ERG, K_VLQT1 (also known as KCNQ1) and minK and they observed decreased mRNA levels of all these factors and suggested that this could explain the postnatal decrease in the beating rate and increase of action potential duration (Allah et al., 2011).

Ca-handling in cardiomyocytes also changes during embryonic development. According to ultrastructural studies, the sarcoplasmic reticulum is not completely developed at the early developmental stages and therefore neonatal cardiomyocytes are suggested to be more dependent on transsarcolemmal Ca^{2+} influx than sarcoplasmic Ca^{2+} release (Brook et al., 1983, Nakanishi et al., 1987, Nassar et al., 1987, Klitzner & Friedman, 1989). Therefore Na^+/Ca^{2+} exchanger (NCX) have been suggested to have a important role in excitation-contraction coupling during the early developmental stages (Klitzner et al., 1991, Wetzel et al., 1991, Wetzel et al., 1991, Huynh et al., 1992) . Indeed, NCX gene and protein expression, in addition to NCX current have been shown to be enhanced at the early developmental stages (Artman, 1992, Artman et al., 1995, Chin et al., 1997, Haddock et al., 1997, Gershome et al., 2011).

Asp and colleagues compared the cardiac marker and ion channel expression of human embryonic stem cell derived cardiomyocyte (hESC-CM) clusters to human fetal, neonatal and adult atrial and ventricular origin heart tissue samples (Asp et al., 2010). They found the beating frequencies between hESC-CM clusters to vary substantially. They could identify two groups, one having slow (< 50 beats per minute[bpm]) and the other high (> 50 bmp) beating rate and they suggested these could represent ventricular and atrial type of cardiac cells, respectively. They also demonstrated that hESC-CMs had higher *NKX2.5* and cardiac muscle actin mRNA expression levels than the heart samples. The *NKX2.5* expression level, however, decreased over time in culture finally approaching that of the heart samples. Cardiac troponin T was more strongly expressed in ventricular samples and in hESC-CMs compared to atrial samples. The levels of cardiac troponin T mRNA also decreased over time in hESC-CMs. Phospholamban was expressed less in the atrial samples and hESC-CMs compared to ventricle samples. α-myosin heavy chain, which is normally mostly expressed in atrial tissue, was more strongly expressed in hESC-CMs with beat rates over 50 bpm and in adult atrial tissue samples whereas β-myosin heavy chain was more expressed in the ventricular heart samples and less in all the other heart preparations of hESC-CMs. The α-myosin heavy chain mRNA levels increased with increasing age of the hESC-CMs. Across all the heart tissue and hESC-CM samples cardiac RyR2, L-type calcium channel, and $Na_{V1.5}$ sodium channel mRNA were similarly expressed. HERG mRNA expression in hESC-CMs was similar to neonatal and adult atrial samples. *HCN2* was expressed in a more comparable way to the ventricular samples. Only *HCN4* expression differed between the hESC-CMs, with those having the beating rate of less than 50 bpm having lower expression. Overall, it was concluded that the difference between slow beating and fast beating hESC-CMs paralleled the human atrial and ventricular tissues (Asp et al., 2010). Despite small differences in expression levels, the conclusion from this study was that stem cell -derived cardiac cells share many similarities with human heart tissue and thus stem cell -derived cardiac cells are a good cellular model for human heart.

5. Electrophysiology of human pluripotent stem cell derived cardiomyocytes

The electrical properties of pluripotent stem cell derived cardiac cells have been studied principally either with patch clamp analysis of single cells or with microelectrode array (MEA) platform using beating cell aggregates.

5.1 Patch clamp analysis

Patch clamp method has been developed to study ion channels in excitable membranes. (Sakmann & Neher, 1984). In this technique micropipette is attached to the cell membrane by a giga seal and this can be exploited to measure current changes and voltage across the membrane. This technique has been widely used in detailed electrical analysis of pluripotent stem cell derived cardiomyocytes.

Key cardiac ion channel types (and respective currents in brackets) involved in the human ventricular action potential include $Na_{V1.5}$ (I_{Na}), $K_{V4.3}$ (I_{to}), $Ca_{V1.2}$ ($I_{Ca,L}$) $K_{V11.1}$ (I_{Kr}), $K_{V7.1}$ (I_{Ks}), and $K_{ir2.X}$ (I_{K1}) (Pollard et al., 2010). These ion channels mediate the complex interaction between the currents and result in the characteristic action potential shape which can be divided into five different phases (Figure 2). Phase 0 of the action potential is the depolarization of the cardiomyocytes from the negative membrane potential to positive, called the upstroke. This is followed by phase 1, the short transient repolarization that is followed by phase 2, the plateau at slightly less positive membrane potential than the

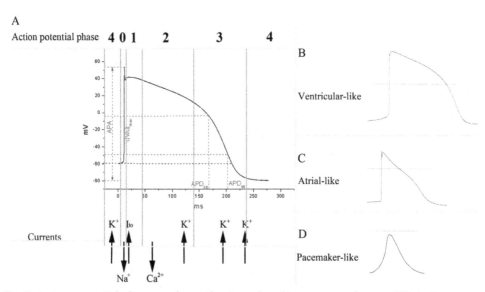

Fig. 2. Action potential phases and specification of cardiomyocyte subtypes. (A) Action potential (AP) parameters: Action potential amplitude (APA), maximum rate of rise of the action potential (dV/dtmax), action potential delay (ADP) and membrane diastolic potential (MDP). AP phase 0 is a rapid depolarization phase when the sodium channels are activated and membrane permeability is increased to Na+. Rapid depolarisation is followed by rapid repolarization phase 1 and plateau phase 2, where Ca2+ ions are entered to the cell throught L-type calcium channels. At phase 3, calcium channels are inactivated and repolarization is caused by outward potassium currents. Repolarization is due to the currents carried mainly by the slow Iks and rapid Ikr components of the delayed rectifier potassium channels. The Ikr current is produced by hERG channel (encoded by the human ether-à-go-go-related gene). By contrast, inward potassium current contributes to the maintenance of the resting membrane potential, phase 4. B-D. Classification of ventricular (B), atrial (C) an pacemaker-like (D) action potentials. Ventricular action potential has a prominent plateau phase whereas atrial action potential is more triangularly shaped. Pacemaker-like cells are characterized by slower upstroke velocity and amplitude if compared to ventricular and atrial type of cells.

maximal upstroke value. Phase 2 is followed by phase 3, which is the repolarization back to the resting membrane potential. The resting state of the membrane potential is phase 4 (Nerbonne & Kass, 2005).

Sartiani and co-workers have investigated the expression of different ion channel proteins and respective ion currents with patch clamp technique in undifferentiated hESCs and in their early- (days 15 to 40) and late-stage (days 50-110) cardiomyocyte derivates using the EB differentiation method (Sartiani et al., 2007). Some ion currents were present readily in the undifferentiated cells (I_{Kr}, I_f, $I_{ca,L}$). The properties of these currents were modified during hESC-CM development and some new currents (I_{to} and I_{K1}) were introduced, so the cardiomyocytes achieved maturation over time. With regard to the I_{to}, transient outward potassium current, the two isoforms $K_{v1.4}$ and $K_{v4.3}$ were differentially expressed in the developing cardiomyocytes at mRNA level. The shorter $K_{v4.3}$ splice variant was expressed in over 57-days-old cardiomyocytes whereas the longer one was expressed in the earlier cardiomyocytes. The $K_{v1.4}$ isoform is expressed at least from day 25 onward. Despite $K_{v4.3}$ mRNA expression in hESCs I_{to} current was not present in them. I_{to} could be detected using patch clamp on day 12 in the developing hESC-CMs and it was higher in later-stage (57 days old) cardiomyocytes compared to earlier ones (Sartiani et al., 2007).

Another repolarizing current (I_{Kr}), encoded by the human ether-a-go-go related gene (*HERG*) channel is also expressed in hESCs as well as the developing cardiomyocytes. However, the shorter splice variant *HERG1b* mRNA was only expressed in the developing hESC-CMs. Using patch clamp an outward K^+-current sensitive to E-4031, a selective blocker of the I_{Kr} current, could also be recorded in hESCs. *HCN* isoforms encode the I_f depolarization current. *HCN1* and *HCN4* were expressed more strongly in the undifferentiated hESCs and early cardiomyocytes than in late cardiomyocytes. *HCN4* was also expressed in the adult heart, whereas *HCN1* was not. *HCN2* was expressed in the adult heart as well as strongly in hESCs and early and late hESC-CMs. Voltage clamp experiments revealed I_f currents in hESCs and early and late developing cardiomyocytes. However, during cardiomyocyte maturation, the I_f activation rate decreased. With regard to another depolarization current I_{K1}, the $K_{ir2.1}$ mRNA was already present in hESCs but the current could only be measured from the developing cardiomyocytes (Sartiani et al., 2007).

Voltage-dependent Ca^{2+} current ($I_{ca,L}$) is mediated by α1C subunit of the calcium channel in many tissues and this subunit is encoded by *CACNA1C* gene. Sartiani and co-workers demonstrated mRNA expression of *CACNA1C* to be present both in undifferentiated hESCs and in the cardiomyocytes. Also, the $I_{ca,L}$ current could be recorded from hESCs as well as the hESC-CMs. During hESC-CM development the action potential upstroke velocity and action potential duration increased significantly. The beating rate on the other hand decreased during cardiomyocyte maturation and the diastolic depolarization rate flattened in the late cardiomyocytes. Pharmacological interventions also demonstrated intact ion channel function and expected responses were obtained with E4031 and $BsCl_2$ (I_{K1} blockers), zatebradine (I_f blocker), and lacidipine ($I_{ca,L}$ blocker). Finally, stimulation with isoprenaline proved intact β-adrenergic signalling in the stem cell derived cardiomyocyte (Sartiani et al., 2007).

Taken together, the cardiomyocytes seem to achieve a more mature cardiac phenotype over time in cell culture, even though this has not been confirmed in all studies (Pekkanen-Mattila et al., 2010). The I_{to} and I_{K1} currents could serve as markers for hESC cardiac differentiation (Sartiani et al., 2007) since they appear only later in cardiac differentiation. I_{to} current has also been shown to increase in postnatal rat cardiomyocytes (Guo et al., 1996,

Shimoni et al., 1997) and I_{K1} current has been shown to stabilize the diastolic potential in myocytes (Silva & Rudy, 2003).

With regard to the EB and END-2 co-culture differentiation methods our own experiments demonstrated that the EB method produces slightly more cardiomyocytes with consistent beating rate and more cardiomyocytes with ventricular type action potentials. The EB method also produced cardiomyocytes with significantly more hyperpolarized MDP (Pekkanen-Mattila et al., 2010). Low expression of I_{K1} current in developing hESC-CMs seems to be responsible, at least in part, for their low MDP (Sartiani et al., 2007). Cardiomyocytes produced with both methods did not differ in their upstroke velocity (Pekkanen-Mattila et al., 2010a).

Dolnikov and colleagues studied mechanical functions of hESC derived cardiac cells. They found that hESC-CMs have a negative force-frequency relation, whereas mature human myocardium the relationship is positive (Dolnikov et al., 2005). They also found that blocking the ryanodine receptor or the sarcoplasmic-endoplasmic reticulum Ca^{2+} -ATPase did not affect the hESC-CM contraction as it usually does in mature cardiomyocytes. Furthermore, caffeine did not result in increase of intracellular calcium concentration. However, in subsequent studies caffeine-indused release of intracellular Ca^{2+} has been documented both in hESC and hiPSC -derived cardiac cells (Satin et al., 2008, Itzhaki et al., 2011). Both RyR mediated release of intracellular Ca^{2+} stores as well as the reuptake of Ca^{2+} by SERCA into endoplasmic reticulum were reported to occur the same way as in cardiac tissue. These results indicate that Ca^{2+} handling in both hESC and hiPSC-derived cardiac cells are functional and further indicate the potential of these cardiac cells in the future applications in basic research as well as in translational cardiac research.

5.2 Microelectrode array platform

In addition to the more traditional patch clamp (Hamill et al., 1981) studies the MEA platform (Reppel et al., 2004) offers an easy and convenient medium-throughput technique to assess the electrical properties of the differentiated cardiomyocytes (Reppel et al., 2005). Action and field potential curves achieved by patch clamp and by MEA are represented in Figure 3. The MEA platform presents an advantageous additional tool for cardiac safety studies in addition to the more traditional Langendorff heart organ model, conventional patch clamp electrophysiology studies and heterologous expression systems of ion channels, especially the hERG potassium channel (Meyer et al., 2004)..

The MEA system allows examination of multicellular cardiac syncythia, thus enabling electrocardiogram-like mapping of their field potential properties. Cardiac repolarization in hESC-CMs can be therefore investigated with MEAs and it has been demonstrated that drug effects can be investigated using this platform (Reppel et al., 2005). With MEA system, Caspi and co-workers were able to investigate drug effects on hESC-CMs. E-4031 is a compound that blocks I_{Kr} repolarizing current and this effect can be seen as prolongation of the cardiac field potential (FP) cycle in the electrocardiogram. The authors were able to demonstrate a dose-dependent effect where the field potential duration (FPD) prolonged by escalating concentrations of E-4031. Sotalol, a class III antiarrhythmic agent, also increased FPD as did quinidine and procainamide, both class IA antiarrhythmic agents. Cisapride, a gastrointestinal prokinetic drug that was withdrawn for the market due to adverse cardiac side effects, prolonged the FPD as well, as seen on the MEA recordings (Caspi et al., 2009, Liang et al., 2010).

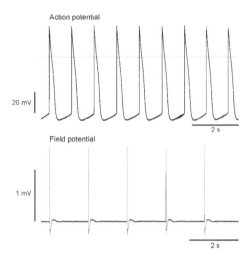

Fig. 3. Action and field potentials recorded from human embryonic stem cell –derived cardiomyocytes. Action potentials can be measured from single cardiomyocytes in current clamp mode using the patch clamp technique. Field potentials can be measured from a multicellular cardiac syncytium with microelectrode arrays.

To assess the practicality of using hESC-CMs in conjunction with the MEA platform in pharmacotoxicological testing, Braam and colleagues investigated the effects of various drugs on the FPD of cardiomyocytes derived from human ES cells (Braam et al., 2010). They tested 12 compounds for their potential in prolonging repolarization (FPD) in hESC-CMs. Despite the relatively lower maturation of hESC-CMs compared to mature cardiomyocytes, they could be used in predicting the clinically observed cardiotoxic effects. Blocking of sodium, calcium and *HERG* potassium channels by lidocaine, nifidipine, and E-4031, respectively, had expected effects on hESC-CM field potential properties. Quinidine and sotalol, both used clinically to prolong repolarization, increased hESC-CM FPD at concentrations near the unbound effective therapeutic plasma concentration (ETCP unbound). They also tested drugs which have been known to prolong the QT interval in patients and noticed that the FPD prolongations too place at concentrations that were not as near the ECTP unbound range. The varying FP shapes in hESC-CM recordings did not affect the results, meaning that FPD changes in these cardiomyocytes can be reliably detected despite the large variety of FP shapes (Braam et al., 2010). The study provided, for the first time, data on the effects of large number of tested compound over a high concentration range on the FP properties of hESC-CM.

6. Applications for pluripotent stem cell-derived cardiomyocytes

6.1 Human model for development of cardiomyocytes and cardiac electrophysiology
The amount of data about electrophysiological changes during human cardiac differentiation is limited. Data is mostly based on animal models, but due to the physiological differences between species this data cannot be always applied directly to humans. Human pluripotent stem cells differentiate into functional cardiomyocytes and these cells also mature in culture (Sartiani et al., 2007). Therefore they provide a good model

to study development of complex network of cardiac ion channels involved in signal transduction and cardiomyocyte contraction.

6.2 Drug screening and safety pharmacology

Many cardiac and also non-cardiac drugs have been withdrawn from the market because of toxic effects on heart and its function. Even though all new chemical entities (NCE) are tested according to requirements during drug development process, unforeseen effects such as syncope, arrhythmia, sudden death, polymorphic ventricular tachycardia (Torsade de pointes [TdP]) are occasionally seen only in clinical trials or when the drug is already on the market (Redfern et al., 2003, Roden, 2004, Lexchin, 2005). Pharmaceutical regulatory authorities have specified and expanded the requirements for safety testing and recommend that tests are done with two mammalian species, one rodent and other nonrodent species. Tests include electocardiographic recordings and also histological studies of the heart (ICH, 2005, ICH, 2005, EMEA, 2008).

With regard to proarrhythmic potential, the QT interval is the cornerstone of the guidelines for the assessment of new chemical compounds (ICH, 2005, ICH, 2005). A number of drugs can potentially prolong the QT interval (Fenichel et al., 2004, Roden, 2004), and it is also a leading cause for use restriction and market withdrawal (Roden, 2004), the International Conference of Harmonization has defined the evaluation of this risk for new chemical entities as standard preclinical process (Bode & Olejniczak, 2002, Cavero & Crumb, 2005).

Delayed rectifier potassium current (I_{Kr}) is responsible in part for the repolarization of the action potential (Vandenberg et al., 2001, Pollard et al., 2008). Inhibition of this hERG channel ($K_{V11.1}$) and the subsequent inhibition of the I_{Kr}, is the predominant basis of drug-induced QT prolongation and TdP (Hancox et al., 2008; Redfern et al., 2003). Currently a number of preclinical models and assays have been employed by pharmaceutical companies (Carlsson, 2006, Pollard et al., 2008). These assays include in vivo QT assays, such as ECG telemetry of conscious dogs (Miyazaki et al., 2005), and in vitro assays, such as repolarization assay, which detects changes in the action potential delay (APD) of cardiac tissues (isolated animal Purkinje fibres, papillary muscles or cardiomyocytes) or the hERG channel assay where hERG current expressed in heterologous cell system (such as CHO or HEK293 cells) or native I_{Kr} is characterized (Finlayson et al., 2004, Martin et al., 2004). However, current methods are not fully adequate (Redfern et al., 2003, Lu et al., 2008). They are costly and the in vivo assays are ethically questionable because of the large number of animals used. Therefore there is a need for an in vitro method based on human cardiac cells that would bring additional value and reliability for testing novel pharmaceutical agents. Cardiomyocytes derived both from hESC and iPS cells have many potential applications in the pharmaceutical industry including target validation, screening and safety pharmacology. These cells would serve as an inexhaustible and reproducible human model system and preliminary reports of the validation of hESC-CM system already exist (Braam et al., 2010, Mandenius et al., 2011).

6.3 Disease modelling with induced pluripotent stem cell –derived cardiomyocytes

The hiPSC technology (Takahashi et al., 2007, Yu et al., 2007) presents a great opportunity to investigate diseases in cell culture that would otherwise be challenging to study. Although the full potential of this method is still to be realized in cardiac research, some preliminary results provide encouragement to investigate this path further.

One condition that is challenging to study in patients in terms of underlying molecular mechanisms is the long QT syndrome (LQTS). This condition can be either genetic or acquired as a side effect of using certain therapeutic drugs. The first LQTS modelling using hiPSCs was reported in 2010 (Moretti et al., 2010). Pluripotent stem cells were reprogrammed from fibroblasts of two family members having LQTS type 1, and cardiac cells derived from these hiPSCs with LQT1 genotype had prolonged action potential. Additionally increased arrhythmogenicity could be demonstrated with isoproterenol. Similar findings have been reported about LQTS type 2 (Itzhaki et al., 2011, Matsa et al., 2011).

Cardiomyocytes have also been derived from hiPSCs from a patient with Timothy syndrome (Yazawa et al., 2011). These patients have mutation in the *CACNA1C* gene that encodes the $Ca_V1.2$ calcium ion channel in humans. The cardiomyocytes having Timothy syndrome genotype exhibited irregular contractions and excessive calcium influx as well as action potential prolongation, irregularities in the electrical activation and abnormal calcium transients in the ventricular-type cardiomyocytes (Yazawa et al., 2011).

Taken together these results provide optimism for modelling different cardiac disease phenotypes in cell culture conditions. This allows for more detailed dissection of the pathological pathways and molecular interactions within and between the cells. An additional benefit is also the fact that these studies can be now carried out in patient-specific cells which provide suitable genomic backgrounds for more optimal comparison between the clinical disease phenotype and results obtained *in vitro*.

7. Challenges in pluripotent stem cell research

While human pluripotent stem cells represent a promising new tool for pharmacological and toxicological testing and hopefully also for regenerative therapies in the future some hurdles remain to be cleared before we can achieve those goals efficiently. With regards to hiPSC a question remains how close these cells are to hESCs in their properties. While they fulfil the criteria required for pluripotent stem cells, some recent studies suggest that they retain some aberrant epigenetic reprogramming compared to ES cells (Lister et al., 2011). Both cell types have similar global methylomes, but the reprogrammed iPS cell seem to retain some memory of the somatic cell DNA methylation patterns in addition to the methylation patterns that are specific for iPSCs (Lister et al., 2011). However, the cardiomyocytes differentiated from hiPSCs and hESCs seem to have very similar global transcriptomes (Gupta et al., 2010).

Another issue with both, hESCs and hiPSCs, are the currently suboptimal differentiation protocols for desired differentiated cell types. Cardiomyocytes are no exception in this case and several protocols for more efficient differentiation have been experimented with. Recently, increased yields of cardiomyocytes have been obtained by stage-specific optimization of the activin/nodal and bone morphogenetic protein (BMP) signalling (Kattman et al., 2011). The directed differentiation protocol of hESC-CMs in a monolayer, with activin A and BMP4 supplementation, represents another step forward in creating more efficient differentiation methods (Laflamme et al., 2007). In hiPS reprogramming omission of c-Myc from the four factor Yamanaka cocktail has been shown to enhance their cardiogenic potential (Martinez-Fernandez et al., 2010).

To achieve better cardiomyocyte differentiation efficiencies with pluripotent stem cells we need to gain more insight into the lineage-specification steps that govern the transformation of pluripotent stem cells to committed progenitors and finally to mature differentiated cardiomyocytes. For example, ISL1+ cardiac progenitors are able to give rise to cardiomyocytes, smooth muscle, and endothelial cell lineages and these progenitor populations can be expanded in cell culture (Bu et al., 2009). KDR+ cells derived from human embryonic stem cells have also been shown to give rise to cardiac progenitor cells (Yang et al., 2008).

8. Conclusion

In conclusion, human pluripotent stem cell derived cardiomyocytes have very similar electrophysiological properties as human heart tissue and, thus, they have a great potential in the future to benefit pharmaceutical and toxicological industry. Additionally, with these cells we are closer than ever before to individualized, patient-specific treatments. However, a lot of basic research is still required before we can utilize the full advantage of human pluripotent stem cell –derived cardiac cells.

9. References

Allah, E.A., Tellez, J.O., Yanni, J., Nelson, T., Monfredi, O., Boyett, M.R. & Dobrzynski, H. (2011). Changes in the expression of ion channels, connexins and Ca2+-handling proteins in the sino-atrial node during postnatal development. *Exp Physiol,* Vol. 96, No. 4, (Apr), pp. 426-38

Artman, M. (1992). Sarcolemmal Na(+)-Ca2+ exchange activity and exchanger immunoreactivity in developing rabbit hearts. *Am J Physiol,* Vol. 263, No. 5 Pt 2, (Nov), pp. H1506-13

Artman, M., Ichikawa, H., Avkiran, M. & Coetzee, W.A. (1995). Na+/Ca2+ exchange current density in cardiac myocytes from rabbits and guinea pigs during postnatal development. *Am J Physiol,* Vol. 268, No. 4 Pt 2, (Apr), pp. H1714-22

Asp, J., Steel, D., Jonsson, M., Ameen, C., Dahlenborg, K., Jeppsson, A., Lindahl, A. & Sartipy, P. (2010). Cardiomyocyte clusters derived from human embryonic stem cells share similarities with human heart tissue. *J Mol Cell Biol,* Vol. 2, No. 5, (October 2010), pp. 276-283

Beqqali, A., Kloots, J., Ward-Van Oostwaard, D., Mummery, C. & Passier, R. (2006). Genome-wide transcriptional profiling of human embryonic stem cells differentiating to cardiomyocytes. *Stem Cells,* Vol. No. (May 4, 2006), pp. 2006-0054

Bettiol, E., Sartiani, L., Chicha, L., Krause, K.H., Cerbai, E. & Jaconi, M.E. (2007). Fetal bovine serum enables cardiac differentiation of human embryonic stem cells. *Differentiation,* Vol. 75, No. 8, (Oct), pp. 669-81

Bode, G. & Olejniczak, K. (2002). ICH Topic: The draft ICH S7B step 2: Note for guidance on safety pharmacology studies for human pharmaceuticals. *Fundamental & Clinical Pharmacology,* Vol. 16, No. 2, (April 2002), pp. 105-118

Braam, S.R., Tertoolen, L., Van De Stolpe, A., Meyer, T., Passier, R. & Mummery, C.L. (2010). Prediction of drug-induced cardiotoxicity using human embryonic stem cell-derived cardiomyocytes. *Stem Cell Research,* Vol. 4, No. 2, (March 2010), pp. 107-116

Braam, S.R., Tertoolen, L., Van De Stolpe, A., Meyer, T., Passier, R. & Mummery, C.L. (2010). Prediction of drug-induced cardiotoxicity using human embryonic stem cell-derived cardiomyocytes. *Stem Cell Res*, Vol. 4, No. 2, (Mar), pp. 107-16

Brook, W.H., Connell, S., Cannata, J., Maloney, J.E. & Walker, A.M. (1983). Ultrastructure of the myocardium during development from early fetal life to adult life in sheep. *J Anat*, Vol. 137 (Pt 4), No. (Dec), pp. 729-41

Bu, L., Jiang, X., Martin-Puig, S., Caron, L., Zhu, S., Shao, Y., Roberts, D.J., Huang, P.L., Domian, I.J. & Chien, K.R. (2009). Human ISL1 heart progenitors generate diverse multipotent cardiovascular cell lineages. *Nature*, Vol. 460, No. 7251, (July 2009), pp. 113-117

Buckingham, M., Meilhac, S. & Zaffran, S. (2005). Building the mammalian heart from two sources of myocardial cells. *Nat Rev Genet*, Vol. 6, No. 11, (Nov), pp. 826-35

Burridge, P.W., Anderson, D., Priddle, H., Barbadillo Munoz, M.D., Chamberlain, S., Allegrucci, C., Young, L.E. & Denning, C. (2007). Improved human embryonic stem cell embryoid body homogeneity and cardiomyocyte differentiation from a novel V-96 plate aggregation system highlights interline variability. *Stem Cells*, Vol. 25, No. 4, (Apr), pp. 929-38

Carlsson, L. (2006). In vitro and in vivo models for testing arrhythmogenesis in drugs. *J Intern Med*, Vol. 259, No. 1, (Jan), pp. 70-80

Caspi, O., Itzhaki, I., Kehat, I., Gepstein, A., Arbel, G., Huber, I., Satin, J. & Gepstein, L. (2009). In vitro electrophysiological drug testing using human embryonic stem cell derived cardiomyocytes. *Stem Cells and Development*, Vol. 18, No. 1, (February 2009), pp. 161-172

Cavero, I. & Crumb, W. (2005). ICH S7B draft guideline on the non-clinical strategy for testing delayed cardiac repolarisation risk of drugs: a critical analysis. *Expert Opinion on Drug Safety*, Vol. 4, No. 3, (May 2005), pp. 509-530

Chin, T.K., Christiansen, G.A., Caldwell, J.G. & Thorburn, J. (1997). Contribution of the sodium-calcium exchanger to contractions in immature rabbit ventricular myocytes. *Pediatr Res*, Vol. 41, No. 4 Pt 1, (Apr), pp. 480-5

Dolnikov, K., Shilkrut, M., Zeevi-Levin, N., Danon, A., Gerecht-Nir, S., Itskovitz-Eldor, J. & Binah, O. (2005). Functional properties of human embryonic stem cell-derived cardiomyocytes. *Annals of the New York Academy of Sciences*, Vol. 1047, No. (June 2005), pp. 66-75

Dolnikov, K., Shilkrut, M., Zeevi-Levin, N., Gerecht-Nir, S., Amit, M., Danon, A., Itskovitz-Eldor, J. & Binah, O. (2006). Functional properties of human embryonic stem cell-derived cardiomyocytes: intracellular Ca2+ handling and the role of sarcoplasmic reticulum in the contraction. *Stem Cells*, Vol. 24, No. 2, (Feb), pp. 236-45

Fabiato, A. (1983). Calcium-induced release of calcium from the cardiac sarcoplasmic reticulum. *Am J Physiol*, Vol. 245, No. 1, (Jul), pp. C1-14

Fenichel, R.R., Malik, M., Antzelevitch, C., Sanguinetti, M., Roden, D.M., Priori, S.G., Ruskin, J.N., Lipicky, R.J., Cantilena, L.R. & Independent Academic Task, F. (2004). Drug-Induced Torsades de Pointes and Implications for Drug Development. *Journal of Cardiovascular Electrophysiology*, Vol. 15, No. 4, (April 2004), pp. 475-495

Finlayson, K., Witchel, H.J., Mcculloch, J. & Sharkey, J. (2004). Acquired QT interval prolongation and HERG: implications for drug discovery and development. *Eur J Pharmacol*, Vol. 500, No. 1-3, (Oct 1), pp. 129-42

Freund, C., Ward-Van Oostwaard, D., Monshouwer-Kloots, J., Van Den Brink, S., Van Rooijen, M., Xu, X., Zweigerdt, R., Mummery, C. & Passier, R. (2008). Insulin redirects differentiation from cardiogenic mesoderm and endoderm to neuroectoderm in differentiating human embryonic stem cells. *Stem Cells*, Vol. 26, No. 3, (Mar), pp. 724-33

Fujiwara, M., Yan, P., Otsuji, T.G., Narazaki, G., Uosaki, H., Fukushima, H., Kuwahara, K., Harada, M., Matsuda, H., Matsuoka, S., Okita, K., Takahashi, K., Nakagawa, M., Ikeda, T., Sakata, R., Mummery, C.L., Nakatsuji, N., Yamanaka, S., Nakao, K. & Yamashita, J.K. (2011). Induction and enhancement of cardiac cell differentiation from mouse and human induced pluripotent stem cells with cyclosporin-a. *PLoS ONE*, Vol. 6, No. 2, pp. e16734

Gershome, C., Lin, E., Kashihara, H., Hove-Madsen, L. & Tibbits, G.F. (2011). Colocalization of voltage-gated Na+ channels with the Na+/Ca2+ exchanger in rabbit cardiomyocytes during development. *Am J Physiol Heart Circ Physiol*, Vol. 300, No. 1, (Jan), pp. H300-11

Graichen, R., Xu, X., Braam, S.R., Balakrishnan, T., Norfiza, S., Sieh, S., Soo, S.Y., Tham, S.C., Mummery, C., Colman, A., Zweigerdt, R. & Davidson, B.P. (2008). Enhanced cardiomyogenesis of human embryonic stem cells by a small molecular inhibitor of p38 MAPK. *Differentiation*, Vol. 76, No. 4, (Apr), pp. 357-70

Guo, W., Kamiya, K. & Toyama, J. (1996). Modulated expression of transient outward current in cultured neonatal rat ventricular myocytes: comparison with development in situ. *Cardiovascular Research*, Vol. 32, No. 3, (September 1996), pp. 524-533

Gupta, M.K., Illich, D.J., Gaarz, A., Matzkies, M., Nguemo, F., Pfannkuche, K., Liang, H., Classen, S., Reppel, M., Schultze, J.L., Hescheler, J. & Saric, T. (2010). Global transcriptional profiles of beating clusters derived from human induced pluripotent stem cells and embryonic stem cells are highly similar. *BMC Developmental Biology*, Vol. 10, No. (September 2010), pp. 98

Haddock, P.S., Coetzee, W.A. & Artman, M. (1997). Na+/Ca2+ exchange current and contractions measured under Cl(-)-free conditions in developing rabbit hearts. *Am J Physiol*, Vol. 273, No. 2 Pt 2, (Aug), pp. H837-46

Hamill, O.P., Marty, A., Neher, E., Sakmann, B. & Sigworth, F.J. (1981). Improved patch-clamp techniques for high-resolution current recording from cells and cell-free membrane patches. *European Journal of Physiology*, Vol. 391, No. 2, (August 1981), pp. 85-100

He, J.-Q., Ma, Y., Lee, Y., Thomson, J.A. & Kamp, T.J. (2003). Human Embryonic Stem Cells Develop Into Multiple Types of Cardiac Myocytes: Action Potential Characterization. *Circ Res*, Vol. 93, No. 1, (July 11, 2003), pp. 32-39

Huang, X., Yang, P., Du, Y., Zhang, J. & Ma, A. (2007). Age-related down-regulation of HCN channels in rat sinoatrial node. *Basic Res Cardiol*, Vol. 102, No. 5, (Sep), pp. 429-35

Huynh, T.V., Chen, F., Wetzel, G.T., Friedman, W.F. & Klitzner, T.S. (1992). Developmental changes in membrane Ca2+ and K+ currents in fetal, neonatal, and adult rabbit ventricular myocytes. *Circ Res*, Vol. 70, No. 3, (Mar), pp. 508-15

Itskovitz-Eldor, J., Schuldiner, M., Karsenti, D., Eden, A., Yanuka, O., Amit, M., Soreq, H. & Benvenisty, N. (2000). Differentiation of human embryonic stem cells into embryoid bodies compromising the three embryonic germ layers. *Mol Med*, Vol. 6, No. 2, (Feb), pp. 88-95

Itzhaki, I., Maizels, L., Huber, I., Zwi-Dantsis, L., Caspi, O., Winterstern, A., Feldman, O., Gepstein, A., Arbel, G., Hammerman, H., Boulos, M. & Gepstein, L. (2011). Modelling the long QT syndrome with induced pluripotent stem cells. *Nature*, Vol. 471, No. 7337, (March 2011), pp. 225-259

Kattman, S.J., Witty, A.D., Gagliardi, M., Dubois, N.C., Niapour, M., Hotta, A., Ellis, J. & Keller, G. (2011). Stage-Specific Optimization of Activin/Nodal and BMP Signaling Promotes Cardiac Differentiation of Mouse and Human Pluripotent Stem Cell Lines. *Cell Stem Cell*, Vol. 8, No. 2, (February 2011), pp. 228-240

Kehat, I., Kenyagin-Karsenti, D., Snir, M., Segev, H., Amit, M., Gepstein, A., Livne, E., Binah, O., Itskovitz-Eldor, J. & Gepstein, L. (2001). Human embryonic stem cells can differentiate into myocytes with structural and functional properties of cardiomyocytes. *The Journal of Clinical Investigation*, Vol. 108, No. 3, (August 2001), pp. 407-414

Kehat, I., Kenyagin-Karsenti, D., Snir, M., Segev, H., Amit, M., Gepstein, A., Livne, E., Binah, O., Itskovitz-Eldor, J. & Gepstein, L. (2001). Human embryonic stem cells can differentiate into myocytes with structural and functional properties of cardiomyocytes. *J Clin Invest*, Vol. 108, No. 3, (Aug), pp. 407-14

Klitzner, T.S., Chen, F.H., Raven, R.R., Wetzel, G.T. & Friedman, W.F. (1991). Calcium current and tension generation in immature mammalian myocardium: effects of diltiazem. *J Mol Cell Cardiol*, Vol. 23, No. 7, (Jul), pp. 807-15

Klitzner, T.S. & Friedman, W.F. (1989). A diminished role for the sarcoplasmic reticulum in newborn myocardial contraction: effects of ryanodine. *Pediatr Res*, Vol. 26, No. 2, (Aug), pp. 98-101

Laflamme, M.A., Chen, K.Y., Naumova, A.V., Muskheli, V., Fugate, J.A., Dupras, S.K., Reinecke, H., Xu, C., Hassanipour, M., Police, S., O'sullivan, C., Collins, L., Chen, Y., Minami, E., Gill, E.A., Ueno, S., Yuan, C., Gold, J. & Murry, C.E. (2007). Cardiomyocytes derived from human embryonic stem cells in pro-survival factors enhance function of infarcted rat hearts. *Nature Biotechnology*, Vol. 25, No. 9, (September 2007), pp. 1015-1024

Laflamme, M.A., Chen, K.Y., Naumova, A.V., Muskheli, V., Fugate, J.A., Dupras, S.K., Reinecke, H., Xu, C., Hassanipour, M., Police, S., O'sullivan, C., Collins, L., Chen, Y., Minami, E., Gill, E.A., Ueno, S., Yuan, C., Gold, J. & Murry, C.E. (2007). Cardiomyocytes derived from human embryonic stem cells in pro-survival factors enhance function of infarcted rat hearts. *Nat Biotechnol*, Vol. 25, No. 9, (Sep), pp. 1015-24

Lexchin, J. (2005). Drug withdrawals from the Canadian market for safety reasons, 1963-2004. *Cmaj*, Vol. 172, No. 6, (Mar 15), pp. 765-7

Liang, H., Matzkies, M., Schunkert, H., Tang, M., Bonnemeier, H., Hescheler, J. & Reppel, M. (2010). Human and murine embryonic stem cell-derived cardiomyocytes serve together as a valuable model for drug safety screening. *Cell Physiol Biochem*, Vol. 25, No. 4-5, (March 2010), pp. 459-466

Lister, R., Pelizzola, M., Kida, Y.S., Hawkins, R.D., Nery, J.R., Hon, G., Antosiewicz-Bourget, J., O'malley, R., Castanon, R., Klugman, S., Downes, M., Yu, R., Stewart, R., Ren, B., Thomson, J.A., Evans, R.M. & Ecker, J.R. (2011). Hotspots of aberrant epigenomic reprogramming in human induced pluripotent stem cells. *Nature*, Vol. 471, No. 7336, (March 2011), pp. 68-73

Lough, J. & Sugi, Y. (2000). Endoderm and heart development. *Dev Dyn*, Vol. 217, No. 4, (Apr), pp. 327-42

Lu, H.R., Vlaminckx, E., Hermans, A.N., Rohrbacher, J., Van Ammel, K., Towart, R., Pugsley, M. & Gallacher, D.J. (2008). Predicting drug-induced changes in QT interval and arrhythmias: QT-shortening drugs point to gaps in the ICHS7B Guidelines. *Br J Pharmacol*, Vol. 154, No. 7, (Aug), pp. 1427-38

Mandenius, C.F., Steel, D., Noor, F., Meyer, T., Heinzle, E., Asp, J., Arain, S., Kraushaar, U., Bremer, S., Class, R. & Sartipy, P. (2011). Cardiotoxicity testing using pluripotent stem cell-derived human cardiomyocytes and state-of-the-art bioanalytics: a review. *J Appl Toxicol*, Vol. 31, No. 3, (Apr), pp. 191-205

Martin, R.L., Mcdermott, J.S., Salmen, H.J., Palmatier, J., Cox, B.F. & Gintant, G.A. (2004). The utility of hERG and repolarization assays in evaluating delayed cardiac repolarization: influence of multi-channel block. *J Cardiovasc Pharmacol*, Vol. 43, No. 3, (Mar), pp. 369-79

Martinez-Fernandez, A., Nelson, T.J., Ikeda, Y. & Terzic, A. (2010). c-MYC independent nuclear reprogramming favors cardiogenic potential of induced pluripotent stem cells. *Journal of Cardiovascular Translational Research*, Vol. 3, No. 1, (February 2010), pp. 13-23

Matsa, E., Rajamohan, D., Dick, E., Young, L., Mellor, I., Staniforth, A. & Denning, C. (2011). Drug evaluation in cardiomyocytes derived from human induced pluripotent stem cells carrying a long QT syndrome type 2 mutation. *Eur Heart J*, Vol. 32, No. 8, (April 2011), pp. 952-962

Meyer, T., Boven, K.H., Gunther, E. & Fejtl, M. (2004). Micro-electrode arrays in cardiac safety pharmacology: a novel tool to study QT interval prolongation. *Drug Safety*, Vol. 27, No. 11, (n.d.), pp. 763-72

Miyazaki, H., Watanabe, H., Kitayama, T., Nishida, M., Nishi, Y., Sekiya, K., Suganami, H. & Yamamoto, K. (2005). QT PRODACT: sensitivity and specificity of the canine telemetry assay for detecting drug-induced QT interval prolongation. *J Pharmacol Sci*, Vol. 99, No. 5, pp. 523-9

Moretti, A., Bellin, M., Welling, A., Jung, C.B., Lam, J.T., Bott-Flugel, L., Dorn, T., Goedel, A., Hohnke, C., Hofmann, F., Seyfarth, M., Sinnecker, D., Schomig, A. & Laugwitz, K.L. (2010). Patient-specific induced pluripotent stem-cell models for long-QT syndrome. *N Engl J Med*, Vol. 363, No. 15, (October 2010), pp. 1397-1409

Mummery, C., Ward-Van Oostwaard, D., Doevendans, P., Spijker, R., Van Den Brink, S., Hassink, R., Van Der Heyden, M., Opthof, T., Pera, M., De La Riviere, A.B., Passier,

R. & Tertoolen, L. (2003). Differentiation of human embryonic stem cells to cardiomyocytes: role of coculture with visceral endoderm-like cells. *Circulation,* Vol. 107, No. 21, (Jun 3), pp. 2733-40

Nakanishi, T., Okuda, H., Kamata, K., Abe, K., Sekiguchi, M. & Takao, A. (1987). Development of myocardial contractile system in the fetal rabbit. *Pediatr Res,* Vol. 22, No. 2, (Aug), pp. 201-7

Nassar, R., Reedy, M.C. & Anderson, P.A. (1987). Developmental changes in the ultrastructure and sarcomere shortening of the isolated rabbit ventricular myocyte. *Circ Res,* Vol. 61, No. 3, (Sep), pp. 465-83

Nerbonne, J.M. & Kass, R.S. (2005). Molecular physiology of cardiac repolarization. *Physiol Rev,* Vol. 85, No. 4, (October 2005), pp. 1205-1253

Passier, R., Oostwaard, D.W., Snapper, J., Kloots, J., Hassink, R.J., Kuijk, E., Roelen, B., De La Riviere, A.B. & Mummery, C. (2005). Increased cardiomyocyte differentiation from human embryonic stem cells in serum-free cultures. *Stem Cells,* Vol. 23, No. 6, (Jun-Jul), pp. 772-80

Pekkanen-Mattila, M., Chapman, H., Kerkela, E., Suuronen, R., Skottman, H., Koivisto, A.P. & Aalto-Setala, K. (2010). Human embryonic stem cell-derived cardiomyocytes: demonstration of a portion of cardiac cells with fairly mature electrical phenotype. *Experimental Biology and Medicine,* Vol. 235, No. 4, (April 2010), pp. 522-530

Pekkanen-Mattila, M., Kerkela, E., Tanskanen, J.M., Pietila, M., Pelto-Huikko, M., Hyttinen, J., Skottman, H., Suuronen, R. & Aalto-Setala, K. (2009). Substantial variation in the cardiac differentiation of human embryonic stem cell lines derived and propagated under the same conditions--a comparison of multiple cell lines. *Ann Med,* Vol. 41, No. 5, pp. 360-70

Pekkanen-Mattila, M., Kerkelä, E., Tanskanen, J.M.A., Pietilä, M., Pelto-Huikko, M., Hyttinen, J., Skottman, H., Suuronen, R. & Aalto-Setälä, K. (2009). Substantial variation in the cardiac differentiation of human embryonic stem cell lines derived and propagated under the same conditions: a comparison of multiple cell lines. *Annals of Medicine,* Vol. 41, No. 5, (n.d.), pp. 360-370

Pekkanen-Mattila, M., Pelto-Huikko, M., Kujala, V., Suuronen, R., Skottman, H., Aalto-Setala, K. & Kerkela, E. (2010). Spatial and temporal expression pattern of germ layer markers during human embryonic stem cell differentiation in embryoid bodies. *Histochem Cell Biol,* Vol. 133, No. 5, (May), pp. 595-606

Pera, M.F. & Trounson, A.O. (2004). Human embryonic stem cells: prospects for development. *Development,* Vol. 131, No. 22, (Nov), pp. 5515-25

Pollard, C.E., Abi Gerges, N., Bridgland-Taylor, M.H., Easter, A., Hammond, T.G. & Valentin, J.P. (2010). An introduction to QT interval prolongation and non-clinical approaches to assessing and reducing risk. *British Journal of Pharmacology,* Vol. 159, No. 1, (January 2010), pp. 12-21

Pollard, C.E., Valentin, J.P. & Hammond, T.G. (2008). Strategies to reduce the risk of drug-induced QT interval prolongation: a pharmaceutical company perspective. *Br J Pharmacol,* Vol. 154, No. 7, (Aug), pp. 1538-43

Redfern, W.S., Carlsson, L., Davis, A.S., Lynch, W.G., Mackenzie, I., Palethorpe, S., Siegl, P.K., Strang, I., Sullivan, A.T., Wallis, R., Camm, A.J. & Hammond, T.G. (2003).

Relationships between preclinical cardiac electrophysiology, clinical QT interval prolongation and torsade de pointes for a broad range of drugs: evidence for a provisional safety margin in drug development. *Cardiovasc Res*, Vol. 58, No. 1, (Apr 1), pp. 32-45

Reppel, M., Pillekamp, F., Brockmeier, K., Matzkies, M., Bekcioglu, A., Lipke, T., Nguemo, F., Bonnemeier, H. & Hescheler, J. (2005). The electrocardiogram of human embryonic stem cell-derived cardiomyocytes. *Journal of Electrocardiology*, Vol. 38, No. 4, Supplement 1, (October 2005), pp. 166-170

Reppel, M., Pillekamp, F., Lu, Z.J., Halbach, M., Brockmeier, K., Fleischmann, B.K. & Hescheler, J. (2004). Microelectrode arrays: A new tool to measure embryonic heart activity. *Journal of Electrocardiology*, Vol. 37, No. Supplement 1, (October 2004), pp. 104-109

Roden, D.M. (2004). Drug-Induced Prolongation of the QT Interval. *New England Journal of Medicine*, Vol. 350, No. 10, (March 2004), pp. 1013-1022

Roden, D.M. (2004). Drug-induced prolongation of the QT interval. *N Engl J Med*, Vol. 350, No. 10, (Mar 4), pp. 1013-22

Sakmann, B. & Neher, E. (1984). Patch clamp techniques for studying ionic channels in excitable membranes. *Annual Review of Physiology*, Vol. 46, No. (n.d.), pp. 455-72

Sartiani, L., Bettiol, E., Stillitano, F., Mugelli, A., Cerbai, E. & Jaconi, M.E. (2007). Developmental changes in cardiomyocytes differentiated from human embryonic stem cells: a molecular and electrophysiological approach. *Stem Cells*, Vol. 25, No. 5, (May 2007), pp. 1136-1144

Sartiani, L., Bettiol, E., Stillitano, F., Mugelli, A., Cerbai, E. & Jaconi, M.E. (2007). Developmental changes in cardiomyocytes differentiated from human embryonic stem cells: a molecular and electrophysiological approach. *Stem Cells*, Vol. 25, No. 5, (May), pp. 1136-44

Satin, J., Itzhaki, I., Rapoport, S., Schroder, E.A., Izu, L., Arbel, G., Beyar, R., Balke, C.W., Schiller, J. & Gepstein, L. (2008). Calcium handling in human embryonic stem cell-derived cardiomyocytes. *Stem Cells*, Vol. 26, No. 8, (August 2008), pp. 1961-1972

Satin, J., Itzhaki, I., Rapoport, S., Schroder, E.A., Izu, L., Arbel, G., Beyar, R., Balke, C.W., Schiller, J. & Gepstein, L. (2008). Calcium handling in human embryonic stem cell-derived cardiomyocytes. *Stem Cells*, Vol. 26, No. 8, (Aug), pp. 1961-72

Shimoni, Y., Fiset, C., Clark, R.B., Dixon, J.E., Mckinnon, D. & Giles, W.R. (1997). Thyroid hormone regulates postnatal expression of transient K+ channel isoforms in rat ventricle. *Journal of Physiology*, Vol. 500, No. 1, (April 1997), pp. 65-73

Silva, J. & Rudy, Y. (2003). Mechanism of Pacemaking in IK1-Downregulated Myocytes. *Circulation Research*, Vol. 92, No. 3, (February 2003), pp. 261-263

Snir, M., Kehat, I., Gepstein, A., Coleman, R., Itskovitz-Eldor, J., Livne, E. & Gepstein, L. (2003). Assessment of the ultrastructural and proliferative properties of human embryonic stem cell-derived cardiomyocytes. *Am J Physiol Heart Circ Physiol*, Vol. 285, No. 6, (Dec), pp. H2355-63

Sperelakis, N. & Shigenobu, K. (1972). Changes in membrane properties of chick embryonic hearts during development. *J Gen Physiol*, Vol. 60, No. 4, (Oct), pp. 430-53

Takahashi, K., Tanabe, K., Ohnuki, M., Narita, M., Ichisaka, T., Tomoda, K. & Yamanaka, S. (2007). Induction of Pluripotent Stem Cells from Adult Human Fibroblasts by Defined Factors. *Cell*, Vol. 131, No. 5, (November 2007), pp. 861-872

Thomson, J.A., Itskovitz-Eldor, J., Shapiro, S.S., Waknitz, M.A., Swiergiel, J.J., Marshall, V.S. & Jones, J.M. (1998). Embryonic stem cell lines derived from human blastocysts. *Science*, Vol. 282, No. 5391, (November 1998), pp. 1145-1147

Toda, N. (1980). Age-related changes in the transmembrane potential of isolated rabbit sino-atrial nodes and atria. *Cardiovasc Res*, Vol. 14, No. 1, (Jan), pp. 58-63

Tran, T.H., Wang, X., Browne, C., Zhang, Y., Schinke, M., Izumo, S. & Burcin, M. (2009). Wnt3a-induced mesoderm formation and cardiomyogenesis in human embryonic stem cells. *Stem Cells*, Vol. 27, No. 8, (Aug), pp. 1869-78

Vandenberg, J.I., Walker, B.D. & Campbell, T.J. (2001). HERG K+ channels: friend and foe. *Trends Pharmacol Sci*, Vol. 22, No. 5, (May), pp. 240-6

Wetzel, G.T., Chen, F., Friedman, W.F. & Klitzner, T.S. (1991). Calcium current measurements in acutely isolated neonatal cardiac myocytes. *Pediatr Res*, Vol. 30, No. 1, (Jul), pp. 83-8

Wetzel, G.T., Chen, F. & Klitzner, T.S. (1991). L- and T-type calcium channels in acutely isolated neonatal and adult cardiac myocytes. *Pediatr Res*, Vol. 30, No. 1, (Jul), pp. 89-94

Xu, X.Q., Graichen, R., Soo, S.Y., Balakrishnan, T., Rahmat, S.N., Sieh, S., Tham, S.C., Freund, C., Moore, J., Mummery, C., Colman, A., Zweigerdt, R. & Davidson, B.P. (2008). Chemically defined medium supporting cardiomyocyte differentiation of human embryonic stem cells. *Differentiation*, Vol. 76, No. 9, (Nov), pp. 958-70

Yang, L., Soonpaa, M.H., Adler, E.D., Roepke, T.K., Kattman, S.J., Kennedy, M., Henckaerts, E., Bonham, K., Abbott, G.W., Linden, R.M., Field, L.J. & Keller, G.M. (2008). Human cardiovascular progenitor cells develop from a KDR+ embryonic-stem-cell-derived population. *Nature*, Vol. 453, No. 7194, (May 22), pp. 524-8

Yang, L., Soonpaa, M.H., Adler, E.D., Roepke, T.K., Kattman, S.J., Kennedy, M., Henckaerts, E., Bonham, K., Abbott, G.W., Linden, R.M., Field, L.J. & Keller, G.M. (2008). Human cardiovascular progenitor cells develop from a KDR+ embryonic-stem-cell-derived population. *Nature*, Vol. 453, No. 7194, (May 2008), pp. 524-528

Yazawa, M., Hsueh, B., Jia, X., Pasca, A.M., Bernstein, J.A., Hallmayer, J. & Dolmetsch, R.E. (2011). Using induced pluripotent stem cells to investigate cardiac phenotypes in Timothy syndrome. *Nature*, Vol. 471, No. 7337, (March 2011), pp. 230-234

Yu, J., Vodyanik, M.A., Smuga-Otto, K., Antosiewicz-Bourget, J., Frane, J.L., Tian, S., Nie, J., Jonsdottir, G.A., Ruotti, V., Stewart, R., Slukvin, I.I. & Thomson, J.A. (2007). Induced Pluripotent Stem Cell Lines Derived from Human Somatic Cells. *Science*, Vol. 318, No. 5858, (December 2007), pp. 1917-1920

Zhang, J., Wilson, G.F., Soerens, A.G., Koonce, C.H., Yu, J., Palecek, S.P., Thomson, J.A. & Kamp, T.J. (2009). Functional cardiomyocytes derived from human induced pluripotent stem cells. *Circ Res*, Vol. 104, No. 4, (Feb 27), pp. e30-41

Zhang, J., Wilson, G.F., Soerens, A.G., Koonce, C.H., Yu, J., Palecek, S.P., Thomson, J.A. & Kamp, T.J. (2009). Functional cardiomyocytes derived from human induced pluripotent stem cells. *Circulation Research*, Vol. 104, No. 4, (February 2009), pp. e30-e41

Zwi, L., Caspi, O., Arbel, G., Huber, I., Gepstein, A., Park, I.H. & Gepstein, L. (2009). Cardiomyocyte differentiation of human induced pluripotent stem cells. *Circulation*, Vol. 120, No. 15, (October 2009), pp. 1513-1523

10

Human Pluripotent Stem Cells in Cardiovascular Research and Regenerative Medicine

Ellen Poon[1], Chi-wing Kong[1-3] and Ronald A. Li[1-5]
[1]Stem Cell & Regenerative Medicine Consortium,
[2]Heart, Brain, Hormone & Healthy Aging Research Center,
[3]Departments of Medicine and [4]Physiology,
LKS Faculty of Medicine, University of Hong Kong
[5]Center of Cardiovascular Research, Mount Sinai School of Medicine, New York, NY,
[1,2,3,4]Hong Kong
[5]USA

1. Introduction

Heart disease is one of the leading causes of mortality worldwide. Because adult cardiomyocytes (CMs) lack the ability to regenerate, malfunctions or significant loss of CMs due to disease or aging can lead to cardiac arrhythmias, heart failure, and subsequently death. Heart transplantation for patients with end stage heat failure is limited by the number of donor organs available. Cell-based therapies offer a promising alternative for myocardial repair, but there are significant challenges involved. The transplantation of human CMs, eg fetal CMs, is difficult for practical and ethical reasons, thus cells of non-cardiac lineage, such as skeletal myoblasts (Murry et al., 1996; Menasche et al., 2003) and mesenchymal stem cells (Shake et al., 2002; Toma et al., 2002), have been considered as alternatives. Animal studies and clinical trials involving these cells have yielded conflicting results. Transplanted non-cardiac cells such as bone marrow-derived hematopoietic cells do not transdifferentiate into the cardiac lineage (Balsam et al., 2004; Murry et al., 2004). They also do not integrate into the host myocardium. For instance, the lack of electrical integration of skeletal myoblasts after their autologous transplantation into the myocardium resulted in the generation of malignant ventricular arrhythmias, which led to the premature termination of clinical trials involving skeletal myoblasts (Menasche et al., 2003; Smits et al., 2003). Therefore, an alternative cell source is needed.

2. Human embryonic stem cells and induced pluripotent stem cells

Human embryonic stem cells (hESCs), isolated from the inner cell mass of blastocysts, can self-renew while maintaining their pluripotency to differentiate into all cell types (Thomson et al., 1998), including CMs (Kehat et al., 2001; Mummery, C. et al., 2002; Xu, C. et al., 2002; Xue et al., 2004; Mummery, C. et al., 2003). Therefore, hESCs may provide an unlimited *ex vivo* source of CMs for cell-based heart therapies. The laboratories of Yamanaka (Takahashi et al., 2007) and Thomson (Yu et al., 2007) showed that adult somatic cells can be reprogrammed to become pluripotent hES-like cells (a.k.a. induced pluripotent stem cells or iPSCs) via the forced expression of four pluripotency genes (Oct4, Sox2, c-Myc, and Klf4 *or* Oct4, Sox2, Nanog, and Lin28) (Takahashi and Yamanaka, 2006; Takahashi et al., 2007; Aasen et al., 2008). More recent studies have further demonstrated the successful use of less pluripotency factors (Huangfu et al., 2008; Kim, J. B. et al., 2008; Nakagawa et al., 2008) and non-viral methods (e.g., with synthetic modified RNA (Warren et al., 2010)) to reprogram somatic cells into iPSCs. Although concerns such as induced somatic coding mutations (Gore et al., 2011) have yet to be fully addressed, hiPSCs have morphology, gene expression profile, epigenetic status, *in vitro* and *in vivo* differentiation capacities similar to hESCs (Takahashi et al., 2007; Yu et al., 2007).

3. Differentiation of hESC into CMs

Previous studies studies have demonstrated that hESCs and hiPSCs can spontaneously differentiate into CMs when they aggregate in suspension to form embryoid bodies (Xu, C. et al., 2002; Zwi et al., 2009). Recent studies have focused on improving the yield and purity of CM differentiation. For instance, hESC differentiation into the CM lineage can be enhanced by coculture with visceral endoderm-like cells (Mummery, C. et al., 2003; Mummery, C. L. et al., 2007). Recently, an effective protocol for cardiac differentiation has been successfully developed by the Keller laboratory involving the stage-specific addition of growth factors, including BMP4, Activin-A, DKK, bFGF etc, to drive sequential differentiation into the epiblast, mesoderm and CMs, resulting in greatly increased yield of up to 50%, as gauged by the proportion of cells that express cardiac troponin T (Yang et al., 2008). Other approaches have also been pursued, utilizing different extracellular matrices, serum (Passier et al., 2005) and insulin elimination (Xu, X. Q. et al., 2008). Besides improving the yield of CM differentiation, the isolation of a pure population of CMs is also important in order to prevent malignancy and arrhythmias. Various purification methods have been developed including Percoll gradient centrifugation (Xu, C. et al., 2002), optical signatures (Chan, J. W. et al., 2009) and genetic selection based on the expression of a reporter protein under the transcriptional control of a cardiac-restricted promoter (e.g., α-myosin heavy chain (α-MHC) (Anderson et al., 2007), ventricular myosin light chain (MLC-2v) (Huber et al., 2007; Fu et al., 2010)).

4. Properties of hESC-derived CMs (hESC-CMs)

4.1 Human ESC-CMs have molecular and structural properties of CMs

Gene expression profiles have been examined for hESC-CMs cultured in different laboratories using different differentiation protocols and from different hESC lines (Kehat et al., 2001; Xu, C. et al., 2002; Snir et al., 2003; Norstrom et al., 2006). There is now consensus that hESC-CMs express transcription factors and structural proteins specific to human cardiomyocytes (Kehat et al., 2001; Xu, C. et al., 2002; Snir et al., 2003; Norstrom et al., 2006). Human ESC-CMs express cardiac-specific transcription factors such as NKx2.5, GATA4 and Mef-2 (Kehat et al., 2001; Xu, C. et al., 2002), which are expressed in the precardiac mesoderm but persist in the heart during development. Structural components of the myofibers can also be detected in hESC-CMs. These include α−, β- and sarcomeric-myosin heavy chain (MHC), atrial and ventricular forms of myosin light chain (MLC-2a and –2v), tropomyosin, α-actinin and desmin (Kehat et al., 2001; Xu, C. et al., 2002; Norstrom et al.,

2006). Two members of the troponin complex, cardiac tropinin T, which binds to tropomyosin, and cardiac tropinin I, which regulates Ca^{2+}-sensitive muscle contraction, are also present in hESC-CMs (Kehat et al., 2001; Xu, C. et al., 2002; Norstrom et al., 2006). At the ultrastructural level, hESC-CMs show clearly identifiable sarcomeres and intercalated discs (Kehat et al., 2001; Snir et al., 2003). Morphologically, single hESC-CMs show spindle, round, and tri- or multiangular morphologies, rather than the more defined rod shape of mature cells (Xu, C. et al., 2002). Sarcomeric striations are organized in separated bundles, reminiscent of the pattern seen in human fetal CMs, and rather than the highly organized parallel bundles seen in human adult CMs (Mummery, C. et al., 2003). These data suggest that hESC-CMs display molecular and structural properties consistent with immature human CMs.

4.2 Human ESC-CMs have immature Ca^{2+} handling properties
4.2.1 Mechanism of Ca^{2+}-induced Ca^{2+}-release and Ca^{2+} transient
The contractile apparatus of CMs is dependent on the rise and decay of intracellular Ca^{2+}, known as the Ca^{2+} transient. During an action potential (AP) of adult CMs, Ca^{2+} entry into the cytosol through sarcolemmal L-type Ca^{2+} channels triggers the release of Ca^{2+} from the intracellular Ca^{2+} stores (sarcoplasmic reticulum or SR) via the ryanodine receptors (RyR). This process, the so-called Ca^{2+}-induced Ca^{2+}-release (Bers, 2002), escalates the cytosolic Ca^{2+} ($[Ca^{2+}]i$) to activate the contractile apparatus for contraction. For relaxation, elevated $[Ca^{2+}]i$ gets pumped back into the SR by the sarco/endoplasmic reticulum Ca^{2+}-ATPase (SERCA) and extruded by the Na^+-Ca^{2+} exchanger (NCX) to return to the resting $[Ca^{2+}]i$ level. Such a rise and subsequent decay of $[Ca^{2+}]i$ is known as Ca^{2+} transient. Given the central importance of Ca^{2+}-induced Ca^{2+}-release in cardiac excitation-contraction coupling, proper Ca^{2+} handling properties of hESC-CMs are crucial for their successful functional integration with the recipient heart after transplantation. Indeed, abnormal Ca^{2+} handling, as in the case of heart failure, can even be arrhythmogenic.

4.2.2 Human ESC-CMs have functional SRs
Dolnikov et al (2006) were the first to study the Ca^{2+}-handling properties of hESC-CMs in detail (Dolnikov et al., 2006). They reported that Ca^{2+} transients recorded from spontaneously beating or electrically stimulated hESC-CMs respond to neither caffeine nor ryanodine; hESC-CMs recorded as beating clusters also displayed a negative force-frequency relationship that is different from adult CMs. Based on these observations, the authors concluded that hESC-CMs are immature, do not express functional SRs, and that their contractions result from trans-sarcolemmal Ca^{2+} influx (rather than Ca^{2+} release from the SR). Given the paucity of related data, our laboratory performed a comprehensive analysis to better define the Ca^{2+} handling properties of hESC-CMs by comparing Ca^{2+} transients from hESC-CMs and human fetal left ventricular (LV) CMs (16–18 weeks) (Figure 1, adopted with permission from Liu et al 2007 *Stem Cells* Vol. 25, No. 12: pp.3038-3044). Upon electrical stimulation, all of hESC-CMs and fetal LV-CMs generated similar Ca^{2+} transients. However, caffeine induced Ca^{2+} release in 65% of fetal LVCMs and 38% of hESC-CMs. Ryanodine significantly reduced the electrically evoked Ca^{2+} transient amplitudes of caffeine-responsive but not -insensitive hESC-CMs and slowed their upstroke; thapsigargin, which inhibits SERCA, reduced the amplitude of only caffeine-responsive hESC-CMs and slowed the decay (Liu et al., 2007). The discrepancy between our findings and those of Dolnikov et al can be largely attributed to the newly identified caffeine-responsive population.

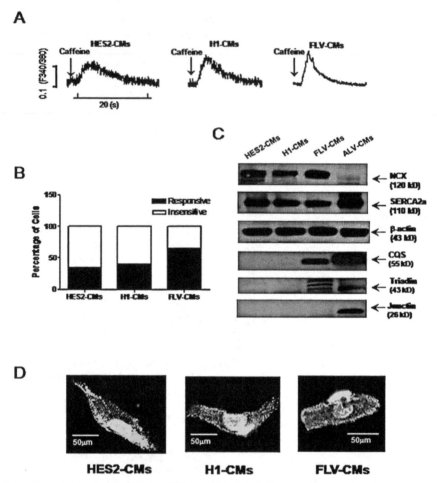

Fig. 1. Ca²⁺ handling properties of hESC-CMs
A) Representative tracings caffeine-induced Ca²⁺ transients of hESC-CMs (HES2-, H1-CMs) and fetal (F) LV-CMs. B) % of caffeine-responsive and -insensitive cells. C) Expression of various Ca²⁺ handling proteins. β-actin was used as the loading control. D) Immunostaining of RyRs. Adopted with permission from Liu et al 2007 *Stem Cells* Vol. 25, No. 12: pp.3038-3044.

4.2.3 Differential expression of Ca²⁺ handling proteins

While hESC-CMs express functional SRs, their Ca²⁺ handling properties are immature and are similar to those of fetal CMs. The functional immaturity of hESC-CMs may be attributed to the expression pattern of Ca²⁺ handling proteins (Figure 1C) (summarized in Table 1, adopted with permission from Kong et al 2010 *Thromb Haemost* Vol. 104, No. 1: pp.30-38). Compared to adult CMs, hESC-CMs express significantly lower levels of RyR, SERCA, phospholamban, calsequestrin and higher levels of calreticulin and NCX (Liu et al., 2007). The regulatory proteins junctin, triadin, and calsequestrin (CSQ) are expressed in adult LV-CMs but are completely absent in hESC-CMs (Liu et al., 2007).

		hESC-CMs	Fetal LVCMs	Adult LVCMs
Expression levels of Ca²⁺-handling proteins.	RyR	++	++	++++
	SERCA	+++	+++	++++
	Phospholamban	-	++	++++
	CSQ/Triadin/Junctin	-	+	++++
	Calreticulin	++++	++++	+
	NCX	+++	++++	+
Ca²⁺ transient properties	Basal [Ca²⁺]$_i$	++	+++	++++
	Amplitude	++	++	++++
	Decay	++	++	++++
	Upstroke	++	++	++++

Table 1. Ca^{2+} handling properties of hESC-CMs, fetal and adult LVCMs.
Adopted with permission from Kong et al 2010 *Thromb Haemost* Vol. 104, No. 1: pp.30-38.

4.2.4 T-Tubules are absent in hESC-CMs

Transverse (t) tubules are invaginations in the sarcolemmal membrane that concentrate dihydropyridine receptors and bring them spatially close to RyRs residing on the SR membrane located deeper in the cytoplasm (Brette and Orchard, 2003; Brette and Orchard, 2007). By physically minimizing the diffusion distance, RyRs in CMs can participate in Ca^{2+}-induced Ca^{2+}-release without a lag. The result is a synchronized, faster, and greater transient $[Ca^{2+}]i$ increase from the peripheries to the center, creating a uniform Ca^{2+} wavefront across the transverse section with simultaneous recruitment of all SR. Fast and synchronized activation of RyRs translates into a greater Ca^{2+} transient amplitude, recruitment of more actin–myosin cross-bridge cycling, and generation of greater contractile force. The presence of t-tubules is therefore crucial to the mature Ca^{2+} handling of CMs. Lieu et al used fluorescent staining (Figure 2A and C, adopted with permission from Lieu et al 2009 *Stem Cells Dev* Vol. 18, No. 10: pp.1493-1500) and atomic force microscopy (Figure 2B and D) to detect the presence of t-tubules and showed that the latter is absent in hESC-CMs. Consistent with CMs deficient of t-tubules, hESC-CMs also exhibit a U-shaped Ca^{2+} wavefront that is caused by a delayed Ca^{2+} increase in the central region of the cell relative to the peripheral region (Lieu et al., 2009) (Figure 2E).

4.2.5 Attempts to improve Ca²⁺-handling properties by genetic modification

We hypothesize that the differential expression of key CM proteins underpins the immaturity of hESC-CMs relative to adult CMs. We tested this idea by overexpressing CSQ in hESC-CMs. CSQ is the most abundant, high-capacity but low-affinity, Ca^{2+}-binding protein in the SR that is anchored to the RyR. The cardiac isoform CSQ2 can store up to 20 mM Ca^{2+} while buffering the free SR $[Ca^{2+}]$ at ~1 mM. This allows repetitive muscle contractions without rundown. While CSQ is robustly expressed in adult CMs, it is completely absent in hESC-CMs (Liu et al., 2007). We hypothesized that forced expression of CSQ in hESC-CMs would induce functional improvement of SR. We tested this hypothesis by transduction of hESC-CMs with the recombinant adenovirus Ad-CMV-CSQ-IRES-GFP (Ad-CSQ) and demonstrated that Ad-CSQ significantly increased the transient amplitude, upstroke velocity, and transient decay compared with the control and a truncated mutant (Liu et al., 2009) (Figure 3, adopted with permission from Liu et al 2009 *Am J Physiol Cell*

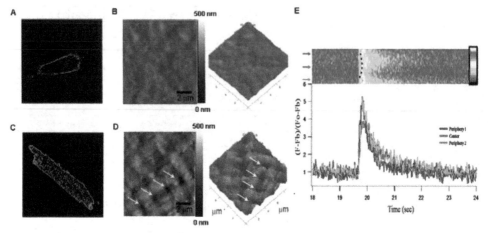

Fig. 2. T-tubule imaging of a hESC-CM and a mature ventricular CM.
Confocal microscopic images of a hESC-CM (A) did not show intracellular fluorescent spots
like those in an adult guinea pig ventricular CM (C) suggesting the absence of t-tubules.
The absence of t-tubules in ESC-CMs was further confirmed by atomic force microscopy
imaging of an adult ventricular cardiomyocyte (D) showing regularly spaced pores in the
sarcolemma that coincide with the Z-lines, while hESC-CM (B surface showed
comparatively smoother topology with no presence of invaginations that are indicative of t-
tubules. E) Electrically induced Ca^{2+} transient in hESC-CMs. Top: Time progression
linescans of pseudo-colored transient increase in intracellular Ca^{2+} across the mid-plane of a
hESC-CM showed a U-shaped wavefront. Bottom: Quantified Ca^{2+} transient of linescans of
the top panel. Adopted with permission from Lieu et al 2009 *Stem Cells Dev* Vol. 18, No. 10:
pp.1493-1500.

Physiol Vol. 297, No. 1: pp.C152-159). These results showed that immature Ca^{2+}-handling
properties of hESC-CMs can be rescued by genetic modification and improved our
understanding of CM maturation.

4.3 Human ESC-CMs demonstrate immature electrophysiological properties similar to 'embryonic' CMs

He et al (2003) were the first to study the electrophysiological properties of hESC-CMs (He
et al., 2003). They characterized the contractions and action potentials (APs) from beating EB
outgrowths cultured for 40 to 95 days and showed that hESC can differentiate into a
heterogeneous mixture of CMs, with APs classified as 'nodal-like', 'embryonic ventricular-
like' and 'embryonic atrial-like', analogous to CM specification into pacemaker, ventricular
and atrial CMs. The latter two classes are considered 'embryonic' based on their Maximum
diastolic potential and more depolarized resting membrane potential, and "slow" type APs
based on low dV/dt_{max}. Unlike adult CMs, which are normally electrically silent yet are
excitable upon stimulation, the majority of hESC-CMs fire spontaneously, exhibiting a high
degree of automaticity. Our laboratory examined triggered activity and found that
'embryonic ventricular-like' CMs exhibit delayed after depolarization, suggesting that
hESC-CMs can be arrhythmogenic.

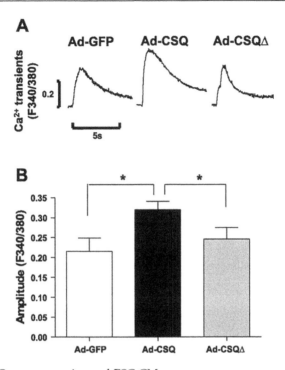

Fig. 3. Effect of CSQ overexpression on hESC-CMs.
A) Representative electrically-induced Ca^{2+} transient tracings for Ad-GFP (n=12) and Ad-CSQ (n=29) and Ad-CSQΔ (truncated mutant) (n=14) transduced hESC-CMs. B) Bar graphs of amplitude.* P < 0.05, ** P < 0.01. Adopted with permission from Liu et al 2009 *Am J Physiol Cell Physiol Vol. 297, No. 1*: pp.C152-159.

Subsequent studies were done to assess if hESC-CMs mature over time to acquire electrophysiological properties that are comparable to those of adult CMs and results are conflicting. Sartiani et al (2007) examined the AP of CMs over 3 months of culture and concluded that the molecular and functional expression of ion channels in hESC-CMs change over time, although they still do not reach the phenotype typical of adult VCMs (Sartiani et al., 2007). This is in contrast to findings by Pekkanen-Mattila et al (2010), which show that although one third of hESC-CMs exhibit a more mature phenotype, these changes are not correlated with time in culture (Pekkanen-Mattila et al., 2010). Taken together, these data suggest that hESC-CMs are functionally immature and present an arrhythmogenic risk. Therefore, facilitated *in vitro* maturation is important for the translation of hESC-CMs to the clinic and other applications (such as disease modeling, drug discovery and cardiotoxicity screening).

Our group sought to define the immature proarrhythmic electrophysiological properties observed in hESC-CMs by examining the role of different currents in automaticity (Azene et al., 2005; Siu et al., 2006; Xue et al., 2007; Lieu et al., 2008; Chan, Y. C. et al., 2009). I_{K1} (the inward-rectifier K^+ current encoded by Kir2.1), which stabilises a negative resting membrane potential, is important for suppressing automaticity and we hypothesize that its absence in hESC-CMs may underlie their immature phenotype. Consistent with this, forced Kir2.1 expression alone sufficed to render the electrical phenotype indistinguishable from that of primary adult ventricular cells (Lieu DK, Fu JD and Li RA, unpublished data). These proof-of-concept experiments show that developmentally arrested Ca^{2+} and electrophysiological phenotypes of hESC-CMs can be rescued. We are currently developing a non-genetic, non-pharmacologic method to drive global maturation, by targeting the microenvironmental niches and other non-cell autonomous means.

5. The use of hESC-CMs for myocardial repair and bioartificial pacemakers

Myocardial infarction is the major worldwide cardiovascular disorder in humans and is the leading cause of death in many parts of the world. Immediately after a heart attack, oxygen starvation of myocardial tissues leads to cell death, often resulting in irreversible and permanent damage to the heart. Despite some improvements in short term management of acute myocardial infarction, long term prognosis remains poor. Sudden cardiac death due to ventricular arrhythmias remains a leading cause of morbidity and mortality in the industrialised world, claiming well over 300,000 lives annually in the United States alone. After myocardial infarction, the heart undergoes hypertrophy in an attempt to compensate for loss of CMs, and cardiac fibroblasts secrete collagen and other extracellular matrix proteins during scar formation, leading to impaired cardiac function. Since terminally differentiated CMs have very limited potential for regeneration, transplantation is the only treatment for end-stage heart failure. However, this is hampered by the lack of suitable donor organs and tissues. Cell-based therapy is thus a promising option for myocardial repair. A range of cell sources have been considered, including bone marrow cells, skeletal myoblasts and smooth muscle cells, but their non-cardiac identity has presented major problems. They either do not differentiate into the cardiac lineage or they do not integrate well into the host myocardium (Menasche et al., 2003; Smits et al., 2003; Balsam et al., 2004; Murry et al., 2004). As discussed in previous sections, hESC-CMs have functional and structural properties very similar to human embryonic/fetal CMs and is therefore a very promising cell source. Transplantation of hESC-CMs to mouse/rat hearts showed that the cells survived, formed myocardial tissue and promoted functional improvement in rat models of myocardial infarction (Laflamme et al., 2007; Mignone et al., 2010). More detailed studies into the maturation of hESC-CMs, as well as the electropysiological consequences of hESC-CM transplantation are required before these early successes can be translated into clinical therapies.

Normal rhythms originate in the SA node (SAN), a specialized cardiac tissue consisting of only a few thousands pacemaker cells. Malfunction of cardiac pacemaker cells due to disease or aging can cause rhythm generation disorders. Current treatments include pharmacological intervention and/or implantation of electronic pacemakers, but they are associated with significant shortcomings (e.g. increased susceptibility to infection, haemorrhage, lung collapse and death infection, finite battery life, patient discomfort related to the permanent implantation of a foreign device, and lack of intrinsic responsiveness to neural and hormonal regulation). Therefore 'bioartificial-pacemakers', made up of transplanted cells with pacemaker properties, may be a desirable alternative.

There are two major strategies for creating bioartificial-pacemakers. The first is to confer pacemaker ability on cells that are normally silent. For instance, adult atrial and ventricular

CMs are electrically silent unless they are stimulated by signals transmitted from the SAN. This is due to the absence of I_f, encoded by the HCN channel family, and the presence of I_{K1}. Several gene-based approaches have been pursued to induce pacemaker activity in these normally silent cells. Our group took a protein engineering approach to define criteria important for pacing and created a bioengineered construct of HCN (Lesso and Li, 2003; Tsang et al., 2004; Tsang et al., 2004; Tse et al., 2006; Xue et al., 2007). This engineered-construct was shown to produce pacing *in vitro* and *in vivo* (Tse et al., 2006; Xue et al., 2007). In a sick sinus syndrome porcine model, pacing of the heart was restored and originated from the site of focal transduction in the left atrium with HCN-construct injection (Tse et al., 2006). Somatic gene transfer to create such a gene-based bioartificial pacemaker significantly reduces the dependence on device-supported pacing by electronic pacemaker from 85% to 15%. Alternatively, hESCs can be differentiated into pacemaker-like derivatives for transplantation to recreate a cell-based bioartificial pacemaker (Kehat et al., 2004; Xue et al., 2005). Of note, the construction of cell-based bioartificial-pacemakers requires much fewer cells (several thousands) than myocardial transplantation (hundreds of millions). Furthermore, the spherical SAN is structurally less complex than the left ventricular myocardium. Our group is currently exploring the possibility of using nodal progenitors. We are also testing non-invasive catheter-based delivery techniques for implantation as well as long-term safety and efficacy.

6. Creation of engineered cardiac tissue constructs

The ventricular myocardium is a highly complex structure consisting of aligned, connected CMs, stromal cells and a vascular network systematically embedded in a mesh of extracellular matrix. Indeed, hESC-CMs differentiated *in vitro* lack the sub-cellular organization and higher order structural 2- or 3-dimensionality seen in adult heart. To more closely recapitulate the *in vivo* environment of the heart, various groups have used different approaches to manipulate the surface and geometry of the culture platform, cell and matrix composition. For instance, Luna et al used a tunable culture platform comprised of biomimetic wrinkles to simulate the heart's complex anisotropic and multiscale architecture and showed that the hESC-CMs cultured on these 'microgrooved' substrates display the typical tropomyosin banding pattern consistent with organized sarcomeric structure patterns (Luna et al., 2011) (Figure 4, adopted with permission from Luna et al 2011 *Tissue Eng Part C Methods* Vol. 17, No. 5: pp.579-588). Quantitative assessment based on nuclei shape and actin organization show that the hESC-CMs exhibit increased alignment on microgrooved substrates compared with controls. Functionally, aligned monolayers of hESC-CMs display anisotropic conduction properties with distinct longitudinal and transverse velocities, a signature characteristic of the native heart, not seen in control randomly organized monolayers (Lieu, Wang, Khine and Li, unpublished data). In another approach to mimic the structure of the heart, the Costa lab was among the first to construct 3-D engineered cardiac tissue constructs including cardiac papillary-like muscle strips as well as ventricle-like "organoid" chambers that exhibit key characteristics of cardiac physiology by ejecting fluid and displaying force-frequency and pressure-volume relationships (Kim, Do Eun et al., 2006; Lee et al., 2008). These studies were originally performed using rat cardiac myocytes but are now being applied to hESC/iPSC-CMs. Further optimization of hESC/iPSC-based cardiac tissue constructs will not only provide powerful tools for disease modeling, drug/cardiotoxicity screening and clinical translations, but physiologic 3D environment also promises to reveal novel insights not possible with conventional rigid 2D culture systems.

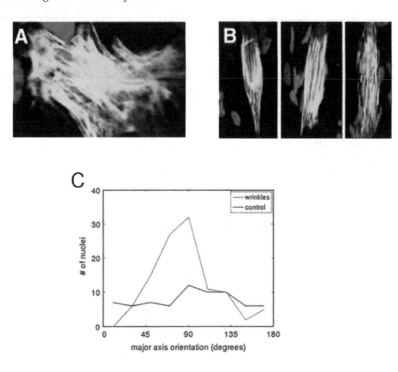

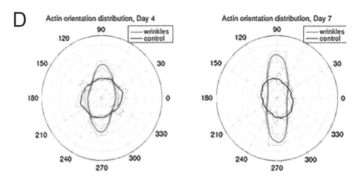

Fig. 4. Confocal micrographs of hESC-derived CMs alignment on wrinkles.
Human ESC-CMs were isolated and cultured on flat substrate (A) and wrinkle substrates (B) for 8 days. Green indicates tropomyosin staining, blue nuclear staining DAPI.
C) Image processing was used to detect the orientation of the DAPI-labeled nuclei. D) Anisotropy analysis of control (black) versus green (on wrinkles) showing that 90° is direction of wrinkles. The thinner lines indicate the standard deviations. Adopted with permission from Luna et al 2011 *Tissue Eng Part C Methods* Vol. 17, No. 5: pp.579-588.

7. Pharmacological testing using hESC-CMs

Adverse cardiac side effects is one of the most frequent reasons that cause drugs to be removed from the market. For instance, Vioxx, a once widely used COX-2 inhibitor prescribed to patients with arthritis and other conditions causing acute and chronic pain, was withdrawn from the market due to unexpected cardiotoxicity. Therefore, cardiotoxicity screening is necessary to test the efficacy and safety of new drug treatments. Cardiotoxicity arises from various mechanisms, including the modulation of signaling pathways and/or interference with the I_{Kr} current. The hERG channel, which produces the I_{Kr} current, is robustly blocked by a large class of drugs. This current has a major role in cardiac repolarization, so it affects the length of the action potential and the QT interval (the duration of ventricular depolarization and subsequent repolarization). QT prolongation may lead to arrhythmias, e.g. torsade de pointes, with potentially lethal consequences. Since adult CMs do not proliferate, animal CMs, isolated hearts or non-cardiac cells, which express cardiac ion channels are used although their non-human origin and instability in culture greatly limit their usefulness. Human ESC and hiPSC may provide an unlimited cell source for cardiotoxicity screening. Preliminary studies have already established that hESC-CMs/hiPSC-CMs do express the hERG mRNA (Sartiani et al., 2007; Tanaka et al., 2009), and display an outward 'I_{Kr}-like' current that is sensitive to selective blockers of I_{Kr} and canonical long QT-inducing inhibitors including E4031, sotalol, and cisapride (Sartiani et al., 2007; Caspi et al., 2009). When treated with a range of cardiac and non-cardiac drugs, hESC-CM also exhibit dose responses predictive of clinical effects (Braam et al., 2010). These suggest that hESC-CMs may be a suitable model for cardiotoxicity testing, although issues of CM purity and maturation should be considered in the design of future experiments, as already discussed elsewhere. It is hoped that high-throughput pharmacological systems involving hESC/hiPSC-CMs will soon be developed.

8. Human ESC-CMs/hiPSC-CMs as models of cardiovascular diseases

The use of hESC-/hiPSC-CMs as models of cardiac disorders is an exciting area of research. Previously, transgenic mouse models were used to study human cardiac diseases, but these mouse models do not always fully recapitulate the same phenotypes as those seen in humans. For instance, electrophysiologically, mice also have shorter action potential duration and higher heart rate compared to humans (Danik et al., 2002), limiting their usefulness as models of some disorders such as arrhythmias. Human pluripotent stem cell derived CMs are therefore logical suitable alternative. Reprogramming technology pioneered by Yamanaka and Thomson has led to the creation of disease- or patient-specific iPSCs. The derivation of hiPSC from patients with a range of diseases including adenosine deaminase deficiency-related severe combined immunodeficiency, Shwachman-Bodian-Diamond syndrome, Gaucher disease type III, Duchenne and Becker muscular dystrophy, Parkinson disease, Huntington disease, juvenile-onset, type 1 diabetes mellitus, Down Syndrome/trisomy 21, and the carrier state of Lesch-Nyhan syndrome has been reported (Park et al., 2008). More recently, Ebert et al (2009) reported the generation of hiPSC line from a patient of spinal muscular atrophy and these cells maintained the disease genotype and generated motor neurons that showed selective deficits compared to those derived from the patient's unaffected mother (Ebert et al., 2009). Some advances have also been made in the area of cardiovascular research. For instance, hiPSC models of long-QT syndrome type 1 and type 2 were generated (Moretti et al., 2010; Itzhaki et al., 2011). CMs differentiated from these hiPSC recapitulated the electrophysiological features of the disorders such as prolongation of AP and arrhythmogenicity and enabled the groups to study the pathogenesis of the diseases. Itzhaki et al (2011) also used the hiPSC-CMs to evaluate the potency of existing and novel pharmacological agents that may either aggravate or ameliorate the long-QT syndrome type 2 disease phenotype. These studies illustrate the potential of human iPSC technology to model the abnormal functional phenotype of inherited cardiac disorders and to identify potential new therapeutic agents.

9. Conclusion

Adult CMs lack the potential to regenerate. Human ESC and hiPSCs, with their potential for unlimited self-renewal and differentiation, offer an exciting means of generating human CMs for research and regenerative medicine. Concentrated effort by research groups worldwide has resulted in higher efficiency of cardiogenic differentiation and better characterization of hESC-/hiPSC-CMs. Experiments using animal models have demonstrated functional improvement after hESC-CM transplantation. However, substantial hurdles have to be overcome before hESC-/hiPSC-CMs can be translated into clinical applications. For instance, hESC-CMs are functionally immature, limiting their use for transplantation and as disease models. More studies are required to evaluate the long term effect of hESC-/hiPSC-CMs transplantation. Nonetheless, there is much reason to believe that hESC and hiPSC technology will bring significant benefit to cardiac research and treatment.

10. References

Aasen, T., A. Raya, et al., (2008). Efficient and rapid generation of induced pluripotent stem cells from human keratinocytes. *Nat Biotechnol* Vol. 26, No. 11: pp.1276-1284.

Anderson, D., T. Self, et al., (2007). Transgenic enrichment of cardiomyocytes from human embryonic stem cells. *Mol Ther* Vol. 15, No. 11: pp.2027-2036.

Azene, E. M., T. Xue, et al., (2005). Non-equilibrium behavior of HCN channels: insights into the role of HCN channels in native and engineered pacemakers. *Cardiovasc Res* Vol. 67, No. 2: pp.263-273.

Balsam, L. B., A. J. Wagers, et al., (2004). Haematopoietic stem cells adopt mature haematopoietic fates in ischaemic myocardium. *Nature* Vol. 428, No. 6983: pp.668-673.

Bers, D. M., (2002). Cardiac excitation-contraction coupling. *Nature* Vol. 415, No. 6868: pp.198-205.

Braam, S. R., L. Tertoolen, et al., (2010). Prediction of drug-induced cardiotoxicity using human embryonic stem cell-derived cardiomyocytes. *Stem Cell Res* Vol. 4, No. 2: pp.107-116.

Brette, F. and C. Orchard, (2003). T-tubule function in mammalian cardiac myocytes. *Circ Res* Vol. 92, No. 11: pp.1182-1192.

Brette, F. and C. Orchard, (2007). Resurgence of cardiac t-tubule research. *Physiology (Bethesda)* Vol. 22, No. 167-173.

Caspi, O., I. Itzhaki, et al., (2009). In vitro electrophysiological drug testing using human embryonic stem cell derived cardiomyocytes. *Stem Cells Dev* Vol. 18, No. 1: pp.161-172.

Chan, J. W., D. K. Lieu, et al., (2009). Label-free separation of human embryonic stem cells and their cardiac derivatives using Raman spectroscopy. *Anal Chem* Vol. 81, No. 4: pp.1324-1331.

Chan, Y. C., C. W. Siu, et al., (2009). Synergistic effects of inward rectifier (I) and pacemaker (I) currents on the induction of bioengineered cardiac automaticity. *J Cardiovasc Electrophysiol* Vol. 20, No. 9: pp.1048-1054.

Danik, S., C. Cabo, et al., (2002). Correlation of repolarization of ventricular monophasic action potential with ECG in the murine heart. *Am J Physiol Heart Circ Physiol* Vol. 283, No. 1: pp.H372-381.

Dolnikov, K., M. Shilkrut, et al., (2006). Functional properties of human embryonic stem cell-derived cardiomyocytes: intracellular Ca2+ handling and the role of sarcoplasmic reticulum in the contraction. *Stem Cells* Vol. 24, No. 2: pp.236-245.

Ebert, A. D., J. Yu, et al., (2009). Induced pluripotent stem cells from a spinal muscular atrophy patient. *Nature* Vol. 457, No. 7227: pp.277-280.

Fu, J. D., P. Jiang, et al., (2010). Na+/Ca2+ exchanger is a determinant of excitation-contraction coupling in human embryonic stem cell-derived ventricular cardiomyocytes. *Stem Cells Dev* Vol. 19, No. 6: pp.773-782.

Gore, A., Z. Li, et al., (2011). Somatic coding mutations in human induced pluripotent stem cells. *Nature* Vol. 471, No. 7336: pp.63-67.

He, J. Q., Y. Ma, et al., (2003). Human embryonic stem cells develop into multiple types of cardiac myocytes: action potential characterization. *Circ Res* Vol. 93, No. 1: pp.32-39.

Huangfu, D., K. Osafune, et al., (2008). Induction of pluripotent stem cells from primary human fibroblasts with only Oct4 and Sox2. *Nat Biotechnol* Vol. 26, No. 11: pp.1269-1275.

Huber, I., I. Itzhaki, et al., (2007). Identification and selection of cardiomyocytes during human embryonic stem cell differentiation. *FASEB J* Vol. 21, No. 10: pp.2551-2563.

Itzhaki, I., L. Maizels, et al., (2011). Modelling the long QT syndrome with induced pluripotent stem cells. *Nature* Vol. 471, No. 7337: pp.225-229.

Kehat, I., D. Kenyagin-Karsenti, et al., (2001). Human embryonic stem cells can differentiate into myocytes with structural and functional properties of cardiomyocytes. *J Clin Invest* Vol. 108, No. 3: pp.407-414.

Kehat, I., L. Khimovich, et al., (2004). Electromechanical integration of cardiomyocytes derived from human embryonic stem cells. *Nat Biotechnol* Vol. 22, No. 10: pp.1282-1289.

Kim, D. E., L. Eun Jung, et al. (2006). Engineered Cardiac Tissues for in vitro Assessment of Contractile Function and Repair Mechanisms, *Engineering in Medicine and Biology Society, 2006. EMBS '06. 28th Annual International Conference of the IEEE*, 2006

Kim, J. B., H. Zaehres, et al., (2008). Pluripotent stem cells induced from adult neural stem cells by reprogramming with two factors. *Nature* Vol. 454, No. 7204: pp.646-650.

Kong, C. W., F. G. Akar, et al., (2010). Translational potential of human embryonic and induced pluripotent stem cells for myocardial repair: insights from experimental models. *Thromb Haemost* Vol. 104, No. 1: pp.30-38.

Laflamme, M. A., K. Y. Chen, et al., (2007). Cardiomyocytes derived from human embryonic stem cells in pro-survival factors enhance function of infarcted rat hearts. *Nat Biotechnol* Vol. 25, No. 9: pp.1015-1024.

Lee, E. J., E. Kim do, et al., (2008). Engineered cardiac organoid chambers: toward a functional biological model ventricle. *Tissue Eng Part A* Vol. 14, No. 2: pp.215-225.

Lesso, H. and R. A. Li, (2003). Helical secondary structure of the external S3-S4 linker of pacemaker (HCN) channels revealed by site-dependent perturbations of activation phenotype. *J Biol Chem* Vol. 278, No. 25: pp.22290-22297.

Lieu, D. K., Y. C. Chan, et al., (2008). Overexpression of HCN-encoded pacemaker current silences bioartificial pacemakers. *Heart Rhythm* Vol. 5, No. 9: pp.1310-1317.

Lieu, D. K., J. Liu, et al., (2009). Absence of transverse tubules contributes to non-uniform Ca(2+) wavefronts in mouse and human embryonic stem cell-derived cardiomyocytes. *Stem Cells Dev* Vol. 18, No. 10: pp.1493-1500.

Liu, J., J. D. Fu, et al., (2007). Functional sarcoplasmic reticulum for calcium handling of human embryonic stem cell-derived cardiomyocytes: insights for driven maturation. *Stem Cells* Vol. 25, No. 12: pp.3038-3044.

Liu, J., D. K. Lieu, et al., (2009). Facilitated maturation of Ca2+ handling properties of human embryonic stem cell-derived cardiomyocytes by calsequestrin expression. *Am J Physiol Cell Physiol* Vol. 297, No. 1: pp.C152-159.

Luna, J. I., J. Ciriza, et al., (2011). Multiscale biomimetic topography for the alignment of neonatal and embryonic stem cell-derived heart cells. *Tissue Eng Part C Methods* Vol. 17, No. 5: pp.579-588.

Menasche, P., A. A. Hagege, et al., (2003). Autologous skeletal myoblast transplantation for severe postinfarction left ventricular dysfunction. *J Am Coll Cardiol* Vol. 41, No. 7: pp.1078-1083.

Mignone, J. L., K. L. Kreutziger, et al., (2010). Cardiogenesis from human embryonic stem cells. *Circ J* Vol. 74, No. 12: pp.2517-2526.

Moretti, A., M. Bellin, et al., (2010). Patient-specific induced pluripotent stem-cell models for long-QT syndrome. *N Engl J Med* Vol. 363, No. 15: pp.1397-1409.

Mummery, C., D. Ward-van Oostwaard, et al., (2003). Differentiation of human embryonic stem cells to cardiomyocytes: role of coculture with visceral endoderm-like cells. *Circulation* Vol. 107, No. 21: pp.2733-2740.

Mummery, C., D. Ward, et al., (2002). Cardiomyocyte differentiation of mouse and human embryonic stem cells. *J Anat* Vol. 200, No. Pt 3: pp.233-242.

Mummery, C. L., D. Ward, et al., (2007). Differentiation of human embryonic stem cells to cardiomyocytes by coculture with endoderm in serum-free medium. *Curr Protoc Stem Cell Biol* Vol. Chapter 1, No. Unit 1F 2.

Murry, C. E., M. H. Soonpaa, et al., (2004). Haematopoietic stem cells do not transdifferentiate into cardiac myocytes in myocardial infarcts. *Nature* Vol. 428, No. 6983: pp.664-668.

Murry, C. E., R. W. Wiseman, et al., (1996). Skeletal myoblast transplantation for repair of myocardial necrosis. *J Clin Invest* Vol. 98, No. 11: pp.2512-2523.

Nakagawa, M., M. Koyanagi, et al., (2008). Generation of induced pluripotent stem cells without Myc from mouse and human fibroblasts. *Nat Biotechnol* Vol. 26, No. 1: pp.101-106.

Norstrom, A., K. Akesson, et al., (2006). Molecular and pharmacological properties of human embryonic stem cell-derived cardiomyocytes. *Exp Biol Med (Maywood)* Vol. 231, No. 11: pp.1753-1762.

Park, I. H., N. Arora, et al., (2008). Disease-specific induced pluripotent stem cells. *Cell* Vol. 134, No. 5: pp.877-886.

Passier, R., D. W. Oostwaard, et al., (2005). Increased cardiomyocyte differentiation from human embryonic stem cells in serum-free cultures. *Stem Cells* Vol. 23, No. 6: pp.772-780.

Pekkanen-Mattila, M., H. Chapman, et al., (2010). Human embryonic stem cell-derived cardiomyocytes: demonstration of a portion of cardiac cells with fairly mature electrical phenotype. *Exp Biol Med (Maywood)* Vol. 235, No. 4: pp.522-530.

Sartiani, L., E. Bettiol, et al., (2007). Developmental changes in cardiomyocytes differentiated from human embryonic stem cells: a molecular and electrophysiological approach. *Stem Cells* Vol. 25, No. 5: pp.1136-1144.

Shake, J. G., P. J. Gruber, et al., (2002). Mesenchymal stem cell implantation in a swine myocardial infarct model: engraftment and functional effects. *Ann Thorac Surg* Vol. 73, No. 6: pp.1919-1925; discussion 1926.

Siu, C. W., D. K. Lieu, et al., (2006). HCN-encoded pacemaker channels: from physiology and biophysics to bioengineering. *J Membr Biol* Vol. 214, No. 3: pp.115-122.

Smits, P. C., R. J. van Geuns, et al., (2003). Catheter-based intramyocardial injection of autologous skeletal myoblasts as a primary treatment of ischemic heart failure: clinical experience with six-month follow-up. *J Am Coll Cardiol* Vol. 42, No. 12: pp.2063-2069.

Snir, M., I. Kehat, et al., (2003). Assessment of the ultrastructural and proliferative properties of human embryonic stem cell-derived cardiomyocytes. *Am J Physiol Heart Circ Physiol* Vol. 285, No. 6: pp.H2355-2363.

Takahashi, K., K. Tanabe, et al., (2007). Induction of pluripotent stem cells from adult human fibroblasts by defined factors. *Cell* Vol. 131, No. 5: pp.861-872.

Takahashi, K. and S. Yamanaka, (2006). Induction of pluripotent stem cells from mouse embryonic and adult fibroblast cultures by defined factors. *Cell* Vol. 126, No. 4: pp.663-676.

Tanaka, T., S. Tohyama, et al., (2009). In vitro pharmacologic testing using human induced pluripotent stem cell-derived cardiomyocytes. *Biochem Biophys Res Commun* Vol. 385, No. 4: pp.497-502.

Thomson, J. A., J. Itskovitz-Eldor, et al., (1998). Embryonic stem cell lines derived from human blastocysts. *Science* Vol. 282, No. 5391: pp.1145-1147.

Toma, C., M. F. Pittenger, et al., (2002). Human mesenchymal stem cells differentiate to a cardiomyocyte phenotype in the adult murine heart. *Circulation* Vol. 105, No. 1: pp.93-98.

Tsang, S. Y., H. Lesso, et al., (2004). Critical intra-linker interactions of HCN1-encoded pacemaker channels revealed by interchange of S3-S4 determinants. *Biochem Biophys Res Commun* Vol. 322, No. 2: pp.652-658.

Tsang, S. Y., H. Lesso, et al., (2004). Dissecting the structural and functional roles of the S3-S4 linker of pacemaker (hyperpolarization-activated cyclic nucleotide-modulated) channels by systematic length alterations. *J Biol Chem* Vol. 279, No. 42: pp.43752-43759.

Tse, H. F., T. Xue, et al., (2006). Bioartificial sinus node constructed via in vivo gene transfer of an engineered pacemaker HCN Channel reduces the dependence on electronic pacemaker in a sick-sinus syndrome model. *Circulation* Vol. 114, No. 10: pp.1000-1011.

Warren, L., P. D. Manos, et al., (2010). Highly efficient reprogramming to pluripotency and directed differentiation of human cells with synthetic modified mRNA. *Cell Stem Cell* Vol. 7, No. 5: pp.618-630.

Xu, C., S. Police, et al., (2002). Characterization and enrichment of cardiomyocytes derived from human embryonic stem cells. *Circ Res* Vol. 91, No. 6: pp.501-508.

Xu, X. Q., R. Graichen, et al., (2008). Chemically defined medium supporting cardiomyocyte differentiation of human embryonic stem cells. *Differentiation* Vol. 76, No. 9: pp.958-970.

Xue, T., H. C. Cho, et al., (2005). Functional integration of electrically active cardiac derivatives from genetically engineered human embryonic stem cells with quiescent recipient ventricular cardiomyocytes: insights into the development of cell-based pacemakers. *Circulation* Vol. 111, No. 1: pp.11-20.

Xue, T., C. W. Siu, et al., (2007). Mechanistic role of I(f) revealed by induction of ventricular automaticity by somatic gene transfer of gating-engineered pacemaker (HCN) channels. *Circulation* Vol. 115, No. 14: pp.1839-1850.

Yang, L., M. H. Soonpaa, et al., (2008). Human cardiovascular progenitor cells develop from a KDR+ embryonic-stem-cell-derived population. *Nature* Vol. 453, No. 7194: pp.524-528.

Yu, J., M. A. Vodyanik, et al., (2007). Induced pluripotent stem cell lines derived from human somatic cells. *Science* Vol. 318, No. 5858: pp.1917-1920.

Zwi, L., O. Caspi, et al., (2009). Cardiomyocyte differentiation of human induced pluripotent stem cells. *Circulation* Vol. 120, No. 15: pp.1513-1523.

11

Maintenance Of Calcium Homeostasis in Embryonic Stem Cell-Derived Cardiomyocytes

Iek Chi Lo[1], Chun Kit Wong[1] and Suk Ying Tsang[1,2,3,4*]
[1]School of Life Sciences, The Chinese University of Hong Kong
[2]State Key Laboratory of Agrobiotechnology, The Chinese University of Hong Kong
[3]Stem Cell and Regeneration Program, School of Biomedical Sciences,
The Chinese University of Hong Kong
[4]Key Laboratory for Regenerative Medicine, Ministry of Education,
The Chinese University of Hong Kong
Hong Kong Special Administrative Region

1. Introduction

Myocardial infarction is one of the major causes of morbidity and mortality in many developed countries. A potential method for treatment of such disease is the cell replacement therapy which involves the transplantation of cardiomyocytes (CMs). However, CMs are of very limited supply. Embryonic stem cells (ESCs) isolated from the inner cell mass of blastocysts are capable of self-renewal and can differentiate into all cell lineages, including CMs (He et al., 2003; Kehat et al., 2002; Kehat et al., 2001; Moore et al., 2008; Mummery et al., 2003; Ng et al., 2010; Thomson et al., 1998; Xu et al., 2002; Xue et al., 2005). Therefore, ESCs can be an excellent source of CMs for regenerative medicine.

Calcium (Ca^{2+}) is a universal signaling molecule that regulates a wide variety of cellular functions. In CMs, intracellular Ca^{2+} concentration ($[Ca^{2+}]_i$) plays an important role in the contraction and relaxation of CMs. The $[Ca^{2+}]_i$ is tightly regulated by many proteins, including ion channels, receptors, pumps, and exchangers that are located on the cell surface plasma membrane and on the sarcoplasmic reticulum (SR). The aim of this book chapter is to provide a thorough review on Ca^{2+} handling in ESC-derived CMs.

For each protein of interest, some basic information on the protein was firstly presented. Then, changes in the expression of the protein and their contribution to the Ca^{2+} homeostasis and Ca^{2+} transient as described in human (h) and/or mouse (m) ESC studies were presented. *In vivo* data in mouse embryo studies were also presented for comparison purposes.

The information reviewed in this chapter would be important not only for understanding the basic biology of early differentiating CMs, it would also be important for providing insights into the future uses of ESC-derived CMs for cell replacement therapies.

2. Regulation of intracellular calcium level by voltage-operated calcium channels

Voltage-operated Ca^{2+} channels are typically composed of five subunits, namely α_1, α_2, β, δ and γ (Catterall, 1995; Catterall, 2000; De Waard et al., 1996; Dolphin, 2006; Moreno Davila,

---

* Corresponding author.

1999). The α_1 subunit forms the ion conduction pore of the channels while the other subunits modulate the functions of the channels. The α_1 subunit is itself a tetramer of proteins, each of which consists of six transmembrane segments (S1-S6). This subunit confers all of the major properties to voltage-operated Ca^{2+} channels in that it contains a voltage sensor at segment S4 and forms a Ca^{2+}-selective pore at segments S5-S6. The other subunits are regarded as to providing ancillary functions to the channels. The α_2 and δ subunits are two products of the same gene; the protein is cleaved into two peptides following translation. Subsequent disulfide bond formation anchors the extracellular α_2 subunit to the membrane via the transmembrane δ subunit. The β subunit is a cytoplasmic protein; it contains an α_1-binding pocket, where specific amino acids in the linker region between segments S1 and S2 of the α_1 subunit bind (Richards et al., 2004). The γ subunit is a monomer, which consists of four transmembrane segments (S1-S4). A diverse range of functionally distinct voltage-operated Ca^{2+} channels are formed by the combinations of different isoforms that have been identified for each of these subunits. The α_1 subunit is encoded by a family of ten distinct genes (the Ca_V gene family), which can be divided into three sub-families; Ca_V1 consists of $Ca_V1.1-1.4$, Ca_V2 consists of $Ca_V2.1-2.3$ and Ca_V3 consists of $Ca_V3.1-3.3$ (Catterall et al., 2005). The α_2/δ and β subunits are each encoded by four genes; α_2/δ_{1-4} and β_{1-4} respectively, while the γ subunit is encoded by eight genes; γ_{1-8} (Arikkath and Campbell, 2003; Yang et al., 2011). Voltage-operated Ca^{2+} channels function by regulating the entry of extracellular Ca^{2+} into cells. Two types of voltage-operated Ca^{2+} channels exist in adult CMs (Catterall et al., 2005; Ono and Iijima, 2005). These are T-type Ca^{2+} channels, which open in response to more negative membrane potentials at about >-70mV for very short durations of 0.5 to 2 milliseconds (transient activation), and L-type Ca^{2+} channels, which open in response to less negative membrane potentials at about >-30mV for relatively longer periods of 0.5 to 10 milliseconds (long-lasting activation) (De Waard et al., 1996).

2.1 T-type calcium channels

T-type Ca^{2+} channels could be the simplest type of voltage-operated Ca^{2+} channels known thus far. Its structure was initially predicted *in silico* by homology to other α_1 subunits known at the time (Perez-Reyes, 2006). Since expression of the synthetic products was able to reproduce most of the electrophysiological properties observed in its native form, T-type Ca^{2+} channels were thought to consist of only one α_1 subunit; the other ancillary subunits (α_2, β, δ and γ) were considered absent. Although later co-expression studies could describe a role for the other ancillary subunits in the regulating functions of T-type Ca^{2+} channels *in vitro*, presence of these subunits have not been validated *in vivo* (Dolphin et al., 1999; Dubel et al., 2004; Green et al., 2001; Hobom et al., 2000; Lacinova and Klugbauer, 2004). Therefore, further investigations will be required to ascertain the genuine structure of this type of voltage-operated Ca^{2+} channel.

The α_1 subunit of T-type Ca^{2+} channels is encoded by either one of the three Ca_V3 genes, among which $Ca_V3.1$ and $Ca_V3.2$ are expressed in sinoatrial (SA) nodal cells of the heart (Bohn et al., 2000; Perez-Reyes, 2003). The SA node is the primary site, where spontaneous rhythmic action potentials are initiated. At the beginning of each action potential in an SA nodal cell, an influx of extracellular Na^+ into the cytosol, known as the funny current (I_f), first depolarizes the cell to about -50mV, at which T-type Ca^{2+} channels on the membrane open to allow an influx of extracellular Ca^{2+} into the cytosol. This produces a T-type Ca^{2+} current ($I_{Ca, T}$), which further depolarizes the cell to about -40mV. L-type Ca^{2+} channels on the membrane then open at this membrane potential to allow a greater influx of extracellular

Ca^{2+} into the cytosol and produce an L-type Ca^{2+} current ($I_{Ca, L}$) to a membrane potential until the threshold to produce an action potential is reached. Action potentials generated in the SA nodal cells are conducted to CMs within the working myocardium via gap junctions, ultimately resulting in regular contractions of the adult heart.

$Ca_V3.1$ mRNA and protein were simultaneously detected as early as embryonic day 14 (E14) after the heart has fully matured *in vivo* within mouse embryos (Cribbs et al., 2001). In a separate experiment, the mRNA level of $Ca_V3.1$ was moderately reduced from E18 when compared to its expression at adult stage (Yasui et al., 2005). Ni^{2+} at a high concentration of 100µM could be used to selectively block 50% of $Ca_V3.1$ T-type channels. The application of Ni^{2+} at this concentration was found to reduce $I_{Ca, T}$ by about 40% in CMs derived from mouse embryos at E12.5, indicating that the $Ca_V3.1$ T-type channels were functional by this time-point (Cribbs et al., 2001). In addition, homozygous null $Ca_V3.1^{-/-}$ mice displayed bradycardia, i.e. a reduced rate of cardiac contraction (Mangoni et al., 2006). Expression of $Ca_V3.1$ has also been studied *in vitro*. Its mRNA could be detected as early as day 5 and generally increased up until its last measurement at day 15 post-differrntiation in ht7 mouse ESC- (mESC-) derived CMs (Mizuta et al., 2005). In R1 mESC-derived CMs, however, $Ca_V3.1$ mRNA could only be detected at two copies per cell by day 12, with its expression reaching the highest level at day 23 and declining by day 34 post-differentiation; the expression pattern reflected the amplitudes of $I_{Ca, T}$ measured at these time-points. (Zhang et al., 2003). A reduction of about 46% in $Ca_V3.1$ expression from day 9.5 to day 23.5 post-differentiation was also reported in EMG7 mESC-derived CMs; this down-regulation was found to be associated with a decrease in the contraction rates of the CMs in that $I_{Ca, T}$ was smaller in non-contracting myocytes at day 23.5 when compared to contracting CMs at day 9.5 and that the contraction rate at day 9.5 could be reduced via the application of 10µM efonidipine, an L- and T-type blocker, to the CMs (Yanagi et al., 2007). These data suggested a role for $Ca_V3.1$ in regulating the early contractions observed in the developing embryonic heart; by maintaining these contractions exclusively in developing pacemaker cells, other cells could then develop into non-contracting atrial or ventricular cells.

$Ca_V3.2$ mRNA was detected as early as eight-week gestation in humans (Qu and Boutjdir, 2001). In mouse, the expression of $Ca_V3.2$ was also measured at three time-points; its mRNA was detected as early as E9.5 and then its level was decreased by E18 until it was no longer detected at adult stage (Yasui et al., 2005). Again, $Ca_V3.2$ has been studied *in vitro*. Its mRNA was detected as early as day 5, but peaked at day 6 and gradually declined and was still detectable up until the last measurement at day 15 post-differentiation in ht7 mESC-derived CMs (Mizuta et al., 2005). In line with this finding, $Ca_V3.2$ mRNA level was also found to be down-regulated by about 24% from day 9.5 to day 23.5 post-differentiation in EMG7 mESC-derived CMs (Yanagi et al., 2007). Ni^{2+} at a low concentration of <50µM could be used to selectively block 50% of $Ca_V3.2$ T-type channels. When Ni^{2+} was applied at 40µM to ht7 mESC-derived CMs at day 8 post-differentiation, $I_{Ca, T}$ was found to be evidently decreased by about 60%, which signified the presence of functional $Ca_V3.2$ T-type channels by this time-point. Homozygous null $Ca_V3.2^{-/-}$ mice showed no sign of cardiac arrhythmia, but cardiac fibrosis with age-dependent severity (Chen et al., 2003). These data suggested a role for $Ca_V3.2$ in regulating the growth and maturation of the developing embryonic heart.

2.1.1 L-type calcium channels

L-type Ca^{2+} channels are distinguished from other voltage-operated Ca^{2+} channels that open at high membrane potentials for long periods on the basis of their sensitivity to 1, 4-

dihydropyridines (DHPs) (Hess et al., 1984). DHP-binding sites are contained within the α_1 subunit of L-type Ca^{2+} channels, which are encoded by either one of the four genes of the Ca_V1 sub-family. Among these, $Ca_V1.1$ is expressed predominantly in skeletal myocytes, $Ca_V1.2$ in adult CMs and $Ca_V1.3$ exclusively in SA nodal and atrial cells of the heart (Catterall, 2000; Qu et al., 2005). Unlike T-type, L-type Ca^{2+} channels are typical voltage-operated Ca^{2+} channels, which are made up of five subunits. Together with one of each of the α_2/δ_{1-4}, β_{1-3} and $\gamma_{4, 6-8}$ ancillary subunits, $Ca_V1.2$- and $Ca_V1.3$-encoded α_1 proteins form the functional L-type Ca^{2+} channels that are found within the adult heart (Freise et al., 1999; Hosey et al., 1996; Yang et al., 2011).

$Ca_V1.2$ L-type Ca^{2+} channels are responsible for cardiac excitation-contraction coupling (E-C coupling), a mechanism by which an action potential is transformed into contraction in adult CMs. Upon the arrival of an action potential from SA nodal cells, L-type Ca^{2+} channels, which are clustered at transverse tubules (T-tubules), briefly open at the sarcolemma to allow an influx of extracellular Ca^{2+} into the cytosol of the CMs. This only accounts for about 30% of the increase in cytosolic Ca^{2+}, which is maintained and magnified through a process known as calcium-induced calcium release (CICR) (Bers, 2002). CICR is mediated via ryanodine receptor (RyR) Ca^{2+} release channels, which detect the $I_{Ca, L}$ and open to release Ca^{2+} from its intracellular stores within the SR into the cytosol of the CMs. This rise enhances binding of Ca^{2+} to troponin within the CMs, ultimately bringing about contractions of the adult heart. Conversely, $Ca_V1.3$ L-type Ca^{2+} channels are responsible for producing $I_{Ca, L}$, which constitutes one of the ionic currents to initiate action potentials at the SA node. Hence, these L-type Ca^{2+} channels contribute in maintaining the pacemaker activity of the adult heart (see 'T-type calcium channels' for details).

Consistent with its role in E-C coupling in the adult heart, $Ca_V1.2$ mRNA was detected as early as eight-week gestation in humans, with its level culminating to its maximum at adult stage (Qu and Boutjdir, 2001). $Ca_V1.2$ mRNA was also present *in vitro* at <40 days post-beating in H9.2 human ESC- (hESC-) derived CMs (Satin et al., 2008). In H7 hESC-derived CMs, Ca^{2+} transients that were detected at day 17 post-differentiation could be eliminated by the application of 10μM diltiazem, an L-type specific antagonist; this signified the functionality of L-type channels by this time-point (Zhu et al., 2009). Similar to humans, the expression of $Ca_V1.2$ was also up-regulated from its initial detection at E9.5 when the earliest contractions were observed by about three-fold at E15.5 when the heart has fully matured in mouse embryos; its protein was detected by E12.5 in mouse embryos (Acosta et al., 2004; Xu et al., 2003). In mESCs, patch clamp and Ca^{2+} imaging experiments indicated the functional expression of the $I_{Ca, L}$ starting from differentiation day 7, even before the appearance of spontaneous contractions (Kolossov et al., 1998). The current density of I_{Ca} continued to increase to day 10, the day of beginning of spontaneous contractions in most differentiating embryoid bodies (EBs). Thereafter, similar current density was recorded on day 17, the last day of measurement (Kolossov et al., 1998). Homozygous null $Ca_V1.2^{-/-}$ mice died *in utero* by E14.5, probably due to an absence of CICR-regulated contractions, resulting in reduced oxygen supply to the embryos (Seisenberger et al., 2000). Despite the lethality observed, normal rhythmic contractions were sustained in the $Ca_V1.2^{-/-}$ mice until E12.5. For this reason, CICR was initially thought to be non-essential for regulating the early cardiac contractions observed before E12.5 until later time-points. This conclusion was further supported by the fact that both the contractions and Ca^{2+} oscillations of D3 mESC-derived CMs were insensitive to the application of 50nM nisoldipine, a specific L-type channel blocker, at days 8-11 post-differentiation (Viatchenko-Karpinski et al., 1999). In addition, these cells were insensitive to the application of high K$^+$ when compared to D3 mESC-derived CMs at day 16 post-differentiation; exposure to high K$^+$ at this stage would normally lead to immediate hyper-contraction and death of these cells. Albeit these findings, the notion that $I_{Ca, L}$ was not required at earlier stages of development was overthrown when evidence for the existence of a compensatory mechanism emerged; the expression of Ca$_V$1.3 was eminently up-regulated at E9.5 and E12.5 by four fold to produce a DHPR-insensitive $I_{Ca, L}$ in Ca$_V$1.2$^{-/-}$ mouse embryos when compared to wild-type (Xu et al., 2003). This has not only reinstated the importance of $I_{Ca, L}$ in maintaining cardiac contractions, even at the embryonic stage of the heart, but also appointed a new role for Ca$_V$1.3 to substitute for Ca$_V$1.2 and preserve its role in CICR for E-C coupling in its absence. In contrast with Ca$_V$1.2, Ca$_V$1.3 mRNA was detected by E9.5, with its level elevated only by a modest amount at E15.5 in mouse embryos. Its protein was also detected by E12.5 in mouse embryos (Xu et al., 2003). Analogous to Ca$_V$3.1$^{-/-}$ mice, homozygous null Ca$_V$1.3$^{-/-}$ mice developed bradycardia, consistent with its primary role in regulating the pacemaker activity of the heart (Platzer et al., 2000; Zhang et al., 2002). In R1 mESC-derived CMs, the expression of L-type Ca^{2+} channels could be detected as early as day 7 post-differentiation; given that the application of 1µM nifedipine, an L-type channel-specific antagonist, could eliminate Ca^{2+} transients that were normally observed at early (days 9-11) and intermediate (days 13-15), but only partially inhibit those at late (18-21 days post-differentiation) stages, this indicated that L-type channels were, in fact, playing a more dominant role at earlier developmental stages (Fu et al., 2006b).

2.2 Regulation of intracellular calcium level by ligand-operated calcium release channels

2.2.1 Ryanodine receptor (RyR) calcium release channels

RyR-Ca^{2+} release channels of a molecular mass of greater than two Mega-Daltons probably form the largest ion channels known thus far (Lanner et al., 2010). RyR-Ca^{2+} release channels are composed of homo-tetramers of RyR proteins. Owing to its enormous size, structural elucidation of these channels has been a major challenge. Nonetheless, RyR-Ca^{2+} release channels have been predicted to be largely cytoplasmic, with an ion-conducting pore consisting of around four to twelve transmembrane segments.

Three mammalian isoforms of RyRs exist; RyR1 is predominantly expressed in skeletal myocytes, RyR2 in CMs and RyR3 in astrocytes. The isoforms differ in three particular regions, which have been named domains D1-3 (Ma et al., 2004). As mentioned earlier in this chapter, RyR-Ca^{2+} release channels are induced to open in response to Ca^{2+} influx via L-type Ca^{2+} channels to facilitate E-C coupling in muscle cells. In skeletal myocytes, E-C coupling takes place through direct physical interaction between RyR1 and the D2 region, which is located between segments S2 and S3 of the Ca$_V$1.1-encoded α$_1$ subunit of L-type Ca^{2+} channels. In CMs, however, sequence divergence in the D2 domain between RyR1 and RyR2 means that RyR2 cannot physically interact with the Ca$_V$1.2-encoded α$_1$ subunit of L-type Ca^{2+} channels; E-C coupling can, therefore, only occur via CICR. RyR-Ca^{2+} release channels are, thus, organized into large arrays at junctions between the SR and the sarcolemma, in close proximity to the Ca$_V$1.2 L-type Ca^{2+} channels in adult CMs (Bers, 2004). Localized Ca^{2+} release events are referred to as Ca^{2+} sparks, which are collectively synchronized by $I_{Ca, L}$ to produce large, whole cell Ca^{2+} transients in the CMs.

Release of Ca^{2+} from the SR stores greatly increases the amount of cytosolic Ca^{2+} available to bind troponins in adult CMs. Adult CMs are mostly occupied by bouquets of thick and thin filaments. Thick filaments are composed of myosin II molecules, while thin filaments are made up of troponin, tropomyosin and actin molecules. Troponin is itself a globular complex, which consists of three subunits, namely troponin T (TnT), troponin C (TnC) and troponin I (TnI). The TnT subunit binds tropomyosin, which coils around strands of actin molecules in the thin filament. Binding of Ca^{2+} to the TnC subunit induces a conformational change in the TnI subunit, thereby removing the steric hindrance on actin from tropomyosin. Binding of myosin II to actin can then occur, inducing a conformational change in the complex. This pulls the actin-associated thin filament pass the myosin II-associated thick filament, resulting in a contracting phenomenon in the CMs.

RyR2 protein was present as early as day 17 post-differentiation in H7 hESC-derived CMs (Zhu et al., 2009). In H9.2 hESC-derived CMs, the application of a puff of 10mM caffeine was able to induce Ca^{2+} release from the SR as early as day 2 post-beating; this signified the functionality of RyR-channels in these cells at this early time-point (Satin et al., 2008). In mouse embryos, RyR2 mRNA was detected as early as E8.5, the level of which continued to increase up until its last measurement at E16.5 (Rosemblit et al., 1999). Ca^{2+} release from the SR was inducible by the application of 10mM caffeine, indicating the functionality of RyR2 channels by E8.5 in mouse embryos. In a different study, RyR2 protein was also detected at E18 and the detection persisted until adult stage (Liu et al., 2002). Homozygous null RyR2$^{-/-}$ mice died at E10, displaying morphological abnormalities in the heart tube (Takeshima et al., 1998). RyR2 expression has also been studied in vitro in mESC-derived CMs. RyR2 mRNA and protein were detected as early as day 5 and day 9 post-differentiation in mESC-derived CMs respectively (Boheler et al., 2002; Fu et al., 2006a). Immunohistochemistry revealed a continuous increase in RyR immunofluorescence intensity in differentiation day 15-25 CMs compared with differentiation day 8-11 CMs, suggesting an increasing density of RyRs during cardiac differentiation (Sauer et al., 2001). The application of 10mM caffeine elicited Ca^{2+} transients, the amplitudes of which increased from day 8 to day 17 post-differentiation in mESC-derived CMs (Kapur and Banach, 2007). Hence, RyR2 channels were functional by day 8 post-differentiation in mESC-derived CMs. RyR2$^{-/-}$ knockout R1 mESC-derived CMs exhibited no difference in the amplitudes of Ca^{2+} transients but contractions at a reduced rate from early (days 9-11) to intermediate (days 13- 15) to late (days 18-21 post-differentiation) differentiation stages when compared with wild-type (Fu et al., 2006a; Yang et al., 2002). The applications of 10µM ryanodine and 10mM caffeine were able to inhibit and induce Ca^{2+} release from the SR respectively. Cardiac differentiation was not affected, as indicated by the number of contracting colonies present in the differentiating cultures. Both effects of ryanodine and caffeine were seen to increase with time post-differentiation, indicating that SR Ca^{2+} loads increased during differentiation (Fu et al., 2006a; Sauer et al., 2001). Altogether, these findings suggested a role for RyR to mediate SR Ca^{2+} release, thereby regulating the rate of the earliest contractions observed in the developing embryonic heart, and that this regulation increases with differentiation.

2.2.2 Inositol 1, 4, 5-trisphosphate Receptor (IP₃R) calcium release channels

IP_3R Ca^{2+} release channels represent a type of enigmatic intracellular Ca^{2+} channels in that both its structure and function(s) are not fully understood (Foskett et al., 2007; Taylor et al., 2004; Taylor and Tovey, 2010; Yule et al., 2010). IP_3R-Ca^{2+} release channels can be formed from either homo- or hetero-tetramers of IP_3R proteins. Each subunit of IP_3R proteins contains an IP_3-binding domain at its N-terminus and six transmembrane segments (S1-6) at its C-terminus; the Ca^{2+}-selective pore is formed at segments S5-6. Three mammalian isoforms of IP$_3$R exist, namely IP$_3$R1, IP$_3$R2 and IP$_3$R3. These isoforms differ in their binding affinities for IP$_3$, with IP$_3$R2 being the most and IP$_3$R3 being the least sensitive to the ligand (Iwai et al., 2007; Tu et al., 2005). All three IP$_3$Rs are expressed in human adult CMs, but their subcellular localizations have not been studied (Nakazawa et al., 2011; Uchida et al., 2010). In rat adult CMs, these are expressed at about 50-fold lower than those of RyRs; IP$_3$R1s are localized around the nuclear envelope and SR, both of which are connected, while IP$_3$R2s are dispersed throughout the cytosol in a punctate pattern (Bare et al., 2005; Li et al., 2005; Moschella and Marks, 1993). Thus far, the role of IP$_3$Rs in the adult heart has not been defined, but an up-regulation in their expression has been associated with conditions of cardiac failure in that the mRNA levels of IP$_3$R1 and IP$_3$R2 were increased by 123% and 93% respectively in failing compared with normal heart tissues (Ai et al., 2005; Go et al., 1995).

Activation of IP$_3$R-Ca^{2+} release channels is regulated by both the concentration of cytosolic Ca^{2+} ions and the binding of IP$_3$ to one or more of the IP$_3$-binding domains (Iino, 1990; Taylor and Laude, 2002). Low concentrations of cytosolic Ca^{2+} ions are known to activate pore opening, while high concentrations inhibit it. IP$_3$ is a second messenger that is generated via a G protein-coupled receptor-mediated signal transduction pathway. G protein-coupled receptors are transmembrane receptors that are able to sense external stimuli and relay these signals into the cell via their interactions with cytosolic G proteins. G proteins are heterotrimeric complexes, which consist of a GDP-bound G$_\alpha$ subunit and a G$_{\beta\gamma}$ dimer. G protein-coupled receptors are classified into different types according to the isoform of the G$_\alpha$ subunits contained within their G protein-interacting partners. Generation of IP$_3$ involves the stimulation of a G$_q$ type of G protein-coupled receptors. Upon stimulation with their agonists, a conformational change is induced in the G$_q$ protein-coupled receptors. This causes an exchange of GDP for GTP in the G$_\alpha$ subunits, which then dissociate from their G$_q$ protein complexes. GTP-bound G$_\alpha$ subunits of G$_q$ protein complexes are responsible for activating phospholipase C. It is this enzyme, which hydrolyses phosphatidylinositol 4, 5-bisphosphate (PIP$_2$), a phospholipid component of the plasma membrane, to ultimately yield IP$_3$ and another second messenger, diacylglycerol (DAG). IP$_3$ then binds to and activates IP$_3$R-Ca^{2+} release channels.

IP$_3$R mRNA was present at detectable levels in D3 mESCs at the undifferentiated state (Yanagida et al., 2004). Application of 5μM ATP generated a Ca^{2+} transient in the undifferentiated D3 mESCs, which was inhibited by pre-treatment with 75μM 2-APB, an IP$_3$R blocker. This verified the functionality of IP$_3$R-channels in these cells. In H9.2 hESCs, immunostaining indicated that both IP$_3$R1 and IP$_3$R2 were expressed in hESC-dervied CMs (Sedan et al., 2010; Sedan et al., 2008); and the expression of IP$_3$R2 was shown to gradually decline with maturation as revealed by quantitative RT-PCR (Satin et al., 2008). The expression of IP$_3$R was also tested during development *in vivo*; its mRNA was first measured and detected as early as E5.5 in mouse embryos; it was present at high levels by E8.5 and continued to increase until E16.5 when its level started to drop (Rosemblit et al., 1999). These were demonstrated to be functional at two time-points; application of 5μM of IP$_3$ was able to induce Ca^{2+} release from the SR in CMs derived from mouse embryos at E5.5 and E8.5. Application of 5μM xestospongin C, an IP$_3$R antagonist, to mouse embryos at E10 diminished its Ca^{2+} spiking; washing the drug out allowed slow recovery of this spiking activity (Mery et al., 2005). Likewise, application of 5μM xestospongin C also abrogated the Ca^{2+} spiking activity observed in CGR8 mESC-derived CMs at day 8-10 post-differentiation. In addition, during the whole course of cardiac differentiation of R1 mESCs, 2-APB decreased both the amplitude and upstroke velocity of Ca^{2+} transients, with the inhibitory effect decreased as differentiation proceeded, suggesting that IP_3R contributes to the Ca^{2+} transient and its effect decreases with differentiation (Fu et al., 2006b). In an attempt to discriminate between the roles of RyR- and IP_3R2- channels, $50\mu M$ ryanodine was first used to block RyR-channels before the application of 5-20μM IP_3-AM to CMs derived from mouse embryos at E10 (Rapila et al., 2008). This was able to induce a Ca^{2+} leak from the SR of the CMs in a concentration-dependent manner, whereby the slopes of the Ca^{2+} transients were elevated, despite its frequency stayed unchanged. In the absence of ryanodine, however, application of 10μM IP_3-AM led to an increase in the frequency of Ca^{2+} transients and, hence, increased contractions in the CMs at E10. These data suggested a role for IP_3R in regulating the rate of the earliest contractions observed in the developing embryonic heart, perhaps by providing a source of Ca^{2+} to bind RyRs so as to increase its open probability for greater Ca^{2+} release from the SR, as suggested by Rapila et al. (Rapila et al., 2008) In support of this finding, genetic knockdown of IP_3R in CGR8 mESC-derived pacemaker cells resulted in weak and infrequent contractions, although differentiation was not affected, whilst mice over-expressing the IP_3R2 gene developed mild cardiac hypertrophy by three months of age (Mery et al., 2005; Nakayama et al., 2010).

2.3 Regulation of intracellular calcium level by exchanger and pump

As previously mentioned, upon arrival of cardiac action potential, activation of L-type Ca^{2+} channel followed by CICR increases $[Ca^{2+}]_i$ for the contraction process. Subsequently, the excess Ca^{2+} has to be removed in order to initiate relaxation. In CMs, this Ca^{2+} removal process is mediated by different Ca^{2+} extrusion mechanisms via the action of sodium-calcium exchanger (NCX) and sarcoplasmic/endoplasmic reticulum Ca^{2+}-ATPase (SERCA).

2.3.1 Sodium-calcium exchanger (NCX)

NCX contains 9 transmembrane segments with a large loop at the cytoplasmic side (Philipson and Nicoll, 2000). Mutation experiments demonstrated the importance of α-helices in the transmembrane segments for the transport activity of NCX (Nicoll et al., 1996). The large intracellular loop is found to be not essential for the transport; however, it is important for catalyzing the ion translocation reaction and has important regulatory functions (Philipson and Nicoll, 2000). This loop consists of multiple regulatory sites, including the regulatory Ca^{2+} binding site and the exchanger inhibitory peptide (XIP) region. The activity of NCX is known to be regulated by at least 4 factors, including Ca^{2+} (DiPolo, 1979), Na^+ (Hilgemann et al., 1992), PIP_2 (Hilgemann, 1990), and phosphorylation (Iwamoto et al., 1996). Binding of Ca^{2+} to the Ca^{2+} binding site is required for activating the Na^+-Ca^{2+} exchange activity (Giladi et al., 2010; Ottolia et al., 2004; Wu et al., 2010). On the other hand, the XIP region is responsible for the Na^+-dependent inactivation and is involved in the elimination of the Na^+-dependent inactivation process by PIP_2 (Matsuoka et al., 1997). The activity of NCX is also regulated by phosphorylation, with stronger phosphorylation leading to higher NCX activity (Reppel et al., 2007a). Requirements of direct phosphorylation for up-regulation of NCX function by PKA and PKC are still in debate. A recent study by Wanichawan et al. demonstrated that the PKA phosphorylation site in full-length NCX1 is inaccessible, suggesting that NCX1 is not a direct substrate of PKA (Wanichawan et al., 2011). On the other hand, another study showed that the activity of NCX1 is dependent on PKC, although direct phosphorylation by PKC is not required (Iwamoto et al., 1998). NCX exists in 3 different isoforms, namely NCX1, NCX2 and NCX3.

NCX1 is referred as the cardiac NCX isoform as it is highly expressed in CMs but only in a lesser extent in other tissues such as brain and kidney (Lee et al., 1994).

NCX is classified as a secondary active transporter, which uses the energy stored in the electrochemical gradient in Na^+ to extrude Ca^{2+} out of the cells, while the electrochemical gradient of Na^+ is maintained by the Na^+/K^+-ATPase. Under normal condition, NCX operates in the forward mode in which it constitutively brings 3 Na^+ into the cells and extrudes 1 Ca^{2+} in each translocation cycle. The forward mode is stimulated in response to a rise in $[Ca^{2+}]_i$, and it serves to bring $[Ca^{2+}]_i$ back to normal level. In CMs, the primary role of NCX is to extrude Ca^{2+} after excitation under normal physiological conditions (Philipson and Nicoll, 2000). Some studies also showed that NCX functions in shaping the cardiac action potential. Application of NCX blocker KB-R7943 leads to shortening of plateau phase of cardiac potential (Spencer and Sham, 2003); similarly, CMs from NCX knockout mice also has a shorter AP when compare to wild-type mice (Pott et al., 2005), while induced over-expression of NCX leads to a longer plateau (Wang et al., 2009). On the other hand, NCX also operates in the reverse mode in response to membrane depolarization in CMs. During the depolarization phase of action potential when the $[Ca^{2+}]_i$ has not reached the peak of Ca^{2+} transients, the reverse mode is predominant (Sah et al., 2003). Ca^{2+} influx via the reverse mode of NCX has been suggested to act synergistically with Ca^{2+} influx via L-type Ca^{2+} channels to trigger Ca^{2+} release from the SR as $I_{Ca, L}$ are small at depolarized membrane potential (Sah et al., 2003). In addition, NCX can positively regulate SR Ca^{2+} load via the reverse mode action (Hirota et al., 2007). Interestingly, under pathophysiological conditions such as cardiac failure, NCX also operates in the reverse mode to allow additional Ca^{2+} influx for contraction in order to compensate for the reduction in Ca^{2+} release from SR (Gaughan et al., 1999).

NCX is found to be essential for embryo development. Several studies showed that NCX1 is expressed restrictedly in the embryonic heart during early development. NCX knockout are embryonic lethal at ~9-11 days post coitum with immature heart development (Cho et al., 2000; Koushik et al., 2001; Reuter et al., 2003; Wakimoto et al., 2000). Molecular studies demonstrated that NCX mRNA expresses before the appearance of spontaneously beating mESC-CMs; the expression persists thereafter in the CMs (Fu et al., 2006b). It is suggested that expression of NCX at that early stage is essential for early EC-coupling as SR is not well-developed at that stage, NCX is hence essential for maintaining the proper Ca^{2+} homeostasis even in the very early stage cardiac development (Reppel et al., 2007a; Reppel et al., 2007b).

Two approaches were used to demonstrate the functional expression of NCX in ESC-CM. In Otsu *et al.* (Otsu et al., 2005), function of NCX was indirectly assessed by using high concentration of NCX blocker KB-R7943. Application of KB-R7943 induced sustained elevation of $[Ca^{2+}]_i$, and this elevation increased as differentiation of mESC-CMs proceeded (Otsu et al., 2005). Apart from using pharmacological blocker, direct measurement of NCX activity was performed by using patch-clamping. I_{NCX} was found to be increased as hESC-CMs developed from day 7+40 to day 7+90 (Fu et al., 2010). However, CMs derived from murine embryonic heart at late stage (E16.5) showed a significantly lower I_{NCX} density when compared to CMs at early stage (E10.5) (Reppel et al., 2007a), probably due to the high phosphorylation status of NCX in early stage. Consistently, upon differentiation, the proportion of Ca^{2+} extrusion by NCX declined from day 9 to day 17 in mESC-CMs (Kapur and Banach, 2007). The discrepancy between different studies on the absolute functional expression of NCX as development proceeds is unknown. Nonetheless, it is clear that NCX is important for Ca^{2+} extrusion in differentiating CMs and the decreased contribution by

NCX to Ca^{2+} extrusion as development proceeds may be explained by the gradual development of SERCA on the SR.

In the study by Fu *et al.*, the basal $[Ca^{2+}]_i$ of mESC-CMs in both early and late developmental stages was increased after applying Na^+-free solution, suggesting that NCX is functional in maintaining Ca^{2+} homeostasis (Fu et al., 2006b). Interestingly, Na^+-free solution completely blocked the Ca^{2+} transients in CMs from late developmental stage but not the CMs from early developmental stage, suggesting that NCX starts to regulate Ca^{2+} transients only in the late developmental stage (Fu et al., 2006b). Similar results were obtained from hESC-CMs (Fu et al., 2010). Basal $[Ca^{2+}]_i$ was marginally increased in CMs at day 7+90 after applying Na^+-free solution, but the same was not observed in CMs at day 7+40. In addition, irregular Ca^{2+} transient pattern was observed in day 7+90 CMs treated with Na^+-free solution (Fu et al., 2010). These suggested that the contribution of NCX to Ca^{2+} transients becomes more important as development proceeds in ESC-CMs.

2.3.2 Sarcoplasmic/endoplasmic reticulum Ca^{2+}-ATPase (SERCA)

Details of the structure and function relationship of SERCA have been extensively reviewed (Periasamy et al., 2008; Periasamy and Huke, 2001; Toyoshima, 2008; Toyoshima and Inesi, 2004; Wuytack et al., 2002). SERCA is a single polypeptide with ~1000 amino acid residues located on the ER/SR membrane. It consists of 10 transmembrane (M) domains and 3 cytosolic domains, including actuator (A) domain, phosphorylation (P) domain, and nucleotide-binding (N) domain. A domain regulates the Ca^{2+} binding and release. N domain is connected to the P domain; it contains the adenosine binding site and forms the catalytic site. On the other hand, the γ-phosphate reacts with an amino acid residue in the P domain. SERCA utilizes the energy derived from ATP hydrolysis to pump Ca^{2+} against concentration gradient from the cytosol to the lumen of ER/SR. Two Ca^{2+} are transported by hydrolysis of one ATP in each catalytic cycle.

Regulation of SERCA is mainly achieved by the action of SR membrane proteins phospholamban and sarcolipin (Asahi et al., 2003a; Edes and Kranias, 1987; MacLennan et al., 2002; MacLennan and Kranias, 2003; Simmerman and Jones, 1998; Traaseth et al., 2008). De-phosphorylated form of phospholamban interacts with SERCA and inhibits the pumping activities by decreasing the Ca^{2+} affinity of SERCA. Phospholamban exists in monomeric or pentameric form, while the monomeric form is inhibitory. Phosphorylation of phospholamban favors the formation of pentameric form, which in turns relieves the inhibitory effect on SERCA. Phosphorylation of phospholamban is regulated by cAMP-dependent protein kinase (Schwinger et al., 1998) and Ca^{2+}/calmodulin-dependent kinase (Ji et al., 2003). Sarcolipin is a shorter homolog of phospholamban (Hellstern et al., 2001). Unlike phospholamban, sarcolipin has no obvious phosphorylation site (Odermatt et al., 1997); therefore, the effect of sarcolipin on SERCA inhibition is mainly controlled by altering the expression level of sarcolipin (Odermatt et al., 1998). Sarcolipin interacts directly with SERCA and inhibits its function by decreasing the Ca^{2+} affinity of SERCA. Sarcolipin can also exert its superinhibitory effect on SERCA by forming the tertiary complex phospholamban-sarcolipin-SERCA (Asahi et al., 2002; Asahi et al., 2003b). In addition, sarcolipin stabilizes the SERCA-phospholamban complex in the absence of phospholamban phosphorylation and also inhibits phospholamban phosphorylation (Asahi et al., 2004).

SERCA plays a vital role in Ca^{2+} cycling between SR and cytosol, and this is important for EC-coupling. Over-expression of SERCA2a improved cardiac contractility by increasing SR Ca^{2+} loading and frequency of Ca^{2+} transients (Baker et al., 1998; He et al., 1997; Maier et al.,

2005; Prasad et al., 2004). On the other hand, homozygous SERCA2a knockout mice are embryonic lethal (Periasamy et al., 1999), while heterozygous knockout mice are alive and able to reproduce (Shull et al., 2003). Ji *et al.* has reported that the content of SR Ca^{2+} stores and the amplitude of Ca^{2+} transients were decreased by 40-60% and ~30-40%, respectively, in heterozygous CMs (Ji et al., 2000). Interestingly, heterozygous CMs showed a reduced phospholamban expression, an enhanced phospholamban phosphorylation, and an upregulated NCX expression. However, these changes in Ca^{2+} handling proteins were not sufficient to compensate the effects on contractility by the loss of SERCA2a, indicating that SERCA2a is a critical regulator in controlling the E-C coupling of CMs (Ji et al., 2000). Apart from genetic manipulation of the expression level of SERCA, function of SERCA can also be assessed by using the pharmacological blocker thapsigargin. Acute application of thapsigargin caused the decrease in Ca^{2+} transient amplitude, rate of decay of Ca^{2+} transients, and duration of action potential in isolated ventricular myocytes (Kirby et al., 1992), again suggesting the involvement of SERCA in the E-C coupling of CMs.

In vertebrates, SERCA is encoded by three genes, including the SERCA1, SERCA2, and SERCA3. Alternative splicing of the transcripts from these genes produces more than 10 SERCA isoforms. In CMs, SERCA2a and SERCA2b are expressed, with SERCA2a being the predominant form (Periasamy and Kalyanasundaram, 2007).

SERCA2a mRNA is present before initial contraction of mESC-CMs, but has no obvious change in expression level during further differentiation (Fu et al., 2006b). From embryo studies, SERCA2 protein increased from E9.5 to E18 in mouse heart (Liu et al., 2002). In human, it was reported that SERCA2a protein level remained steady between 8 to 15th week gestation, and started to increase afterwards (Qu and Boutjdir, 2001). Role of SERCA in regulating Ca^{2+} transients in ESC-CMs has been studied by several groups. Zhu *et al.* demonstrated that SERCA inhibitors, including thapsigargin and cyclopiazonic acid, reduced ~70% amplitude of Ca^{2+} transients in hESC-CMs, but had no effect on the time of decay (Zhu et al., 2009). In case of mESC-CMs, thapsigargin reduced both the amplitude and decay of Ca^{2+} transients, but exerted similar inhibitory effect on CMs from the 3 developmental stages (Fu et al., 2006a; Fu et al., 2006b). These findings are therefore consistent with the mRNA expression level of SERCA during mESC-CM differentiation. However, the contribution of Ca^{2+} removal by SERCA is estimated to be more important as differentiation proceeds based on Ca^{2+} imaging experiments (Kapur and Banach, 2007). Therefore, the role of other SR Ca^{2+} handling proteins cannot be neglected. For example, expression level of calsequestrin increases as SR matures (Fu et al., 2006a). This increases the capacity of SR Ca^{2+} load and may account for the requirement of greater contribution of Ca^{2+} removal by SERCA in later developmental stage of mESC-CMs.

To summarize for the whole chapter, Figure 1 represents a summary of the relative contributions of different proteins responsible for regulating Ca^{2+} transients in early differentiating ESC-CMs as development proceeds.

3. Conclusion

In summary, early differentiating ESC-CMs have already developed a scheme for regulating their $[Ca^{2+}]_i$ for E-C coupling. The relative contributions of the proteins that regulate Ca^{2+} transients alter upon the maturation of CMs. By comparing the regulation of $[Ca^{2+}]_i$ in ESC-CMs and that in adult CMs, we can obtain important insights into the potential strategies for 'fine-tuning' ESC-CMs to better-suit different therapeutic and research purposes.

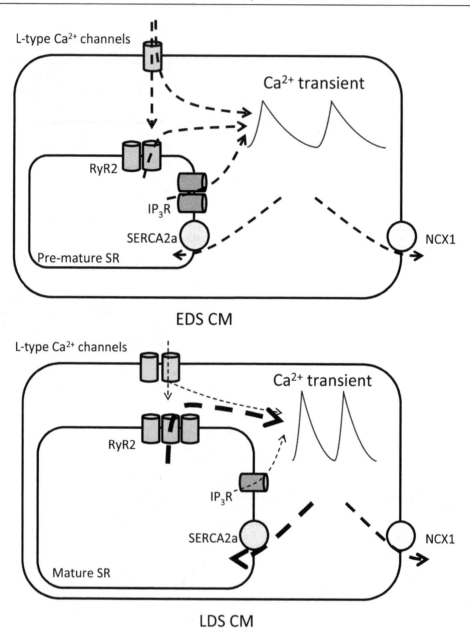

Fig. 1. Summary of the regulation of Ca²⁺ transients in CMs at early differentiation stage (EDS) and late differentiation stage (LDS). Number of a particular protein represents the relative changes in the expression level of that particular protein as differentiation proceeds. Thickness of the arrows represents the relative contribution of a particular path to the Ca²⁺ transients as differentiation proceeds.

4. Acknowledgements

When writing up this book chapter, due to space limitations, we were unable to include all the important studies in the field related to calcium homeostasis in ESC-CMs; we apologize to those investigators whom we may have missed here. I. C. Lo and C. K. Wong contributed equally to this work. I. C. Lo and C. K. Wong were supported by postgraduate studentships from the Chinese University of Hong Kong (CUHK). This work was supported by the Competitive Earmarked Research Grant (474907) from the University Grants Committee of the Hong Kong Special Administrative Region and the Focused Investment Scheme (1901073) from the CUHK.

5. References

Acosta L, Haase H, Morano I, Moorman AF, Franco D. 2004. Regional expression of L-type calcium channel subunits during cardiac development. Dev Dyn 230(1):131-136.

Ai X, Curran JW, Shannon TR, Bers DM, Pogwizd SM. 2005. $Ca2+$/calmodulin-dependent protein kinase modulates cardiac ryanodine receptor phosphorylation and sarcoplasmic reticulum $Ca2+$ leak in heart failure. Circ Res 97(12):1314-1322.

Arikkath J, Campbell KP. 2003. Auxiliary subunits: essential components of the voltage-gated calcium channel complex. Curr Opin Neurobiol 13(3):298-307.

Asahi M, Kurzydlowski K, Tada M, MacLennan DH. 2002. Sarcolipin inhibits polymerization of phospholamban to induce superinhibition of sarco(endo)plasmic reticulum $Ca2+$-ATPases (SERCAs). J Biol Chem 277(30):26725-26728.

Asahi M, Nakayama H, Tada M, Otsu K. 2003a. Regulation of sarco(endo)plasmic reticulum $Ca2+$ adenosine triphosphatase by phospholamban and sarcolipin: implication for cardiac hypertrophy and failure. Trends Cardiovasc Med 13(4):152-157.

Asahi M, Otsu K, Nakayama H, Hikoso S, Takeda T, Gramolini AO, Trivieri MG, Oudit GY, Morita T, Kusakari Y, Hirano S, Hongo K, Hirotani S, Yamaguchi O, Peterson A, Backx PH, Kurihara S, Hori M, MacLennan DH. 2004. Cardiac-specific overexpression of sarcolipin inhibits sarco(endo)plasmic reticulum $Ca2+$ ATPase (SERCA2a) activity and impairs cardiac function in mice. Proc Natl Acad Sci U S A 101(25):9199-9204.

Asahi M, Sugita Y, Kurzydlowski K, De Leon S, Tada M, Toyoshima C, MacLennan DH. 2003b. Sarcolipin regulates sarco(endo)plasmic reticulum $Ca2+$-ATPase (SERCA) by binding to transmembrane helices alone or in association with phospholamban. Proc Natl Acad Sci U S A 100(9):5040-5045.

Baker DL, Hashimoto K, Grupp IL, Ji Y, Reed T, Loukianov E, Grupp G, Bhagwhat A, Hoit B, Walsh R, Marban E, Periasamy M. 1998. Targeted overexpression of the sarcoplasmic reticulum $Ca2+$-ATPase increases cardiac contractility in transgenic mouse hearts. Circ Res 83(12):1205-1214.

Bare DJ, Kettlun CS, Liang M, Bers DM, Mignery GA. 2005. Cardiac type 2 inositol 1,4,5-trisphosphate receptor: interaction and modulation by calcium/calmodulin-dependent protein kinase II. J Biol Chem 280(16):15912-15920.

Bers DM. 2002. Cardiac excitation-contraction coupling. Nature 415(6868):198-205.

Bers DM. 2004. Macromolecular complexes regulating cardiac ryanodine receptor function. J Mol Cell Cardiol 37(2):417-429.

Boheler KR, Czyz J, Tweedie D, Yang HT, Anisimov SV, Wobus AM. 2002. Differentiation of pluripotent embryonic stem cells into cardiomyocytes. Circ Res 91(3):189-201.

Bohn G, Moosmang S, Conrad H, Ludwig A, Hofmann F, Klugbauer N. 2000. Expression of T- and L-type calcium channel mRNA in murine sinoatrial node. FEBS Lett 481(1):73-76.

Catterall WA. 1995. Structure and function of voltage-gated ion channels. Annu Rev Biochem 64:493-531.

Catterall WA. 2000. Structure and regulation of voltage-gated Ca2+ channels. Annu Rev Cell Dev Biol 16:521-555.

Catterall WA, Perez-Reyes E, Snutch TP, Striessnig J. 2005. International Union of Pharmacology. XLVIII. Nomenclature and structure-function relationships of voltage-gated calcium channels. Pharmacol Rev 57(4):411-425.

Chen CC, Lamping KG, Nuno DW, Barresi R, Prouty SJ, Lavoie JL, Cribbs LL, England SK, Sigmund CD, Weiss RM, Williamson RA, Hill JA, Campbell KP. 2003. Abnormal coronary function in mice deficient in alpha1H T-type Ca2+ channels. Science 302(5649):1416-1418.

Cho CH, Kim SS, Jeong MJ, Lee CO, Shin HS. 2000. The Na+ -Ca2+ exchanger is essential for embryonic heart development in mice. Mol Cells 10(6):712-722.

Cribbs LL, Martin BL, Schroder EA, Keller BB, Delisle BP, Satin J. 2001. Identification of the t-type calcium channel (Ca(v)3.1d) in developing mouse heart. Circ Res 88(4):403-407.

De Waard M, Gurnett CA, Campbell KP. 1996. Structural and functional diversity of voltage-activated calcium channels. Ion Channels 4:41-87.

DiPolo R. 1979. Calcium influx in internally dialyzed squid giant axons. J Gen Physiol 73(1):91-113.

Dolphin AC. 2006. A short history of voltage-gated calcium channels. Br J Pharmacol 147 Suppl 1:S56-62.

Dolphin AC, Wyatt CN, Richards J, Beattie RE, Craig P, Lee JH, Cribbs LL, Volsen SG, Perez-Reyes E. 1999. The effect of alpha2-delta and other accessory subunits on expression and properties of the calcium channel alpha1G. J Physiol 519 Pt 1:35-45.

Dubel SJ, Altier C, Chaumont S, Lory P, Bourinet E, Nargeot J. 2004. Plasma membrane expression of T-type calcium channel alpha(1) subunits is modulated by high voltage-activated auxiliary subunits. J Biol Chem 279(28):29263-29269.

Edes I, Kranias EG. 1987. Regulation of cardiac sarcoplasmic reticulum function by phospholamban. Membr Biochem 7(3):175-192.

Foskett JK, White C, Cheung KH, Mak DO. 2007. Inositol trisphosphate receptor Ca2+ release channels. Physiol Rev 87(2):593-658.

Freise D, Himmerkus N, Schroth G, Trost C, Weissgerber P, Freichel M, Flockerzi V. 1999. Mutations of calcium channel beta subunit genes in mice. Biol Chem 380(7-8):897-902.

Fu JD, Jiang P, Rushing S, Liu J, Chiamvimonvat N, Li RA. 2010. Na+/Ca2+ exchanger is a determinant of excitation-contraction coupling in human embryonic stem cell-derived ventricular cardiomyocytes. Stem Cells Dev 19(6):773-782.

Fu JD, Li J, Tweedie D, Yu HM, Chen L, Wang R, Riordon DR, Brugh SA, Wang SQ, Boheler KR, Yang HT. 2006a. Crucial role of the sarcoplasmic reticulum in the developmental regulation of Ca2+ transients and contraction in cardiomyocytes derived from embryonic stem cells. FASEB J 20(1):181-183.

Fu JD, Yu HM, Wang R, Liang J, Yang HT. 2006b. Developmental regulation of intracellular calcium transients during cardiomyocyte differentiation of mouse embryonic stem cells. Acta Pharmacol Sin 27(7):901-910.

Gaughan JP, Furukawa S, Jeevanandam V, Hefner CA, Kubo H, Margulies KB, McGowan BS, Mattiello JA, Dipla K, Piacentino V, 3rd, Li S, Houser SR. 1999. Sodium/calcium exchange contributes to contraction and relaxation in failed human ventricular myocytes. Am J Physiol 277(2 Pt 2):H714-724.

Giladi M, Boyman L, Mikhasenko H, Hiller R, Khananshvili D. 2010. Essential role of the CBD1-CBD2 linker in slow dissociation of Ca2+ from the regulatory two-domain tandem of NCX1. J Biol Chem 285(36):28117-28125.

Go LO, Moschella MC, Watras J, Handa KK, Fyfe BS, Marks AR. 1995. Differential regulation of two types of intracellular calcium release channels during end-stage heart failure. J Clin Invest 95(2):888-894.

Green PJ, Warre R, Hayes PD, McNaughton NC, Medhurst AD, Pangalos M, Duckworth DM, Randall AD. 2001. Kinetic modification of the alpha(1I) subunit-mediated T-type Ca(2+) channel by a human neuronal Ca(2+) channel gamma subunit. J Physiol 533(Pt 2):467-478.

He H, Giordano FJ, Hilal-Dandan R, Choi DJ, Rockman HA, McDonough PM, Bluhm WF, Meyer M, Sayen MR, Swanson E, Dillmann WH. 1997. Overexpression of the rat sarcoplasmic reticulum Ca2+ ATPase gene in the heart of transgenic mice accelerates calcium transients and cardiac relaxation. J Clin Invest 100(2):380-389.

He JQ, Ma Y, Lee Y, Thomson JA, Kamp TJ. 2003. Human embryonic stem cells develop into multiple types of cardiac myocytes: action potential characterization. Circ Res 93(1):32-39.

Hellstern S, Pegoraro S, Karim CB, Lustig A, Thomas DD, Moroder L, Engel J. 2001. Sarcolipin, the shorter homologue of phospholamban, forms oligomeric structures in detergent micelles and in liposomes. J Biol Chem 276(33):30845-30852.

Hess P, Lansman JB, Tsien RW. 1984. Different modes of Ca channel gating behaviour favoured by dihydropyridine Ca agonists and antagonists. Nature 311(5986):538-544.

Hilgemann DW. 1990. Regulation and deregulation of cardiac Na(+)-Ca2+ exchange in giant excised sarcolemmal membrane patches. Nature 344(6263):242-245.

Hilgemann DW, Matsuoka S, Nagel GA, Collins A. 1992. Steady-state and dynamic properties of cardiac sodium-calcium exchange. Sodium-dependent inactivation. J Gen Physiol 100(6):905-932.

Hirota S, Pertens E, Janssen LJ. 2007. The reverse mode of the Na(+)/Ca(2+) exchanger provides a source of Ca(2+) for store refilling following agonist-induced Ca(2+) mobilization. Am J Physiol Lung Cell Mol Physiol 292(2):L438-447.

Hobom M, Dai S, Marais E, Lacinova L, Hofmann F, Klugbauer N. 2000. Neuronal distribution and functional characterization of the calcium channel alpha2delta-2 subunit. Eur J Neurosci 12(4):1217-1226.

Hosey MM, Chien AJ, Puri TS. 1996. Structure and regulation of L-type calcium channels a current assessment of the properties and roles of channel subunits. Trends Cardiovasc Med 6(8):265-273.

Iino M. 1990. Biphasic Ca2+ dependence of inositol 1,4,5-trisphosphate-induced Ca release in smooth muscle cells of the guinea pig taenia caeci. J Gen Physiol 95(6):1103-1122.

Iwai M, Michikawa T, Bosanac I, Ikura M, Mikoshiba K. 2007. Molecular basis of the isoform-specific ligand-binding affinity of inositol 1,4,5-trisphosphate receptors. J Biol Chem 282(17):12755-12764.

Iwamoto T, Pan Y, Nakamura TY, Wakabayashi S, Shigekawa M. 1998. Protein kinase C-dependent regulation of Na+/Ca2+ exchanger isoforms NCX1 and NCX3 does not require their direct phosphorylation. Biochemistry 37(49):17230-17238.

Iwamoto T, Pan Y, Wakabayashi S, Imagawa T, Yamanaka HI, Shigekawa M. 1996. Phosphorylation-dependent regulation of cardiac Na+/Ca2+ exchanger via protein kinase C. J Biol Chem 271(23):13609-13615.

Ji Y, Lalli MJ, Babu GJ, Xu Y, Kirkpatrick DL, Liu LH, Chiamvimonvat N, Walsh RA, Shull GE, Periasamy M. 2000. Disruption of a single copy of the SERCA2 gene results in altered Ca2+ homeostasis and cardiomyocyte function. J Biol Chem 275(48):38073-38080.

Ji Y, Li B, Reed TD, Lorenz JN, Kaetzel MA, Dedman JR. 2003. Targeted inhibition of Ca2+/calmodulin-dependent protein kinase II in cardiac longitudinal sarcoplasmic reticulum results in decreased phospholamban phosphorylation at threonine 17. J Biol Chem 278(27):25063-25071.

Kapur N, Banach K. 2007. Inositol-1,4,5-trisphosphate-mediated spontaneous activity in mouse embryonic stem cell-derived cardiomyocytes. J Physiol 581(Pt 3):1113-1127.

Kehat I, Gepstein A, Spira A, Itskovitz-Eldor J, Gepstein L. 2002. High-resolution electrophysiological assessment of human embryonic stem cell-derived cardiomyocytes: a novel in vitro model for the study of conduction. Circ Res 91(8):659-661.

Kehat I, Kenyagin-Karsenti D, Snir M, Segev H, Amit M, Gepstein A, Livne E, Binah O, Itskovitz-Eldor J, Gepstein L. 2001. Human embryonic stem cells can differentiate into myocytes with structural and functional properties of cardiomyocytes. J Clin Invest 108(3):407-414.

Kirby MS, Sagara Y, Gaa S, Inesi G, Lederer WJ, Rogers TB. 1992. Thapsigargin inhibits contraction and Ca2+ transient in cardiac cells by specific inhibition of the sarcoplasmic reticulum Ca2+ pump. J Biol Chem 267(18):12545-12551.

Kolossov E, Fleischmann BK, Liu Q, Bloch W, Viatchenko-Karpinski S, Manzke O, Ji GJ, Bohlen H, Addicks K, Hescheler J. 1998. Functional characteristics of ES cell-derived cardiac precursor cells identified by tissue-specific expression of the green fluorescent protein. J Cell Biol 143(7):2045-2056.

Koushik SV, Wang J, Rogers R, Moskophidis D, Lambert NA, Creazzo TL, Conway SJ. 2001. Targeted inactivation of the sodium-calcium exchanger (Ncx1) results in the lack of a heartbeat and abnormal myofibrillar organization. FASEB J 15(7):1209-1211.

Lacinova L, Klugbauer N. 2004. Modulation of gating currents of the Ca(v)3.1 calcium channel by alpha 2 delta 2 and gamma 5 subunits. Arch Biochem Biophys 425(2):207-213.

Lanner JT, Georgiou DK, Joshi AD, Hamilton SL. 2010. Ryanodine receptors: structure, expression, molecular details, and function in calcium release. Cold Spring Harb Perspect Biol 2(11):a003996.

Lee SL, Yu AS, Lytton J. 1994. Tissue-specific expression of Na(+)-Ca2+ exchanger isoforms. J Biol Chem 269(21):14849-14852.

Li X, Zima AV, Sheikh F, Blatter LA, Chen J. 2005. Endothelin-1-induced arrhythmogenic Ca2+ signaling is abolished in atrial myocytes of inositol-1,4,5-trisphosphate(IP3)-receptor type 2-deficient mice. Circ Res 96(12):1274-1281.

Liu W, Yasui K, Opthof T, Ishiki R, Lee JK, Kamiya K, Yokota M, Kodama I. 2002. Developmental changes of Ca(2+) handling in mouse ventricular cells from early embryo to adulthood. Life Sci 71(11):1279-1292.

Ma J, Hayek SM, Bhat MB. 2004. Membrane topology and membrane retention of the ryanodine receptor calcium release channel. Cell Biochem Biophys 40(2):207-224.

MacLennan DH, Abu-Abed M, Kang C. 2002. Structure-function relationships in Ca(2+) cycling proteins. J Mol Cell Cardiol 34(8):897-918.

MacLennan DH, Kranias EG. 2003. Phospholamban: a crucial regulator of cardiac contractility. Nat Rev Mol Cell Biol 4(7):566-577.

Maier LS, Wahl-Schott C, Horn W, Weichert S, Pagel C, Wagner S, Dybkova N, Muller OJ, Nabauer M, Franz WM, Pieske B. 2005. Increased SR Ca2+ cycling contributes to improved contractile performance in SERCA2a-overexpressing transgenic rats. Cardiovasc Res 67(4):636-646.

Mangoni ME, Traboulsie A, Leoni AL, Couette B, Marger L, Le Quang K, Kupfer E, Cohen-Solal A, Vilar J, Shin HS, Escande D, Charpentier F, Nargeot J, Lory P. 2006. Bradycardia and slowing of the atrioventricular conduction in mice lacking CaV3.1/alpha1G T-type calcium channels. Circ Res 98(11):1422-1430.

Matsuoka S, Nicoll DA, He Z, Philipson KD. 1997. Regulation of cardiac Na(+)-Ca2+ exchanger by the endogenous XIP region. J Gen Physiol 109(2):273-286.

Mery A, Aimond F, Menard C, Mikoshiba K, Michalak M, Puceat M. 2005. Initiation of embryonic cardiac pacemaker activity by inositol 1,4,5-trisphosphate-dependent calcium signaling. Mol Biol Cell 16(5):2414-2423.

Mizuta E, Miake J, Yano S, Furuichi H, Manabe K, Sasaki N, Igawa O, Hoshikawa Y, Shigemasa C, Nanba E, Ninomiya H, Hidaka K, Morisaki T, Tajima F, Hisatome I. 2005. Subtype switching of T-type Ca 2+ channels from Cav3.2 to Cav3.1 during differentiation of embryonic stem cells to cardiac cell lineage. Circ J 69(10):1284-1289.

Moore JC, Tsang SY, Rushing SN, Lin D, Tse HF, Chan CW, Li RA. 2008. Functional consequences of overexpressing the gap junction Cx43 in the cardiogenic potential of pluripotent human embryonic stem cells. Biochem Biophys Res Commun 377(1):46-51.

Moreno Davila H. 1999. Molecular and functional diversity of voltage-gated calcium channels. Ann N Y Acad Sci 868:102-117.

Moschella MC, Marks AR. 1993. Inositol 1,4,5-trisphosphate receptor expression in cardiac myocytes. J Cell Biol 120(5):1137-1146.

Mummery C, Ward-van Oostwaard D, Doevendans P, Spijker R, van den Brink S, Hassink R, van der Heyden M, Opthof T, Pera M, de la Riviere AB, Passier R, Tertoolen L. 2003. Differentiation of human embryonic stem cells to cardiomyocytes: role of coculture with visceral endoderm-like cells. Circulation 107(21):2733-2740.

Nakayama H, Bodi I, Maillet M, DeSantiago J, Domeier TL, Mikoshiba K, Lorenz JN, Blatter LA, Bers DM, Molkentin JD. 2010. The IP3 receptor regulates cardiac hypertrophy in response to select stimuli. Circ Res 107(5):659-666.

Nakazawa M, Uchida K, Aramaki M, Kodo K, Yamagishi C, Takahashi T, Mikoshiba K, Yamagishi H. 2011. Inositol 1,4,5-trisphosphate receptors are essential for the development of the second heart field. J Mol Cell Cardiol.

Ng SY, Wong CK, Tsang SY. 2010. Differential gene expressions in atrial and ventricular myocytes: insights into the road of applying embryonic stem cell-derived cardiomyocytes for future therapies. Am J Physiol Cell Physiol 299(6):C1234-1249.

Nicoll DA, Hryshko LV, Matsuoka S, Frank JS, Philipson KD. 1996. Mutation of amino acid residues in the putative transmembrane segments of the cardiac sarcolemmal Na+-Ca2+ exchanger. J Biol Chem 271(23):13385-13391.

Odermatt A, Becker S, Khanna VK, Kurzydlowski K, Leisner E, Pette D, MacLennan DH. 1998. Sarcolipin regulates the activity of SERCA1, the fast-twitch skeletal muscle sarcoplasmic reticulum Ca2+-ATPase. J Biol Chem 273(20):12360-12369.

Odermatt A, Taschner PE, Scherer SW, Beatty B, Khanna VK, Cornblath DR, Chaudhry V, Yee WC, Schrank B, Karpati G, Breuning MH, Knoers N, MacLennan DH. 1997. Characterization of the gene encoding human sarcolipin (SLN), a proteolipid associated with SERCA1: absence of structural mutations in five patients with Brody disease. Genomics 45(3):541-553.

Ono K, Iijima T. 2005. Pathophysiological significance of T-type Ca2+ channels: properties and functional roles of T-type Ca2+ channels in cardiac pacemaking. J Pharmacol Sci 99(3):197-204.

Otsu K, Kuruma A, Yanagida E, Shoji S, Inoue T, Hirayama Y, Uematsu H, Hara Y, Kawano S. 2005. Na+/K+ ATPase and its functional coupling with Na+/Ca2+ exchanger in mouse embryonic stem cells during differentiation into cardiomyocytes. Cell Calcium 37(2):137-151.

Ottolia M, Philipson KD, John S. 2004. Conformational changes of the Ca(2+) regulatory site of the Na(+)-Ca(2+) exchanger detected by FRET. Biophys J 87(2):899-906.

Perez-Reyes E. 2003. Molecular physiology of low-voltage-activated t-type calcium channels. Physiol Rev 83(1):117-161.

Perez-Reyes E. 2006. Molecular characterization of T-type calcium channels. Cell Calcium 40(2):89-96.

Periasamy M, Bhupathy P, Babu GJ. 2008. Regulation of sarcoplasmic reticulum Ca2+ ATPase pump expression and its relevance to cardiac muscle physiology and pathology. Cardiovasc Res 77(2):265-273.

Periasamy M, Huke S. 2001. SERCA pump level is a critical determinant of Ca(2+)homeostasis and cardiac contractility. J Mol Cell Cardiol 33(6):1053-1063.

Periasamy M, Kalyanasundaram A. 2007. SERCA pump isoforms: their role in calcium transport and disease. Muscle Nerve 35(4):430-442.

Periasamy M, Reed TD, Liu LH, Ji Y, Loukianov E, Paul RJ, Nieman ML, Riddle T, Duffy JJ, Doetschman T, Lorenz JN, Shull GE. 1999. Impaired cardiac performance in heterozygous mice with a null mutation in the sarco(endo)plasmic reticulum Ca2+-ATPase isoform 2 (SERCA2) gene. J Biol Chem 274(4):2556-2562.

Philipson KD, Nicoll DA. 2000. Sodium-calcium exchange: a molecular perspective. Annu Rev Physiol 62:111-133.

Platzer J, Engel J, Schrott-Fischer A, Stephan K, Bova S, Chen H, Zheng H, Striessnig J. 2000. Congenital deafness and sinoatrial node dysfunction in mice lacking class D L-type Ca2+ channels. Cell 102(1):89-97.

Pott C, Philipson KD, Goldhaber JI. 2005. Excitation-contraction coupling in Na+-Ca2+ exchanger knockout mice: reduced transsarcolemmal Ca2+ flux. Circ Res 97(12):1288-1295.

Prasad V, Okunade GW, Miller ML, Shull GE. 2004. Phenotypes of SERCA and PMCA knockout mice. Biochem Biophys Res Commun 322(4):1192-1203.

Qu Y, Baroudi G, Yue Y, El-Sherif N, Boutjdir M. 2005. Localization and modulation of {alpha}1D (Cav1.3) L-type Ca channel by protein kinase A. Am J Physiol Heart Circ Physiol 288(5):H2123-2130.

Qu Y, Boutjdir M. 2001. Gene expression of SERCA2a and L- and T-type Ca channels during human heart development. Pediatr Res 50(5):569-574.

Rapila R, Korhonen T, Tavi P. 2008. Excitation-contraction coupling of the mouse embryonic cardiomyocyte. J Gen Physiol 132(4):397-405.

Reppel M, Fleischmann BK, Reuter H, Sasse P, Schunkert H, Hescheler J. 2007a. Regulation of the Na+/Ca2+ exchanger (NCX) in the murine embryonic heart. Cardiovasc Res 75(1):99-108.

Reppel M, Sasse P, Malan D, Nguemo F, Reuter H, Bloch W, Hescheler J, Fleischmann BK. 2007b. Functional expression of the Na+/Ca2+ exchanger in the embryonic mouse heart. J Mol Cell Cardiol 42(1):121-132.

Reuter H, Henderson SA, Han T, Mottino GA, Frank JS, Ross RS, Goldhaber JI, Philipson KD. 2003. Cardiac excitation-contraction coupling in the absence of Na(+) - Ca2+ exchange. Cell Calcium 34(1):19-26.

Richards MW, Butcher AJ, Dolphin AC. 2004. Ca2+ channel beta-subunits: structural insights AID our understanding. Trends Pharmacol Sci 25(12):626-632.

Rosemblit N, Moschella MC, Ondriasa E, Gutstein DE, Ondrias K, Marks AR. 1999. Intracellular calcium release channel expression during embryogenesis. Dev Biol 206(2):163-177.

Sah R, Ramirez RJ, Oudit GY, Gidrewicz D, Trivieri MG, Zobel C, Backx PH. 2003. Regulation of cardiac excitation-contraction coupling by action potential repolarization: role of the transient outward potassium current (I(to)). J Physiol 546(Pt 1):5-18.

Satin J, Itzhaki I, Rapoport S, Schroder EA, Izu L, Arbel G, Beyar R, Balke CW, Schiller J, Gepstein L. 2008. Calcium handling in human embryonic stem cell-derived cardiomyocytes. Stem Cells 26(8):1961-1972.

Sauer H, Theben T, Hescheler J, Lindner M, Brandt MC, Wartenberg M. 2001. Characteristics of calcium sparks in cardiomyocytes derived from embryonic stem cells. Am J Physiol Heart Circ Physiol 281(1):H411-421.

Schwinger RH, Bolck B, Munch G, Brixius K, Muller-Ehmsen J, Erdmann E. 1998. cAMP-dependent protein kinase A-stimulated sarcoplasmic reticulum function in heart failure. Ann N Y Acad Sci 853:240-250.

Sedan O, Dolnikov K, Zeevi-Levin N, Fleishmann N, Spiegel I, Berdichevski S, Amit M, Itskovitz-Eldor J, Binah O. 2010. Human embryonic stem cell-derived cardiomyocytes can mobilize 1,4,5-inositol trisphosphate-operated [Ca2+]i stores:

the functionality of angiotensin-II/endothelin-1 signaling pathways. Ann N Y Acad Sci 1188:68-77.

Sedan O, Dolnikov K, Zeevi-Levin N, Leibovich N, Amit M, Itskovitz-Eldor J, Binah O. 2008. 1,4,5-Inositol trisphosphate-operated intracellular Ca(2+) stores and angiotensin-II/endothelin-1 signaling pathway are functional in human embryonic stem cell-derived cardiomyocytes. Stem Cells 26(12):3130-3138.

Seisenberger C, Specht V, Welling A, Platzer J, Pfeifer A, Kuhbandner S, Striessnig J, Klugbauer N, Feil R, Hofmann F. 2000. Functional embryonic cardiomyocytes after disruption of the L-type alpha1C (Cav1.2) calcium channel gene in the mouse. J Biol Chem 275(50):39193-39199.

Shull GE, Okunade G, Liu LH, Kozel P, Periasamy M, Lorenz JN, Prasad V. 2003. Physiological functions of plasma membrane and intracellular Ca2+ pumps revealed by analysis of null mutants. Ann N Y Acad Sci 986:453-460.

Simmerman HK, Jones LR. 1998. Phospholamban: protein structure, mechanism of action, and role in cardiac function. Physiol Rev 78(4):921-947.

Spencer CI, Sham JS. 2003. Effects of Na+/Ca2+ exchange induced by SR Ca2+ release on action potentials and afterdepolarizations in guinea pig ventricular myocytes. Am J Physiol Heart Circ Physiol 285(6):H2552-2562.

Takeshima H, Komazaki S, Hirose K, Nishi M, Noda T, Iino M. 1998. Embryonic lethality and abnormal cardiac myocytes in mice lacking ryanodine receptor type 2. EMBO J 17(12):3309-3316.

Taylor CW, da Fonseca PC, Morris EP. 2004. IP(3) receptors: the search for structure. Trends Biochem Sci 29(4):210-219.

Taylor CW, Laude AJ. 2002. IP3 receptors and their regulation by calmodulin and cytosolic Ca2+. Cell Calcium 32(5-6):321-334.

Taylor CW, Tovey SC. 2010. IP(3) receptors: toward understanding their activation. Cold Spring Harb Perspect Biol 2(12):a004010.

Thomson JA, Itskovitz-Eldor J, Shapiro SS, Waknitz MA, Swiergiel JJ, Marshall VS, Jones JM. 1998. Embryonic stem cell lines derived from human blastocysts. Science 282(5391):1145-1147.

Toyoshima C. 2008. Structural aspects of ion pumping by Ca2+-ATPase of sarcoplasmic reticulum. Arch Biochem Biophys 476(1):3-11.

Toyoshima C, Inesi G. 2004. Structural basis of ion pumping by Ca2+-ATPase of the sarcoplasmic reticulum. Annu Rev Biochem 73:269-292.

Traaseth NJ, Ha KN, Verardi R, Shi L, Buffy JJ, Masterson LR, Veglia G. 2008. Structural and dynamic basis of phospholamban and sarcolipin inhibition of Ca(2+)-ATPase. Biochemistry 47(1):3-13.

Tu H, Wang Z, Nosyreva E, De Smedt H, Bezprozvanny I. 2005. Functional characterization of mammalian inositol 1,4,5-trisphosphate receptor isoforms. Biophys J 88(2):1046-1055.

Uchida K, Aramaki M, Nakazawa M, Yamagishi C, Makino S, Fukuda K, Nakamura T, Takahashi T, Mikoshiba K, Yamagishi H. 2010. Gene knock-outs of inositol 1,4,5-trisphosphate receptors types 1 and 2 result in perturbation of cardiogenesis. PLoS One 5(9).

Viatchenko-Karpinski S, Fleischmann BK, Liu Q, Sauer H, Gryshchenko O, Ji GJ, Hescheler J. 1999. Intracellular Ca2+ oscillations drive spontaneous contractions in cardiomyocytes during early development. Proc Natl Acad Sci U S A 96(14):8259-8264.

Wakimoto K, Kobayashi K, Kuro OM, Yao A, Iwamoto T, Yanaka N, Kita S, Nishida A, Azuma S, Toyoda Y, Omori K, Imahie H, Oka T, Kudoh S, Kohmoto O, Yazaki Y, Shigekawa M, Imai Y, Nabeshima Y, Komuro I. 2000. Targeted disruption of Na+/Ca2+ exchanger gene leads to cardiomyocyte apoptosis and defects in heartbeat. J Biol Chem 275(47):36991-36998.

Wang J, Chan TO, Zhang XQ, Gao E, Song J, Koch WJ, Feldman AM, Cheung JY. 2009. Induced overexpression of Na+/Ca2+ exchanger transgene: altered myocyte contractility, [Ca2+]i transients, SR Ca2+ contents, and action potential duration. Am J Physiol Heart Circ Physiol 297(2):H590-601.

Wanichawan P, Louch WE, Hortemo KH, Austbo B, Lunde PK, Scott JD, Sejersted OM, Carlson CR. 2011. Full-length cardiac Na+/Ca2+ exchanger 1 protein is not phosphorylated by protein kinase A. Am J Physiol Cell Physiol 300(5):C989-997.

Wu M, Le HD, Wang M, Yurkov V, Omelchenko A, Hnatowich M, Nix J, Hryshko LV, Zheng L. 2010. Crystal structures of progressive Ca2+ binding states of the Ca2+ sensor Ca2+ binding domain 1 (CBD1) from the CALX Na+/Ca2+ exchanger reveal incremental conformational transitions. J Biol Chem 285(4):2554-2561.

Wuytack F, Raeymaekers L, Missiaen L. 2002. Molecular physiology of the SERCA and SPCA pumps. Cell Calcium 32(5-6):279-305.

Xu C, Police S, Rao N, Carpenter MK. 2002. Characterization and enrichment of cardiomyocytes derived from human embryonic stem cells. Circ Res 91(6):501-508.

Xu M, Welling A, Paparisto S, Hofmann F, Klugbauer N. 2003. Enhanced expression of L-type Cav1.3 calcium channels in murine embryonic hearts from Cav1.2-deficient mice. J Biol Chem 278(42):40837-40841.

Xue T, Cho HC, Akar FG, Tsang SY, Jones SP, Marban E, Tomaselli GF, Li RA. 2005. Functional integration of electrically active cardiac derivatives from genetically engineered human embryonic stem cells with quiescent recipient ventricular cardiomyocytes: insights into the development of cell-based pacemakers. Circulation 111(1):11-20.

Yanagi K, Takano M, Narazaki G, Uosaki H, Hoshino T, Ishii T, Misaki T, Yamashita JK. 2007. Hyperpolarization-activated cyclic nucleotide-gated channels and T-type calcium channels confer automaticity of embryonic stem cell-derived cardiomyocytes. Stem Cells 25(11):2712-2719.

Yanagida E, Shoji S, Hirayama Y, Yoshikawa F, Otsu K, Uematsu H, Hiraoka M, Furuichi T, Kawano S. 2004. Functional expression of Ca2+ signaling pathways in mouse embryonic stem cells. Cell Calcium 36(2):135-146.

Yang HT, Tweedie D, Wang S, Guia A, Vinogradova T, Bogdanov K, Allen PD, Stern MD, Lakatta EG, Boheler KR. 2002. The ryanodine receptor modulates the spontaneous beating rate of cardiomyocytes during development. Proc Natl Acad Sci U S A 99(14):9225-9230.

Yang L, Katchman A, Morrow JP, Doshi D, Marx SO. 2011. Cardiac L-type calcium channel (Cav1.2) associates with gamma subunits. FASEB J 25(3):928-936.

Yasui K, Niwa N, Takemura H, Opthof T, Muto T, Horiba M, Shimizu A, Lee JK, Honjo H, Kamiya K, Kodama I. 2005. Pathophysiological significance of T-type Ca2+

channels: expression of T-type Ca2+ channels in fetal and diseased heart. J Pharmacol Sci 99(3):205-210.

Yule DI, Betzenhauser MJ, Joseph SK. 2010. Linking structure to function: Recent lessons from inositol 1,4,5-trisphosphate receptor mutagenesis. Cell Calcium 47(6):469-479.

Zhang YM, Shang L, Hartzell C, Narlow M, Cribbs L, Dudley SC, Jr. 2003. Characterization and regulation of T-type Ca2+ channels in embryonic stem cell-derived cardiomyocytes. Am J Physiol Heart Circ Physiol 285(6):H2770-2779.

Zhang Z, Xu Y, Song H, Rodriguez J, Tuteja D, Namkung Y, Shin HS, Chiamvimonvat N. 2002. Functional Roles of Ca(v)1.3 (alpha(1D)) calcium channel in sinoatrial nodes: insight gained using gene-targeted null mutant mice. Circ Res 90(9):981-987.

Zhu WZ, Santana LF, Laflamme MA. 2009. Local control of excitation-contraction coupling in human embryonic stem cell-derived cardiomyocytes. PLoS One 4(4):e5407.

12

Myogenic Differentiation of ES Cells for Therapies in Neuromuscular Diseases: Progress to Date

Camila F. Almeida, Danielle Ayub-Guerrieri
and Mariz Vainzof
University of São Paulo, Human Genome Research Center
Brazil

1. Introduction

The neuromuscular disorders are a heterogeneous group of genetic diseases characterized by progressive degeneration and impaired regeneration of skeletal muscle, resulting in weakness. The mobility of patients is very reduced, leading, depending on the disease severity, to wheelchair dependency and reduced life expectancy and quality.

Currently there are no proven treatments for these diseases, except for palliative measures to improve a patient's quality of life. Nevertheless, cell therapy using embryonic or somatic stem cells is considered to offer the best potential for success, and many projects are now being undertaken to evaluate the therapeutic possibilities of this approach.

Theoretically, due to their pluripotency, embryonic stem cells can give rise to any type of tissue, and raises the possibility of successfully treating many diseases. However, a simple injection of ES cells into various body locations in model organisms often leads to formation of undesirable teratomas and not to healthy new tissues. Accordingly, ES cells must be partially differentiated and selected prior to injection to increase the likelihood of implantation and growth of tissue exhibiting differentiation of the desired type.

Although some modest advances have been achieved, to date the use of ES cells for therapy of neuromuscular disorders still remains a distant goal. In this review we mainly consider the role of embryonic stem cells in neuromuscular therapeutic approaches.

2. Muscular dystrophies

The neuromuscular disorders form a heterogeneous group of genetic diseases characterized by progressive loss of muscular strength caused by defects in or absence of muscle proteins and also to imbalance between rates of tissue degeneration and regeneration. There is great clinical variability, ranging from extremely mild to severe forms (Emery, 2002).

More than 30 genetically defined forms are recognized, and in the last decade, mutations in several genes coding for the sarcolemmal, sarcomeric, cytosolic or nuclear muscle proteins have been reported. Deficiencies or loss of function of these proteins leads to variable degrees of progressive muscle degeneration, which in turn results in progressive loss of motor ability (Vainzof et al., 2003). The principle proteins involved occupy specific niches in muscle cells: dystrophin (*Dmd*), sarcoglycan (*Sgca*) and dysferlin (Dysf) are sarcolemmal or peri-sarcolemmal proteins; laminin alpha 2 (*Lama2*) and collagen type VI (*Col6*) are extracellular matrix proteins; telethonin (Tcap) and actin alpha 1 (*Acta1*) are sarcomeric proteins; calpain 3 (*Capn3*) and FKRP (Fkrp) are cytosolic enzymes; and emerin (Emd) and lamin A/C (*Lmna/c*)are nuclear proteins (Figure 1).

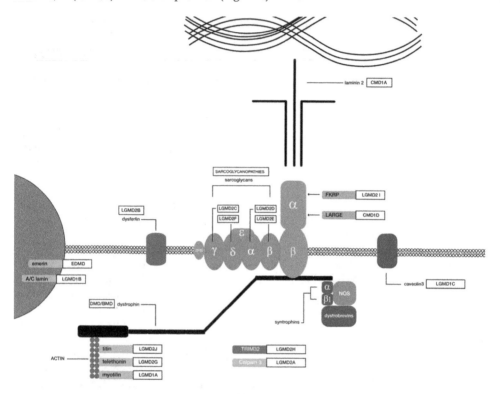

Fig. 1. Schematic representation of proteins involved in the process of muscle degeneration in neuromuscular disorders, localized at the sarcolemma, the sarcomere, the cytosol and the nucleus. The boxes contain the disease name associated with the protein. LGMD – limb-girdle muscular dystrophy; EDMD- Emery-Dreifuss muscular dystrophy; FKRP – fukutin-related protein; NOS – nitric oxide synthase.

Defects in components of the dystrophin-glycoprotein complex (DGC) are known to be an important cause of different forms of muscular dystrophies (Ervasti & Campbell, 1993; Yoshida & Ozawa, 1990). The DGC is an oligomeric complex connecting the subsarcolemmal cytoskeleton to the extracellular matrix. The DGC consists of dystroglycan (α- and β-DG), sarcoglycan (α, β-, γ-, δ- and ε-SG) and syntrophin/dystrobrevin sub-complexes. The intracellular link of the DGC is the protein dystrophin that plays an important structural role in muscle fibers. Mutations in the dystrophin gene cause the most common form of neuromuscular disorder, namely X-linked Duchenne muscular dystrophy (DMD) (Hoffman et al., 1987) with a frequency of 1 in 3000 males in most populations studied. Further, this disease epitomises the severe need for efficient treatment modalities, since 1/3rd of all patients arise from new mutations and the disease frequency can never be modulated efficiently by genetic counselling approaches.

Mutations in the genes coding the four SG proteins cause severe forms of limb-girdle muscular dystrophies type LGMD2D, 2E, 2C and 2F. The peripheral membrane glycoprotein α-DG, a receptor for the heterotrimeric basement membrane protein laminin-2, binds to β-DG and so completes the connection from the inside to the outside of the cell (Straub and Campbell, 1997). Mutations in the *Lama2* gene, encoding the α2 chain of laminin-2, cause α2-laminin deficiency, and a severe form of congenital muscular dystrophy (CMD1A) linked to human chromosome 6q (Tomé et al., 1994). In addition, some forms of muscular dystrophy have recently been associated with genes encoding putative or known glycosyltransferases. Muscle protein analysis in these patients shows a hypoglycosilation of α-dystroglycan and a consequent reduction of numerous ligands components of the extracellular matrix, such as laminin 2 (Muntoni et al., 2004). Other milder forms of muscular dystrophy are caused by mutations in genes coding the enzyme calpain 3 (*Capn3*), the sarcolemmal protein dysferlin (*Dysf*), and the sarcomeric protein telethonin (*Tcap*) (Vainzof & Zatz, 2003).

2.1 Animal models for neuromuscular diseases

Several animal models, manifesting phenotypes observed in neuromuscular diseases have been identified in nature or generated in laboratory. These models generally present physiological alterations observed in human patients, and can be used as important tools for genetic, clinical and histopathological studies (Vainzof et al., 2008).

The *mdx* mouse is the most widely used animal model for Duchenne muscular dystrophy (DMD) (Bulfield et al., 1984). Although it is a good genetic and biochemical model, presenting total deficiency of dystrophin in muscle, this mouse is not useful for clinical comparisons, because of its very mild phenotype. The canine golden retriever MD model presents a more clinically relevant model for DMD in humans due to the much larger size of the animals, significant muscle weakness progression and premature lethality.

Models for autosomal recessive limb-girdle MD include the *SJL/J* mice that develop spontaneous myopathy resulting from a mutation in the Dysferlin gene, which is a specific model for LGMD2B (Bittner et al., 1999). For the human sarcoglycanopathies (SG), the BIO14.6 hamster is the spontaneous animal model for δ-SG deficiency, while some canine models with deficiency of SG proteins have also been identified (Straub et al., 1998). More recently, using homologous recombination in embryonic stem cells, several mouse models have been developed with null mutations in each one of the four SG genes. All sarcoglycan-null animals display a progressive muscular dystrophy of variable severity, and share the property of a significant secondary reduction in the expression of the other members of the sarcoglycan subcomplex, and other components of the Dystrophin-glycoprotein complex.

Mouse models for congenital MD include the *dy/dy* (dystrophia-muscularis) mouse, and the allelic mutant *dy2J/dy2J* mouse, both presenting a significant reduction of α2-laminin in the muscle and a severe phenotype. The myodystrophy mouse (*Largemyd*), harbors a mutation in the glycosyltransferase Large, which leads to altered glycosylation of α-DG, and a severe phenotype (Grewal et al., 2001).

Other informative models for muscle proteins include the knockout mouse for myostatin, demonstrating that this protein is a negative regulator of muscle growth (Patel & Amthor, 2005). Additionally, the stress syndrome in pigs, caused by mutations in the porcine *Ryr1* gene, helped to localize the gene causing malignant hyperthermia and Central Core myopathy in humans (Yang et al., 2006).

The study of animal models for genetic neuromuscular diseases, in spite of some differences with their equivalent human disease phenotypes, can provide important clues to understanding the pathogenesis of these disorders in humans and are also very valuable for testing strategies for cellular therapeutic approaches.

3. Muscle development

Activating key genes in a sequence similar to that occurring in the normal organism is a reasonable approach to obtain differentiated muscle cells in vitro. This depends on understanding the gene pathways leading to myogenic differentiation.

Skeletal muscle development can be divided into a number of principal stages: determination of the cell fate (myoblast formation); myoblasts proliferation; alignment and fusion of myoblasts; formation of myotubes; maturation of myotubes and muscle fibre formation (Figure 2). Different molecular factors regulate each step in a particular and very ordered manner.

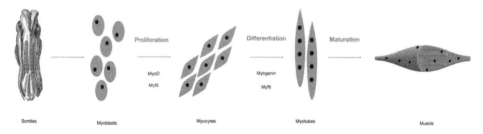

Fig. 2. Schematic of the myogenic cascade

3.1 Anatomy of embryonic myogenesis – Myotome formation

The majority of skeletal myogenic progenitors arise from somites, which are transitory condensations of paraxial mesoderm on either side of the neural tube and notochord. As the maturation of somites progresses, myogenic progenitor cells are confined to the epithelium of the dermomyotome, which give rise to the dermis and the skeletal muscle of the trunk and limbs (Buckingham, 2006).

The dermomyotome is subdivided into the hypaxial dermomyotome – the source of the lateral trunk muscles and limb muscles – and the epaxial dermomyotome – the source of the deep back musculature (Parker et al., 2003). In this structure, it is possible to distinguish two lips: the hypaxial and epaxial lips, from which cells delaminate and migrate under the dermomyotome, forming the myotome, an intermediate structure (Buckingham, 2001) (Figure 3).

3.2 Molecular markers and regulatory factors

Pax3 and *Pax7* are markers for cells derived from the dermomyotome and recently formed muscle masses. *Pax3* expression is involved in progenitor muscle cell formation and is essential for the definition and migration of these cells to their proper location in the body. *Pax3* acts mainly during embryogenesis, while *Pax7* is more important in adult myogenesis.

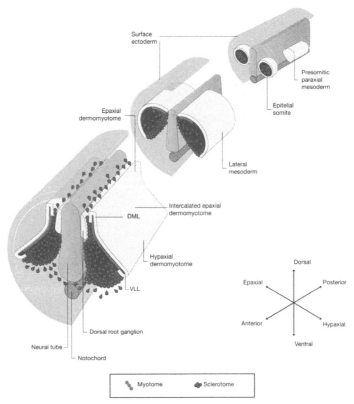

Fig. 3. The origin of different muscles in the embryo. VLL – ventral lateral lip. DML – dorsal medial lip. (Adapted from Buckingham, 2001).

The induction of myogenesis in the cells of somites is conducted by factors secreted by the notochord and neural tube: various members of the *Wnt* family and *Shh*, are responsible for the activation of MRFs (myogenic regulatory factors). Expression of *Ctnnb1* (β-catenin) dependent *Wnt6* signalling is important for the maintenance of the epithelial structure of the dermomyotome that is essential for the ordered progression of myogenesis. In epaxial muscle, *Wnt* family members are involved in *Myf5* and *MyoD* regulation through a complex cascade of gene regulation that includes the action of *Shh* as a positive regulator of *Myf5* (Parker et al., 2003) (Figure 4 A).

The MRFs concerned are *MyoD*, *Myf5*, myogenin and *Myf6* (*Mrf4*) and each one has a defined role in regulating skeletal muscle development and differentiation, directing the expression of genes responsible for the formation of the contractile machinery of the muscle (Bryson-Richardson & Currie, 2008). All have a homologous bHLH domain, required for DNA binding and dimerization with transcription factors of the E-protein family. The complexes of MRF-E proteins bind to a specific consensus sequence found in the promoters of many muscle-specific genes.

In hypaxial muscle, the MRFs are up-regulated by *Pax3*, which in turn, is regulated by family members of the sine oculis homeobox (*Six*) and eyes absent (*Eya*) genes (Bryson-Richardson & Currie, 2008) (Figure 4 B).

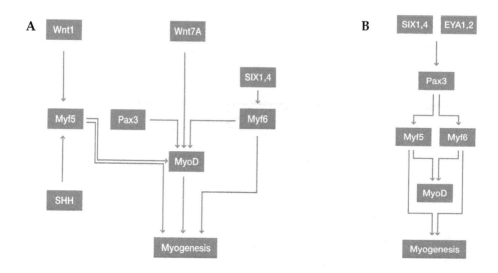

Fig. 4. Gene regulatory networks in A- epaxial muscle (left) and in B- hypaxial muscle (right).

Another important family of transcription factors is the myocyte enhancer factor-2 (*Mef2*), also involved in the expression of many muscle-protein genes in mouse (Naya & Olson, 1999). The *Mef2* family acts in conjunction with MRFs, especially *Myf6* and *Myog* (myogenin), to coordinate myoblast terminal differentiation.

3.3 Myogenesis in the adult – muscle regeneration

The cells responsible for regeneration in adult muscle are the satellite cells, localized under the basal lamina of muscle fibers. The satellite cells are partially undifferentiated myogenic precursor cells capable of both self-renew and differentiation into new myogenic cells (Relaix & Marcelle, 2009).

In response to injury, and under the stimulus of several myogenic factors, these cells are activated, start to proliferate and differentiate, fuse to pre-existing fibers (hypertrophy), or generate new fibers (hyperplasia) in a process recapitulating muscle development (Hawke & Garry, 2001). Myogenic determinants involve the components of the family of transcription factors called muscle regulatory factors (MRFs), include: a) *Myf5* and *Myod1*, responsible for muscle-cell type determination and satellite-cells activation; b) *Myf6* (also called *Mrf4*) and *Myog*, responsible for muscle differentiation (Brand-Saberi & Christ, 1999).

In addition to satellite cells, there are other cell types that contribute to muscle regeneration: bone-marrow derived cells (Ferrari et al., 1998), muscle side-population cells (Gussoni et al., 1999), CD34+/Sca1+ cells (Torrente et al., 2001; Lee et al., 2000) and cells of vascular origin (Figure 5).

The regenerative capacity of the satellite cells, however, is finite, and the exhaustion of the pool of precursor cells is an important factor contributing to the progressive muscle deterioration observed in human and murine muscular dystrophy. In fact, the exhaustion of satellite cells is the primary cause of onset of symptoms in Duchenne muscular dystrophy.

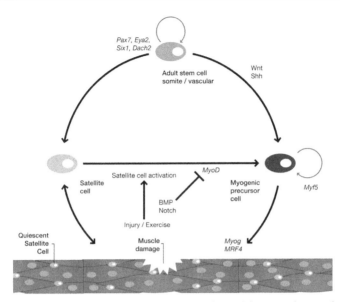

Fig. 5. Adult myogenesis and precursors cell types. Adapted from Parker et al., 2003.

Thus, cell therapies for muscular dystrophies can also focus on the re-establishment of the muscle's satellite cell pool, which reduces rapidly when there are excessive cycles of degeneration and regeneration.

4. ES cells in myogenic differentiation

Any attempt to direct the differentiation of ES cells must be designed so that the majority of cells will start to differentiate, as far as possibly, simultaneously into the desired cell type with avoidance of teratoma formation caused by non-committed pluripotent stem cells. Induction of appropriate myogenesis is a relatively difficult task given the unique architecture of muscle tissue.

There are three main potential approaches to directed differentiation of ES cells into muscle: the use of muscle specific growth and differentiation factors, genetic modifications and use of genetically modified feeder cells (Grivennikov, 2008). The first two have already been tested for myogenic induction, but to date, there are no reports on the use of modified feeder cells for this purpose.

For the differentiation of ES cells into different cell lineages, the cells must be cultivated in aggregates called embryoid bodies (EBs) by the hanging drop method (Figure 6), in which the 3-dimensional structure of the embryoid bodies, in combination with application of growth factors favouring myogenesis, encourages the stem cells to differentiate into myoblasts. The ES cells are first cultivated in drops of medium containing an exact number of cells leading to formation of EBs within 2 days, following which, the EBs are transferred into suspension cultures for some additional days resulting in adhesion of the EBs onto the bottom of tissue culture plates. The medium for EB cultivation is changed for one supporting myogenic differentiation at the time of EB adhesion. Studies suggest that the EBs need to be cultivated for five days in the suspension phase to obtain maximal differentiation into skeletal muscle cells.

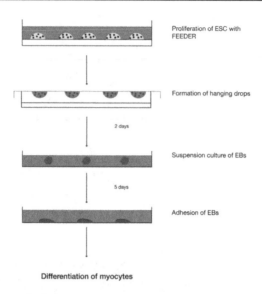

Fig. 6. Hanging drop method

4.1 *In vitro* induction of myogenesis

The use of chemical compounds to induce differentiation is a quite simple approach based on media supplementation. In some cases, different cell types can be obtained from the same compound according to the substance's concentration. For instance, 1μM retinoic acid causes neuronal differentiation, while 25nM retinoic acid enhances skeletal myogenesis (Kennedy et al., 2009).

One of the first reports of myogenic differentiation of ES cells was reported by Rohwedel et al. (1994), based on protocols developed by Wobus et al. in 1988 (2002), which depend on a prior differentiation in embryoid bodies followed by a posterior treatment with 1% DMSO (dimethyldisulfoxide) or 10^{-8}M retinoic acid. The myogenic cells obtained in this work were identified as myoblasts and myotubes by hematoxylin-eosin staining. The first myosin-positive and desmin-positive skeletal muscle cells appeared four days after EB adhesion. Myogenin-positive myocytes were identified after six days and fusion into myotubes on the seventh day. Neuronal cells also appeared mostly before the differentiation of skeletal muscle cells, which reached a maximum in nine days. However, some EB outgrowths containing ES cells, which decreased with prolonged time of differentiation. Using RT-PCR the authors detected expression of the myogenic regulatory factors myogenin, *Myf5*, *Myf6* and *Myod1*, indicating that ES myogenic differentiation *in vitro* resembles myogenesis *in vivo* (Rohwedel et al., 1994).

Retinoic acid (RA) is a derivate of vitamin A and has different roles in various processes in embryonic development and regulates the expression of several hundreds of genes (Blomhoff & Blomhoff, 2006), including MRFs. In stem cells and myoblast cells lines, RA enhances skeletal myogenesis at low concentrations (Edwards & McBurney, 1983; Halevy & Lerman, 1993; Albagli-Curiel et al., 1993, as cited in Kennedy et al., 2009). In the work of Kennedy et al. (2009), mouse ES cells and P19 cells (pluripotent embryonal carcinoma cells) were differentiated with various RA concentrations, ranging from zero to 50 nM and 1%DMSO, that promotes skeletal myogenesis, but not cardiogenesis. They detected increasing transcript levels of *Meox1, Pax3* and *Myod1* (all skeletal muscle markers) in the presence of various concentrations of RA by RT-PCR and showed that transcription peaked at a concentration of 25nM.

Prelle et al. (2000) overexpressed the *Igf2* gene (*insulin-like growth factor 2*) in mouse embryonic stem cells to evaluate this protein as a stimulator of myogenesis. *Igf2* was identified as an autocrine differentiation factor in myoblasts (Stewart et al., 1996, as cited in Prelle et al., 2000). It is also a survival factor during the transition from proliferation to differentiation in myoblasts and overexpression of *Igf2* in myoblasts results in enhanced differentiation characterized by accelerated expression of myogenin mRNA and extensive myotube formation (Stewart & Rotwein, 1996, as cited in Prelle et al., 2000). Embryoid bodies were formed by overexpression of *Igf2* in ES cells and myocytes were observed three days after adhesion, with myotube formation four days later and commencement of myotube contraction after ten days. They also detected the expression of the myogenic proteins titin and sarcomeric *Myhc* (myosin heavy chain). On the last day of differentiation (day 23), the large contracting myotubes showed a regular sarcomeric organization of both titin and myosin proteins.

By semi-quantitative RT-PCR, the expression onset and intensity of the skeletal muscle-specific genes *Myf5, Myod1* and *Myog* showed an increase in EB outgrowths overexpressing *Igf2*, with a similar pattern of expression to that occurring in vivo. Compared with non-transformed cells, the cells overexpressing *Igf2* showed an accelerated myogenic differentiation, associated with enhanced expression of MRFs, without effects in the sarcomeric structural organization.

We recently tested different factors for differentiating murine embryonic stem cells into muscle. In terms of morphology, the cells obtained are very similar to myoblasts in primary culture. The cells obtained also express mRNA from some proteins typical of the process of myogenesis, but proteins of mature muscle were not detected. To induce myogenesis in mES cells, EBs were cultured in media with 1%DMSO or 5μL of 10^{-7}M *Igf2*. After 13 days, cells were harvested for mRNA and protein analysis. Cells treated with *Igf2* visually seemed to differentiate more rapidly and with a larger proportion of cells morphologically similar to myoblasts than the cells treated with DMSO (data not published) (Figure 7).

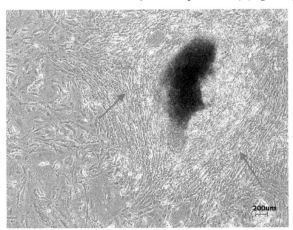

Fig. 7. Embryoid body from mES cells treated with Igf2 twelve days after adhesion. Cells indicated by the arrows are similar in morphology to myoblasts.

4.2 *In vivo* experiments and potential of therapies for NMD

Due to the lack of any available therapy for NMDs, cell therapy has been suggested as a promising alternative. Several attempts to use adult stem cells have been carried out, but with limited results. However, due to their greater pluripotency, ES cells show a greater potential for cell therapy, but can also form teratomas, when simply injected into the organism without predifferentiation, which must be avoided. Methods must be developed for inducing differentiation of the ES cells into the desired cell type before therapy, in such a way as to obtain a uniform population of differentiated cells, and, ideally, without the presence of undifferentiated ES cells.

Although there are a reasonable number of articles describing derivation of cell lines with some skeletal muscle features, the functional results are far from ideal and more basic research into *in vitro* culturing procedures is required. The skeletal muscle tissue has a unique architecture, and it is very complicated to reproduce this *in vitro*, rendering it impossible to obtain totally differentiated cells prior to transplantation. Accordingly, transplants are best made with cells that are already committed to differentiating into the myogenic lineage but have not yet completed the process, which will occur *in vivo* following transplantation.

Co-culturing of muscle stem/precursor cells from skeletal muscle with EB outgrowths can induce myogenic differentiation in vivo. This was achieved by Bhagavati & Xu, (2005) by obtaining muscle from normal mice and deriving ES cells by pre-plating muscle fragments and culturing EBs over them. The myogenic differentiation obtained in this manner is probably due to the myogenic stem/precursor cells being provided an optimal developmental environment by inductive signals for the EBs. Alternatively, it is possible that the occasional cell fusion between ES cells and myogenic precursor cells, results in the reprogramming of a limited number of ES cells. To test the potential of these cells to form skeletal muscle *in vivo*, the ES cells derived from co-culturing were injected into *mdx* mice via intramuscular injection. The muscles were analyzed after two weeks by immunohistochemical and *in situ* hybridization analyses. Dystrophin positive fibers that were lying on the surface of recipient muscle fibres were observed in 2 out of 8 injected mice. However, no functional evaluation was performed to test whether this newly derived muscle tissue was functionally normal (Bhagavati & Xu, 2005).

Zheng et al. (2006) used three different media, and treatment with 10mM 5-azacytidine in some experiments, to induce myogenic differentiation in EBs derived from hES cells. The 5-azacytidine treatment reduced cell proliferation and caused the cells to elongate. The expression analysis showed that the drug decreased the expression of *Met* and *Pax3*, but increased the expression of *Pax7* and *Myod1*. The expression of *Myf5*, *Des* (desmin), *Myhc*, *Tnni1* (troponin I), *Ncam1* was observed under all culture conditions, but occurred in the absence of myotube and myofiber formation. This indicates that, although the treated cells had the potential to initiate myogenic gene expression, they were not yet committed to complete the process and form muscle cells. The transplantation of the human ES-derived precursors to NOD-SCID mice injured with cardiotoxin and irradiation resulted in the incorporation of approximately 28% of cells into host myofibers. In the adult environment, hES cells derived precursors followed the same sequence of muscle development as during embryogenesis: myoblasts expressed muscle-specific structural proteins, fused together to form myotubes and to mature into myofibers. Hybrid regenerated myofibers displayed striated myofibrils and expressed desmin, actinin, troponin I, dystrophin (human) and myosin heavy chain. The transplanted hES cells also gave rise to satellite cells, which can provide a semi-permanent source of donor cells (Zheng et al., 2006).

A mouse ES cell line (ZHTc6-MyoD) was established by Ozasa et al. (2007) by introducing a *Myod1* transgene controlled by a Tet-Off system. This cell line is feeder-free, proliferates indefinitely and has the potential to differentiate almost exclusively into the myogenic lineage in the absence of doxycycline, and without pre-differentiation into embryoid bodies. To start the differentiation process, doxycycline is removed and a differentiation medium containing 4% fetal bovine serum (FBS) is used. Although other FBS concentrations were tested, the best one for differentiation was found to be 4%. The morphology of ZHTc6-MyoD cells in an undifferentiated state is round, but after changing to differentiation medium, they became elongated. After seven days, they started to fuse into myotubes, and occasional light muscle contractions were observed. Besides *Myod1* expression, the expression of desmin (day 4), myogenin (day 4) and dystrophin (day 8) was detected by Western blotting. *Pax7*, *Myod1*, desmin, myosin heavy chain and dystrophin expression was assayed by immuno-histochemical analysis. The cell's potential to differentiate into myofibers *in vivo* was also investigated by intramuscular injections into mdx mice and clusters of dystrophin-positive myofibers were detected in the injected area (Ozasa et al., 2007).

The use of hES cells in regenerative medicine requires pure cell populations, so that specific precursors are isolated; this is important to control cell differentiation into the desired lineage and avoid problems, such as teratomas. Barberi et al. (2007) developed a feeder-free induction system in monolayer culture to derive mesenchymal precursors from hES cells. The isolation of mesenchymal precursors was made using FACS (fluorescent activated cell sorting) of CD73+ cells, from which skeletal myoblasts were isolated by selecting for the expression of *Ncam1* (neural cell adhesion molecule 1) in another round of cell sorting. When induced with N2 medium, these skeletal myoblasts underwent terminal differentiation and formed contractile myotubes. The majority of *Ncam1*+ cells expressed *Myod1* and *Myog* in both undifferentiated and differentiated condition; however, the expression of mature muscle protein markers, such as myosin heavy chain 2a, desmin, skeletal muscle actin and sarcomeric myosin were present only in cells in terminal differentiation. After transplantation into a muscle injury model, long-term engraftment of hES cell-derived skeletal myoblasts was observed (Barberi et al., 2007).

One of the reasons for the difficulty in obtaining skeletal muscle progenitors from ES cells is the scarcity of paraxial mesoderm formation in the embryoid body, due to the lack of signals from the neural tube and notochord that are only present in the embryo. Enhancement of paraxial mesoderm formation was achieved by Darabi et al. (2008) by inducing *Pax3* by doxycyclin and sorting EBs for the presence of the PDGF-α receptor (*Pdgfr1*) a paraxial mesoderm marker, and absence of *Flk1* (synonymous with *VEGFR* in humans), which is a lateral plate mesoderm marker. The PDGFαR+Flk1- (*Pdgfr1+/Flk1-*) cell population is enriched under *Pax3* induction for doxycycline, once paraxial mesoderm expansion is *Pax3* dependent in the embryo; this population shows proliferative capacity and myogenic potential. However, terminal muscle differentiation occurs only when *Pax3* expression is removed and the cells exposed to a differentiation medium containing 2% horse serum. When transplanted into the tibialis anterior muscle of *Rag2-/-γc-/-* mice injured with cardiotoxin, the *Pdgfr1+/Flk1-* cells do not form teratomas and show muscle regeneration without the necessity of continuous *Pax3* induction. In *mdx* mice, these cells exhibited significant engraftment and better functional properties (Darabi et al., 2008).

The majority of transplantation experiments have been carried out in recessive models of muscular dystrophy, so it is unknown whether the same cellular therapies would produce equivalent results in dominant models. To address this question, Darabi et al. (2009) tested the therapeutic potential of the *Pax3* induced *Pdgfr1+/Flk1-* cells in *Frg1* transgenic mice, a model for the dominant facioscapulohumeral muscular dystrophy (FSHD). Consistent with the results of the previous work, these cells showed appropriate engraftment and brought amelioration to muscle contractile properties, especially in males, perhaps due to gender differences. This work confirms the therapeutic potential of stem cells to treat both recessive and dominant forms of muscular dystrophy.

According to Sakurai et al. (2008) the *Pdgfr1*+ population, when either positive or negative for *Flk1*, clearly consisted of paraxial mesoderm precursors, confirmed by the expression *Msgn1* (mesogenin), *Mesp2* and *Tbx6*. However, myotome and myogenic markers are not expressed by *Pdgfr1*+ cells, indicating that these cells have progressed to an early somatic stage, but are not yet completely committed to a specific lineage. When transplanted into the injured quadriceps femoris muscle of *KSN* nude mice, the *Pdgfr1*+ mesodermal progenitors are localized in the interstitial zone of muscles, adjacent to the myofibers. This localization suggests that these progenitor cells differentiated into satellite cells, which is confirmed by the expression of *Pax7* and *Cd34*. Some progenitor nuclei are found in the center of myofibers, indicating the contribution of *Pdgfr1*+ cells to muscle regeneration (Sakurai et al., 2008).

The culture of EBs in a differentiation medium composed by DMEM, 0.1 mM nonessential amino acids, 0.1 mM 2-mercaptoethanol, 5% horse serum and 10% fetal bovine serum, gives rise to cells expressing *Pax7*, but not *Myod1*, indicating the presence of quiescent satellite cells (Chang et al., 2009). These *Pax7* positive cells were enriched by fluorescense activated sorting using the surface marker SM/C-2.6 antibody, typical of quiescent adult and neonatal mouse satellite cells. The SM/C-2.6 positive cells represented 15.7% of the EB derived cells. The SM/C-2.6 positive population showed myogenic potential both *in vitro* and *in vivo* experiments. *In vivo*, GFP+SM/C-2.6-positive cells were injected directly into cardiotoxin damaged muscles of mdx mice and were localized between the basal lamina and the muscle cell plasma membrane, which is the same location as satellite cells. After a second injury, a contribution of the injected cells to regeneration was observed, evidenced by the presence of GFP positive muscle fibers with central nuclei. In addition, the GFP+SM/C-2.6-positive cells were able to proliferate, and to replace recipient satellite cells that were still present 24 weeks after transplantation, which is important for a continuous regeneration of the surrounding tissue (Chang et al., 2009).

A summary of all published experiments to date are in table 1.

ES cell type	Strategy	Animal models	Markers	Delivery	Reference
mESC	media supplementation with DMSO	only in vitro experiments	none	only in vitro experiments	Rohwedel et al., 1994
mESC	IGF-II overexpression	only in vitro experiments	none	only in vitro experiments	Prelle et al., 2000
mESC	co-culture with muscle cells culture	mdx mice/ Rag2-/-γc-/- mice	none	intramuscular	Bhagavati & Xu, 2005
hESC	media supplementation 5-azacytidine	NOD-SCID mice	none	intramuscular	Zheng et al., 2006
ZHTc6 mESC	MyoD gene-inducible system	mdx nude mice	Sca+/c-kit+/CD34-	intramuscular	Ozasa et al., 2007
hESC	FACS of mesenchymal precursors	SCID/Beige mice	CD73+/CD56+	intramuscular	Barberi et al., 2007
mESC	Pax3 induction/ FACS	mdx mice/ Rag2-/-γc-/- mice	PDGFαR+/Flk1-	intramuscular/systemic	Darabi et al., 2008
mESC	FACS of paraxial mesoderm precursors	KSN nude mice	PDGFαR+/Flk1- or Flk+	intramuscular	Sakurai et al., 2008
mESC	media supplementation DMSO and RA	only in vitro experiments	none	only in vitro experiments	Kennedy et al., 2009
mESC	Pax3 induction/ FACS	Frg1 mice	PDGFαR+/Flk1-	intramuscular/systemic	Darabi et al., 2009
mESC	media composed of 5% HS and 10% FBS	mdx mice	SM/C-2.6+	intramuscular	Chang et al., 2009

Table 1. Summary of experiments testing the myogenic potential of ES cells.

5. Conclusion

Several attempts to achieve appropriate differentiation of ES cells and implantation into model organisms have been tested with mixed results. The differentiation into the muscular lineage could be successfully obtained *in vitro*, as evidenced by the expression of myogenic markers. However, despite attempts to direct *in vivo* differentiation, to date few reports have documented successful long term therapeutic results using these procedures. Strategies, such as selecting subpopulations of undifferentiated or partially differentiated embryonic stem cells before any kind of implantation treatment is undertaken, are emerging and should result in more homogenous cell populations and, diminish the frequency of maturation of stem cells into undesired cell types. In fact, the combination of several approaches, including cell sorting, genetic modification, and prior *in vitro* induction will probably be necessary to obtain successful therapeutic outcomes with ES cells.

6. Acknowledgment

The authors would like to thank the following researchers, for scientific and technical support: Dr. Mayana Zatz, Dr. Lydia Yamamoto, Dr. Lygia da Veiga Pereira. The authors also thank Dr P. L. Pearson, a visiting professor to Brazil for his contributions to both the grammar and scientific content of this work. This work was supported by Fundação de Amparo a Pesquisa do Estado de São Paulo - Centro de Pesquisa, Inovação e Difusão (FAPESP-CEPID), Conselho Nacional de Desenvolvimento Científico e Tecnológico (CNPq), and Instituto Nacional de Ciencia e Tecnologia (INCT), FINEP, and Associação Brasileira de Distrofia Muscular (ABDIM).

7. References

Barberi, T.; Bradbury, M.; Dincer, Z.; Panagiotakus, G.; Socci, N. D. & Studer, L. (2007). Derivation of engraftable skeletal myoblasts from human embryonic stem cells. *Nature Medicine,* Vol.13, No.5, (May, 2007), pp.642-648

Bhagavati, S. & Xu, W. (2005). Generation of skeletal muscle from transplanted embryonic stem cells in dystrophic mice. *Biochemical and Biophysical Research Communications,* Vol.333, No.2, (June, 2005), pp.644-649

Bittner, R. E.; Anderson, L. V.; Burkhardt, E.; Bashir, R.; Vafiadaki, E.; Ivanova, S.; Raffelsberger, T.; Maerk, I.; Höger, H.; Jung, M.; Karbasiyan, M.; Storch, M.; Lassmann, H.; Moss, J. A.; Davison, K.; Harrison, R.; Bushby, K.M. & Reis, A. (1999). Dysferlin deletion in SJL mice (SJL-Dysf) defines a natural model for limb girdle muscular dystrophy 2B. *Nature Genetics,* Vol.23, No.2, (October, 1999), pp.141-142

Blomhoff, R. & Blomhoff, H.F. (2006). Overview of retinoid metabolism and function. *Journal of Neurobiology,* Vol.66, No.7, (June, 2006), pp.606-630

Brand-Saberi, B. & Christ, B. (1999). Genetic and epigenetic control of muscle development in vertebrates. *Cell Tissue Research,* Vol.296, No.1, (April, 1999), pp.199-212

Bryson-Richardson, R.J. & Currie, P. D. (2008). The genetics of vertebrate myogenesis. *Nature Reviews Genetics,* Vol.9, No.8, (August, 2008), pp.632-646

Buckingham, M. (2006). Myogenic progenitor cells and skeletal myogenesis in vertebrates. *Current Opinion in Genetics & Development*, Vol.16, No.5, (October, 2006), pp. 525-532

Buckingham, M. (2001). Skeletal muscle formation in vertebrates. *Current Opinion in Genetics & Development*, Vol.11, No.4, (August, 2001), pp.440-448

Bulfield, G.; Siller W. G.; Wight, P. A. & Moore, K. J. (1984). X Chromosome-Linked Muscular Dystrophy (mdx) in the Mouse. *Proceedings of the National Academy of Sciences*, Vol.81, No.4, (February, 1984), pp.1189-1192

Chang, H.; Yoshimoto, M.; Umeda, K.; Iwasa, T.; Mizuno, Y.; Fukada, S.; Yamamoto, H.; Motobashi, N.; Suzuki, Y. M.; Takeda, S.; Heike, T. & Nakahata, T. (2009). Generation of transplantable, functional satellite-like cells from mouse embryonic stem cells. *The FASEB Journal*, Vol.23, No.6, (June, 2009), pp.1907-1919

Darabi, R.; Gehlbach, K.; Bachoo, R. M.; Kamath, S.; Osawa, M.; Kamm, E. K.; Kyba, M. & Perlingeiro, R. C. R. (2008). Functional skeletal muscle regeneration from differentiating embryonic stem cells. *Nature Medicine*, Vol.14, No.2, (February, 2008), pp.134-143

Darabi, R.; Baik, J.; Clee, M.; Kyba, M.; Tupler, R. & Perlingeiro, R. C. R. (2009). Engraftment of embryonic stem cell-derived myogenic progenitors in a dominant model of muscular dystrophy. *Experimental Neurology*, Vol.220, No.1, (August, 2009), pp.212-216

Emery, A. E. H. (2002). The muscular dystrophies. *The Lancet*, Vol.359, No.9307, (February, 2002), pp.687-695

Ervasti, J. M. & Campbell, K. P. (1993). A role for the dystrophin-glycoprotein complex as a transmembrane linker between laminin and actin. *Journal of Cell Biology*, Vol.122, No.4, (August, 1993), pp.809-823

Ferrari, G.; Cusella-De Angelis, G.; Coletta, M.; Paolucci, E.; Stornaiuolo, A.; Cossu, G. & Mavilio, F. (1998). Muscle regeneration by bone marrow-derived myogenic progenitors. *Science*, Vol.279, No.5356, (March, 1998), pp.1528-1530

Grivennikov, I. A. (2008). Embryonic stem cells and the problem of directed differentiation. *Biochemistry (Moscow)*, Vol.73, No.13, (February, 2008), pp.1438-1452

Gussoni, E.; Soneoka, Y.; Strickland, C. D.; Buzney, E. A.; Khan, M. K.; Flint, A. F.; Kunkel, L. M. & Mulligan R. C. (1999). Dystrophin expression in the mdx mouse restored by stem cell transplantation. *Nature,* Vol.401, No.6751, (September, 1999), pp.390-394

Hawke, T.J. & Garry, D.J. (2001). Myogenic satellite cells: physiology to molecular biology. *Journal of Applied Physiology*, Vol.91, No.2, (August, 2001), pp.534-551

Hoffman, E. P.; Brown, R. H. Jr & Kunkel, L. M. (1987). Dystrophin: the protein product of the Duchenne muscular dystrophy locus. *Cell*, Vol.51, No.6, (December, 1987), pp.919-928

Kennedy, K. A. M.; Porter, T.; Mehta, V.; Ryan, S. D.; Price, F.; Peshdary, V.; Karamboulas, C.; Savage, J.; Drysdale, T. A.; Li, S.; Bennett, S. A. L. & Skerjanc, I. L. (2009). Retinoic acid enhances skeletal muscle progenitor formation and bypasses inhibition by bone morphogenetic protein 4 but not dominant negative β-catenin. *BMC Biology*, Vol.7, (October, 2009), pp.67-88

Lee, J. Y, Qu-Petersen, Z.; Cao, B. ; Kimura, S. ; Jankowski, R. ; Cummins, J. ; Usas, A. ; Gates, C. ; Robbins, P. ; Wernig, A. & Huard, J. (2000). Clonal isolation of muscle-derived cells capable of enhancing muscle regeneration and bone healing. *Journal of Cell Biology*, Vol.150, No.5, (September, 2000), pp.1085-1100

Muntoni, F.; Brockington, M.; Torelli, S. & Brown, S. C. (2004). Defective glycosylation in congenital muscular dystrophies. *Current Opinion in Neurology*, Vol.17, No.2, (April, 2004), pp.205-209

Naya, F. S. & Olson, E. (1999). MEF2: a transcriptional target for signaling pathways controlling skeletal muscle growth and differentiation. *Current Opinion in Cell Biology*, Vol.11, No.6, (December, 1999), pp.683-688

Ozasa, S.; Kimura, S.; Ito, K.; Ueno, H.; Ikezawa, M.; Matsukura, M.; Yoshioka, K.; Araki, K.; Yamamura, K.; Abe, K.; Niwa, H. & Miike, T. (2007). Efficient conversion of ES cells into myogenic lineage using the gene-inducible system. *Biochemical and Biophysical Research Communications*, Vol.357, No.4, (April, 2007), pp.957-963

Parker, M. H.; Seale, P. & Rudnicki, M.A. (2003). Looking back to the embryo: defining transcriptional networks in adult myogenesis. *Nature Reviews Genetics*, Vol.4, No.7, (July 2003), pp. 495-507

Patel, K. & Amthor, H. (2005). The function of Myostatin and strategies of Myostatin blockade - new hope for therapies aimed at promoting growth of skeletal muscle. *Neuromuscular Disorders*, Vol.15, No.2, (February, 2005), pp.117-126

Prelle, K.; Wobus, A. M.; Krebs, O.; Blum, W. F. & Wolf, E. (2000). Overexpression of insulin-like growth factor-II in mouse embryonic stem cells promotes myogenic differentiation. *Biochemical and Biophysical Research Communications*, Vol.277, No.3, (September, 2000), pp.631-638

Relaix, F. & Marcelle, C. (2009). Muscle stem cells. *Current Opinion in Cell Biology*, Vol.21, No.6, (December, 2009), pp.748-753

Rohwedel, J.; Maltsev, V.; Bober, E.; Arnold, H. H.; Hescheler, J. & Wobus, A. M. (1994). Muscle cell differentiation of embryonic stem cells reflects myogenesis in vivo: developmentally regulated expression of myogenic determination genes and functional expression of ionic currents. *Developmental Biology*, Vol.164, No.1, (February, 1994), pp.87-101

Sakurai, H.; Okawa, Y.; Inami, Y.; Nishio, N. & Isobe, K. (2008). Paraxial mesodermal progenitors derived from mouse embryonic stem cells contribute to muscle regeneration via differentiation into muscle satellite cells. *Stem Cells*, Vol.26, No.7, (May, 2008), pp.1865-1873

Straub, V. & Campbell, K. P. (1997). Muscular dystrophies and the dystrophin-glycoprotein complex. *Current Opinion in Neurology*, Vol.10, No.2, (April, 1997), pp.168-175

Straub, V.; Duclos, F.; Venzke, D. P.; Lee, J. C.; Cutshall, S.; Leveille, C. J. & Campbell, K. P. (1998). Molecular pathogenesis of muscle degeneration in the delta-sarcoglycan-deficient hamster. *American Journal of Pathology*, Vol.153, No.5, (November, 1998), pp.1623-1630

Tome, F. M.; Evangelista, T.; Leclerc, A.; Sunada, Y.; Manole, E., Estournet, B.; Barois, A.; Campbell, K. P. & Fardeau, M. (1994). Congenital muscular dystrophy with merosin deficiency. *Comptes Rendus De l'Academie des Sciences III*, Vol.317, No.4, (April, 1994), pp.351-357

Torrente, Y.; Tremblay, J. P.; Pisati, F.; Belicchi, M.; Rossi, B.; Sironi, M.; Fortunato, F.; El Fahime, M.; D'Angelo, M. G.; Caron, N. J.; Constantin, G.; Paulin, D.; Scarlato, G. & Bresolin, N. (2001). Intraarterial injection of muscle-derived CD34(+) Sca-1(+) stem cells restores dystrophin in mdx mice. *Journal of Cell Biology*, Vol.152, No.2, (January, 2001), pp.335-348

Vainzof, M.; Passos-Bueno, M.R. & Zatz, M. (2003). Immunological methods for the analysis of protein expression in neuromuscular diseases. *Methods Molecular Biology*, Vol.217, pp.355-378.

Vainzof, M. & Zatz, M. (2003).Protein defects in neuromuscular diseases. *Brazilian Journal of Medical and Biological Research*, Vol.36, No.5, (May, 2003), pp.543-555

Vainzof, M.; Ayub-Guerrieri, D.; Onofre, P.C.G.; Martins, P.C.M.; Lopes, V.F.; Zilberztajn, D.; Maia, L.S.; Sell, K. & Yamamoto, L.U. (2008). Animal Models for genetic neuromuscular diseases. *Journal of Molecular Neuroscience*, Vol.34, No.3, (March, 2008), pp.241-248

Wobus, A. M.; Guan, K.; Yang, H. T. & Boheler, K. R. (2002). Embryonic stem cells as a model to study cardiac, skeletal muscle and vascular smooth muscle cell differentiation. *Methods in Molecular Biology*, Vol.185, pp.127-156

Yang, T.; Riehl, J.; Esteve, E.; Matthael, K. I.; Goth, S.; Allen, P. D.; Pessah, I. N. & Lopez, J. R. (2006). Pharmacologic and functional characterization of malignant hyperthermia in the R163C RyR1 knock-in mouse. *Anestesiology*, Vol.105, No.6, (December, 2006),pp.1164-1175

Yoshida, M. & Ozawa, E. (1990). Glycoprotein complex anchoring dystrophin to sarcolemma. *Journal of Biochemistry*, Vol.108, No.5, (November, 1990), pp.748-752

Zheng, J. K.; Wang, Y.; Karandikar, A.; Wang, Q.; Gai, H.; Liu, A. L.; Peng, C. & Sheng, H. Z. (2006). Skeletal myogenesis by human embryonic stem cells. *Cell Research*, Vol.16, No.8, (August, 2006), pp.713-722

Permissions

The contributors of this book come from diverse backgrounds, making this book a truly international effort. This book will bring forth new frontiers with its revolutionizing research information and detailed analysis of the nascent developments around the world.

We would like to thank Michael S. Kallos, for lending his expertise to make the book truly unique. He has played a crucial role in the development of this book. Without his invaluable contribution this book wouldn't have been possible. He has made vital efforts to compile up to date information on the varied aspects of this subject to make this book a valuable addition to the collection of many professionals and students.

This book was conceptualized with the vision of imparting up-to-date information and advanced data in this field. To ensure the same, a matchless editorial board was set up. Every individual on the board went through rigorous rounds of assessment to prove their worth. After which they invested a large part of their time researching and compiling the most relevant data for our readers. Conferences and sessions were held from time to time between the editorial board and the contributing authors to present the data in the most comprehensible form. The editorial team has worked tirelessly to provide valuable and valid information to help people across the globe.

Every chapter published in this book has been scrutinized by our experts. Their significance has been extensively debated. The topics covered herein carry significant findings which will fuel the growth of the discipline. They may even be implemented as practical applications or may be referred to as a beginning point for another development. Chapters in this book were first published by InTech; hereby published with permission under the Creative Commons Attribution License or equivalent.

The editorial board has been involved in producing this book since its inception. They have spent rigorous hours researching and exploring the diverse topics which have resulted in the successful publishing of this book. They have passed on their knowledge of decades through this book. To expedite this challenging task, the publisher supported the team at every step. A small team of assistant editors was also appointed to further simplify the editing procedure and attain best results for the readers.

Our editorial team has been hand-picked from every corner of the world. Their multi-ethnicity adds dynamic inputs to the discussions which result in innovative outcomes. These outcomes are then further discussed with the researchers and contributors who give their valuable feedback and opinion regarding the same. The feedback is then collaborated with the researches and they are edited in a comprehensive manner to aid the understanding of the subject.

Apart from the editorial board, the designing team has also invested a significant amount of their time in understanding the subject and creating the most relevant covers. They scrutinized every image to scout for the most suitable representation of the subject and create an appropriate cover for the book.

The publishing team has been involved in this book since its early stages. They were actively engaged in every process, be it collecting the data, connecting with the contributors or procuring relevant information. The team has been an ardent support to the editorial, designing and production team. Their endless efforts to recruit the best for this project, has resulted in the accomplishment of this book. They are a veteran in the field of academics and their pool of knowledge is as vast as their experience in printing. Their expertise and guidance has proved useful at every step. Their uncompromising quality standards have made this book an exceptional effort. Their encouragement from time to time has been an inspiration for everyone.

The publisher and the editorial board hope that this book will prove to be a valuable piece of knowledge for researchers, students, practitioners and scholars across the globe.

List of Contributors

Erhard Bieberich and Guanghu Wang
Georgia Health Sciences University, U.S.A.

Prasenjit Sarkar and Balaji M. Rao
Department of Chemical and Biomolecular Engineering, North Carolina State University, Raleigh, NC, USA

Zoltan Simandi and Laszlo Nagy
University of Debrecen, Hungary

Irina Kerkis and Nelson F. Lizier
Laboratory of Genetics, Butantan Institute and Department of Morphology and Genetics, Federal University of Sao Paulo, Brazil

Mirian A. F. Hayashi
Departament of Pharmacology, Federal University of Sao Paulo, Brazil

Antonio C. Cassola
Department of Physiology and Biophysics, University of Sao Paulo, Brazil

Lygia V. Pereira
Institute of Biosciences, University of Sao Paulo, Brazil

Alexandre Kerkis
Celltrovet (Genética Aplicada), Ltda., Brazil

Siddharth Gupta and Angelo All
Department of Biomedical Engineering, America

Candace Kerr
Department of Obstetrics and Gynecology, America
Institute for Cell Engineering, America

Angelo All
Department of Neurology, Johns Hopkins University School of Medicine, Baltimore, MD, United States of America

Maria Elisabetta Ruaro, Jelena Ban and Vincent Torre
International School for Advanced Studies, (SISSA-ISAS), via Bonomea 265, Trieste, Italy

Rubens Camargo Siqueira
São Paulo University - Ribeirão Preto, Rubens Siqueira Research Center, Retina Cell, Brazil

Diego Franco, Estefania Lozano-Velasco and Amelia Aránega
Cardiovascular Development Group, Department of Experimental Biology, University of Jaén, Jaén, Spain

Ville Kujala, Mari Pekkanen-Mattila and Katriina Aalto-Setälä
University of Tampere, Institute of Biomedical Technology, Tampere, Finland

Ellen Poon, Chi-wing Kong and Ronald A. Li
Stem Cell & Regenerative Medicine Consortium, Hong Kong

Chi-wing Kong and Ronald A. Li
Heart, Brain, Hormone & Healthy Aging Research Center, Hong Kong

Chi-wing Kong and Ronald A. Li
Departments of Medicine, LKS Faculty of Medicine, University of Hong Kong, Hong Kong

Ronald A. Li
Departments of Physiology, LKS Faculty of Medicine, University of Hong Kong
Center of Cardiovascular Research, Mount Sinai School of Medicine, New York, NY, USA

Iek Chi Lo, Chun Kit Wong and Suk Ying Tsang
School of Life Sciences, The Chinese University of Hong Kong

Suk Ying Tsang
State Key Laboratory of Agrobiotechnology, The Chinese University of Hong Kong
Stem Cell and Regeneration Program, School of Biomedical Sciences, The Chinese University of Hong Kong
Key Laboratory for Regenerative Medicine, Ministry of Education, The Chinese University of Hong Kong
Hong Kong Special Administrative Region

Camila F. Almeida, Danielle Ayub-Guerrieri and Mariz Vainzof
University of São Paulo, Human Genome Research Center, Brazil